Introduction to Novel Drug Delivery Systems

SP Vyas PhD Postdoc

Department of Pharmaceutical Sciences
Dr H S Gour University, Sagar (MP) 470003

Roop K Khar PhD

BS Anangpuria Institute of Pharmacy,
Faridabad (Pt B D Sharma University of Health Sciences)
Faridabad District, Alampur, Haryana 121004

Sonal Vyas MBBS MD

Practicing Pathologist
Department of Pharmaceutical Sciences
Dr H S Gour University, Sagar (MP) 470003

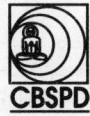

CBSPD

CBS Publishers & Distributors Pvt Ltd

New Delhi • Bengaluru • Chennai • Kochi • Kolkata • Lucknow • Mumbai
Hyderabad • Jharkhand • Nagpur • Patna • Pune • Uttarakhand

Introduction to
Novel Drug
Delivery Systems

ISBN: 978-93-88527-81-1

Copyright © Authors and Publisher

First Edition: 2020
Reprint: 2024

Published by **Satish Kumar Jain** and produced by **Varun Jain** for

CBS Publishers & Distributors Pvt Ltd
4819/XI Prahlad Street, 24 Ansari Road, Daryaganj, New Delhi 110 002, India.
Ph: 011-23289259, 23266861   Website: www.cbspd.com
                                    e-mail: delhi@cbspd.com

Corporate Office: 204 FIE, Industrial Area, Patparganj, Delhi 110 092
Ph: 011-4934 4934   Fax: 011-4934 4935 e-mail: publishing@cbspd.com;publicity@cbspd.com

Branches

- **Bengaluru:** Seema House 2975, 17th Cross, K.R. Road, Banasankari 2nd Stage, Bengaluru 560 070, Karnataka, India
  Ph: +91-80-26771678/79   Fax: +91-80-26771680   e-mail: bangalore@cbspd.com
- **Chennai:** 7, Subbaraya Street, Shenoy Nagar, Chennai 600 030, Tamil Nadu, India
  Ph: +91-44-26680620, 26681266   Fax: +91-44-42032115   e-mail: chennai@cbspd.com
- **Kochi:** 42/1325, 1326, Power House Road, Opp KSEB, Ernakulam 682 018, Kochi, Kerala, India
  Ph: +91-484-4059061-67   Fax: +91-484-4059065   e-mail: kochi@cbspd.com
- **Kolkata:** 147, Hind Ceramics Compound, 1st Floor, Nilgunj Road, Belghoria, Kolkata 700 056, West Bengal, India
  Ph: +91-33-25633055/56   e-mail: kolkata@cbspd.com
- **Lucknow:** Basement, Khushnuma Complex, 7-Meerabai Marg (Behind Jawahar Bhawan), Lucknow 226 001, UP, India
  Ph: +0552-4000032   e-mail:tiwari.lucknowi@cbspd.com
- **Mumbai:** PWD Shed. Gala no. 25/26, Ramchandra Bhatt Marg, Next to JJ Hospital Gate no. 2, Opp. Union Bank of India, Noorbaug, Mumbai 400 009, Maharashtra, India
  Ph: 022-66661880/89   e-mail: mumbai@cbspd.com

Representatives

• **Hyderabad**	0-9885175004	• **Jharkhand**	0-9811541605	• **Nagpur**	0-8692091830
• **Patna**	0-9334159340	• **Pune**	0-9664372571	• **Uttarakhand**	0-9716462459

Printed at: Mudrak, Noida, UP

Preface

Novel Drug Delivery System refers to strategy, technology, formulation based approaches and customized system(s) developed for safe administration and within body transportation of drugs as needed for optimum therapeutic benefits while ensuring minimum to nil toxic effects.

Multidisciplinary approaches and cutting edge technology have been used to develop the carrier modules to deliver the contained drug to the target tissues in a pre-programmed manner. The process desirably modifies the drug distribution and accumulation thereby producing optimum therapeutic effects.

Carrier-mediated drug delivery has emerged as a powerful technology for the treatment of various difficult pathologies.

The therapeutic index of conventional and novel drug is enhanced owing to specificity due to targeting of drug to the particular tissue.

There has been a persistent need of a book which introduces the concept, carrier(s), material, design, novelty, present status and future prospects of various novel drug delivery systems/ carriers. The present book shall be a useful source for the undergraduates and also to all those interested in the working concepts of a system and its performance. The book contains 23 chapters including introduction to novel drug delivery, oral osmotic pumps, bioadhesive and mucoadhesive systems, multiple emulsions, colon-specific drug delivery systems, transdermal drug delivery systems, spherical crystallization, microemulsion, implants and inserts, micellar systems, liposomes, microspheres and microcapsules, nanoparticles, nanospheres and nanocapsules, resealed erythrocytes, transfersomes and ethosomes, organogels, dendrimers, niosomes, solid lipid nanoparticles, drug conjugates, cyclodextrin complexes, multifunctional nanomedicines, and floating drug delivery system(s). Each chapter attempts to discuss introduction, concept, progress, status and future prospects of the concerned novel drug delivery system. Hope the book shall be a useful compilation to the undergraduate, postgraduate, pharmacy students and researchers working in drug delivery research, research and development and National Research Institutes.

I am thankful to my research team that includes Madhu Gupta, Udita Agrawal, Devyani Dubey, Nishi Mody, Surbhi Dubey, Neeraj Mishra and Rajeev Sharma. The inputs and support from them helped enormously in bringing out the book to the presentable and printable shape. I thankfully acknowledge the support of my family who assisted me to their fullest by sparing me from family responsibilities. I place on record the motivation/inspiration of my wife Mrs Vasundhara Vyas during the preparation of this book. My sincere thanks are due to my daughter Dr Sonal, son Himanshu and daughter-in-law Akanksha who have ever been supporting. I am also thankful to CBS Publishers & Distributors Pvt. Ltd., New Delhi for their interest and support in quality printing of the book. I realize that feedback, suggestions and inputs from teachers in pharmacy, researchers and students shall help improving the next edition of the book.

Sagar

SP Vyas

Contents

Preface   *v*

1. Introduction to Novel Drug Delivery   1–30
Drug Delivery 1
Physicochemical Properties 11
Biological Factors 13
Potential Applications of Nanocarriers in Targeted Drug Delivery 23
Future Opportunities and Challenges 29

2. Oral Osmotic Pumps   31–51
Introduction 31
Osmosis: An Overview 31
Classification 33
Rose–Nelson Pump 35
Higuchi–Leeper Osmotic Pump 36
Higuchi–Theeuwes Osmotic Pump 37
Elementary Osmotic Pump 37
General Considerations and Materials Used 41
Modified Multichamber Elementary Osmotic Pump 44
Advantages 47
Disadvantages and Limitations 48

3. Bioadhesive and Mucoadhesive Systems   52–81
Introduction 52
Fundamentals of Bioadhesion 53
Mechanism of Bioadhesion 55
Bioadhesion at Exposed Epithelial Surface 59
Naturally Occurring Bioadhesives 59
Factors Affecting Bioadhesion 60
Modulation of Mucoadhesion 63
Adhesion Promoters 63
Mucoadhesive Polymers Used in the Oral Cavity 64
Evaluation of Bioadhesive Drug Delivery Systems 66
Evaluation of Various Bioadhesion Properties 66
X-ray Studies for Monitoring GI Transit 71
Bioavailability Studies of Radiolabeled Nanoparticles 72
Bioavailability Studies of Drug Encapsulated Bioadhesive Microspheres 72
Challenges 78

4. Multiple Emulsions

82–91

Introduction 82
Formulation Aspects of Multiple Emulsions 83
General Methods of Preparation 83
Applications 88

5. Colon-specific Drug Delivery Systems

92–130

Introduction 92
Anatomic and Physiological Considerations 93
Factors Governing the Colon Drug Delivery 95
Targeting Approaches to Colon 101
Formulations for Colon-specific Drug Delivery 116
Conclusion 126

6. Transdermal Drug Delivery Systems

131–156

Introduction 131
Skin: A Biological Barrier to Drug Transport 133
Mechanistic Aspects of Drug Delivery in TDDS 134
Factors affecting percutaneous absorption 136
Characterization of Transdermal Drug Delivery Systems 142

7. Spherical Crystallization

157–171

Introduction 157
Methods of Spherical Crystallization 157
Applications of Spherical Crystallization in Pharmaceuticals 169

8. Microemulsion

172–195

Introduction 172
Methods of Preparation 172
Structure of Microemulsion 174
Formulation of Microemulsion 175
Preparation of Microemulsions 180
Characterization of Lipid Microemulsion 180

9. Implants and Inserts

196–214

Introduction 196
Classification 196
Classification-based on Mechanisms of Drug Release from Implants 197
Implantable Infusion Pump 199
Implantable Mini-osmotic Pump (ALZET) 201
Ophthalmic Inserts 202
Evaluation of Implantable Polymeric Materials 205
Therapeutic Applications of Implants and Inserts 207
Intra-arterial Catheter Infusion Drug Delivery System 211
Present Status and Future Prospects 213

10. Micellar Systems   215–233

Introduction 215
Formation of Micelles 217
Critical Micellar Concentration (CMC) 218
Stability of Polymer Micelle 219
Application of Micelles in Pharmaceutical Science 225
Conclusion 231

11. Liposomes   234–260

Introduction 234
Mechanism(s) of Liposomes Formation 234
Classification of Liposomes 238
Characterization of Liposomes 251
Therapeutic Applications of Liposomes 252

12. Microspheres and Microcapsules   261–288

Introduction 261
Material(s) Used 261
Prerequisites for Ideal Microparticulate Carriers 262
Methods of Preparation 262
Loading of Drug 267
Drug Release Kinetics 268
Characterization of Microparticles 270
Various Types of Polymeric Microspheres 271
Fate of Microspheres in Body 278
Applications of Microspheres 279
Chemoembolization 284

13. Nanoparticles   289–317

Introduction 289
Preparation Techniques of Nanoparticles 290
Characterization of Nanoparticles 302
Therapeutic Applications of Nanoparticles 304
Magnetic Nanoparticles 312

14. Resealed Erythrocytes   318–341

Introduction 318
Composition of Erythrocytes 318
Erythrocytes Morphology 319
In Vitro Characterization 323
In Vivo Survival and Immunological Consequences 325
Pharmacokinetics of Drugs or Peptides Administered in Loaded Erythrocytes 326
Applications of Carrier Red Cells 327
Other Applications 338

15. Transfersomes and Ethosomes   342–358
Introduction 342
Skin 343
Transfersomes 344
Ethosomes 351

16. Organogels   359–377
Introduction 359
Organogelators 360
Properties of Organogelators 365
Low Molecular Weight Organogelators 367
Organogels as Drug Delivery Vehicles 370

17. Dendrimers   378–392
Introduction 378
Origin of Dendrimers 379
Dendrimers and Polymers: A Comparison 380
Properties of Dendrimers 381
Featured Advantages of Dendrimers as Drug Carrier 381
Classification of Dendrimers 381
Synthesis and Designing of Dendrimers 382
Analytical Methods for Structure Validation of Dendrimers 384
Dendrimer Toxicity 385

18. Niosomes   393–415
Introduction 393
Formulation Aspects 394
Methods of Preparation 399
Characterization of Niosomes 401
Stability of Niosomes 404
Types of Niosomes 405
Applications of Niosomes 409

19. Solid Lipid Nanoparticles   416–439
Introduction 416
Advantages of SLNs as Alternative Particulate Carrier 416
SLNs versus Other Colloidal Drug Carriers 417
Ingredients and Formulation Processes 418
Microemulsion-based SLNs Preparations 420
Influence of Ingredient Composition on Product Quality 424
Characterization of SLNs 425
Toxicity Aspects and *In Vivo* Fate of SLNs 434
Applications of SLNs in Drug Delivery 434

20. Drug Conjugates   440–469

Introduction 440

Bioconjugate Techniques 440

Glutaraldehyde-based Hapten-carrier Conjugation 447

Carbodiimide-based Conjugation to Phosphatidylethanolamine Lipid Derivatives 447

Glutaraldehyde-based Conjugation to Phosphatidylethanolamine Lipid Derivative 447

Avidin-biotin System 448

Preparation of Colloidal Gold-labeled Proteins 449

Radiolabeled Antibodies 450

Antibody-toxin Conjugates 451

Protein Conjugates of Fungal Toxins 452

Poly-L-lysine Conjugates 453

Dextran and Inulin Conjugates as Drug Carriers 456

Lectin as Carrier 456

Glycoproteins as Drug Carriers 457

Galactose Terminated Fetuin as Carriers for Pepstatin 457

Bioconjugates with Protein Drugs 458

Polymer-drug Conjugates 459

Advantages in the Preparation of Bioconjugates with Low Molecular
   Weight Drugs 461

Limitations in the Conjugation of Polymers to Low Molecular Weight Drugs 462

Polyglutamic Acid (PGA)-E-[c(RGDfk)2]-paclitaxel Conjugate 463

N-(2-hydroxypropyl) Methacrylamide (HPMA)-based Polymeric
   Drug Conjugates 465

Polyethylene Glycol (PEG)-based Polymeric Drug Conjugates 467

21. Cyclodextrin Complexes   470–488

Introduction 470

Cyclodextrin-based Products 471

Advantages 472

Limitations 473

Mechanism of Drug Cyclodextrin Complexation 473

Inclusion and Noninclusion Complexes 475

Methods to Enhance the Complexation Efficiency 476

Toxicological Aspects 476

Drug Availability from CD-containing Products 477

Regulatory Status 477

Patents 478

Pharmaceutical Applications of Drug-CD Complexes 479

CD Used in the Design of Delivery Systems 483

22. Multifunctional Nanomedicines 489–509

Introduction 489
Designing of Multifunctional Nanomedicines 490
Applications 493

23. Floating Drug Delivery System(s) 510–527

Introduction 510
Low Density System or Floating Drug Delivery System 511
Classification of FDDS: Classification of Single Unit FDDS 512
Classification of Multiple Unit FDDS 513
Raft Forming Systems 515
Ingredients Used in Preparation of FDDS 515
List of Drugs Explored for Various Floating Dosage Forms 515
Approaches to Design FDDS 516
Formulation Development and Mechanism of FDDS 519
In Vitro and *In Vivo* Evaluation 520
Advantages of FDDS 521
Disadvantages of FDDS 522
Marketed Products of FDDS 522
Applications of FDDS 523
Pharmaceutical Aspects 525
Future Perspectives in FDDS 525

Index 529

■ Introduction to Novel Drug Delivery

1

DRUG DELIVERY

Drug delivery modes, modules and mechanisms essentially involved in the development of controlled or site specific discipline are of vital importance in modern medicine and healthcare discipline. Cotrolled drug delivery seems to improve the bioavailability of drugs by preventing premature degradation, clearance and enhancing uptake; thus maintains drug concentration within the therapeutic window by controlling the drug release rate, vis-a-vis reduces side effects by selective delivery allowing site-specific accumulation of drug into the diseased site or target cells. Innovations in material chemistry have initiated rapid development of drug delivery systems (DDS), providing material option for carrier construction; particularly the materials which are biodegradable, biocompatible, target, and stimulus responsive. Every drug molecule needs a delivery system to carry the drug to the site of action upon administration to the patient. Delivery of the drugs can be achieved using appropriately developed dosage forms including tablets, capsules, creams, ointments, liquids, aerosols, injections, and suppositories. Most of these conventional drug delivery systems are known to provide immediate release of the drug with little or no control over delivery rate. To achieve and maintain therapeutically effective plasma

concentrations, several doses are needed daily, which may cause significant fluctuations in plasma levels. Because of these fluctuations in drug plasma levels, the drug level could fall below the minimum effective concentration (MEC) or may exceed the minimum toxic concentration (MTC). Such fluctuations result in unwanted side effects and intended therapeutic benefit to the patient is denied. Sustained-release and controlled release drug delivery systems can reduce the undesired fluctuations of drug levels, thus minimize side effects while the therapeutic outcomes of the drug are improved. The terms sustained release and controlled release refer to two different types of drug delivery systems, although they are often used interchangeably. Ideally a drug delivery system should deliver a specified amount of medication to the site of action at an appropriate time and rate as desired and demanded by body. Similarly, the effects of dosage forms and dosing intervals on the therapeutic efficacy of drugs have been recognized as important factors which may affect the treatment of disease. As a result of massive distribution of drugs to the nontarget over tissue and body fluids; the amount of drug used in therapeutic doses is exceedingly high than the amount required in the target tissues/organs; as a consequence this leads to serious adverse effects during the

1

course of treatment. Over the past two decades, considerable advances in the understanding of pharmacokinetic and pharmacodynamic behaviors of drugs in humans have offered more scientific approaches for the development of optimal drug delivery systems. Consequently, controlled release formulations with both rate modulation and targeting capabilities will obviously prove to be beneficial. The ultimate goal of pharmacotherapeutics is to maximize the therapeutic efficacy of a drug while minimizing its adverse effects. The realization of this goal is complicated by a number of factors, few of them are presently defined while many others still remain unknown. Intrinsic drug properties represent the most basic issues to be understood and addressed in designing a clinically useful drug product. Other variable factors to be considered include route of administration, dosage regimen, and drug delivery systems.

Historically, drug delivery systems were developed primarily for conventional routes of administration such as oral and intravenous. However, there has been an explosion in research on delivery options for so-called nonconventional routes, such as transdermal (skin), nasal, ocular (eyes), and pulmonary (lung) administration. Drug delivery applications have expanded from traditional drugs to therapeutic peptides, vaccines, hormones, and viral vectors for gene therapy. These systems employ a variety of rate-controlling mechanisms, including matrix diffusion, membrane diffusion, biodegradation and osmosis. To design and produce a new drug delivery system, a bioengineer must fully understand the drug and material properties and also the processing variables that affect the release of the drug from the system, as well as the pharmacokinetic properties of the drug in the body. There are two main objectives of drug delivery systems:

1. **Drug targeting:** To deliver a drug to the desired location in the body.
2. **Controlled release:** To deliver a drug at a desired rate over a desired length of time. Many drug delivery systems attempt either controlled or targeted delivery; while some drug delivery systems attempt to combine both of them.

Rationale of Sustained, Controlled and Targeted Drug Delivery

The drug delivery systems usually cover-up terminology like sustained, controlled, targeted, smart, intelligent, novel, therapeutic and programmed. However, the basic rationale for these varied delivery modules is to alter or manipulate the pharmacokinetic and pharmacodynamics of pharmacologically active moieties by using either novel delivery devices (like liposomes, transdermal patches or matrix or membrane controlled devices), or by modifying the molecular structure (prodrug or chemical delivery system) and/or physiological parameters route of administration specific inherent (like rectal route to avoid first pass metabolism). A drug delivery system may be developed encompassing three components, i.e the drug input function; the pharmacokinetic responses (metabolism) and the pharmacodynamic responses (therapeutic and side effects).

It is important to critically understand and evaluate different terms frequently used under broad category of novel drug delivery systems:

- **Localized drug delivery devices:** Deliver the drug through spatial or temporal control for drug release directly to or in the vicinity of the target.
- **Modified release drug product:** The term modified release drug product is used to describe products that alter the timing or release rate of active drug substance.
- **Extended release dosage forms:** When absorption of drug is greater than its elimination the release is known as extended release. A dosage form should allow at least a twofold reduction in dosage frequency as compared to that drug presented as an immediate release (conventional) dosage form. Examples of extended-release dosage forms include

controlled release, sustained release and long-acting drug products.

• **Sustained release:** It includes the drug delivery systems that achieve and ensure slow release of drugs over an extended/ prolonged period of time or at a constant release (zero order) rate to attain and maintain therapeutically effective levels of drug concentration in the circulation. Here the absorption rate is equal to the elimination rate over an extended period of time.

• **Controlled release:** It includes any drug delivery system from which the drug is delivered at a predetermined rate over a prolong period of time.

• **Delayed release dosage form:** A dosage form that releases a discrete fraction of drug at a time or times other than administration, although one portion may be released immediately after administration, e.g. enteric-coated dosage forms.

• **Targeted release drug products:** A dosage form that releases drug at or near the intended physiologic site of action. Targeted release dosage forms may have either immediate or extended release characteristics. Targeted drug delivery is implicated by using carriers either meant for passive-preprogrammed or active-preprogrammed or self-programmed drug release approach. Thus, they are usually appended with suitable site-directing molecules, which recognize their receptor or molecular determinants at the target.

• **Repeat-action dosage forms:** It is a type of modified-release drug product that is designed to release one dose or drug initially followed by a second dose of drug at a latter time.

• **Prolonged action dosage forms:** They release the drug slowly and provide a continuous supply of drug over an extended period of time.

Targeted drug delivery, sometimes called smart drug delivery, is a method of delivering medication to a patient in a manner that increases the concentration of the medication in target sites of the body relative to others. This helps to maintain the required drug levels in the targeted tissue or organ in the body. Therefore, avoids any damage to the healthy tissue due to the drug. It is developed to optimize regenerative techniques. The drug delivery system is developed using integrated approaches and requires the involvement of various disciplines, such as chemists, biologist and engineers, to join, design and develop the system with precise performance. In case of conventional drug delivery system, the drug is absorbed across a biological membrane, whereas the targeted drug delivery implicates the release of drug to the target site after the delivery system reaches and localizes at or within the target tissues/organ. It is pivotal while designing a particular delivery system to understand, whether the behavior of the drug in its delivery system or the behavior of the delivery system (containing drug) will be crucial factor in biodistribution of the drug. For conventional drug delivery systems, the rate limiting step is the bioavailability (rate and extent of absorption) of drug across a biological membrane. Several factors affect the absorption of the drug from the conventional drug delivery devices (Table 1.1).

Table 1.1: Factors affecting the drug absorption from a delivery system
Physicochemical factors affecting liberation and absorption rate pH-partition, drug dissolution and dissolution rate, polymorphism and pseudopolymorphism, complexation and adsorption, viscosity, drug stability in body fluids, incompatibility formulation factors affecting drug liberation and absortion solutions, disperse systems, capsules, tablets, dosage forms for administrations in body cavities, dosage form for topical administration, modified release dosage forms, targeted drug delivery systems, physiological factors affecting absorption, distribution, metabolism and excretion of drug.

Contd.

Table 1.1: Factors affecting the drug absorption from a delivery system *(Contd.)*

Membrane physiology, gastrointestinal physiology, skin physiology, pulmonary physiology, eye physiology, physiology of the respiratory system.

However, in a sustained and controlled release formulation, the release of drug from the delivery device is the rate-limiting step. Thus, drug availability is controlled by the kinetics of drug release rather than absorption. This limits the drugs with specific features which can be designed for sustained and controlled drug delivery (Table 1.2).

Table 1.2: Unsuitable features of drugs for sustained and controlled delivery

- Short or large elimination half-life
- Narrow therapeutic index
- Larger doses
- Extensive first pass clearance
- Low or slow solubility
- Poor absorption
- Active absorption
- Pharmacological effect and circulation time course incompatible

However, in targeted drug delivery systems, the carrier design of drug contained in the majority of the cases dominates the biofate of the drug. The interplay between physicochemical properties of the drug and the characteristics of the delivery systems determines the spatial or temporal pattern of the drug release as well as target tissue distribution (Table 1.3).

These events are extremely complex and determine the fate of the drug during its transit and transportation to the target tissue as well as in the biofluids. Availability of the drug thus relies upon the pharmacokinetics of the drug as well as the characteristics of the carrier system. As with sustained and controlled delivery systems where a drug has to possess some characteristics to be a candidate, targeted drug delivery could also be used to deliver a drug to the therapeutic levels in the general circulation. Nevertheless, in such cases carriers are designed to target the carrier sampling ports of absorption site for improved uptake followed by an access to systemic circulation.

Advantages of Controlled Drug Delivery Systems

1. Better patient compliance
2. Employ less total drug
   a. Minimize or eliminate local side effects
   b. Minimize or eliminate systemic side effects
   c. Obtain less potentiation or reduction in drug activity with chronic use.
   d. Minimize drug accumulation with chronic dosing.
3. Improve efficiency in treatment
   a. Cure or control the disease more promptly.
   b. Reduce fluctuation in drug level.
   c. Improve bioavailability of some drugs.
4. Economy, i.e. reduction in health care costs. The average cost of treatment over an extended time period may be less, due to less frequency of dosing, enhanced therapeutic benefits and reduced side effects. The time required for health care personnel to dispense, administer the drug and monitor patient is also reduced.
5. Allow safe administration of cytotoxic drugs
6. Avoidance of nontargeted receptors

Disadvantages

1. Decreased systemic availability in comparison to immediate release conventional dosage forms, may be due to incomplete release, increased first-pass metabolism, increased instability, insufficient residence time for complete release, site specific absorption, pH-dependent stability, etc.

Table 1.3: Various sustained and controlled release delivery strategies

Sustained or controlled release mechanism	Comments
Rate-controlled mechanism	Drug is enclosed within device in such a way that the rate of drug release is controlled by its permeation through a membrane wall.
Diffusion controlled	Reservoir devices: Diffusion through membrane
	Monolithic devices: Diffusion through bulk polymer
Water penetration controlled	Osmotic systems: Osmotic transport of water through semipermeable membrane
	Swelling systems: Water penetration into glassy polymer
Chemically controlled	Monolithic systems: Either pure polymer erosion (surface erosion) or combination of erosion and diffusion (bulk erosion)
	Pendant chain systems: Combination of hydrolysis of pendant group and diffusion from bulk polymer
Polymer matrix diffusion-controlled DDS	Active agent is homogeneously dispersed throughout a rate-controlling polymer matrix and the rate of drug release is controlled by diffusion throught the polymer matrix.
Activation-modulated DDS	In these systems the release of drug is activated by some physical, chemical or biochemical process or facilitated by energy supplied externally. Rate is then controlled by regulating the process applied or energy.
Physical means	Osmotic pressure, hydrodynamic pressure, vapor-pressure activated, mechanically-activated, sonophoresis-activated, iontophoresis-activated, hydration-activated
Chemical means	pH, ion-activated, hydrolysis-activated
Biochemical means	Enzyme-activated, small molecule-activated
Regulated systems	Magnetic or ultrasound: External application of magnetic field or ultrasound to facilitate the release of drug from the device.
	Chemical: Use of competitive desorption or enzyme-substrate reactions. Rate control is built into device
	Implantable infusion pumps for long term applications.
	Electrically-activated iontophoresis, pH-activated systems
Feedback-controlled systems	Bio-responsive, DDS-glucose triggered insulin system.

2. Poor in *in vitro–in vivo* correlation.

3. Possibility of dose dumping due to food, physiologic or formulation related variables or chewing or grinding of oral formulations by the patient and thus, increased risk of toxicity.

4. Retrieval of drug is difficult in case of toxicity, poisoning or hypersensitivity reactions.

5. Limited options for dose and dosage adjustment of drugs normally administered in varying strengths.

Phases of Drug Action

The overall effect of any drug occurs in a sequence of three distinct yet interdependent stages as listed in Table 1.4. Ideally, a thorough understanding of each of these stages for a given drug is essential for achieving its most

Table 1.4: Various phases of drug action

Phases	Effect
• Pharmaceutical phase	Release from a dosage form
• Pharmacokinetic phase (PK phase)	Absorption, distribution, metabolism and excretion
• Pharmacodynamic phase (PD phase)	Drug interaction with receptors

effective therapeutic efficacy in patients. The pharmaceutical (PC) phase describes the process of a drug's conversion from a chemical form into a dosage form. Included in this phase are the characterization of physico-chemical drug profiles, design and production of dosage forms, and biopharmaceutical evaluation of drug products. The PC phase can initially influence the pharmacokinetic (PK) phase, which is measured by blood level versus time profiles. The PK phase then directly affects the pharmacodynamic (PD), or efficacy phase. Because the extent of pharmacological activity of a drug is closely related to the plasma drug concentration, it is usually desirable from the standpoint of pharmacodynamics to maintain the drug concentration in the blood at a constant level and within a therapeutic concentration range. Blood level versus time profiles are primarily governed by the pharmaceutical and pharma-cokinetic processes occurring after drug administration.

By controlling the concentrations at which a drug exists in the blood at any given time, the therapeutic efficacy of drugs can be maximized.

The relationship between the PC and PK phases is relatively simple to study compared with the relationship between the PK and PD phases, and more is known about the PC and PK phases than is known about the PD phase of drug action for most commonly used drugs. Nevertheless, a clear understanding and interrelationship of the three phases of drug action can play a critical role in developing an optimal drug delivery system of a given pharmacological agent. The efficacy of a drug also depends on the dosage regimen, the manner in which a drug is administered. The dosage regimen represents the standard protocol for the administration of drugs. In developing such a protocol, three components of the dosage regimen must be considered—dose, dosage interval, and duration of treatment. Additionally, the chosen drug delivery system will affect each component of a dosage regimen and thus contributes to the overall success of pharmacotherapeutics.

The dose and dosage interval combined with elimination half-life will determine the blood level versus time profile of a drug. Differing blood level profiles in turn could affect drug efficacy profiles. Therefore, the optimal dosing interval needed may likely vary widely among different drugs, some requiring continuous administration, others perhaps requiring once per day or longer dosing intervals. Many drugs are administered using 3 times a day or 4 times a day schedules, which were mostly decided during clinical studies for the simplicity of dosing and for the consideration of enhancing patient compliance. However, for most drugs, thera-peutically optimal concentration/time profiles have not been clearly established.

Furthermore, it is likely that concentration/time profiles and elimination half-lives may vary greatly among the drugs. The assumption that steady-state blood concentrations during treatment produce optimal clinical improve-ment should be questioned.

For most therapeutic drugs, the relationship between drug concentration and its effect on the progression of disease remains largely unknown. Thus, it is a reasonable possibility that more sophisticated and variable dosing regimens might greatly enhance the thera-peutic benefits of drugs. In addressing this possibility, detailed studies of the long-term relationship between the pharmacokinetic and pharmacodynamic phases of drug action are needed.

Modern drugs are rarely administered in pure chemical form. Rather, they are prepared in a vehicle called a drug delivery system. Depending on the mode of administration and therapeutic needs, the vehicle can be of different physical states, shapes, or dosage types, as shown in Table 1.5. Most conventional dosage forms function merely to place a drug at the site of administration and pay no regard to the regulation of release and absorption or the duration or targeting of drug in the body.

Design and Formulation of Oral Sustained Release Drug Delivery System

The oral route of administration is the most preferred route due to spectrum of available dosage forms, easy to design and assures patient compliance. But here one has to take into consideration, the various pH that the dosage form would encounter during its transit to or through the gastrointestinal tract, the enzyme system and its influence on the drug as well as the dosage form. The majority of oral sustained release systems rely on dissolution, diffusion or a combination of both mechanisms, to generate slow release of drug to the gastrointestinal milieu. Theoretically and desirably a sustained release delivery device, should release the drug following a zero-order kinetics which would result in a blood-level time profile similar to that obtained after intravenous constant rate infusion. Plasma drug concentration-profiles

for conventional tablet or capsule formulation, a sustained release formulation, and a zero order sustained release formulation are shown in Figures 1.1 and 1.2.

Sustained (zero-order) drug release has been achieved, by following classes of sustained drug delivery system.

a. Diffusion sustained system
- Reservoir type
- Matrix type

b. Dissolution sustained system
- Reservoir type
- Matrix type

c. Methods using ion exchange

d. Methods using osmotic pressure

e. pH-independent formulations

f. Altered density formulations

Methods to Achieve Oral Sustained Drug Delivery

There are various methods employed for the

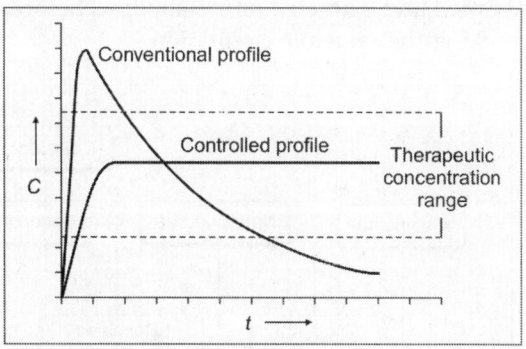

Fig.1.1: Comparison between conventional and controlled release systems

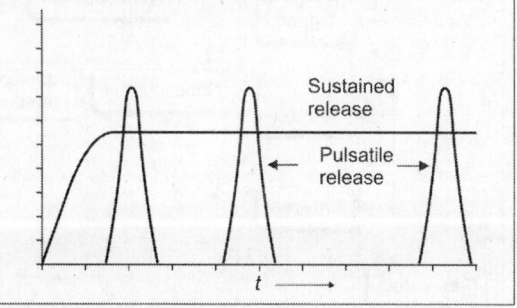

Fig.1.2: Dosage regimen for conventional and controlled release systems

Table 1.5: Drug delivery systems and their market share

Types	Market share
Conventional dosage forms	
Solids, liquids, semisolids	90%
Controlled release	
Sustained release, prolonged release, pulse-release, constant release	10%
Novel delivery systems	
Targeted, self-regulated, biofeedback, biological carriers	<1%

fabrication of oral sustained release delivery systems. Ritschel has given a detailed report of these techniques. These are as follows:

a. Hydrophilic matrix
b. Plastic matrix
c. Barrier resin beads
d. Fat embedment
e. Repeat action
f. Ion exchange resin
g. Soft gelatin depot capsules
h. Drug complexes

Design and Formulation of Parenteral Sustained Release Drug Delivery System

Parenteral drug delivery seeks to optimize therapeutic index by providing immediate drug to the systemic pool in required quantity to treat emergency clinical episode(s) such as cardiac attack(s), respiratory arrests or to administer drugs which are extensively sampled and extracted or metabolized before reaching the systemic circulation.

The carrier systems are invariably ought to be colloidal stable dispersions of particulates or vesicular structure. The parenteral drug delivery is mainly meant for drug concentration maintenance in systemic pool or other site of action(s). The release pattern from such systems may be to sustain the pharmacodynamic effect or to target the drug at the site of its action. The target-oriented systems are generally programmed to release the contents at target vicinity or intra-target locus or molecular levels. The drug is delivered in an explosive burst fashion or following a controlled or regulated release pattern. In the latter case drug release regulation could be monitored through bio-responsive behavior of the system or it may be modulated from some external level using appropriate physical means, i.e. pH variation, magnetic field application or photo irradiation, etc. (Fig. 1.3).

The preparation(s) with different pH should, however ensure that on parenteral administration drug or carrier precipitation or

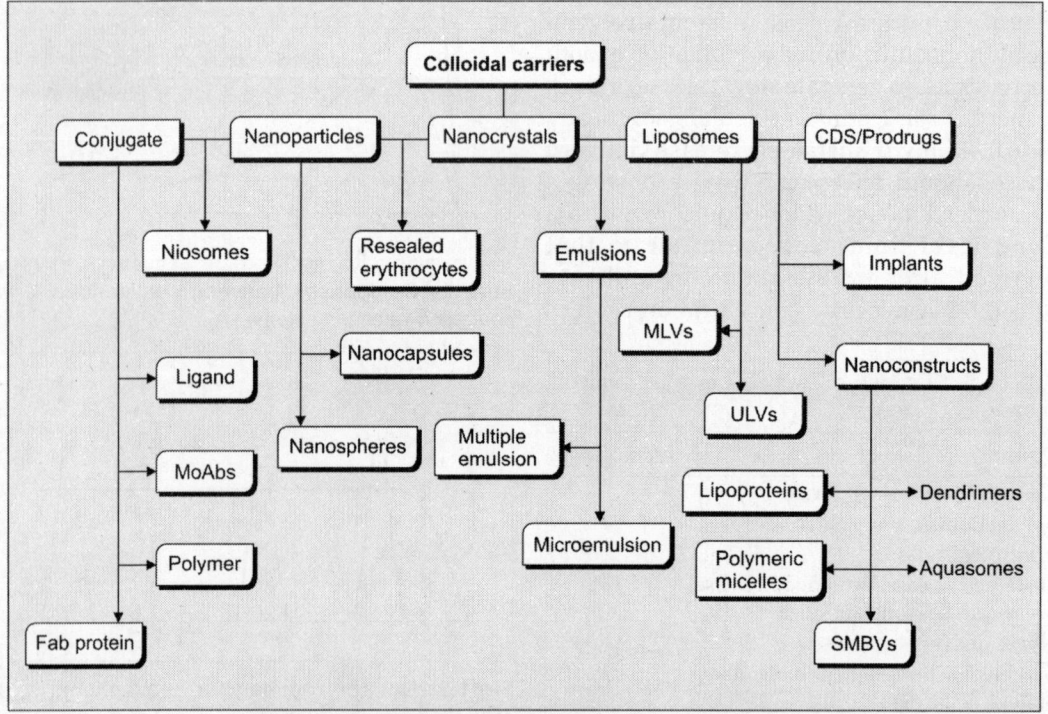

Fig.1.3: Schematic representation of different types of carriers

peptization should not occur. The *in vivo* behavior and instability of carrier composite may drastically affect overall disposition kinetics of drug in an unpredictable manner.

The parenteral drug delivery systems (PDDS) need to meet the basic requirements of parenteral products, i.e. sterility, apyrogenicity, reproducibility in performance, safety and efficacy. Nevertheless, complete removal of bioburden via aseptic filtration may offer working solution to the problem.

It is appreciated that to reach extravascular compartment the carrier must avoid opsonization and should be small enough in size. Furthermore, to be actively targetable it should be designed for site specificity using appropriate ligands. The release of drug may follow various patterns. The bystander explosive release is well exemplified by target sensitive immunoliposomes. Pharmacokinetic profiles of drugs in tissues of varying degree

of blood perfusion are shown in Fig. 1.5. The system is typically based on conventional lipid with a derivatized lipid component, i.e. phosphatidylethylamine lined site-specific immunoglobulin (PE-IgG). This conjugate participates in film structuring as one of the accessory lipids.

Cytosolic-sustained drug release is based on strategy where a carrier construct enters a cellular target via receptor-mediated endocytosis and categorically changes the pH of endosome. Due to change in pH the carrier loaded endosome does not fuse with lysosome thus remains as a cargo and releases drug contents slowly in to the cytosol(s). While another class of drug colloidal carrier(s) exploits/manipulates pH of endolysosomes and leaks intact in to the cytosol. Thus it serves to constitute a cytosolic intracellular cargo for drug, which releases the contents in a controlled manner. The targeted drug delivery

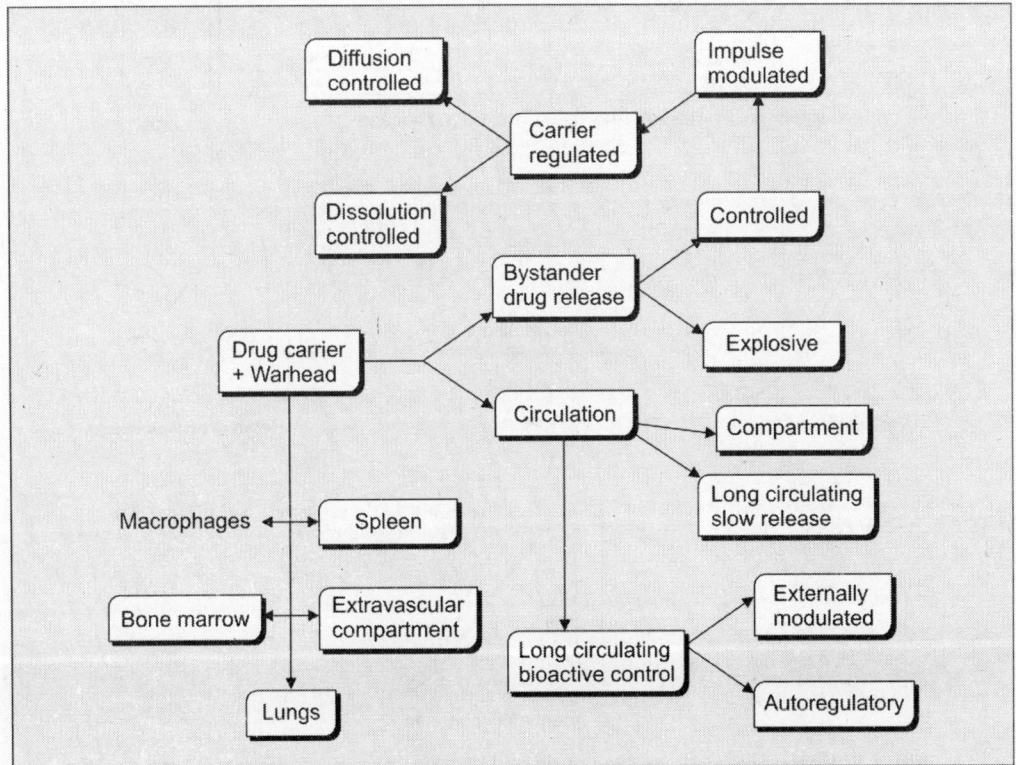

Fig. 1.4: Release profile(s) and biofate of intravenously administered system(s)

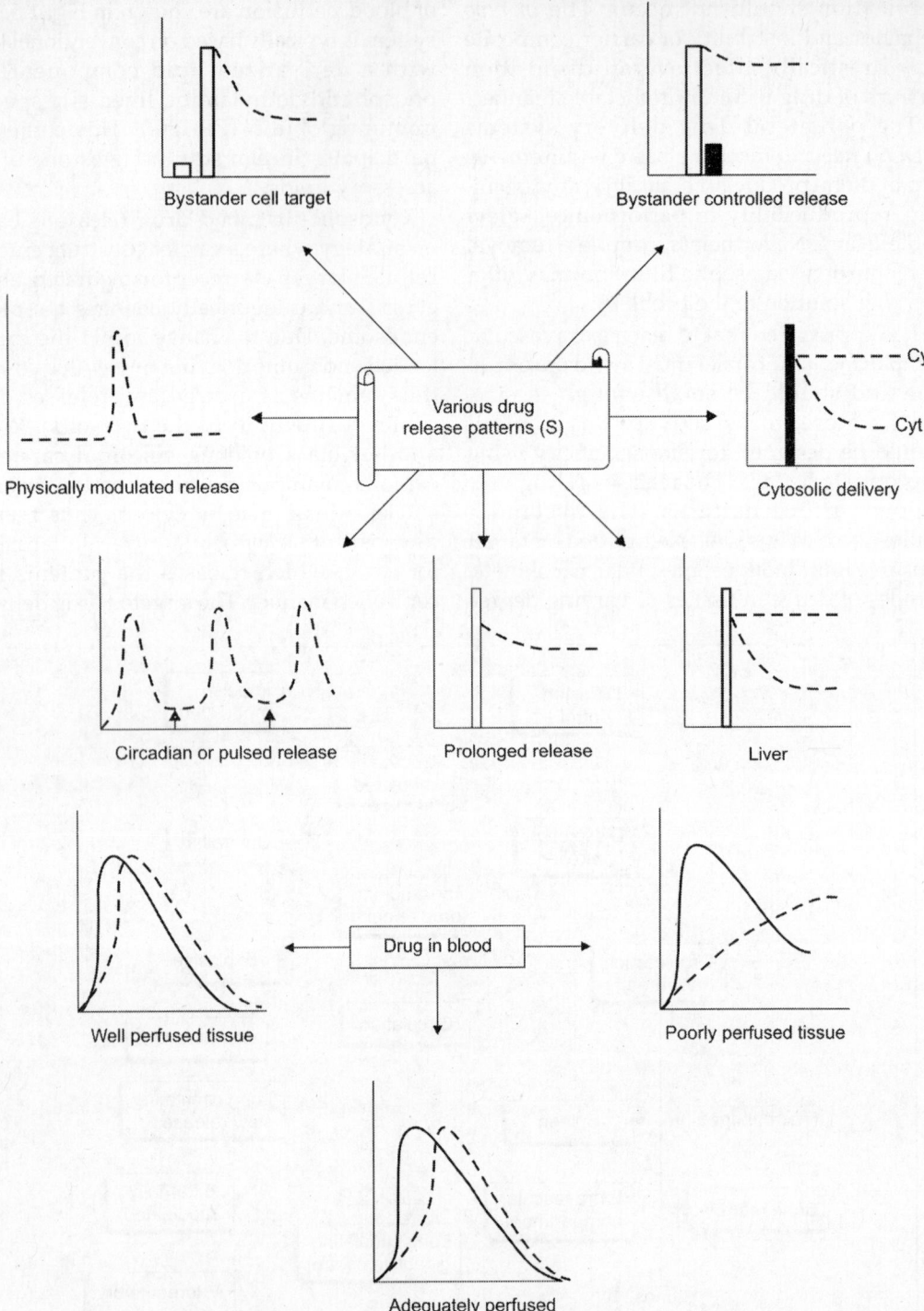

Fig. 1.5: Pharmacokinetic profiles of drugs in tissues of varying degree of blood perfusion

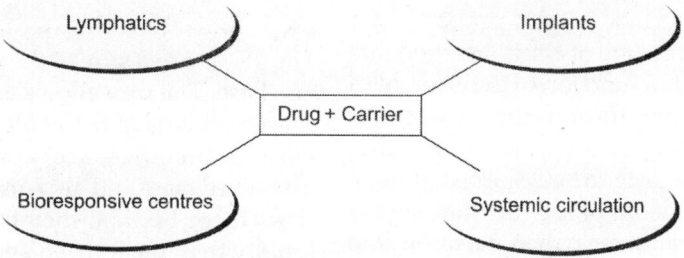

Fig. 1.6: Biofate of intramuscularly administered system

to extracellular compartment is possible via extravasation of carrier, and also the system should be engineered properly to span entire body, avoiding RES uptake and to reach the site where it is retained due to receptor-ligand interaction. The circulating carrier could be arrested by site-specific ligands for ECM or cellular receptors.

Similarly, on intramuscular administration (biofate of intramuscularly administered system is shown in Fig. 1.6) preferably into deltoid, triceps, pectoral, and vastus lateralis muscles, the systemic availability depends on drug perfusion or diffusion into the blood vascular system. Thus degree of site perfusion, nature of blood capillaries and volume of administered dose may affect drug diffusion out of the delivery system and into body tissue. Other than these, drugs related parameter(s) might equivocally affect systemic availability of drug(s). Thus it can be presented schematically as follows:

As it is known for controlled and novel drug delivery, they have various alternative route(s) of administration. The field of drug delivery and targeting has been revolutionized with the advent of a plethora of carrier systems that can be used either parenterally, topically, orally or by implantation. However, parenteral drug delivery remains the leading area of research, which led to the development of sophisticated systems that could allow drug targeting and the sustained or controlled release of parenteral medicines. Intravenous and intra-arterial administration particularly

exploits blood as vehicle for transportation of carrier to the site(s). The colloidal carrier may remain in systemic circulation as a long circulating unit for controlled and prolonged drug release profile(s) and biofate of intravenously administered system(s) is shown in Fig. 1.4.

Factors influencing design of sustained release/controlled release dosage forms:

The therapeutic efficacy of drug under clinical conditions is not simply a function of its intrinsic pharmacological activity but also depends upon the path followed by the drug molecule especially from the site of administration to the target site. Different conditions encountered by the drug molecule while traversing the path of distribution may alter either the effectiveness of the drug or may affect the amount of the drug ultimately reaching the receptor site.

PHYSICOCHEMICAL PROPERTIES

Molecular Size and Diffusivity

The ability of a drug to diffuse within and out of polymers is termed as diffusivity (diffusion coefficient D). It is a function of its molecular size (or molecular weight). A drug must diffuse through a variety of biological membranes during its time course in the body. In addition to diffusion through these biological membranes, drugs administered in the form of many extended release systems must diffuse through a rate-controlling polymeric membrane or matrix in order to be available for *in vivo* diffusion and distribution.

Aqueous Solubility

Solubility is a thermodynamic property of a compound. The fraction of drug absorbed into the portal blood is a function of the amount of drug in the solution form in the GI tract, i.e, this is referred to as the intrinsic permeability of the drug. For a drug to be absorbed, it must dissolve in the aqueous phase surrounding the site of administration and then partition into or across the absorbing membrane. The aqueous solubility of a drug influences its dissolution rate, which in turn establishes the concentration of absorbable fraction in solution and, hence, the driving force for diffusion across biomembranes. Drugs are classified on the basis of solubility and the classification system is known as basic chemical structure (BCS). According to it the drugs are classified as:

Class I: High solubility–high permeability

Class II: Low solubility–high permeability

Class III: High solubility–low permeability

Class IV: Low solubility–low permeability

High solubility: Largest dose dissolved in 250 ml of water over a pH range 1–8.

High permeability: Extent of absorption is >90%.

Class III and class IV drugs are poor candidates for sustained release/controlled release delivery. Compound with solubility below 0.1 mg/ml encounters significant solubilization obstacles and compound with solubility below 10 mg/ml present difficulties related to solubilization during formulation. A drug with very low solubility and a slow dissolution rate will exhibit dissolution-limited absorption and may yield sustained blood level on account of intrinsic characteristics. The pH-dependent solubility, particularly in the physiological pH range would be another crucial factor for consideration in designing of sustained release/controlled release formulation; because of the variation in the pH throughout the gastrointestinal tract, the dissolution rate accordingly varies.

Example—Phenytoin

pK$_a$—Ionization Constant

The pK$_a$ is a measure of the strength of an acid or a base. The pKa allows us to determine the charge on a drug molecule at any given pH. Drug molecules are active only in the unionized state and also unionized molecules cross these lipoidal membranes much more rapidly than the ionized species. The amount of drug that exists in unionized form is a function of dissociation constant of a drug at a pH of fluid at absorption site. For a drug to be absorbed, it must be in unionized form at the absorption site. Drugs which exist in ionized form at the absorption site are poor candidates for sustained/controlled dosage forms since they have poor intrinsic absorption characteristic. Most drugs are weak acids or bases. Since the unchanged form of a drug preferentially permeates across lipid membranes, it is important to note the relationship between the pK$_a$ of the compound and the pH of absorptive environment exists predominantly. Presenting the drug in an unchanged form is advantageous for drug permeation. Unfortunately, the situation is made more complex by the fact that the aqueous solubility of the drug generally decreases on conversion to an unchanged form. Delivery systems that are dependent on diffusion or dissolution will likewise be dependent on the solubility of the drug in aqueous media. These dosage forms must function in an environment of changing pH, the stomach being acidic and the small intestine more neutral, hence the effect of pH on the release process must be defined.

Partition Coefficient (the Solvent: Water Quotient of Drug Distribution)

When a drug is administered to the GI tract, it must cross a variety of biological membranes to produce a therapeutic effect in different bio-areas of the body. It is common to consider that these membranes are lipidic, therefore the partition coefficient of oil-soluble drugs becomes important in determining the effectiveness of membrane barrier penetration. Compounds which are lipophilic in nature with high partition coefficient are poorly aqueous soluble and they are retained in the lipophilic tissue for the longer time. In case of compounds with very low partition coefficient, it is very difficult for them to penetrate the membrane, resulting in poor bioavailability. Furthermore, partitioning effects apply equally to diffusion through polymer membranes. Partition coefficient influences not only the permeation of drug across the biological membranes but also diffusion within and across the rate-controlling membrane or matrix. A major criterion in evaluation of the ability of a drug to penetrate these lipid membranes, (i.e. its membrane permeability) is its apparent oil/water partition coefficient, defined as, $K = C_o/C_w$, where, C_o is the equilibrium concentration of all forms of the drug in an organic phase at equilibrium, and C_w the equilibrium concentration of all forms in an aqueous phase. In general, drugs with extremely large values of K are very oil soluble and will partition into membranes quite readily. The relationship between tissue permeation and partition coefficient for the drug generally is defined by the Hansch correlation, which describes a parabolic relationship between the logarithm of the activity of a drug or its ability to be absorbed and the logarithm of its partition coefficient.

Stability

Orally administered drugs are subjected to both acid–base hydrolysis and enzymatic degradation. Degradation proceeds at a slow rate for drugs in solid state; therefore, this is the preferred state of delivery. One important factor for the loss of drug is through acid hydrolysis and/or metabolism in the GIT when administered orally. It is possible to significantly improve the relative bioavailability of a drug that is unstable in GI tract by placing it in a slowly available controlled release form. For those drugs which are unstable in the stomach, the most appropriate controlling unit would be one that releases its content only in the intestine. The drug release in the cases which are unstable in the environment of the intestine, the most appropriate means of controlling the release rate and supporting better availability of drug is considered to be gastro-retentive and gastric-drug releasing systems. So, drugs with significant stability problems in any particular area of the GI tract are less suitable for formulation into controlled release systems that release the contents uniformly over the length of GIT.

BIOLOGICAL FACTORS

Absorption

The rate, extent and uniformity of absorption of a drug are important considerations for its formulation into modified release system. Absorption of a drug is a critical factor in case of oral administration. Assuming that the transit time of drug through the absorptive area of gastrointestinal tract is between 9–12 hours, the maximum absorption half-life should be 3–4 hours. This corresponds to a minimum absorption rate constant K_a value of 0.17–0.23/hr that is necessary to ensure for about 80–95% absorption of drug over a 9–12 hours transit time.

Drugs absorbed by active transport system are unsuitable for sustained/controlled drug delivery system, e.g. methotrexate, enalapril, nicotinamide, fexofenadine.

Drugs absorbed through amino acid transporters in the intestine, e.g. cephalosporines, gabapentine, baclofen, methyl-dopa, levodopa are not suitable to be formulated as slow sustained release system.

Drugs transported through oligopeptide transporters, e.g. captopril, lisinopril, cephalexine, cefadroxil, cefixime are not suitable for sustained/modified release formulations.

Drugs required to exert a local therapeutic action in the stomach are not suitable for sustained drug delivery, e.g. mesoprostol, 5-fluorouracil, antacids.

Metabolism

Drugs those are significantly metabolized before absorption, either in the lumen or in the tissue of the intestine, can exhibit decreased bioavailability from their slower release dosage form. For a drug to be a candidate for sustained release dosage form, it should have low half-life (<5 hours), larger therapeutic window, absorbed throughout the GIT. The metabolism of a drug can either inactivate an active drug or convert an inactive drug into an active metabolite. Complex metabolic patterns would make the sustained release/controlled release design much more difficult particularly when biological activity is wholly or partly due to a metabolite as in case isosorbide 2, 5-dinitrate.

Regional Delivery and Targeting

The benefit of a drug can be greatly enhanced if it can be targeted to its preferred site of action and kept away from sites associated with toxicity. Localization can occur at the organ, tissue, cellular, and subcellular compartment or organelle level. Direct injection of drug carriers into solid tumors or wound sites provides another example. As a third example, the growth, integration, and vascularization of surgically implanted tissue engineered constructs may require the localized and well-timed release of growth and angiogenesis factors. To specify delivery at the cellular level, it is necessary to coat the carrier surface with ligands which bind to specific cell surface features, such as polysaccharides or receptor proteins. Antibodies raised against molecular determinants expressed at the cell surface are the most obvious targeting ligands, but in recent years peptide ligands have been designed based on other known interactions between cell surface receptors and both soluble and extracellular matrix proteins. Since tumor cells express multiple drug resistance transporters, release of drug from the carrier at the cell surface may not result in increased drug uptake in target cells. The drug/nanocarrier combination is likely to be more effective if it can be brought into the cell by active processes, such as coated pit-mediated endocytosis. Once within the cell, the drug needs to dissociate from the carrier and exit the endosome, in either order. Further for targeting of drug to an organelle, an organelle specific 'address label' is conjugated to the drug/carrier, e.g. gene and protein delivery to the nucleus may require that a nuclear localization sequence be conjugated to the active biomolecule in order to carry and transports the drugs through nuclear pores into the nucleus.

Development of Controlled and Novel Delivery Systems

Clearly, the development of better delivery systems in conjunction with the discovery of novel pharmacological compounds will lead to significant improvements in pharmacotherapeutics. However, given the medicated cost of developing new drugs and the reduced number of novel compounds that gain approval for marketing each year, interest in developing new drug delivery devices has been intensified in recent years (Table 1.6). As a result, existing drugs that can be made more efficacious and safe using improved delivery systems represent both promising marketing opportunities for pharmaceutical companies and advances in the effective treatment of a disease by clinicians.

Table 1.6: Reasons for intense interest in developing new DDS

- For improving efficacy of conventional dosage form of drug which exists in clinical practice.
- Optimally addressing the pharmacodynamic and toxicity related issues of exisiting drugs is viable and cost effective compared to new drug discovery.
- Bioengineered medicines need specialized drug delivery.

Effect of Tolerance/Resistance/Sensitization

Among the compounds that currently are undergoing extensive clinical trials, many fall under the classification of bioengineered compounds such as peptides, proteins, hormones, and nucleic acids. The successful clinical application of these new agents will largely depend on the availability of effective delivery systems. Therefore, it appears that the development of novel delivery approaches will immensely contribute to improved therapies for both currently existing and yet-to be developed pharmacological compounds. A major obstacle to this point in the development of optimal delivery systems is the lack of more specific pharmacokinetic and pharmacodynamic correlation for most of the drugs used today.

Answering some of the fundamental questions such as the relevance of concentration/time profiles to efficacy, linear/nonlinear drug behavior, effects of active metabolite, time-dependent changes in PK/PD properties, and similarly related issues, during the early stages of drug development will bring about a more complete understanding of the variables that affect dosage form design and drug efficacy. These data can also be applied to optimize the therapeutic efficacy of drugs after reevaluating the limitations of currently available dosage regimen and delivery systems for a given drug. Similarly, such specific data could serve to guide the development of improved or novel delivery systems needed to optimize clinical usefulness of a drug. Therefore, a more precise information and understanding of PK/PD profiles of drugs will be necessary for future advances in drug delivery research and should become an integral part of drug development from the earliest stages.

At present, the process of drug development can be divided into three major stages—discovery of new compounds, clinical studies, and formulation of delivery systems.

Pharmaceutical companies traditionally have spent the majority of their time and financial resources in the discovery of new compounds. Despite these efforts, fewer new drugs have received approval for marketing in recent years. The existing trend further enhances the potential for great scientific and economic benefits for developing a novel drug delivery system that can improve drug therapy.

Economic interests at the expense of scientific inquiry have often influenced clinical studies those are primarily funded by pharmaceutical companies. As a result, drugs are commonly tested in clinical settings consisting of a limited number of selected patients and using unsophisticated formulations that produce high blood concentrations for maximal initial effect over a short period of time. These types of studies often do not consider the long-term effects of such varying peak and valley plasma/drug concentration profiles. These studies also preclude careful consideration of a wide variety of dosage regimens and drug delivery options available for drugs under investigation.

The efforts for innovative drug delivery systems developments by pharmaceutical companies to this point have received minimal priority and have been applied primarily to prepare controlled release formulations to simply extend dosing intervals for the sake of convenience in dosing. The lack of sophistication and relatively inexpensive cost of current delivery systems reflect manufacturers' low level of commitment to the development of novel delivery systems. Different novel carrier systems are shown in Fig. 1.7.

Various nanocarriers for the drug delivery are:

- *Floating drug delivery system:* Floating systems do float over the gastric contents owing to their lower bulk density. The use of various film-coating techniques and incorporation of a floating chamber filled with harmless gas or a liquid that gasifies at body temperature are some sophisticated

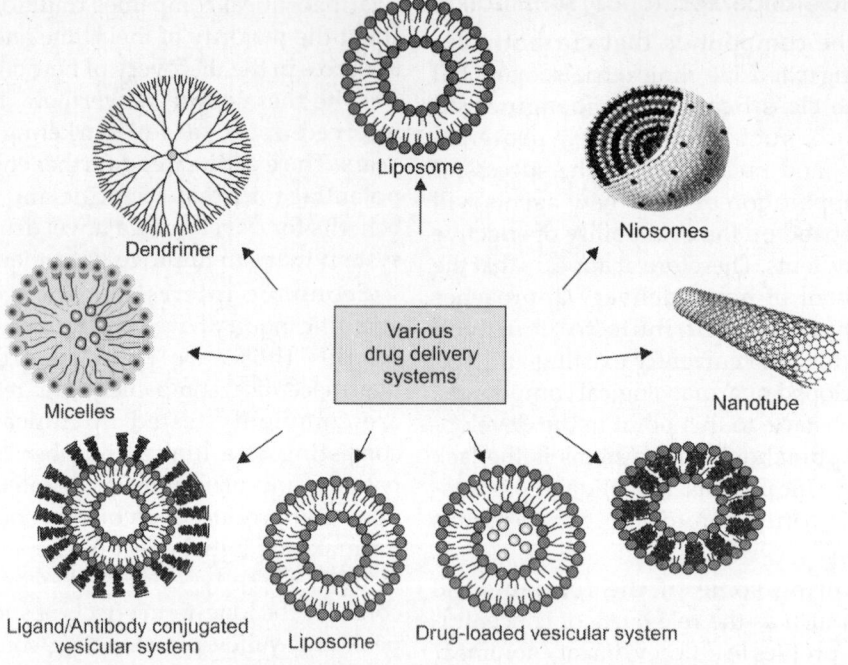

Fig 1.7: Different novel carrier systems

techniques used to develop floating drug delivery system (FDDS). These forms are often called 'hydrodynamically balanced systems (HBS)' as they can maintain low density and keep floating even after hydration. When a floating dosage form is administered with food, the device remains buoyant on the surface of the gastric contents in the upper part of the stomach and moves down toward the pyloric sphincter when the meal empties. The reported gastric retention time (GRT) of such floating devices varies from 4 to 10 hours. The active drug is progressively released from the formulation matrix and gets introduced into the proximal intestine where it can be absorbed.

• *Osmotic drug delivery system:* Osmotic pumps are controlled drug delivery devices based on the principle of osmosis. Osmosis is well known phenomenon, which is

exploited for development of delivery systems with every desirable property of an ideal controlled drug delivery system. Osmotic pumps offer many advantages like they are easy to formulate and simple in operation, improved patient compliance with reduced dosing frequency, more consistent and prolonged therapeutic effect is obtained with constant and uniform blood concentration. Furthermore, they are inexpensive and their industrial adaptability vis-a-vis production scale up is easy. In principle, this delivery system dispenses drug continuously at a zero order rate until the concentration of the osmotically active salt in the system decreases below the saturation solubility, where upon a non-zero order release is followed.

• *Bioadhesive drug delivery system:* Bioadhesive is the term that describes the adhesion of a polymer to a biological substrate. More specifically, when adhesion is restricted to the mucous layer lining of the mucosal surface, it is termed as mucoadhesion. This has gained considerable interest since the localization of drug carrying particles at the mucosal surface would result in prolonged residence time at the site of action or absorption, drug localization, increase in the drug concentration gradient and direct contact with intestinal mucosa. Bioadhesion can be obtained by building either nonspecific interactions, which are driven by the physicochemical properties of the particles and the intestinal surfaces or through specific interactions when a ligand appended on to the particle is used for the recognition and attachment to a specific site at the mucosal surface.

- *Multiple/micro-emulsions:* The complex system containing dispersed droplets themselves contain smaller dispersed droplets. These systems known as multiple emulsions are easily prepared by the reemulsification of simple primary O/W or W/O system to provide O/W/O or W/O/W emulsions. Microemulsion can be defined in general as thermodynamically stable isotropically clear dispersion of two immiscible liquids, consisting of microdomains of one or both liquids stabilized by interfacial films of surface active molecules.

- *Colon-specific drug delivery system:* The site-specific delivery of the drugs to the colon possesses the potential to reduce the side effects and to improve the pharmacological response. However, for successful colonic drug delivery, many physiological barriers must be overcome, the major one being absorption or degradation of the active drug in the upper part of the GI tract. The disease state also can potentially alter the delivery and absorption characteristics of drug from the colon. The drug targeting to colon is also exploited for systemic administration of active drugs. Colon-specific drug delivery systems are able to protect peptide drugs from hydrolysis and enzymatic degradation in the duodenum and jejunum, and eventually release the drugs in the ileum or colon, as a summation of affects it leads to greater systemic bioavailability. This specific release in the colon also gives a time delay between administration and onset of action, which can be useful for diseases with varied degrees of severity, such as asthma and arthritis.

- *Transdermal drug delivery systems:* Transdermal drug delivery systems (TDDS) are specifically designed to obtain systemic blood levels. A TDDS is designed to release the drugs at a predetermined rate continuously, avoiding unnecessarily high peaks and subtherapeutic troughs in plasma drug levels. Transdermal permeation, or percutaneous absorption, can be defined as the passage of a substance, such as a drug, from the outside of the skin through its various layers into the blood stream. Due to frequent pricking, need of constant medical supervision and lack in patient compliance in case of parenteral administration, the transdermal route has been introduced as an alternative to parentral system.

- *Spherical crystallization:* It is a particle design technique, by which crystallization and agglomeration can be carried out simultaneously in one step. The spherical crystallization technique also involves the use of a bridging liquid that improves compressibility by acting as granulating fluid. Thus spherical crystallization is a method that helps achieve good flow ability and compressibility. The steps involved in the process of crystallization include flocculation zone, zero growth zone, fast growth zone and constant size zone.

- *Implantable drug delivery systems:* Implanted or placed in the body like in the ocular, vaginal cavities or subdermally. They are free of limitations associated with oral, intravenous or topical drug administration.

Additionally, subcutaneous implants devices offer one unique advantage of a retrievable or withdrawal opportunity. This feature enables a readily termination of drug administration whenever required.

- *Micellelar system:* Surfactants have the ability to self-associate to form micelles. Micelles consist of surfactant molecules aggregated/packed in a space-filling manner at the critical micellization concentration (CMC). The main driving force for micelle formation in aqueous solution is the effective interaction between the hydrophobic parts of the surfactant molecules, whereas interaction opposing micellization may include electrostatic repulsive interaction between charged head groups of ionic surfactants, repulsive osmotic interactions between chain-like polar head groups, such as oligoethylene oxide chains, or steric interaction between bulky head groups. The way surfactant molecules aggregate is mainly determined by the attraction between the hydrophobic tails and electrostatic repulsions of the hydrophilic head groups, which are present in the surfactant molecules.

- *Liposomes:* Liposomes are concentric bilayered vesicles in which an aqueous core is entirely enclosed by a membranous lipid bilayer mainly composed of natural and synthetic phospholipids. The lipid molecules are usually phospholipids-amphipathic moieties with a hydrophilic head group and two hydrophilic lipidic tails. On addition of excess water, such lipidic moieties spontaneously orient to give the most thermodynamically stable conformation, in which polar head groups face outwards the aqueous medium, and the lipidic chains turn inwards to avoid the water phase, giving rise to double layer or bilayer lamellar structures. In the assembled geometry (structure) both water and lipid soluble drugs can be entrapped into the liposomes.

- *Microspheres:* They in technical sense are spherical polymeric particles. The microspheres are physically free flowing powders consisting of proteins or synthetic polymers, which may or may not be biodegradable in nature, and ideally have average particle size less than 200 μm. Solid biodegradable microspheres incorporating a drug dispersed or dissolved throughout particle matrix have the potential for the controlled release of drug. These carriers have received much attention not only for prolonged release but also for the targeting of the anticancer drugs to the tumor.

- *Nanoparticles:* They are submicrosized colloidal structures composed of synthetic or semisynthetic polymers. The continual quest and maneuvering towards physical stability improvement of liposomes resulted into development of solid core nanoparticles as an alternative drug carrier. The colloidal carriers based on biodegradable and biocompatible polymeric systems have largely influenced the controlled and targeted drug delivery concepts. The nanoparticles loaded bioactives not only deliver drug(s) to specific organs within the body but also the drug delivery can be designed to be rate bystander, burst, controlled, pulsatile or modulated.

- *Resealed erythrocytes:* The developing RBC has the capacity to synthesize hemoglobin; however, adult RBCs do not have this capacity and serve as carriers for hemoglobin. The prime function of these RBCs is to transport gases for respiratory processes. The carrier potential of these cells is exploited for the delivery of bioactives/peptides. Moreover, RBCs can be uniquely poised to modulate the properties of blood vascular components. The idea of using red blood cells as drug containers (erythrocyte encapsulation), whereby biologically active entities can be entrapped within the cell, continues to be explored as a means of drug delivery and targeting.

• *Transfersomes:* They are complex, most often, vesicular aggregate optimized to attain extremely flexible and self-regulating membrane; this makes the vesicle flexibly deformable. The vesicles therefore can cross microporous barrier very efficiently, even when available passage are much smaller than their average (aggregate) size. Similar to liposomes, transfersomes have a lipid bilayer that surrounds an aqueous core, however in contrast to liposomes, transfersomes contain at least one component that soften the membrane and makes them as well as skin more flexible. This also allows easy and rapid changes in or on transfersome shape.

Organogels: A simple working definition of the term 'gel' is a soft, solid or solid-like material, which contains both solid and liquid components, where the solid component (the gelator) is usually present as a mesh/network of aggregates, which traps and immobilizes the liquid component. The solid network prevents the liquid from flowing, primarily due to surface tension. The gel is said to be a hydrogel or an organogel depending on the nature of the liquid component viz.; water in case hydrogels and an organic solvent in case of organogels. Organogels can be distinguished from hydrogels by their predominantly organic continuous phase and can then be further subdivided on the basis of nature of the gelling molecule accordingly they may be polymeric or low molecular weight (LMW) organogelators.

Dendrimers: Dendritic polymers have tree-like structures and consist of hyper-branched polymers commonly referred to as dendrigrafts, dendrons and dendrimers. Each of these four classes reflects the structural features of these complex macromolecular architectures. Dendrimers are monodispersed macromolecules with a regular and highly branched three-dimensional architecture. They are produced in an iterative sequence of reaction steps, in which each iteration leads to a higher generation. They are highly branched symmetrical macromolecules of nano-sized dimensions, have well-defined molecular mass and geometry consist of a central core, repeating units and terminal functional groups.

Niosomes: They are nonionic surfactants based vesicles that result on account of the self-assembly of hydrated surfactant monomers. Nonionic surfactants of a wide structural variation have been found to be useful alternatives to phospholipids in the fabrication of vesicular systems. Niosomes possess physical properties, which are similar to liposomes, which are formed from phospholipids. Nonionic surfactant vesicles are prepared by incorporation of components containing nonionic surfactants. However, they may also posseses various ionic amphiphiles such as dicetyl-phosphate, stearylamine, etc. in order to achieve a stable vesicular suspension. The chemical stability as well as the relatively low cost of the materials used to prepare niosomes make this vesicle more attractive than liposomes for industrial productions both for pharmaceutical and cosmetic applications.

Solid lipid nanoparticles: Solid lipid nanoparticles (SLNs), made from solid lipids are particulate systems with mean particle size ranging from 50 to 1000 nm. SLNs have attracted significant interest by various researchers because of their physical stability, controlled drug release, protection of incorporated drugs from degradation, and excellent tolerability. Depending on their route of administration, SLNs are synthesized by various techniques, which include high-pressure homogenization, solvent emulsification-evaporation or diffusion, water-in-oil-in-water (W/O/W) double-emulsion method, high speed stirring, and/or ultrasonication. Analogous to other nanocarriers, SNPs can be modified for guided drug delivery. A major advantage of this formulation is that SNPs can be prepare to provide controlled drug release.

Intelligent Controlled Release Drug Delivery Systems Stimuli Controlled Nanocarriers

Site-specific Drug Release

Targeting of drugs to the specific site of their action offers several advantages. They mainly, include prevention of side effects of drugs on healthy tissues and enhancement of the drug uptake by targeted cells. Enhancing drug uptake by specific cells not only permits the internalization of drug molecules with low cellular permeability, but also allows for the maintenance of low blood-to-cell concentration ratio, thus reducing therapy-limiting adverse effects.

Responsive or triggered delivery systems are those that act responding an external signal or change in the surrounding environment. The response includes phase separation, shape alteration, dissolution, precipitation, degradation, and collapsing, swelling, change in hydrophilic and hydrophobic balance (Schmaljohann, 2006). These responsive systems may be both metals and polymers, but here polymeric drug delivery systems have been discussed which are able to distinguish biovariants and accordingly alter the delivery of a drug responding to localized changes in pH, or concentration of oxidizing molecules.

* *Temperature-responsive nanocarriers:* Nanocarriers that release the drug at a specific temperature or respond to the changes in the temperature are referred as temperature-responsive delivery systems. Poly (N-isopropylacrylamide) (PNIPAAm) has been most commonly used in the formulation of temperature-responsive drug delivery systems because it has got a lower critical solution temperature (LCST) of about 30–34°C. Below the LCST temperature, the polymer is soluble in water, while above it the polymer becomes insoluble. This behavior can be exploited for controling the delivery of therapeutic

agents from thermosensitive drug delivery systems and a hydrophobic polymer. Above the LCST, the micellar structure is deformed as the PNIPAAm, initially present in the nanoparticle shell when comes in contact with the aqueous environment, becomes insoluble and disorders the equilibrium of the core-shell configuration. Such a property can be utilized, if the LCST of the polymer is above 37°C then, the drug will not be released and the micelle will remain in its intact form until the temperature is increased above 37°C. This has been exploited for the agents which have a number of side effects and are intended to be released only at the site of action as in the case of antitumor agents which for instance have large number of systemic side effects, their cytotoxic properties are desired only at the site of the tumor. Contrary to this, for materials with LCST lower than normal body temperature, their thermoresponsive behavior can be used for delivery of drugs to the regions of low temperature such as hypoxic tissue (Patton et al., 2005). It is imperative to note that the LCST of polymers such as PNIPAAm can be increased or decreased upon polymerization with a hydrophobic or hydrophilic copolymer, respectively (Schmaljohann, 2006). One example of temperature-responsive drug delivery is thermoresponsive polymeric micelle that has been prepared from amphiphilic block copolymers consisting of N-isopropylacrylamide (NIPAAm) as outer shell and styrene (St) as hydrophobic inner core. When the temperature was increased above 32°C, i.e. the transition temperature, the outer shell chains dehydrated and collapsed, allowing aggregation between micelles supporting binding interactions with cell membrane surfaces. Moreover, the changes were reversible. Hydrophobic molecules were incorporated into the inner hydrophobic core of the thermoresponsive micelles and consequently, these were found to be valuable for site-specific delivery of drugs using target site borne changes in temperature (Cammas et al., 1997).

- *pH-responsive nanocarriers:* Similar to temperature, pH sensitivity has also been exploited to trigger the drug release at a particular site. This includes the polymers that undergo conformational changes depending upon the pH of the surrounding environment. For instance, they can precisely deliver chemotherapeutic agents at the site of a tumour due to the acidic pH found in its interstitium (Wike-Hooley et al., 1984), while keeping the rest of the body free from the systemic toxicity of these drugs (Schmaljohann, 2006). Additionally, these systems can be designed to delay release of a specific drug till the drug reaches at an intracellular site after endocytosis and is exposed to lower pH of the endolysosomal compartments (Schmaljohann, 2006). Systems have been designed which by means of their pH responsiveness are turned off due to configurational changes that permit them to preferentially come in contact with the organelle membrane (Panyam et al., 2002). pH-responsive systems have also been studied for applications in oral drug delivery (Schmaljohann, 2006). Such carriers also offer an advantage of protecting labile drugs like copolymers of poly (undecylenic acid) (PUA) and poly (N-isopropylacrylamide) (PNIPAAm) from the harsh acid environment of the stomach while promoting their absorption in the small intestine. Some of the examples of recently developed pH-responsive nanosystems are discussed here. Nanoparticles of poly (beta-amino ester) (PbAE) conjugated with poloxamers, triblock copolymers of poly (ethylene oxide)-poly (propylene oxide)-poly(ethylene oxide), were fabricated for the delivery of hydrophobic drugs to the acidic environment of tumors and other intracellular acidic organelles (Potineni et al., 2003; Shenoy et al., 2005). Studies revealed the successful delivery of paclitaxel by pH-responsive PbAE to SKOV-3 ovarian cancer cells in *in vitro*, and also reported the higher paclitaxel accumulation at the tumor site as compared to free drug administration (in solution) or in pH-insensitive paclitaxel nanoparticles *in vivo*. Further, *in vivo* studies demonstrated that paclitaxel-loaded PbAE nanoparticles resulted in higher therapeutic efficacy as compared to free drug and paclitaxel PCL in mice xenografts of ovarian cancer, and did not result in any noticeable systemic toxicity (Devalapally et al., 2007).

The pH-responsive nanoparticles design based on block copolymers of poly [2-(N,N-diethylamino) ethyl methacrylate] (PDEA) and poly (ethylene glycol) (PEG) has been reported (Xu et al., 2006). These were about 80 nm in diameter with a pH-sensitive core. The pH-responsive nanoparticles were fabricated in such a way so as to release the drug in a very short period of time upon being endocytosed by the target cancer cells and subsequently being exposed to the acidic conditions of the lysosomal compartments. Such rapid release was due to the ability of the PDEA-PEG nanoparticles to solublize in the aqueous biological environment when the pH drops below 6. Cisplatin was used to evaluate the potential of this system to overcome MDR in SKOV-3 cancer cells in *in vitro* and *in vivo* in nude mice xenografts (Xu et al., 2006). Results revealed that PDEA-PEG nanoparticles were internalized by cells into lysosomes and resulted in appreciably higher cellular growth inhibition when compared to free cisplatin. Recently, concept of block ionic complexes (BIC) has been introduced, the BIC are formed by ionic interactions between hydrophilic block copolymers comprising of ionic and nonionic regions with an oppositely charged molecule. These responsive systems undergo changes in response to the environmental conditions (Oh et al., 2006). As the core consists of electrostatically bound polyion-counterion complexes, the encapsulation takes place via hydrophobic or electrostatic interactions. For instance, family of polymer-surfactant complexes formed between block ionomers and oppositely charged surfactants have been evaluated. Complexes between cationic copolymer poly (ethylene oxide)-g-polyethyleneimine (PEO-g-PEI) and sodium salt of oleic acid, a natural nontoxic surfactant, were prepared and characterized. They formed micelles in the size range of 50–60 nm which exhibited the potential to encapsulate hydrophobic drug moieties like paclitaxel. They also demonstrated the use of the biologically active surfactants as co-components of block ionomer complexes. On the whole, these studies suggested that block ionomer complexes could be used to prepare a variety of stable formulations of biologically active compounds, and have a great application potential as drug delivery systems (Bronich et al., 1999). Still another attractive concept has been developed for the pH-sensitive drug delivery system which utilized pH-induced cleavable bonds to modify the surface and cause subsequent release of the drug. These copolymers are consisted of a biocompatible hydrophilic poly (ethylene oxide) (PEO) block and a hydrophobic block (allyl glycidyl ether) (PEO-PAGE) containing covalently bound doxorubicin. The block copolymers were prepared by anionic ring opening polymerization using allyl glycidyl ether as functional monomer and sodium salt of poly (ethylene oxide) monomethyl ether as macroinitiator. The copolymers were subjected to covalent modification by the addition of methyl sulfanylacetate. The consequential ester then reacted with hydrazine hydrate giving polymer hydrazide. The hydrazide was coupled with the drug yielding pH-sensitive hydrazone bonds between it and the carrier. The resulting conjugate encapsulated 3% w/w

doxorubicin. After incubation in buffers at 37°C drug released faster at pH 5.0 which is close to the pH of endosomes and about 43% was released within 24 hours, further at pH 7.4, i.e. pH of blood plasma only about 16% of doxorubicin was released within 24 hours. Continuous cleavage of hydrazone bonds between doxorubicin and carrier was observed even after plateau in drug release profile from micelles incubated in aqueous solutions was reached (Hrubý et al., 2004). Recently, preparation of pH-responsive nanoparticles for oral delivery of proteins has also been reported (Sajeesh et al., 2005). These were formed by ionic complexation of poly (methacrylic acid)-chitosan-poly (ethylene glycol) prepared by free radical polymerization reaction. Loading of the drug occurred through diffusion absorption thus allowing the drug to get into the polymeric system. Regardless of their uneven morphology, these nanoparticles exhibited properties useful for oral delivery of labile molecules. Release of model protein was considerably delayed at a pH of 1.2 (representative of the stomach) compared to pH 7.4. Only about 10% of loaded insulin was released from the nanoparticles at the acidic pH as compared to (about 90%) at pH 7.4 (Sajeesh et al., 2005). Complete release of the protein was noted at pH 7.4 that is pertinent to the residence time of the particles in the small intestine. The pH-dependent release behavior may attributed to the ability of the PMAA polymer to swell or shrink with the increase or decrease in pH due to the protonation and deprotonation of carboxylic acid groups, respectively. When used for oral delivery, the nanoparticles protected the therapeutic agent from degradation in the acidic environment of the stomach, however released it in the small intestine as a result of swelling of nanoparticle.

- *Temperature and pH-responsive combo nanocarriers:* Thermosensitive polymers such as PNIPAAm are successful only if the

LCST of the polymer is above the body temperature so that they remain soluble or in their intact form at physiological fluids, whereas if the LCST is below the body temperature, then on administration into the body, it will deform and the drug well released out. So, the best option at hand is to fabricate the polymer with LCST higher than the body temperature and then artificially heating using an external source to cause the release of the drug. In order to overcome this problem, new delivery systems have been designed with both temperature and pH sensitivity. One such system that has been designed consisted of core-shell nanoparticles of poly (N-isopropylacrylamide-co-N, N-dimethylacrylamide-co-10-undecenoic acid) (PNIPAAm-co-DMAAm-co-UA). In this system, UA constituted the hydrophobic and pH-sensitive core while PNIPAAm constituted the shell at the surface in contact with the aqueous environment. DMMAm, being a hydrophilic polymer, increased the LCST of PNIPAAm to a higher temperature, the degree of shift depended on the molar composition of the copolymers: the higher the molecular weight of the DMMAm, the higher was the LCST of the copolymer. Soppimath et al, prepared a copolymer that had an LCST greater than body temperature (38.6°C) at physiological pH 7.4, and lower than body temperature (35.5°C) at a pH of 6.6 (Soppimath et al., 2005). As a result, nanoparticles from this copolymer could easily deliver drugs selectively to the acidic pH in tumours while remained stable and hence could prevent normal site from toxic effects. The pH dependence of the LCST is ascribed to the protonation and subsequent decrease of hydrophobicity of the UA core with rising pH, which leads to a rise in the LCST for the copolymer.

- *Oxidation-responsive nanocarriers:* Use of oxidation-sensitive materials attracts the attention of many researchers for its use in the drug delivery systems for application in inflamed tissues which are rich in oxidizing substances. For this purpose, vesicles of amphiphilic copolymer PEG-poly (propylene sulfide)-PEG (PEG-PPS-PEG) were fabricated. PPS constitutes the oxidation-sensitive block of the polymeric system which upon exposure to an oxidative environment, is transformed into hydrophilic poly (propylene sulfoxide) and poly (propylene sulfone), converting the vesicles into worm-like and spherical micelles of continuously decreasing size that can eventually be eliminated from the body by glomerular filtration. Another similar oxidation-responsive nanocarrier design is consisted of crosslinked poly (propylene sulfide) nanoparticles synthesised by emulsion polymerization of propylene sulfide in an aqueous phase containing pluronic F-127 followed by reaction with a bifunctional molecule.

POTENTIAL APPLICATIONS OF NANOCARRIERS IN TARGETED DRUG DELIVERY

Tumor Targeting

One of the major applications of nanotechnology is in the selective and effective delivery of various anticancer agents based on extravagation owing to nanosize of the carrier and its subsequent retention due to non-availability of lymphatic drainage system. The microvasculature of healthy tissue varies by tissue type, but in most tissues including the heart, brain, and lung, there are tight intercellular junctions with less than 10 nm intercellular space, however tumor microvasculature contains pores, fenestrae ranging from 100 to 1000 nm in diameter. Therefore, tumor within these tissues can be selectively targeted by creating drug delivery systems of size greater than the intercellular gap of the healthy tissue but smaller than the pores found in tumor vasculature (Hughes, 2005). Therefore, the nanocarriers of size ranging from 10–1000 nm are considered to be appropriate for targeted delivery of various anticancer drugs. The accumulation of liposomes or large macromolecules in tumors is a result of a 'leaky' microvasculature and an impaired lymphatic supporting the tumor area (also known as 'enhanced permeability and retention effect'). The principal pathway for the movement of liposomes into the tumor interstitium is extravasation through the discontinuous endothelium of the tumour microvasculature. Even the size of the liposomes in passive targeting approach determines the degree or extent of extravasation from the normal vasculature (Fig. 1.8). Once in the tumors, non-targeted liposomes are localized in the interstitium surrounding the tumour cells. However, a limited distribution of liposomes within the tumor interstitium results due to typically high interstitial pressure (which though helps in trapping the liposomes within the tumor area but prevents the access of drug into the necrotic zone) and a large interstitial space compared with normal body tissues.

Further, to increase the specificity and to decrease the toxicity of anticancer drugs, these have been modified or functionalized with a homing device which carries these drug-loaded carriers to the particular cells overexpressing corresponding complement receptors on the surface, i.e cancer cells. Various ligands such as folic acid, transferrin, RGD peptide, autacoids, HER-2, antibody etc. have been chemically attached to the surface of nanocarriers in order to deliver the drug to the cancer cells (Fig. 1.9). It was demonstrated that the unique affinity of long circulating and targeted liposomes could be combined in one preparation in which antibodies or other specific binding molecules are attached to PEG chains exposed to dispersion medium.

Targeted Drug Delivery to Central Nervous System

Drug delivery to the central nervous system still remains a challenge because of unique barrier properties of BBB which segregates the brain from the circulating blood and effectively limits the drug solute(s) entry into the brain (Patel et al., 2009). The BBB is a system of vascular cellular structures, mainly represented by tight junctions between endothelial cells, and an ensemble of enzymes, receptors, transporters, and efflux pumps the multidrug resistance (MDR) pathways which control and limit the access of molecules to the brain, either by paracellular or transcellular pathways (Fig. 1.10). Other barrier for brain delivery is barrier which separates the blood from the cerebrospinal fluid (CSF) that runs in the subarachnoid space surrounding the brain. This barrier is located at the choroid plexus, and it is formed by epithelial cells held together at their apices by tight junctions, which limit paracellular flux.

As a result high dose is required for the therapeutic benefit which at the same time

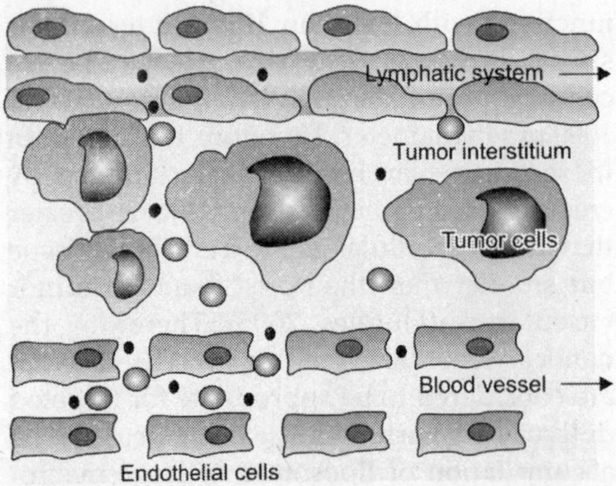

Fig. 1.8: Enhanced permeability and retention effects

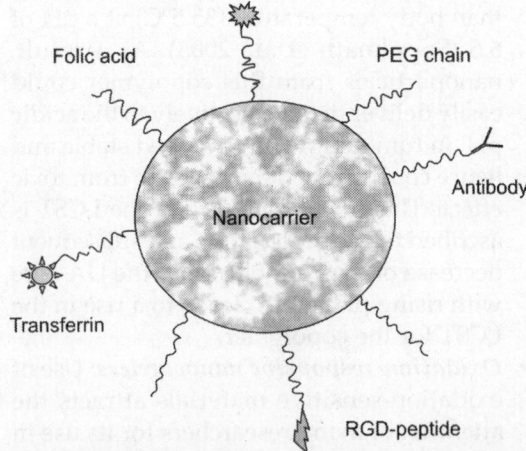

Fig. 1.9: Functionalized carrier for targeted cancer therapy

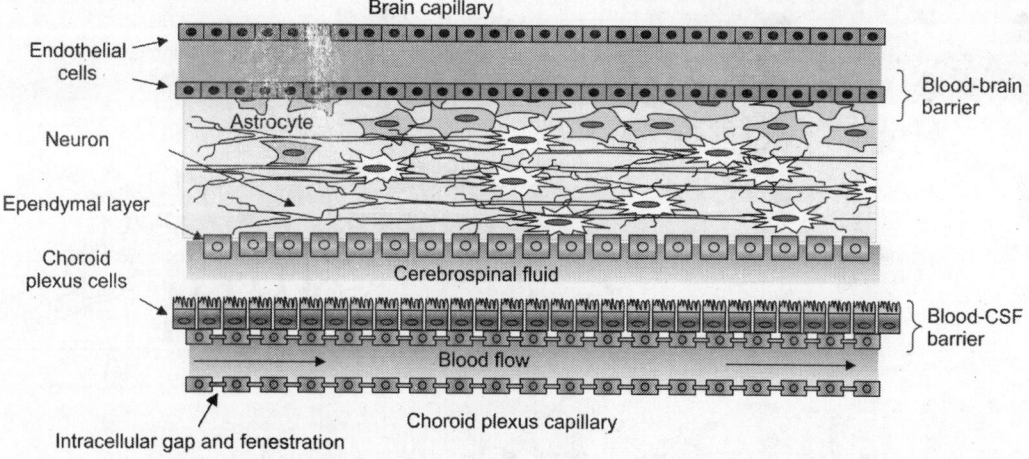

Fig. 1.10: Barriers in the targeted drug delivery to central nervous system

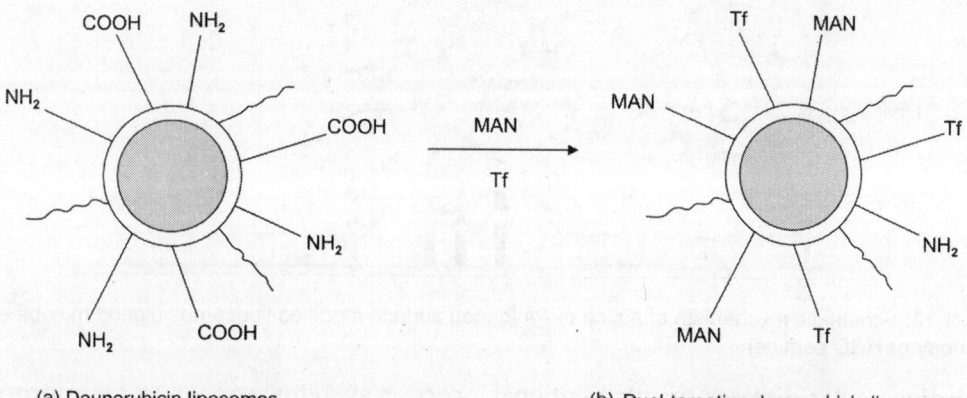

(a) Daunorubicin liposomes

(b) Dual-targeting daunorubicin liposomes

Fig. 1.11: Dual-targeting liposomes for the delivery of anticancer drug

increases risks of adverse effects. Only small, lipophilic drugs are believed to transverse across the BBB. Small colloidal nanocarriers such as liposomes and nanoparticles have been suggested as potential carriers for selective delivery of drugs to the brain (Fig. 1.11).

Small unilamellar vesicles (SUVs) appended with brain-specific transport vectors such as amino acids, insulin, transferrin and mannose may be transported through the BBB through receptor-mediated or absorptive transcytosis. Coating of nanocarriers with surfactant such as polysorbate 80 is another possible approach that increases the concentration of drug inside the brain. SLNs have also been investigated for improved drug delivery to the brain.

Conjugation of ligands on the surface of colloidal carriers, either by covalent or noncovalent linkage, increases selectivity for brain cancers. The future of developments of means and modules for transporting anti-cancer agents across the BBB for the treatment of brain cancers will largely rely on the development of targeting and dynamically transport-enhancing nanocarriers.

Cardiovascular System Targeted Drug Delivery

Targeted drug delivery is a clinically desirable and therapeutically rewarding mode for the treatment of vascular injury-associated thrombotic and occlusive events caused due

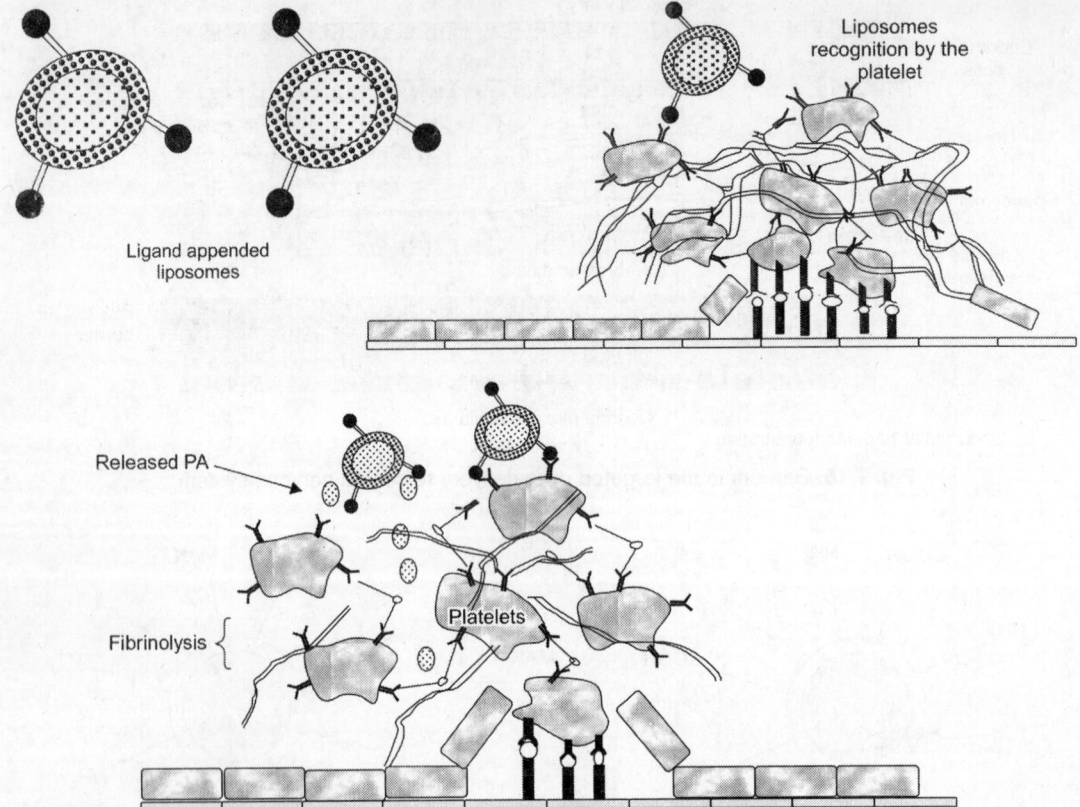

Liposomes recognition by the platelet

Ligand appended liposomes

Released PA

Fibrinolysis

Platelets

Fig. 1.12: Schematic mechanism of action of PA loaded surface modified liposomes (ligand may be either antibody or RGD peptide)

to cardiovascular diseases or interventional procedure. Current strategies for targeted delivery, i.e. transcatheter or drug eluting stent techniques are expensive and known to suffer from limitation of early drug washout, reduced control on drug concentration and late-stage thrombosis.

The short half-life of thrombolytic drugs, usually between 3 and 20 min, necessitates the administration of high dosages of these agents in systemically active forms over an extended period of time, which in turn, increases the risk of side effects such as uncontrolled hemorrhage. For optimal drug delivery, delivery systems should be localized at the site of thrombus as well as should maintain a reservoir which could avoid drug uptake into normal nontarget tissues. To fulfill such requirements nanotechnology-based

carrier systems appear to be appropriate options.

Small size of nanocarriers allows rapid incorporation of drug into the thrombus interior. Encapsulation of immunogenic thrombolytics such as streptokinase in the liposomes may also decrease the immunogenicity of the streptokinase. Thus by using engineered nanocarriers-based formulations it could be possible to treat such diseases more effectively and safely.

Further, to increase the targeting potential of thrombolytic agent to the specific site of thrombus, ligand-receptor based approach has been used by various research groups. Thrombus-targeted RGD peptide conjugated urokinase liposomes were prepared and observed for thrombolytic efficacy on a rat model (Fig. 1.12).

Intracellular Drug Delivery: Mitochondrial Targeting

During the last decade, intracellular drug delivery has become an area of high interest to the researchers in the medical and pharmaceutical fields. Many therapeutic agents such as drugs and DNA/oligonucleotides can be delivered not just to the cells but also to a particular organ compartment to achieve better activity, e.g. proapoptotic drugs to the mitochondria, antibiotics and enzymes to the lysosomes and various anticancer drugs and gene to the nucleus. Mitochondrial research is one of the most exciting areas of research in the field of biomedicine (Weissig et al., 2005, 2006; Paliwal et al., 2007). Studies have shown that mitochondria play a major role in apoptosis and it has been found that various apoptosis inducers act by interacting with the mitochondrial permeability transition pore complex of the mitochondrial membrane (Li et al., 2002). To induce apoptosis in the cancer cell, drugs should be targeted to the mitochondrial membrane. This demands systems which have an affinity for mitochondria. In 1998, Weissig and associates reported for the first time a liposome like vesicular systems, DQAsomes, that have endosomolytic properties and can release plasmid DNA upon contact with the outer mitochondrial membrane *in vitro* (Weissig et al., 2001; D'Souza et al., 2003). DQAsome is a vesicular system prepared by sonicating the dispersion of dequalinium chloride, a dicationic amphiphilic compound, in the aqueous phase (Weissig et al., 1998). It is reported that cancer cells possess an elevated mitochondrial and a higher plasma membrane potential compared to normal cells, and also DQAsomes may be suitable carriers for double targeting, i.e. both on the cellular level (cancer cell *vs.* normal cells) and on the subcellular level (mitochondria vs. rest of the cells). The hypothetical mechanism of action of paclitaxel-loaded DQAsomes is summarized in Fig. 1.13. When DQAsomes reach the endosome by the process of endocytosis they disrupt the endosomal membrane and attracted towards the mitochondrial membrane. The DQAsomes are then destabilized following interaction with the mitochondrial membrane releasing the paclitaxel. The released paclitaxel acts on the mitochondrial membrane resulting in the release of cytochrome C which as a result induces apoptosis and ultimately the cell death. Further, to improve the effectiveness of the DQAsomal paclitaxel, Vaidya et al., (2009) modified the surface of DQAsomes by using folic acid as a ligand. Folic acid delivers the carrier specifically to the cancer cells over-

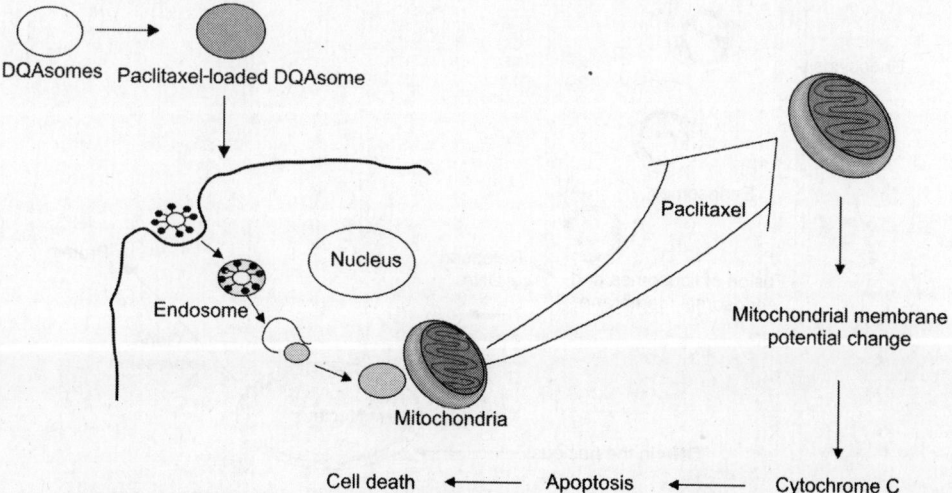

Fig. 1.13: Schematic diagram of hypothetical mechanism of action of paclitaxel-loaded DQAsomes

expressing folate receptors and helps to increase the endosomal uptake of the drug-loaded carrier. Following endosomal escape, DQAsomes selectively release drug at the mitochondrial membrane interfaced with cytosol. It was found that folic acid modified DQAsomes demonstrated higher anticancer activity as compared to plain DQAsomal formulation as well as liposomal formulation.

Gene Delivery

The ability to transfect target genes into cells with their subsequent expression is a leading practical emergence of human gene therapy, wherein, functionally active genes are putatively inserted into the (somatic) cells of a person requiring the expression of a given protein. Here genes would act like 'drugs', generating a product with a specific pharmacological effect. In simple terms, gene therapy involves insertion of genetic material into a patient's cells to make them capable of producing therapeutic protein.

Over the last decade, many molecular targets for genetic disorder have been identified and evaluated using preclinical and clinical trials for genetic diseases such as cancer, autoimmune diseases, and cystic fibrosis. With the discovery of disease causative gene, it can be possible to treat genetic diseases and achieve a desired intracellular effect by either blocking a gene that is being overexpressed or by substituting or replacing a copy of a malfunctioning gene. However, due to the sensitivity of DNA to enzymatic degradation genetic material can not be introduced unprotected *in vivo* (Fig. 1.14). To achieve effective transfection, various vectors are employed as a means of delivering the genetic material. At present, majority of the approved clinical trials on gene therapy in human subjects have involved viral transfection using viral vector-mediated transfer. Among non-viral carriers, cationic liposome, cationic polymers-based carriers etc., have exhibited excellent transfection activity and

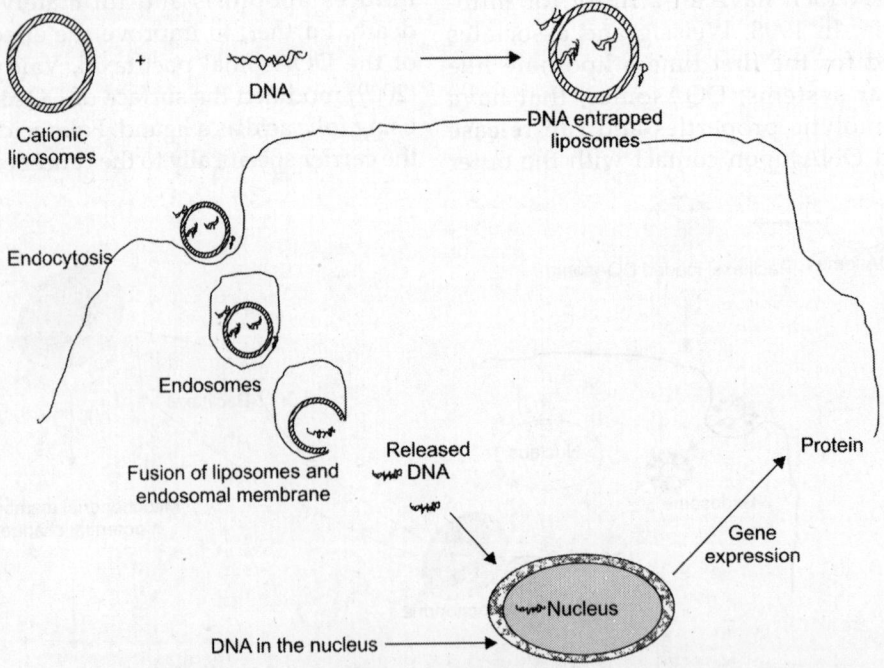

Fig. 1.14: Schematic mechanism of cationic liposomes-mediated DNA delivery

hence are accepted as useful tool for gene therapy.

Vaccine Delivery

Another area of research in the field of material sciences and nanocarrier construct is the delivery of antigens through oral route for the induction of mucosal immunity. Mucosal immunization not only could induce immune response at the systemic site but also induces immune response at other mucosal sites. Nanocarriers such as liposomes, PLGA nanoparticles etc., have potential to stabilize the antigen and protect them from the harsh environment of gastric fluid and increase the uptake of antigen especially through M cells for subsequent presentation to the antigen presenting cells (APCs). Owing to their small size and functional exterior nanocarriers can ameliorated to be amenable for targeting, vis-a-vis controlled drug delivery. Such approaches could be applied in imaging of deep-localized site(s); improving therapeutic indices and minimizing the side effects. Some carriers can even be engineered in such a way so that they get activated in response to pH; temperature; oscillating magnetic field or target site biochemistry. Such modifications not only provide particulate integrity en route to the site of action, moreover simultaneously control the release of carried drug. Conclusively, nanocarriers provide for a cutting edge technique that could judiciously be employed to improve the therapeutic index of potent drugs, to increase the solubility of poorly water-soluble drugs and for the targeted delivery of therapeutics to the diseased cells of the organ which are deprived of the direct blood circulation. However, the potential of these emerging nanotechniques-based formulations has yet to be realised. Toxicological studies of the nanocarriers in human need to be fully studied, evaluated and established before they can become a clinical reality.

FUTURE OPPORTUNITIES AND CHALLENGES

Nanoparticles and nanoformulations have already been applied as drug delivery systems with great success; and nanoparticulate drug delivery systems have still greater potential for many applications, including antitumor therapy, gene therapy, AIDS therapy, radiotherapy, in the delivery of proteins, antibiotics, virostatics, vaccines and as vesicles to pass the blood-brain barrier. Nanoparticles provide massive advantages in drug targeting, controlled drug delivery and release and, with their additional potential to combine diagnosis and therapy, they emerge as one of the major tools in nanomedicine. The main goals are to improve their stability in the biological environment, to mediate the biodistribution of active compounds, improve drug loading, targeting, transport, release, and permeation across or through the biological barriers. The cytotoxicity of nanoparticles or their degradation products remains a major problem, and improvements in biocompatibility obviously are main concerns of future research.

There are many technological challenges to be met, in developing the following techniques:

- Nanodrug delivery systems that deliver large but highly localized quantities of drugs to specific areas to be released in controlled ways;
- Controllable release profiles, especially for sensitive drugs;
- Materials for nanoparticles that are biocompatible and biodegradable;
- Architectures/structures, such as biomimetic polymers, nanotubes;
- Technologies for self-assembly;
- Functions (active drug targeting, on-demand delivery, intelligent drug release devices/bioresponsive triggered systems, self-regulated delivery systems, systems interacting with the body, smart delivery);
- Virus-like systems for intracellular delivery;
- Nanoparticles to improve devices such as implantable devices/nanochips for nanoparticle release, or multi-reservoir drug delivery-chips;
- Nanoparticles for tissue engineering, e.g. for the delivery of cytokines to control cellular growth and differentiation, and

stimulate regeneration; or for coating implants with nanoparticles in biodegradable polymer layers for sustained release;

- Advanced polymeric carriers for the delivery of therapeutic peptide/proteins (biopharmaceuticals);
- Combined therapy and medical imaging, e.g. nanoparticles for diagnosis and manipulation during surgery (e.g. thermotherapy with magnetic particles);
- Universal formulation schemes that can be used as intravenous, intramuscular or peroral drugs;
- Cell and gene targeting systems;
- User-friendly lab-on-a-chip devices for point-of-care and disease prevention and control at home;
- Devices for detecting changes in magnetic or physical properties after specific binding of ligands on paramagnetic nanoparticles that can correlate with the amount of ligand;
- Better disease markers in terms of sensitivity and specificity.

SUGGESTED READINGS

1. Brannon-Peppas, L, Blanchette, JO, 2004. *Adv. Drug Deliv. Rev.* 56, 1649–59.
2. Brigger, IN, Dubernet, C, Couvreur, P, 2002. *Adv. Drug Deliv. Rev.* 54, 631–651.
3. Batrakova, EV, Kabanov, AV, 2008. *J. Control Rel.*, 130(2), 98–106.
4. Boddapati, SV, Tongcharoensirikul, P, Hanson, RN, D'Souza, GG, Torchilin, VP, Weissig, V, 2005. Mitochondriotropic liposomes. *J Liposome Res.*, 15, 49–58.
5. Cheng, SM, Pabba, S, Torchilin, VP, Fowle, W, Kimpfler, A, Schubert, R, Weissig, V, 2005. *J Drug Del Sci Technol.*, 15, 81–6.
6. Chung, JE, Yokoyama, M, Yamato, M, Aoyagi, T, Sakurai, Y, Okano, T, 1999. *J Control Rel.*, 62, 11.
7. D'Souza, GG, Rammohan, R, Cheng, SM, Torchilin, VP, Weissig, V, 2003. *J Control Rel.*, 92, 189–97.
8. Devarakonda, B, Hill, RA, de Villiers, MM, 2004. *Int J Pharm.*, 284 (1–2), 133–40.
9. Dugan, MA, Kazar, JL, Ganse, G, et al., 1972. *J Nucl Med Concise Commun.*, 14, 233–4.
10. Erdogan, S, Özer Dr, AY, Volkan, B, et al., 2006. *Drug Deliv.*, 13, 303–9.
11. Felgner, PL, Gadek, TR, Holm, M., et al., 1987. *Proc Natl Acad Sci USA.*, 84, 7413–7417.
12. Fang J et al., (2011) *Adv Drug Deliv Rev.* 63(3); 136–51.
13. Gemeinhart, RA, Luo, D, Saltzman, WM, 2005. *Biotechnol Prog.*, 21, 532–7.
14. Goyal, AK, Khatri, K, Mishra, N, Mehta, A, Vaidya, B, Tiwari, S, et al., 2005. *Drug Dev Ind Pharm.*, 34(12), 1297–305.
15. Goyal, AK, Rawat, A, Mahor, S, Gupta, PN, Khatri, K, Vyas, SP, 2006. *Int J Pharm.*, 309 (1–2), 227–33.
16. Gupta, AS, Huang, G, Lestini, BJ, et al., 2005. *Thromb Haemost.*, 93, 106–14.
17. Fang J, Nakamura H, Maeda H (2011). *Adv Drug Deliv Rev* 63(3): 136–51.
18. Hardman JG, Limbird LE. Godman and Gilman's 'The Pharmacological Basis of Therapeutics'. 10th ed. New York:
19. Laila F AA, Chandran S, *J Pharm Pharm Sci*, 2006, 9(3): 327–38.
20. Hughes, GA, 2005. *Nanomedicine*, 1, 22–30.
21. Kaur, IP, Bhandari, R, Bhandari, S, Kakkar, V, 2008. *J Control Rel.*, 127(2), 97–109.
22. Le Garrec, D, Taillefer, J, VanLier, JE, Lenaerts, V, Leroux, JC, 2002. *J Drug Target.*, 10, 429.
23. Lestini, BJ, Sagnella, SM, Xu, Z, et al., 2002. *Surface J Control Rel.*, 78, 235–47.
24. Li, S, Ma, Z, 2001. Nonviral gene gherapy. *Curr Gene Ther.*, 1, 201–26.
25. Paliwal, R, Rai, S, Vaidya, B, et al., 2007. *Curr Drug Deliv.*, 4, 211–24.
26. Patel, MM, Goyal, BR, Bhadada, SV, Bhatt, JS, Amin, AF, 2009. *CNS Drugs.*, 23(1), 35–8.
27. Peek, LJ, Middaugh, CR, Berkland, C, 2008. *Adv Drug Deliv Rev.*, 60, 915–28.
28. Quintana, A, Raczka, E, Piehler, L, Lee, I., Myc, A, Majoros, I, et al., 2002. *Pharm Res.*, 19, 1310–1316. McGraw Hill; 2001.

2

Oral Osmotic Pumps

INTRODUCTION

Osmotic pumps are controlled drug delivery devices based on the principle of osmosis. Wide spectrum of osmotic devices are in existence, out of them osmotic pumps are unique, dynamic and widely employed in clinical practice. Osmosis is an aristocratic phenomenon, which is exploited for development of delivery systems with every desirable property of an ideal controlled drug delivery system. Osmotic pumps offer many advantages like they are easy to formulate and simple in operation, improved patient compliance with reduced dosing frequency, more consistent and prolonged therapeutic effect is obtained with uniform blood concentration and moreover they are inexpensive and their industrial adaptability vis-a-vis production scale up is easy.

Elementary osmotic pumps essentially contain an active agent having suitable osmotic pressure, contained into a tablet, coated with a semipermeable membrane usually of cellulose acetate. A small orifice is drilled through the coating by using LASER or high-speed mechanical drill. In fact, this system represents a coated tablet with an aperture. When exposed to an aqueous environment, the osmotic pressure of the soluble drug within the tablet draws water through the semipermeable coating, resulting in formation of a saturated aqueous drug solution within the device. The membrane is nonextensible and increase in volume due to imbibition of water raises inner hydrostatic pressure, eventually leading to flow of saturated solution of active agent out of the device through small orifice. Solubility of drug in water plays a critical role in functioning of osmotic pump. Typically the solubility of drug to be delivered by these pumps should be at least 10 to 15% w/v.

The drug is pumped out of the system through an orifice at a controlled rate dm/dt, which is equal to the multiple of volume flow rate of water (dv/dt) into the core and drug concentration Cs.

$$dm/dt = (dv/dt)\,Cs$$

In principle, this delivery system dispenses drug continuously at a zero order rate until the concentration of the osmotically active salt in the system decreases below saturation solubility, whereupon a non-zero order release pattern results. Recently, controlled release oral osmotic pumps of naproxen sodium and ibuprofen have been developed.

OSMOSIS: AN OVERVIEW

Osmosis refers to the process of movement of solvent from lower concentration of solute towards higher concentration of solute across a semipermeable membrane.

Abbe Nollet first reported osmotic effect in 1748, but Pfeffer is considered to be pioneer of quantitative measurement of osmotic effect. He measured the effect in 1877 by using a membrane, which was selectively permeable to water but impermeable to sugar (Fig. 2.1). This membrane separated sugar solution from pure water. A flow of water into the sugar solution was recorded which was halted when a pressure was applied to the sugar solution. It was postulated that this pressure, the osmotic pressure of the sugar solution is directly proportional to the solution concentration and absolute temperature.

Van't Hoff established the analogy between the Pfeffer results and the ideal gas laws by the expression

$$= n_2 RT \qquad (2.1)$$

where n_2 represents the molar concentration of sugar (or other solute) in the solution, R depicts the gas constant, and T the absolute temperature.

The Van't Hoff equation presents a good means for calculating the osmotic pressures of solutes by using perfect semipermeable membranes. The measurements were accurate especially for low-solute concentrations. But in case, the membrane was not completely semipermeable and permitted the passage for solute along with solvent, the osmotic pressure calculated by equation (2.1) tends to be more, as compared with experimental value. Concentrated solutions also showed deviations from these ideal equations. A number of researchers have subsequently discussed, modified and as a result a more accurate expression of this equation has been brought about.

Another method of obtaining a good approximation of osmotic pressure is measurement of vapour pressure by using the expression:

$$= RT \ln (P_o/P) \qquad (2.2)$$

where P_o represents the vapour pressure of the pure solvent, P is the vapour pressure of the solution, and is the molar volume of the solvent. As vapour pressures can be measured with less effort than osmotic pressure, this expression is frequently used.

Osmotic pressure for soluble solutes are extremely high, as shown in Table 2.1, it enlists the osmotic pressures of solutes commonly used in controlled release pharmaceutical

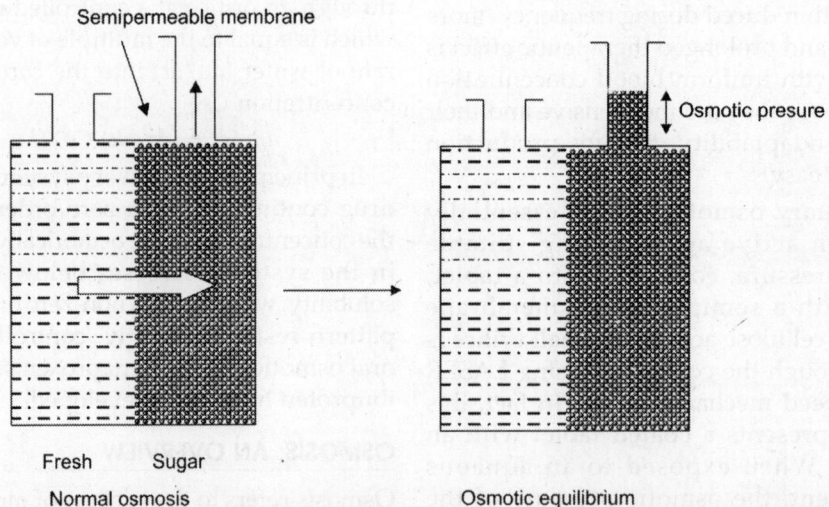

Semipermeable membrane

Osmotic presure

Fresh   Sugar

Normal osmosis

Osmotic equilibrium

Fig. 2.1: A schematic illustrating osmotic flow and the attainment of osmotic equilibrium

Table 2.1: Osmotic pressures of saturated solutions of common pharmaceutical solutes

S.No.	Compound or mixture	Osmotic pressure (atm)
1.	Sodium chloride	356
2.	Fructose	355
3.	Potassium chloride	245
4.	Sucrose	150
5.	Malonic acid	117
6.	Potassium Phosphate	105
7.	Xylitol	104
8.	Sorbitol	84
9.	Dextrose	82
10.	Citric acid	69
11.	Tartaric acid	67
12.	Potassium sulfate	39
13.	Mannitol	38
14.	Sodium phosphate (tribasic)	36
15.	Sodium phosphate (dibasic)	31
16.	Sodium phosphate (monobasic)	28
17.	Lactose	23
18.	Fumaric acid	10

formulations. This high osmotic pressure is largely responsible for high water flow across semipermeable membrane.

The water flow dictated by osmotic pressure can be given by the equation:

$$dV/dt = A/l \qquad (2.3)$$

where dV/dt represents the water flow across the membrane area A and thickness l with permeability. This depicts the difference in osmotic pressure between the two solutions on either side of the membrane.

This equation is strictly applicable for a perfect semipermeable membrane, which is completely impermeable to solute. Staverman reflection coefficient is included in equation to account for any deviation from complete semipermeable character of a membrane.

CLASSIFICATION

The oral osmotic pumps can be conveniently classified into following major types:

Single chamber osmotic pump

1. Elementary osmotic pump

Multichamber osmotic pump

1. Push-pull osmotic pump.
2. Osmotic pump with nonexpanding second chamber.

Specific types

1. Controlled porosity osmotic pump.
2. Monolithic osmotic systems.
3. Osmotic bursting osmotic pump.
4. OROS-CT.
5. Multi-particulates delayed release systems (MPDRS).
6. Liquid oral osmotic system (L-OROS).

Unitary-core Osmotic Systems

Unitary-core osmotic systems represent two-thirds of the marketed oral osmotically driven systems (OODS) products. Four techniques are mainly employed in their preparation. They are as follows:

- The elementary osmotic pump (EOP)
- The single-composition osmotic pump (SCOT)
- The controlled-porosity osmotic pump (CPOP)
- The self-emulsified unitary-core osmotic pump (SEOP/SCPOP)

EOP, CPOP and SCOT have been used primarily to deliver freely water soluble drugs, representing about 71% of the formulated freely soluble drugs, whereas slightly soluble or practically insoluble drugs are at large formulated as SEOP. The design of the unitary-core osmotic system was described by Theeuwes. It is composed of a tablet core surrounded by a semipermeable membrane. EOP and CPOP, however differ only in regard to mode of drug delivery. For the EOP, drug is delivered through a laser-drilled passage-way, while for the CPOP, the drug is released through pores in the membrane. The objective in formulating such a system is to deliver maximum fraction of the drug following zero-order kinetics, the maximum drug fraction over a fixed duration, varying mostly from 4 to 24 hours. The tablet-core composition is considered to be the primary influencer of the drug delivery following a zero-order release rate, whereas the membrane characteristics are thought to control the overall drug release rate.

Thus, the tablet-core composition may be formulated in such a way that both core osmotic pressure and density are maximized. If the drug has sufficient osmotic pressure, such as metformin hydrochloride, single-composition osmotic tablets (SCOT) could be effectively formulated and used, delivering, i.e. 75 to 90% in a constant manner. Even in this case, single osmotic agent or a sugar mixture may be added to the tablet-core composition to obtain a zero-order delivery pattern, which is independent of the external osmolarity. Additional tableting and bulk excipients may be needed to simplify the tableting process, but soluble and finely milled grade is preferred. Furthermore, drug release may be retarded by adding appropriate polymers or solubility modulators. This approach presents the additional advantage of preventing burst effects observed in the event of membrane rupture. In the case of slightly soluble or practically insoluble drugs, self-emulsifying agents are added to the tablet-core composition. Independent of the tablet core, the drug release kinetics from these systems can be modulated by varying the membrane thickness or composition.

All osmotic systems are coated at an appropriate stage of production using spray film-coating technique. Organic solvents such as an acetone-water mixture are used for generating cellulose-based membranes, e.g. cellulose acetate or ethylcellulose, with high mechanical resistances. In production, the high amount of solvent required may become problematic and costly. Therefore, aqueous coatings such as methacrylic polymers in aqueous dispersion are recommended or proposed as an alternative to organic coatings, in order to avoid the solvent recycling as seen in large-scale product manufacturing. Plasticizers are added to improve the membrane physical properties, independent of the polymer selected. The water soluble plasticizers (PEG, HPMC) may be preferred for fast creation of porous structure, thus reducing the latency lag time to drug delivery. Water-insoluble plasticizers, such as castor oil, have also been reported to produce an effect in addition to allow a more constant drug delivery from a single-core based system. Finally, an orifice can be drilled on the coated tablet. Various drilling techniques have been developed depending on the scale using either manual-drilling, laser-drilling, or indentation techniques consisting of a double-cylinder punch making a central hole in a face of the pump (tablet).

Multilayer-core Osmotic Systems

Two main multilayer designs are marketed by Alza, namely the push-pull and push-stick osmotic pumps (PPOP and PSOP). The multilayer-core osmotic systems are composed of a bi-or tri-layer tablet core, surrounded by a semipermeable membrane with a laser-drilled orifice. Developed to deliver drugs independently of their solubility, the tablet-core composition contains mainly polymers and drugs. It allows drug delivery through the orifice either as a solution or dispersion under the hydrodynamic pressure generated on swelling of the so-called 'push-layer'. As for the unitary-core systems, the drug release composition needs to be optimized for delivering the maximum drug load, whereas the release rate and kinetics are controlled mainly by the membrane characteristics. However, the formulation strategy differs from the unitary-core, due to the polymeric nature of the composition, leading to a viscous microenvironment. Therefore, the strategy needs to develop and formulate the tablet-cores which equally control and balance the hydration kinetics of both the layers, and simultaneously control the polymer viscosity and swelling kinetics. The amount of osmotic agent and polymer grades may be varied and selected to enhance the drug dispersion. Water-soluble excipients are added especially in the drug layer avoiding drug agglomeration. Under these conditions, 30% of loaded drug may release following zero-order kinetics over a prolonged period, i.e. extending from 4 to 24 hours, by varying the membrane characteristics. Because of the dispersed drug delivery as against drug solution, a larger size of passageway or orifice is preferred that is drilled using laser, manual or indentation drilling techniques. More complex designs, such as the COER-24 or push-stick osmotic pumps, have recently been developed to deliver higher dosage in a more complex pattern. A hydrophilic polymer layer, the so-called 'flow-promoting layer', is sprayed between the tablet-core and the semipermeable membrane, avoiding internal drug adhesion. Surrounded by an immediate-drug release layer, the tri-layered tablet core gives an additional flexibility. Adapted for methylphenidate (Concerta TM), an extremely controlled plasma profile was recorded, that allowed drug delivery over the school hours for children with attention deficit hyperactivity disorder (ADHD) and also avoiding tachyphylaxis.

Capsule-based Osmotic Systems

Mainly used as exploratory tools, capsule-based osmotic pumps are developed for site-specific drug delivery to investigate drug pharmacokinetics. For example, Chronset™ osmotic pumps were designed as a pulse-delivery system, releasing mucoadhesive particles containing peptides or proteins. The Osmet™ design was developed as a miniature osmotic pump to deliver a drug as bolus or over 8 hours in the colon. Site-specific deliveries of oxprenolol, nitrendipine enantiomers or lidocaine were acheived using the Osmet™ device. Another capsule-based system, the so-called L-Oros™, was developed to deliver nonaqueous liquid formulations which were found to be suitable for either poorly soluble actives or polypeptides. This design offers the advantage of continuous delivery of the liquid or semisolid composition,

improving the bioavailability of the drug. Moreover, in accordance with the formulation viscosity, soft and hard-capsule L-OROS design may be preferred.

ROSE–NELSON PUMP

The present day osmotic devices are modified versions of Rose–Nelson pump, which was introduced by two Australian physiologists Rose and Nelson, who were interested in the delivery of drugs to the sheep and cattle gut. The original pump proposed by these workers was never patented. The pump is composed of three chambers—a drug chamber, a salt chamber holding solid salt, and a water chamber (Fig. 2.2). A semipermeable membrane separates the salt from water chamber. The difference in osmotic pressure across the membrane drives the water from the water chamber to the salt chamber. Conceivably, volume of salt chamber increases due to water in flux, which distends the latex diaphragm dividing the salt and drug chambers, and hence pumps the drug outside the device. The kinetics of pumping from Rose–Nelson pump is presented by equation:

$$dMt/dt = (dV/dt) \cdot C \qquad (2.4)$$

where dMt/dt is the drug release rate, dV/dt is the volume flow of water into the salt chamber, and C represents the concentration of drug in the drug chamber. Combining equations (2.3) and (2.4), results in

$$dMt/dt = AC/l \qquad (2.5)$$

These basic equations are applicable to the osmotically driven-controlled drug delivery devices.

The saturated salt solution creates a high osmotic pressure as compared to the pressure required for pumping of the suspension of an active agent. Therefore, the rate of water entering into the salt chamber remains constant as long as sufficient solid salt is present in the salt chamber to maintain a saturated solution and thereby a constant osmotic pressure as driving force is generated and maintained. The major problem associated with Rose–Nelson

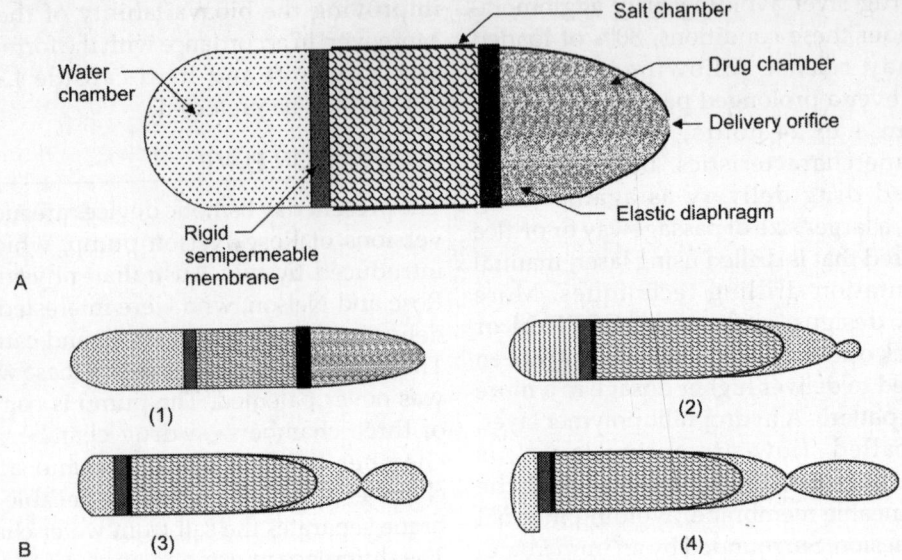

Fig. 2.2: (a) Essential features of the three-chamber Rose–Nelson osmotic pump (b) four stages of drug delivery from Rose–Nelson pump

pumps is that the osmotic action starts whenever water comes in contact with the semipermeable membrane. This reflects that pumps is required to be stored empty and water was ought to be loaded prior to use, an inconvenient and complicated procedure. The Pharmetrix device described in patent 89–1 addressed this drawback. This device is composed of an impermeable membrane placed between the semipermeable membrane and the water chamber. This membrane seal permits the storage of pump in fully loaded condition; the pump is activated when the seal is broken. Water is then drawn by a wick to the membrane surface, and the pumping action begins. This modification allows improved storage of the device, which on demand can be easily activated. There have been a large number of Rose–Nelson patents, most of these patents describe the use of Rose–Nelson pumps as miniature infusion systems to be strapped to the patient, delivering drug via an indwelling catheter. Cyanamid has patented a Rose–Nelson pump 71–1. This patent includes a movable piston instead of elastic diaphragm. This was the first device

described based on osmotic pressure as a driving force.

HIGUCHI–LEEPER OSMOTIC PUMP

Higuchi and Leeper have proposed a series of variations of the Rose–Nelson pump and these designs have been described in US patents 73–1, 73–2 and 73–3, which represent the first series of simplifications of the Rose–Nelson pump made by the Alza corporation. One of these pumps is illustrated in Fig. 2.3. The Higuchi–Leeper pump, has no water chamber, however the activation of the device initiated after imbibition of the water from the surrounding environment. This variation allows the device to be prepared loaded with drug and can be stored for long period prior to use.

Higuchi–Leeper pumps contain a rigid housing, and the semipermeable membrane is supported on a perforated frame. A salt chamber containing a fluid solution with an excess of solid salt is usually incorporated in this type of pump. Higuchi–Leeper pump is widely employed for veterinary use. This type

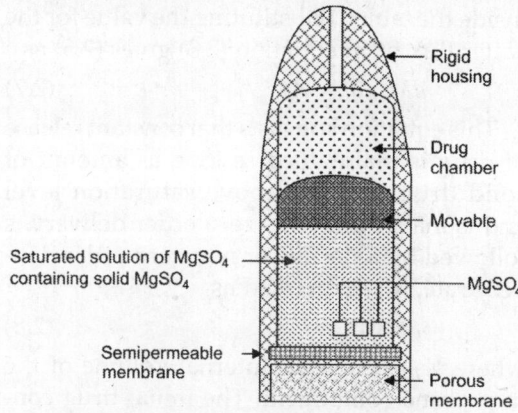

Fig. 2.3: Higuchi–Leeper pump design

of pump is either swallowed or implanted in body of an animal for delivery of antibiotics or growth hormones to animals. This presents advantage over other medications, which ought to be administered repeatedly, and hence is inconvenient particularly in case of animals. This problem is overcome by using this device, which can be loaded with full dose and swallowed once, eventually leads to delivery of full course of medication in the rumen in a controlled manner.

HIGUCHI–THEEUWES OSMOTIC PUMP

Higuchi and Theeuwes in early 1970s developed another variant of the Rose–Nelson pump, even simpler than the Higuchi–Leeper pump. This device is illustrated in Fig. 2.4. In this device, the rigid housing of a semipermeable membrane is provided. This membrane is strong enough to withstand the osmotic pressure developed within the device due to imbibition of water. The desired drug is loaded in the device only prior to its application, which extends an advantage for storage of the device for longer duration. The release of the drug from the device is dictated by the salt and its concentration used in the salt chamber and the permeability characteristics of the outer semipermeable rigid membrane. Small osmotic pumps of this form are available under trade name Alzet. They are used frequently as implantable controlled release

delivery systems in experimental studies requiring continuous administration of drugs. Diffusional loss of the drug from the device could be minimized by making the delivery port in the shape of a long thin tube as shown in Fig. 2.5. One modification of Higuchi–Theeuwes pump utilizes a mixture of citric acid and sodium bicarbonate in the salt chamber (patent 80–2). When contacted with water, the mixture produces carbon dioxide gas, which then exerts a pressure on the elastic diaphragm; eventually leading to drug delivery.

ELEMENTARY OSMOTIC PUMP

Rose–Nelson pump was further simplified in the form of elementary osmotic pump, which made osmotic delivery as a major and simple method of achieving controlled drug release. Elementary osmotic pump essentially contains

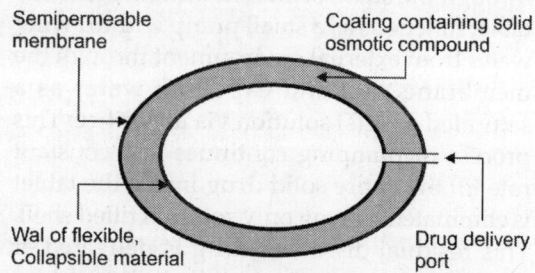

Fig. 2.4: Higuchi–Theeuwes pump design

(a) Pump filled and assembled

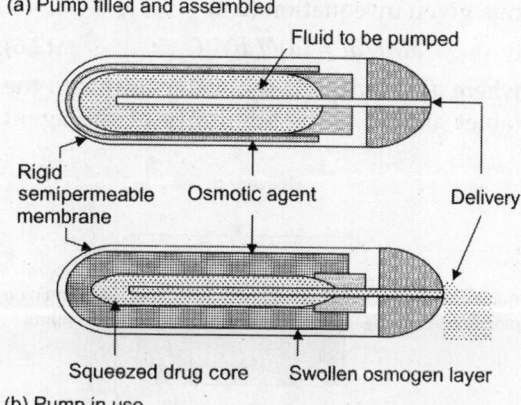

(b) Pump in use

Fig. 2.5: Theeuwes miniature osmotic pump

an active agent having a suitable osmotic pressure, formed into a tablet coated with a semipermeable membrane, usually cellulose acetate. A small orifice is drilled through the membrane coating (Fig. 2.6). This pump eliminates the need of separate salt chamber. This device in fact represents a coated tablet with a hole and perhaps, represents the ultimate simplification of the original Rose Nelson device. When this coated tablet is exposed to an aqueous environment, the osmotic pressure of the soluble drug inside the tablet draws water through the semipermeable coating, resulting in the formation of a saturated aqueous solution inside the device. The membrane is non-extensible and the increase in volume due to imbibition of water raises the hydrostatic pressure inside the tablet, eventually leading to flow of saturated solution of active agents out of the device through the small orifice. In other words, this tablet functions as a small pump withdrawing water from external environment through the membrane wall and expelling water as a saturated drug(s) solution via the orifice. This process of pumping continues at a constant rate till the entire solid drug inside the tablet is eliminated leaving only solution filled shell. This residual dissolved drug is delivered at decline rate to attain equilibrium between external and internal drug solution.

The pump initially releases the drug at a rate given by equation (2.4)

$$dMt/dt = (dV/dt) \cdot C_s \qquad (2.6)$$

where dV/dt depicts the water flow into the tablet and C_s is the solubility of the agent inside the tablet. Substituting the value for the water flux from equation (2.3) gives (2.5) as

$$dMt/dt = A\,C_s/l \qquad (2.7)$$

This equation suggests that constant release of drug is maintained as long as amount of solid drug remains above saturation level and is maximum. This zero order delivery is followed by a decline or non-zero order delivery rate, M_{nz} expressed as

$$M_{nz} = C_s V_p \qquad (2.8)$$

where V_p depicts the internal volume of the membrane component. The initial drug content of the device, M_o, is given by

$$M_o = V_p \qquad (2.9)$$

The fraction of drug delivered at a non-zero order rate is expressed as

$$M_{nz}/M_o = C_s \qquad (2.10)$$

Since M_o represents initial drug content, it must be equal to the drug delivered following zero and non-zero order release kinetics,

$$M_o = M_z + M_{nz} \qquad (2.11)$$

This can further be modified as

$$1 = M_z/M_o + M_{nz}/M_o \qquad (2.12)$$

Substituting values of equation (2.8) in this equation, yields

$$M_z/M_o = 1 - C_s \qquad (2.13)$$

Extinction of last traces of solid drug leads to fall in both C_s and A decline in rate of drug release follows a parabolic pattern. It has been suggested that the non-zero order rate after dissolution of last trace of solid drug can be described by the expression

$$dM/dt = (dM/dt)z/1 + (1/C_sV_p)\,(dM/dt)z\,(t - t_z)^2 \qquad (2.14)$$

where (dM/dt) represents the zero-order rate, V_p depicts the internal volume of the membrane and t_z is the time over which the device delivers drug at a zero-order rate.

Solubility of drug in water, however plays a critical role in functioning of osmotic pump. Typically the solubility of drugs delivered by these pumps are at least 10 to 15 wt%, examples of drugs with this property include

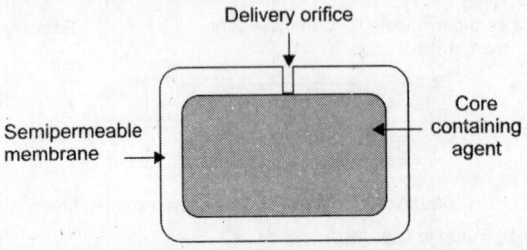

Fig. 2.6: The elementary osmotic pump

sodium indomethacin, potassium chloride, metoprolol and acetamizolamide.

The elementary osmotic pump was developed by Alza under the name OROS, for controlled release oral drug delivery formulations. The conventional high-speed tableting machinery and coating machinery are utilized for production of the devices, and laser-drilling system associated as an accessing of a conventional tablet-labeling machine is used for drilling small hole in coated tablet. Controlled oral drug delivery offers many advantages like they are easy and self-medication can be done, no need of trained personnel, and avoidance of pain, better patient compliance and treatment of some local gastrointestinal infections. Antigen delivery can also be made through oral route, which leads to the elicitation of systemic as well as mucosal immune response. Antigens enter the systemic circulation through M cells present on the Peyer's patches located in the intestinal tract.

The first elementary osmotic pump marketed was Osmosin® (controlled release indomethacin) but withdrawn from the market due to side effects. Subsequently a mega success was attained for controlled release nifedipine (Procardia XL). Other related products include acutrim (phenyl propanolamine), minipress XL (prazosin), and volmax (salbutamol). For OROS tablets, the semipermeable membrane coating the device must be 200–300 microns thick to withstand the pressure generated within the device. These thick coverings lower the water permeation rate, particularly for moderately water-soluble drugs. In general we can predict that these devices with thick coating are suitable for highly water-soluble drugs. The delivery rate attained with moderately soluble drugs is usually low, even with the most water-permeable membranes. Theeuwes has solved this problem by firstly utilizing a coating material with very high water permeability. For example, addition of plasticizers and a water-soluble additive to the cellulose acetate membranes which increases the permeability of latter up to tenfold.

The second approach of Theeuwes involves the use of multilayer composite coating around the tablet (Fig. 2.7).

The first layer is made up of thick microporous film that provides the mechanical strength required to withstand the internal pressure, while second layer is composed of a thin semipermeable membrane that produces the osmotic flux. The support layer is formed by various approaches; one novel approach is based on the coating of the tablets with a layer of cellulose acetate containing 40 to 60% of pore-forming agent such as sorbitol. This layer in turn is coated with the semipermeable layer. When it comes in contact with water, the water-soluble sorbitol leaches out from the membrane, leaving a microporous membrane.

Another variation in the membrane material includes the use of a bioerodable coating, which acts as an enteric coating. One more modification describes the addition of a carbonate or bicarbonate salts to the drug chamber, which eventually leads to effervescence when exposed to water due to formation of carbon dioxide at the stomach pH. This effervescent action prevents the drug precipitation such as of indomethacin, and thus prevents from blocking the delivery passage from the tablet. Moreover, solubility of the drug can be controlled by incorporating buffer compounds in the formulation. the internal pressure, while second layer is composed of a thin semipermeable membrane that produces the osmotic flux.

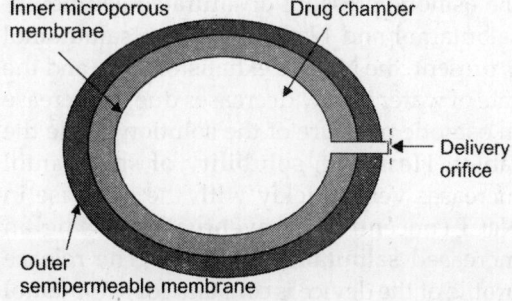

Fig. 2.7: The composite membrane coating used to deliver moderately soluble drugs

The support layer is formed by various approaches; one novel approach is based on the coating of the tablets with a layer of cellulose acetate containing 40 to 60 % of pore-forming agent such as sorbitol. This layer in turn is coated with the semipermeable layer. When it comes in contact with water, the water-soluble sorbitol leaches out from the membrane, leaving a microporous membrane. Another variation in the membrane material includes the use of a bioerodable coating, which acts as an enteric coating. One more modification describes the addition of a carbonate or bicarbonate salts to the drug chamber, which eventually leads to effervescence when exposed to water due to formation of carbon dioxide at the stomach pH. This effervescent action prevents the drug precipitation such as of indomethacin, and thus prevents from blocking the delivery passage from the tablet. Moreover, solubility of the drug can be controlled by incorporating buffer compounds in the formulation. Salbutamol presents unique example of drug with unusual solubility properties.

Patents 88–11 and 89–8 describe an interesting tablet for delivery of salbutamol, which possesses a solubility of 270 mg/ml in pure aqueous media, but upon addition of NaCl, the solubility reduces to 11 mg/ml in a saturated salt solution. The tablet is similar to elementary osmotic pump, containing a mixture of salbutamol and NaCl in the tablet core. When exposed to aqueous environment it imbibes water at a rate that is governed by the osmotic pressure of saturated solution of salbutamol and NaCl. As excess salbutamol is present, the NaCl is exhausted first, and the rate of water inflow decreases due to decrease in osmotic pressure of the solution inside the tablet. However, solubility of salbutamol increases very quickly with the decrease in NaCl concentration, eventually causing an increased salbutamol delivery. The release profile of the device is constant for salbutamol until the sodium chloride becomes exhausted; afterwards the remaining drug is delivered as a large pulse. This release pattern is exploited for nocturnal asthma in which pulsatile delivery of salbutamol is required.

A large number of modifications in simple elementary osmotic pump are discussed in the literature. The simple elementary pump suffers from the disadvantage that it can only deliver relatively soluble drugs, which are capable of developing an osmotic pressure greater than physiological body fluids. Incorporation of water soluble compound into the tablet formulation, serves as osmotic attractants, and overcomes this limitation partially. NaCl, sucrose, fructose or other common tableting adjuvants can be utilized. However, ultimately saturated solution of both the drug and osmotic attractant are left in the device. These constraints the amount of drug delivered at a constant rate. For example, consider a 500 mg tablet containing NaCl as an osmotic attractant (solubility 26 wt%) with drug (solubility 1 wt%). It reflects that the ratio of NaCl to drug in the tablet is 26:1 and the osmotic device would deliver only 18 mg of drug. Osmotic attractant of lower solubility permits for incorporation of more amount of drug into the tablet however the release rate is decreased. Thus, in order to obtain desired or meaningful delivery rates with elementary osmotic pump, solubility of drug must be relatively high.

Delivery of insoluble drug is achieved by a method illustrated in Fig. 2.8. In this approach osmotic agent is incorporated in an elastic, semipermeable film. These particles are then mixed with the insoluble drug substance and the resultant mixture is coated with the rigid semipermeable membrane. Osmotic agent tends to draw water across these two membranes, and hydrostatically forces the insoluble drug out of the orifice made in the device. Several coated tablets have been reported in which the exit hole, through which the drug escapes, is formed following leaching of water soluble component, such as lactose or poly (ethylene glycol), from the coating material. Once the tablet has been

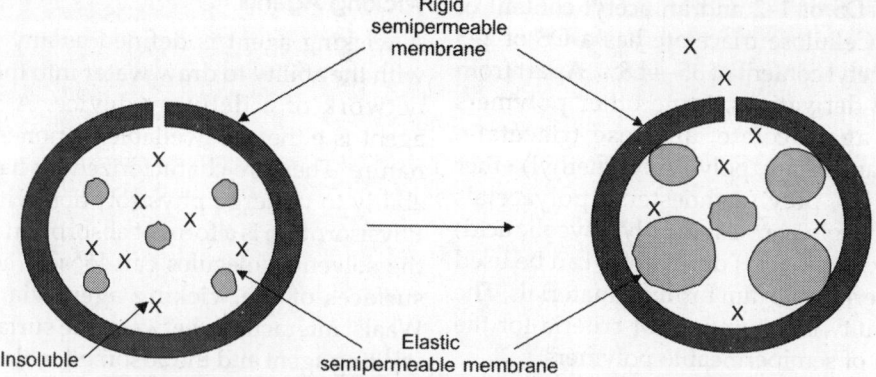

Fig. 2.8: A proposed method of delivering insoluble drugs

swallowed, water-soluble component dissolves in external fluid, resulting in initiation of pumping system. In early 1970s, several slow release tablet formulations were popular, which utilized osmotic principle for the release of the drug.

GENERAL CONSIDERATIONS AND MATERIALS USED

Osmotic pumps essentially contain drug and semipermeable membrane. In this case, drug itself acts as an osmogen and possesses good aqueous solubility (e.g. potassium chloride pumps). If the drug does not possess any osmogenic property, the osmogenic salt and other sugars can be incorporated in the formulation. Osmogens are soluble in water and are capable of producing osmotic pressure. Single osmogen can be used for the formulations and in some case combination of osmogens could be used. Apart from these essential components, other materials such as hydrophilic and hydrophobic polymers and hydrogel (either swellable or non-swellable nature), wicking agents, solubilizing agents and surfactants are used depending on the type of formulations. The coating material of semipermeable membrane usually contains a plasticizer and in some cases surfactants, flux regulating agents and pore-forming agents. Apart from the above materials, common tableting aids such as lubricants, binders,

diluents, glidants, wetting agents etc. can be used for the development of osmotic systems. The wall thickness is kept between 1–1000 µm, however 200–500 µm is desirable. The percentage weight increase of the tablets after coating should be around 10–15%. One aperture is usually made in the system, in some cases more than one delivery passages can be made with the diameter of 200–600 µm.

Semipermeable Membrane

The choice of a rate-controlling membrane is an important aspect in the formulation development of oral osmotic systems. Since the membrane in osmotic systems is semipermeable in nature, any polymer that is permeable to water but impermeable to solute can be selected. Some of the polymers that can be used for above purpose include cellulose esters such as cellulose acetate, cellulose diacetate, cellulose triacetate, cellulose propionate, cellulose acetate butyrate, etc. cellulose ethers like ethyl cellulose and eudragits. Cellulose acetate is a commonly employed semipermeable film forming polymer. It is available in different acetyl content grades. Particularly acetyl content 32 and 38% are widely used. Cellulose acetate is available in various degree of substitution (DS), i.e. the average number of hydroxyl groups on the anhydro-glucose unit of the polymer replaced by substituting group. If it is up to 1, the acetyl content is approximately 21%. Cellulose diacetate is having a DS of 1–2 and an acetyl content of 21–35%. Cellulose triacetate has a DS of 2–3 and an acetyl content of 35–44.8%. Apart from cellulose derivatives, some other polymers such as agar acetate, amylose triacetate, betaglucan acetate, poly (vinyl methyl) ether copolymers, poly (orthoesters), polyacetals and selectively permeable poly (glycolic acid) and poly (lactic acid) derivatives can be used as semipermeable film forming materials. The permeability is the important criteria for the selection of semipermeable polymers.

Hydrophilic and Hydrophobic Polymers

These polymers are used in the formulation development of osmotic regulatory drug delivery systems by entrapping drug in the matrix core of the pumps. The highly water soluble compounds can be entrapped in hydrophobic matrices while moderately water soluble compounds can be entrapped in hydrophilic matrices in order to obtain more controlled release. Generally, mixtures of both hydrophilic and hydrophobic polymers have been used in the development of osmotic pumps of water-soluble drugs. The selection is based on the solubility of the drug as well as the amount of drug that is to be released from the pump. The polymers are either swellable or non-swellable. Mostly swellable polymers have been used for the pumps containing moderately water-soluble drugs, since they increase the hydrostatic pressure inside the pump due to swelling of polymer. The non-swellable polymers are used in case of highly water-soluble drugs. Ionic hydrogels such as sodium carboxymethyl cellulose is preferably used because of its osmogenic nature. More precise controlled release of drugs can be achieved by incorporating these polymers into the formulations. Hydrophilic polymers such as hydroxy ethyl cellulose, carboxy methyl cellulose, hydroxy propyl methyl cellulose, high molecular weight poly (vinyl pyrrolidine) and hydrophobic polymers such as ethyl cellulose and wax materials can be used for this purpose.

Wicking Agents

A wicking agent is defined as any material with the ability to draw water into the porous network of a delivery device. A wicking agent is either of swellable or non-swellable nature. They are characterized by having the ability to undergo physisorption with water. Physisorption is a form of absorption in which the solvent molecules can loosely adhere to surfaces of the wicking agent via van der Waals' interactions between the surface of the wicking agent and the adsorbed molecule. The function of the wicking agent is to carry water from surfaces inside of the core of the tablet, thereby creating channels or a network with increased surface area. For bioactive agents with low solubility in water, the wicking agent aids in the delivery of partially solubilized bioactive agent through the passage way in the semipermeable coating. Materials suitable for acting as wicking agents include colloidal silicon dioxide, kaoline, titanium dioxide, alumina, niacinamide, sodium lauryl sulfate (SLS), low molecular weight poly (vinyl pyrrolidine) (PVP), m-pyrol, bentonite, magnesium aluminum silicate, polyester and polyethylene. SLS, colloidal silica and PVP are non-swellable wicking agents.

Solubilizing Agents

Non-swellable solubilizing agents are classified into three groups:
- Agents that inhibit crystal formation of the drugs or otherwise act by complexation with the drugs, [e.g. PVP, poly (ethylene glycol) (PEG 8000) and, cyclodextrins].
- A high HLB micelle-forming surfactant, particularly anionic surfactants, (e.g. Tween 20, 60 and 80, polyoxyethylene or polyethylene containing surfactants and other long chain anionic surfactants such as SLS)
- Citrate esters and their combinations with anionic surfactants, (e.g. alkyl esters particularly triethyl citrate)

Above all, combinations of complexing agents and anionic surfactants such as PVP with SLS and poly (ethylene glycol) and SLS are often preferred.

Osmogens

Osmogens are essential ingredients of the osmotic formulations. Table 2.2 shows some osmogenic agents commonly used in preparation of osmotic pumps.They include inorganic salts and carbohydrates. Generally, combinations of osmogens are used to achieve optimum osmotic pressure within the system.

Surfactants

Surfactants are particularly useful when added to wall-forming material. They produce an integral composite that is useful for making the operative wall of the device. The surfactants act by regulating the surface energy of materials, improve their blending into the composite and maintain their integrity in the surrounding environment during the drug release period. Typical surfactants such as polyoxyethylenated glyceryl recinoleate, polyoxyethylenated castor oil having ethylene oxide, glyceryl laurates, glycerol (sorbiton oleate, stearate or laurate) etc. are used.

Solvents (Coating Material)

Solvents suitable for manufacturing the wall of the osmotic device include inert inorganic and organic solvents that do not adversely harm the core, wall and other materials. The typical solvents include methylene chloride, acetone, methanol, ethanol, isopropyl alcohol, butyl alcohol, ethyl acetate cyclohexane carbon tetrachloride, water etc. The mixtures of solvents such as acetone-methanol (80:20), acetone-ethanol (80:20), acetone-water (90:10), methylene chloride-methanol (79:21), methylene chloride-methanol-water (75:22:3) etc. can be used and expressed as weight: weight.

Plasticizers

Plasticizers in effect lower the temperature of the second order phase transition of the wall or the elastic modules of the wall and also increase the workability, flexibility and permeability of the fluids. Generally, from 0.001 to 50 parts of a plasticizer or a mixture of plasticizers are incorporated into 100 parts of wall-forming materials. Suitable polymers should have a high degree of solvent power for the materials, compatible with the materials over both the processing and the temperature range, exhibit durability as seen by their strong tendency to remain in the plasticized wall, impart flexibility to the materials and should be non-toxic. Plasticizers include dialkyl phthalates and other phthalates, trioctyl phosphates and other phosphates, alkyl adipates, triethyl citrate and other citrates, acetates, propionates, glycolates, glycerolates, myristates, benzoates, sulfonamides and halogenated phenyls.

Flux Regulators

Flux regulating agent added to a wall forming material, assists in regulating the fluid permeability or flux through wall. This agent

Table 2.2: Characteristics of osmotic pump

Research use	Route of administration	Duration of steady-state delivery (hr)	Fill volume (ml)	Steady-state delivery rate (L/hr)	Distinguishing terminology
Clinical research	Oral	12	0.2	15	Oral pump
Clinical research	Oral	24	0.2	8	Oral pump
Clinical research	Rectal/vaginal	30	2	60	Rectal pump
Animal research	Implant	168	0.2	1	Mini-osmotic pump
Animal research	Implant	336	0.2	0.5	Mini-osmotic pump
Animal research	Implant	168	2	10	Osmotic pump
Animal research	Implant	336	2	5	Osmotic pump

can be pre-selected to increase or decrease the liquid flux. Agents producing a marked increase in permeability to fluid such as water are essentially hydrophilic, while those produce a marked decrease in permeability to fluids (water) are essentially hydrophobic. They also increase the flexibility and porosity of the lamina. Polyhydric alcohols such as poly-alkylene glycols and low molecular weight glycols such as polypropylene, polybutylene and polyamylene etc. can be used as flux regulators. The amount of flux regulator added to a material is generally sufficient to produce the desired permeability, which varies with varying characteristics of lamina forming materials. Usually from 0.001 parts to 50 parts or higher of flux regulator can be used to achieve the desired results.

Pore-forming Agents

These agents are particularly used in the pumps developed for poorly water soluble drugs and in the development of controlled porosity or multi-particulate osmotic pumps. These pore-forming agents cause the formation of microporous membrane. The microporous wall may be formed *in situ* by a pore-former, which is removed on dissolving or leaching during the operation of the system. The pores may also be formed in the wall prior to operation of the system by gas formation within coating polymer solutions which result in voids and pores in the final form of the wall. The pore-formers can be inorganic or organic and solid or liquid in nature. For example, alkaline metal salts such as sodium chloride, sodium bromide, potassium chloride, potassium sulfate, potassium phosphate etc., alkaline earth metals such as calcium chloride and calcium nitrate, carbohydrates such as sucrose, glucose, fructose, mannose, lactose, sorbitol, mannitol and, diols and polyols such as polyhydric alcohols and polyvinyl pyrrolidine can be used as pore-forming agents. Pores may also be formed in the wall by the volatilization of components in a polymer solution or by chemical reactions in

a polymer solution which evolves gases prior to application or during application of the solution to the core mass resulting in the creation of polymer foams serving as the porous wall. The pore formers should be non-toxic, and on their removal, channels are formed which are filled with fluid. The channels become a transport path for fluid. The pH insensitive pore-formers are usually preferred.

MODIFIED MULTICHAMBER ELEMENTARY OSMOTIC PUMP

Elementary osmotic pump is limited to the delivery of relatively soluble drugs, generally with solubilities more than 2–5 wt%. Multi-chamber tablet approach solved the problem practically and commercially proved the worth in the form of major product Procardia XL (controlled release nifedipine). These multichamber tablets can be divided into two major classes based on whether one chamber expands into the other or they have got rigid walls and maintain their volume during the whole course of operation. The classes of tablets with expanding chamber are more important and are frequently employed by manufactures to produce osmotic devices.

Tablets with a Second Expandable Osmotic Chamber

Tablets with two chambers separated by an elastic or movable barrier are particularly interesting and valuable because they allow delivery of poorly soluble drugs. This class of osmotic pump can further be classified into two groups one with internal film that moves from a rest to an expanded state or the volumes of the chambers communicating through opening provided in between. In the tablets with a second expandable osmotic chamber, the water is simultaneously drawn into both the chambers in proportion to the osmotic gradient, resultantly causing an increase in volume of the chamber and subsequently forcing the drug out from the drug chamber. Figure 2.9 illustrates the mechanism of action of these devices. Conceptually, the device is related to Higuchi-Leeper pumps described earlier but in these devices, the semipermeable membrane constitutes the entire shell, and water is drawn simultaneously into both the chambers. The matrix should have sufficient osmotic pressure to draw water through the membrane into the drug chamber. Under hydrated conditions matrix should possess enough fluid to be pushed easily through a small hole by the little pressure generated by the elastic diaphragm.

Among the successful approaches, incorporation of finely dispersed drug in hydrogel is the most valuable alternative. Many of the useful hydrogel polymers were ionic materials such as sodium carboxy methylcellulose, which contain ionizable groups, which contribute most of the osmotic pressure required to draw water through the semipermeable membrane. These polymers possess dual property of being compressed in dry conditions and become fluid gels which are easily extrudable through the small delivery hole of the pump under the hydrated conditions.

The controlled release nifedipine (Procardia XL) device is illustrated in Fig. 2.10. The device contains an external semipermeable membrane made up of cellulose acetate bearing a laser-drilled small orifice. The drug chamber possesses the drug, nifedipine,

hydroxy propyl methylcellulose, polyethylene oxide along with small amount of sodium chloride to assist in drawing water into the chamber. A mixture of poly (ethylene oxide) and hydroxy propyl methyl cellulose constitutes the swellable hydrogel chamber. The two-layered tablet is made with a special tablet press, such as the Manesty Layerpress.

The working principle of the nifedipine osmotic device involves the imbibition of fluid by the drug chamber to form a fluid composition *in situ*, and the delivery of the suspension through the orifice. Concurrently, imbibition of fluid by the hydrogel layer causes this second layer to swell and assists the first composition to drive the drug through the orifice. The osmotic device may be considered as a cylinder, with the second hydrogel composition expanding like the movement of a piston to aid in delivering the drug from the device.

Devices with a Nonexpanding Second Chamber

The second class of multichamber devices comprises of systems containing a non-expanding second chamber. This class can be further divided into two groups, based on the function of the second chamber. In one group of these devices, the second chamber serves for the dilution of the drug solution leaving the device. This is important in the cases where

Before Operation

Semipermeable membrane

Osmotic drug core

During Operation

Delivery orifice

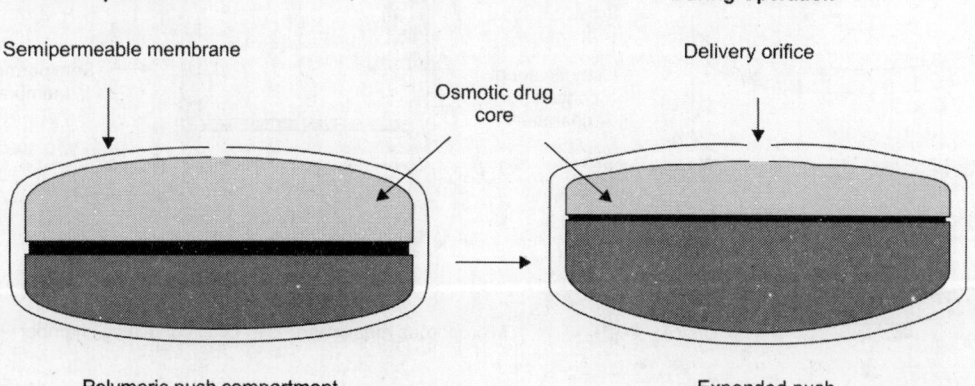

Polymeric push compartment

Expended push

Fig. 2.9: Drug delivery process of two-chamber osmotic tablet

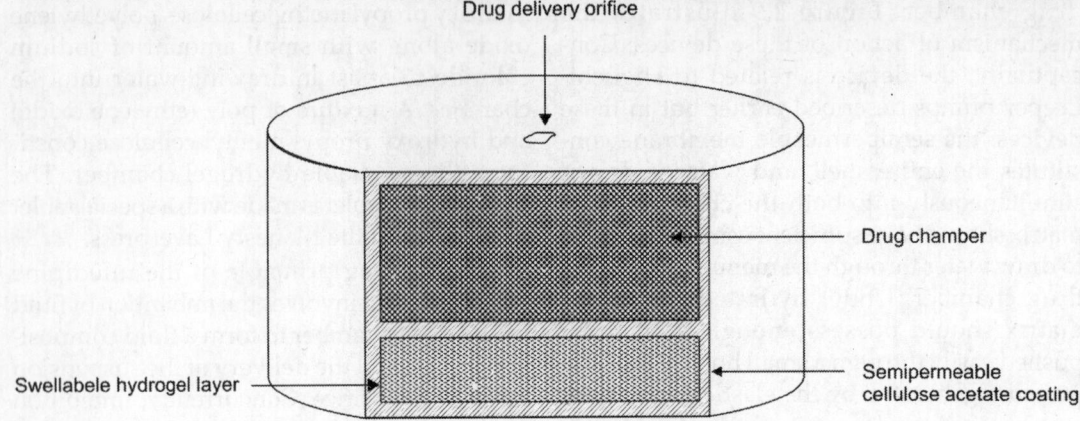

Fig. 2.10: Osmotic tablet of nifedipine

the drug leaves the oral osmotic device as a saturated solution; irritation of the gastro-intestinal tract is a risk. This was the reason behind the withdrawal of Osmosin® (sodium indomethacin). The device essentially contains a normal drug contained in a OROS tablet from which drug is released as a saturated solution. However, before the drug can exit from the device, it must pass through a second chamber. Water is also drawn osmotically into this chamber either due to the osmotic pressure of the drug solution or because the second chamber bears a water-soluble diluents such as sucrose or sodium chloride.

The nonexpanding multichamber devices of second group essentially contain two separate simple OROS tablets formed into a single tablet as shown in Fig. 2.11. Two chambers contain two separate drugs and both are delivered simultaneously. A more sophisticated version of these devices consists of two rigid chambers, one contains biologically

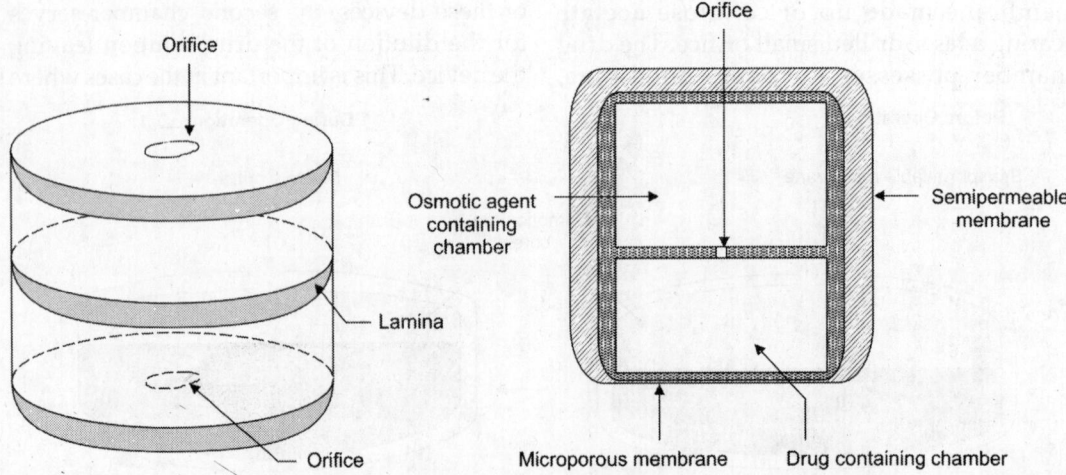

Fig. 2.11: Example of multichamber osmotic devices with chambers separated by rigid nonexpanding walls

inert osmotic agent such as sugar or a simple salt like NaCl, and the second chamber contains the drug. When exposed to aqueous environment, water is drawn into both chambers across the semipermeable membrane as shown in Fig. 2.11. The solution of osmotic agent formed in the first chamber then passes to the drug chamber through the connecting hole where it mixes with the drug solution before escaping through the microporous membrane that forms part of the wall around the drug chamber. Relatively insoluble drug could be delivered using this device. These systems hold promises for research studies. The assessment of the pharmacology and pharmacokinetics of the drug candidates which are to be delivered following controlled release is essential during initial stages of screening and evaluation. Bioavailability studies, therapeutic concentration ranges and clearance measurements are of great value in the design of controlled release systems. A series of osmotic pumps have been developed as shown in Table 2.3, to provide different volumes and delivery rates of incorporated

drug(s). These are useful in evaluating drug pharmacology in the steady state and under conditions of rate-controlled drug inputs. The range of sizes and pumping capabilities is from 0.2 to 2 ml in fill volume; study state pumping rates of 0.5 to 60 µl/hr can be achieved and duration of delivery could be extended from 12 to 336 hours, depending upon the devices fill volume capacity and pumping rate.

Some marketed osmotic delivery system-based formulations are shown in Table 2.4.

ADVANTAGES

There are numerous advantages of oral osmotic pumps which have been listed below:
- Decrease frequency of dosing.
- Reduce the rate of rise of drug concentration in the body.
- Delivery may be pulsed if required.
- Delivery ratio is independent of pH of the environment.
- Delivery is independent of hydrodynamic condition, this suggests that drug delivery is independent of GI motility.

Table 2.3: Patents related to osmotic delivery systems			
Cited patent	Issue date	Original assignee	Title
US4093708	Mar 9, 1977	Alza Corporation	Osmotic releasing device having a plurality of release rate patterns
US4160452	Apr 7, 1977	Alza Corporation	Osmotic system having laminated wall comprising semipermeable lamina and microporous lamina
US4210139	Jan 17, 1979	Alza Corporation	Osmotic device with compartment for governing concentration of agent dispensed from device
US4016880	Mar 4, 1976	Alza Corporation	Osmotically driven active agent dispenser
US4036228	Sep 11, 1975	Alza Corporation	Osmotic dispenser with gas generating means
US4327725	Nov 25, 1980	Alza Corporation	Osmotic device with hydrogel driving member
US4609374	Apr 22, 1985	Alza Corporation	Osmotic device comprising means for governing initial time of agent release therefrom
US4612008	Dec 21, 1984	Alza Corporation	Osmotic device with dual thermodynamic activity
US4765989	Sep 2, 1986	Alza Corporation	Osmotic device for administering certain drugs
US4783337	Sep 29, 1986	Alza Corporation	Osmotic system comprising plurality of members for dispensing drug
US5736159	Apr 7, 1998	Andrx Pharmaceuticals, Inc.	Controlled release formulation for water insoluble drugs in which a passageway is formed in situ
US6110498	Aug 29, 2000	Shire Laboratories, Inc.	Osmotic drug delivery system
US6284276	Sep 4, 2001	Shire Laboratories, Inc.	Soluble form, osmotic dose delivery system
US6361796	Mar 26, 2002	Shire Laboratories, Inc	Soluble form, osmotic dose delivery system

Table 2.4: List of some marketed osmotic delivery system based formulations

Product name	Drug	Delivery system	Developer/marketer
Acutrim	Phenylpropanolamine	Elementry pump	Alza/Heritage
Alpress	Prazosin	Push-pull	Alza/Pfizer
Cardura XL	Doxazosin	Push-pull	Alza/Pfizer
Calan SR	Verapamil		Alza/GD Searle & Co.
Concerta	Methyl phenidate		Alza
Covera HS	Verapamil	Pull-pull time delay	Alza/GD Searle
Ditropan XL	Oxybutinin chloride	Push-pull	Alza/UCB pharma
Dynacirc CR	Isradipine	Push-pull	Alza/Novartis
Efidac 24	Pseudoephedrine	Elementray	Alza/Novartis
Glucotrol XL	Glipizide	Push-pull	Alza/Pfizer
Minipress XL	Prazosin	Push-pull	Alza/Pfizer
Procadia XL	Nifedipine	Push-pull	Alza/Pfizer
Sudafed	Pseudoephedrin	Push-pull	Alza/Pfizer
Teczam	Enaprl and diltiazem	Elementary pump	Merc/Aventis
Tiamate	Diltilazem	Push-pull	Merck/Aventis
Volmax	Albuterol	Push-pull	Alza/Muro Pharm

- Sustained and consistent blood level of drug within the therapeutic window.
- Improved patient compliance.
- High degree of *in vitro–in vivo* correlation is obtained in osmotic system.
- Reduced side effect.
- Delivery rate is also independent of delivery orifice size within the limit.

DISADVANTAGES AND LIMITATIONS

Oral osmotic pumps have produced significant clinical benefit in various therapeutic areas. Some systems have enhanced patient compliance, while other have minimized the side effect of their active compounds. However, some limitations of oral osmotic pump have been reported.

1. Slightly higher cost than matrix tablet or multi particulates capsule dosage forms.
2. Gastrointestinal obstruction cases have been observed with the patient receiving nifedipine GITS tablet.
3. Another case was reported for Osmosin® (indomethacin OROS) which was first introduced in the United Kingdom in 1983. A few months later following its introduction frequent incidences of serious gastrointestinal reactions were observed leading to Osmosin® withdrawal. Various explanations were given based on the toxic effect of KCl used in Osmosin®.
4. Magnetic resonance imaging (MRI) of tablet elucidated that non-uniform coating leads to varied pattern of drug release among the batches.

Evaluation of the Developed Formulations
Drug Release Studies

The developed formulations are subjected to release studies using USP-II dissolution apparatus (Electrolab, India) at 100 rpm. Phosphate buffer containing sodium lauryl sulphate (0.5%) is generally used as a dissolution medium maintained at 37±0.5°C. The samples are withdrawn (10 ml) at 0, 2, 4 6, 8, 10 and 12 hours intervals and replaced with an equivalent amount of fresh medium. The dissolution samples after filtration through 0.45 mm cellulose acetate filter are analyzed using a validated UV spectrophotometric method. Mathematical comparisons of dissolution curves from various formulations provide an opportunity to test the similarity comparative two dissolution profiles.

Burst Strength

Burst strength of the exhausted shells, after dissolution is determined to assure that the pumps would maintain their integrity in the gastrointestinal tract (GIT).

Burst strength is measured by using a texture analyser as the forces required to break/rupture the shells after dissolution studies.

Evaluation of Membrane Variables

- Effect of concentration of pore-forming agent
- Effect of concentration of enteric polymer
- Scanning electron microscopy (SEM)
- Stability studies
- Clinical aspects of OODS

Safety and Precautions

The development of the OODS has been marked by one main safety aspect which must be addressed as a prerequisite. Thus, in the case of the delivery of irritating drug substances, the concern is over the local delivery of the drug from an OODS with impaired transit through the GI tract, which might lead to gut wall irritations. In the worst case, it can result in gut wall perforations, as has been reported from patients receiving the indomethacin OODS, Osmosin®. Thus, Osmosin® was withdrawn from the market after 18 patients died and more than 400 cases of severe intestinal ulcerations were reported. Since 1950s, indomethacin has been a drug known to be irritating the GI system. The risk of irritation was probably aggravated by local drug delivery through the orifice and the potentially prolonged transit time observed with non-degradable systems. Therefore, *in vitro* evaluation of the drug irritation property on GI mucosa was proposed as a standard procedure before human studies. Two precautions must also be considered by the physician before treatment; they relate to the non-degradable nature of OODS. The first precaution is to detect pre-existing GI injury in the patient history that might increase the likelihood of GI narrowing. Thus, the potential hazard of GI occlusion has been reported in about one case for 76 million units. Possible difficulties in swallowing OODS should also be taken into account. Further, physicians must inform the patient that the empty shell may be excreted in the feces, which can disturb fragile patients, such as in the treatment of schizophrenia using paliperidone (Invega®).

Gastrointestinal (GI) Transit and Drug Absorption

Due to non-uniform transit throughout the GI tract, drug absorption remains a key element in the design of the absorption varied from 40 to 80% depending on the transit time, which was due mainly to prolonged residence time in the stomach. Studies on non-disintegrating tablets have been carried out to compare the gastro-intestinal transit of OODS with other modified-release forms, such as erodible matrices or pellets. It appears that the size of the system plays a minor role in the fasted state, as illustrated by comparison of pellets versus large non-disintegrable capsule. However, concomitant administration of food may change the situation. While no significant difference in GI transit was observed for systems with a size lower than 7 mm, large non-disintegrable systems, like Osmet® capsules or 9 mm round tablets, remained of in the stomach for more than 10 hours. Contradictory results for yet larger round tablets with diameters up to 10 mm, carbamazepine SEOP and indomethacin EOP, were reported, with lower gastric retention times of about 3 to 5 hours depending on the meal composition. Despite these controversial results, there is great evidence that the patient-to- patient variability increases with the OODS size. Therefore, efforts to decrease the size of the system should generally pay off. Furthermore, systematic studies on the gastrointestinal transit of nondisintegrating systems may also help to optimize both the drug release rate and the OODS design to satisfy the expected drug absorption.

SUGGESTED READINGS

1. Abrahamsson, B, Alpstrn, M, Bake, B, Jonsson, VE, Eridsson-Lepdowska, M. and Larsson, A. (1998), *J. Control. Rel.* 52(3), 301.

2. Appel LE, Zentner GM: *Pharm Res.* 1991, 8(5): 600–4.

3. A. Schuchert, KH Kuck, Dtsch. Med. Wochenschr. 117 (1992) 607–12.

4. ALZET® Osmotic Pumps, http://www.alzet. com 27-8-2011.

5. Avgerinos, PC, Schurmeyer, TH, Gold, PW, Tomai, TP, Loriaux, DL, Sherins, RJ, Cutler, GB, Jr. and Chrousos, GP (1986), secretory pattern, *J. Clin. Endocrinol. Metab.* 62, 816–21.

6. Chandrasekaran, SK, Theeuwes, F and Yum, SI (1979), *In: Drug Design*, vol. 8, EJ Ariens (Ed.), Academic, New York, 134.

7. CM Rohloff, TR Alessi, B Yang, J Dahms, JP Carr, SD L *J Diab. Sci. Technol.* 2 (2008).

8. DM Fisher, N Kellet, R Lenhardt Anesthesiology 99 (2003) 929–37.

9. DN Soulas, M Sanopoulou, KGJ, *Appl. Polym. Sci.* 113 (2009) 936–49.

10. Eckenhoff, B and Wright, RM (1983), In: *Controlled Drug Delivery*, SD Bruck (Ed.), vol. 2nd, CRC Press, Inc., Florida, 76.

11. Esther, M, van der, Z, Mieneke, CM, Luijendijk, R AH and Adan, SE (2008), *Eur. J. Pharmacol.*, 585, 130–36.

12. Eckenhoff, B, Theeuwes, F and Urquhart, J (1981), *Pharm. Technol.* 5, 35–44.

13. JE Fowler, JE Gottesman, SF Bardot, CF Reid, GL Andriole, PH Bernhard, I. Rivera-Ramirez, JA Libertino, MS Soloway, Urol. 159 (1998) 335.

14. Hill, A, Geißler, S, Weigandt, M and Mäder, K. (2012) *J. Cont. Rel.* 158, 403–12.

15. Kumaravelrajan, R, Narayanan, N, Suba, V and Bhaskar, K, *Int. J. Pharm,* Volume 399, 60–70.

16. MJ Cukierski, PA Johnson, JC Beck, *Int. J. Toxicol.* 20 (2001) 369–81.

17. Mariagrazia, M, Gert, R, Anders, A. (2007) *Int. J. Pharm,* 336, 67–74.

18. JE Fowler, MS Group, J. Urol. 163 (2000) 262–263.

19. JE Fowler, JE Gottesman, CF Reid, GL, J. Urol. 164 (2000) 730–34.

20. JC Wright, J Culwell, J Hadgraft, MS Roberts (Eds.), New York, 2008, pp. 143–49.

21. Liu H, Yang XG, Nie SF, Wei LL, Zhoub LL, Liu H, Tang R, Pan WS, (2007), *International Journal of Pharmaceutics,* 332, 115.

22. Longxiao, L and Xiaocui, W (2008), *Eur. J. Pharm. Biopharm,* 68, 298–302.

23. Longxiao, L and Xiangning, X (2008), *Int. J. Pharm.,* 352, 225–30.

24. Li, H, Yin, X, Ji, J, Sun, L, Shao, Q, York, P, Xiao, T, He, Y and Zhang, J (2012), *Int. J. Pharm.,* 427, 270–75.

25. Ramesh KVRNS, Chowdary KPR: *Ind J Pharm Sci* 1994, 56: 5–12.

26. Singh, K, Bajaj, A, Babul, N and Kao, H (2012), *J. Pain,* 13, S78.

27. SM Herbig, JR Cardinal, RW Korsmeyer, KL Smith, Control. Release 35 (1995) 127–36.

28. Skalko N, Brandl M, Ladan MB, Grid JF, Genjak IJ: *Eur J Pharm Sci* 1996, 4(3): 359–66.

29. Suzuki H, T Tokuda, T Miyagishi, H Yoshida, N Honda, *Sens. Actuators,* B 97 (2004) 90–97.

30. Liversidge, GG, Nishihata, T, Engle, KK and Higuchi, T (1985), *Int. J. Pharmaceut.* 23, 87–95.

31. Lee, VHL, Yamamoto, A and Luo, AM (1988), *Control Rel. Bioact. Mater.* 15, 454–5.

32. M Staples, Wiley Interdiscip. Rev. Nanomed. Nanobiotechnol 2 (2010) 400–417.

33. M Barzegar-Jalali, K Adibkia, G Mohammadi, M. Zeraati, B Bolagh, G Aghaee, A. Drug Deliv. 14 (2007) 461–8.

34. Merkle, HP, Anders, R, Sandow, J and Shurr, W (1985) *Proc. Int. Symp. Control Rel. Bioact. Mater.* 12, 85.

35. Okada, H, Yamazaki, I, Ogawa, Y, Hirai, S, Yashiki, T and Mima, H. (1982) *J. Pharm. Sci.* 71, 1367–71.

36. Ouyang D, Nie S, Li W, Guo H, Liu H, Pan W: *J Pharm Pharmacol.* 2005, 57: 817–20.

37. Pu, F, Rahil, TR, Alan, C, Lee-Yuan, L, Xiaohui, P, John, G, Joseph J MJ, Martin, WA and Toby, KE (2006), *Eur. J. Pharmacol.,* 534, 250–57.

38. Richter A., C. Klenke, K.F. Arndt, A Macromol. Symp. 210 (2004) 377–84.

39. S. Rose, J. Nelson, Aust. J. Exp. Biol. Med. Sci. 33 (1955) 415–21.

40. Santus G, RW Baker, *J. Control. Release* 35 (1995) 1–21.

41. Theeuwes, F and Bayne, W (1981), In: Controlled Release Pharmaceuticals, J. Urquhart (Ed.), American Pharmaceutical Association, Washington, DC, P.

42. Theeuwes, F (1985), *In: Rate Control in Drug Therapy*, LF Prescott and WS Nimmo (Eds.), Churchill Livingstone, Edinburgh, 116.

43. Theeuwes, F, 1984, *Pharm. Int.* 5, 293–6.

44. Theeuwes, F, Yum, SI, 1976. *Ann. Biomed. Eng.* 4, 343–53.

45. T Gosh, A Gosh, *J. Appl. Pharm. Sci.* 1 (2011), 38–49.

46. T. Higuchi, *J. Pharm. Sci.* 52 (1963) 1145–9.

47. Touitou, E, Donbrow, M and Azaz, E (1978) *J. Pharm. Pharmacol.* 30, 662–3.

48. US Pharmacopeia XXXI, 2006. Chlorpheniramine extended-release and isradipine capsule monographs. US Pharmacopeial Convention, 1740 and 2482.

49. UKH Wiegand, J Potratz, H Bonnemeier, F Bode, R Panik, H Haase,W Peters, HA Katus, PACE 23 (2000) 1003–1009.

50. Verma, RK, Mishra, B, Garg, S, 2000. *Dr. Dev. Ind. Pharm.* 26, 695–708.

51. V Malaterre, J Ogorka, N Loggia, R Gurny, Eur *J. Pharm. Biopharm.* 73 (2009) 311–23.

52. Vyas SP and Khar RK (2000), In: Controlled drug delivery, concept and advances, 1st ediion, vallabh prakashan, New Delhi.

53. Wonnemann, M, Schug, B, Schmucker, K, Brendel, E, van Zwieten, PA, Blumel, H, 2006. *Int. J. Clin. Pharm. Ther.* 44, 38–48.

54. Waterman, KC, Goeken, GS, Konagurthu, S, Likar, MD, MacDonald, BC, Mahajan, N and Swaminathan, V (2011), *J. Cont. Rel.*, 152, 264–9.

55. Wright J, Ruminal osmotic bolus, in: E Mathiowitz (Ed.), Encyclopedia of Con-trolled Drug Delivery, Wiley, New York, 1999, pp. 915–20.

56. Waterman KC, BC MacDonald, MC Roy, *J. Control. Release* 134 (3) (2009) 201–206.

57. Yum, SI and Wright RM (1983); In: Controlled Drug Delivery, SD Bruck (Ed.), vol. 2nd, CRC Press, Inc., Florida, 76.

58. Z.R. Xu, CG Yang, CH Liu, Z Zhou, J Fang, JH Wang, Talanta 80 (2010) 1088–1093.

59. Zentner GM, Rork GS, Himmelstein KJ: *J Control Rel* 1985, 1(3): 269–82.

60. Zenter, GM, Rork, GS and Himmelstein, KJ (1985), *J. Control. Rel.* 1, 269.

61. Zentner GM, McClelland GA, Sutton SC, (1991). *J. Control. Release* 16, 237.

62. Zhang, Z, Dong, H, Peng, B, Liu, H, Li, C, Liang, M and Pan, W (2011), *Int. J. Pharm.*, 410, 41–7.

3

Bioadhesive and Mucoadhesive Systems

INTRODUCTION

Interest in controlled and sustained release drug delivery has increased considerably during the past decade and in selected areas it is now possible to employ fairly sophisticated systems which are capable of excellent drug release control. The self regulating insulin delivery systems by using lectin and oral osmotic tablets are illustrative examples. However, for oral administration, all of these systems are limited to some extent because of gastrointestinal (GI) transit. Thus, the duration of most of the oral sustained release products is approximately 8–12 hours due to relatively short GI transit time, and the possibilities to localize a drug delivery system in selected regions of the gastrointestinal tract (GIT) for the purpose of localized drug delivery are under investigation. Several approaches have been suggested to increase GI transit time, addressing the issue of localized drug delivery. Both low and high density drug delivery systems have been suggested as possible approaches to extend transit time, but the results of exploratory studies are equivocal. In another system in which particle size, relative to stomach retropulsion has been suggested as a means to delay stomach emptying and thereby to prolong the transit time. This phenomena is also of relatively

short duration, particularly when the drug delivery system is administered in the absence of food. An alternative approach is to employ bioadhesive polymers that adhere to the mucin/epithelial surface. Such polymer would have to be applied to any mucous membranes and perhaps non-mucous membranes as well. Thus, bioadhesive polymers would find application in the eye, nose, vagina and GIT including the buccal cavity and rectum. In 1986, Longer and Robinson defined the term bioadhesion as the attachment of a synthetic or natural macromolecule to mucus and/or an epithelial surface. The general definition of adherence of a polymeric material to biological surfaces (bioadhesives) or to the mucosal tissue (mucoadhesives) still holds.

Bioadhesives is the term that describes the adhesion of a polymer to a biological substrate. More specifically, when adhesion is restricted to the mucous layer lining of the mucosal surface it is termed as mucoadhesion. This has gained considerable interest since the localization of drug carrying particles at the mucosal surface would result in

- A prolonged residence time at the site of action or absorption
- A localization of the drug delivery system at a given target site

- An increase in the drug concentration gradient due to the contact of the particles with the mucosal surface
- A direct contact with intestinal mucosa is the first step before particle adhesion.

Bioadhesion can be obtained by building of either non-specific interactions, which are driven by the physicochemical properties of the particles and the intestinal surfaces or through specific interactions when a ligand appended on to the particle is used for the recognition and attachment of polymeric particulates to a specific site at the mucosal surface. This chapter focuses on the past development and present status of the various oral and specialized bio/mucoadhesive systems.

Mucoadhesive-controlled release devices can improve the effectiveness of a drug by maintaining the drug concentration between the effective and toxic levels, preventing undesirable dilution of the drug in the body fluids, while allowing targeting and localization of a drug at a specific site. Mucoadhesion also increases the intimacy and duration of contact between a drug containing polymer and a mucous surface. The combined effects of the direct drug absorption and decreased excretion rate (due to prolonged residence time) allow for an increased bioavailability of the drug with a smaller dosage and result in a less frequent administration. Bioadhesive systems can prevent first pass metabolism of certain protein drugs by the liver through the introduction of the drug via this route bypass the digestive tract. Drugs that are absorbed through the mucosal lining of tissues can enter directly into the blood stream and do not undergo enzymatic degradation in the GIT.

FUNDAMENTALS OF BIOADHESION

Development of an adhesive bond between a polymer and biological membrane or its coating can be visualized as a two step process:
- Initial contact between the two surfaces
- Formation of secondary bonds due to non-covalent interactions.

This process of bond formation attributes to the surface (or surface coat) of the biological membrane, surface of the adhesive and the interfacial layer between the two surfaces. Molecular events which take place in the interfacial region depend on properties of the polymer and biomembrane.

Biological Membrane

Membranes of the internal tracts of the body, including the GIT, buccal cavity, eye, ear, nose, vagina and rectum are covered with a thick gel-like structure known as mucin. Therefore, all bioadhesives must primarily interact with mucin layer during the process of attachment. Mucus itself possesses considerable binding property, and thus serves as a link between the adhesive and membrane. Most polymers bind to mucin and never penetrate deep enough to form a bond with the underlying epithelial cells. They are termed as "bioadhesives". Mucin oligosaccharides and glycoproteins are synthesized by goblet cells and special exocrine glands with mucous cell acini. In the total weight of the mucous secreted, only less than 5% contents are glycoproteins. There are about 160–200 oligosaccharide side chains in the glycosylated region of the glycoprotein, each oligosaccharide unit contains 8–10 monosaccharide chains. The terminal end of these oligosaccharides is either sialic acid or L-fucose. At physiological pH, the mucin network has a negative charge due to the presence of sialic acid, which has a pKa of 2.6. Also, the presence of sulfate residues contributing to this negative charge, make the glycoprotein as an anionic polyelectrolyte. Thus, bioadhesive mucin consists of highly hydrated crosslinked, linear, flexible and random coiled glycoprotein molecules with a net negative charge. The cell surface membrane also possesses a net negative charge due to the presence of charged groups. Thus binding of mucin to cell surfaces, through interaction between two surfaces with the same net charge, indicates that the adhesive forces dominate the electrostatic repulsive forces between these two surfaces, i.e mucin and bio cells.

Bioadhesive Polymers

Mucoadhesive polymers are classified into two categories:

1. Polymers that are water soluble, linear and structurally random polymers.
2. Water insoluble, however swellable polymeric compounds networked through some cross-linking agents.

There are so many properties associated with bioadhesive property of the polymers.

Molecular Weight, Chain Length and Crosslinking Density

The bioadhesive strength increases as molecular weight of the polymer increases above 100, 000 and there seems to be a critical molecular weight requirement for significant bioadhesion. For all water-swellable and insoluble polymers, the linear chains are connected via cross-linking agents. For example, polycarbophil, a well-known mucoadhesive, this is poly (acrylic acid) cross-linked with divinyl glycol. Cross-linking density of polycarbophil is expected to influence mucoadhesion by influencing the effective number of poly (acrylic acid) chains in a given volume of their chain segment mobility. The strength of mucoadhesion is found to decrease with an increase in concentration of the cross-linking agent. In fact, an increase in cross-linking density decreases the diffusion coefficient and chain segment-segment flexibility and mobility, thereby reducing the extent of interpenetration.

Charges and Ionization

Polyanionic polymers are preferred over polycationic and neutral polymers when both bioadhesive strength and cellular toxicity are considered. Furthermore, polyanions with carboxyl groups appear to be better candidates than those with sulfates.

Hydrophilic Functional Groups and Hydration

Bioadhesive polymers are usually macromolecules with numerous hydrophilic functional groups that can form hydrogen bonds, e.g. carboxyl, hydroxyl, amide and sulfate groups. The presence of their fixed charges within the macromolecular network establishes a swelling force or swelling pressure or a net osmotic pressure, which drives the solvent into the polymer gel from the more dilute external bulk solution when counterions are added to the hydrating media. They bind to some of the fixed charge groups resulting in a screening effect. Thus the ionic strength and the amount of counterions in solution are important parameters to be considered in mucoadhesive studies. The amount of water at the interface between the interacting adhesive and substrate surface is an important determinant of bioadhesion. Sufficient water is needed to properly hydrate the mucoadhesive to expose the adhesive sites for secondary bond formation, expand the gel to create pores of sufficient size and mobilize all the flexible polymer chains for interpenetration.

Chain Segment Mobility and Expanded Nature of the Network

The ability of the polymer and mucin chains to interpenetrate can be approximated by their ability to diffuse. Over a sufficiently restricted temperature range, the experimental diffusion coefficient, D, shows an exponential temperature dependence of the Arrhenius type,

$$D = D_o \exp (-E/RT)$$

where, the pre-exponential factor D_o is a constant and is independent of temperature over a given temperature range, and E is the experimental activation energy for diffusion or for mobility of the segment chain. At a particular temperature, inter-chain diffusion will increase with chain segment mobility. This chain segment mobility may be increased by an increased degree of hydration, expanded nature of network and reduced degree of cross-linking. The factors which control the strength of mucoadhesion are the effect of expanded nature of the mucin and adhesive network on mucoadhesion, and the pressure applied to the interacting interface. Increasing applied pressure improves the intimacy and intensity of contact and contact area, which promote secondary bond formation and physical entanglement, resulting in greater mucoadhesive strength.

MECHANISM OF BIOADHESION

Various classes of polymers have been investigated for mucoadhesive suitable properties, such as proper hydrogen-bonding functional groups, suitable wetting properties, swelling/water load properties, and sufficient flexibility for entanglement with the tissue mucus network. Derivatives of cellulose (methyl, hydroxypropyl, carboxy methyl cellulose) and poly (acrylic acid) with high molecular weight (polycarbophil, carbomer) have been shown to possess the hydrogel-forming properties, which are necessary for mucoadhesion. Polysaccharides, such as chitosan, are among the newer mucoadhesive polymers. There have also been some recent reports of protein mucoadhesion, in which proteins have been reported to adhere to almost any kind of surfaces non-specifically.

Mucins are highly glucosylated glycoproteins with a large peptide backbone and oligosaccharides as side chains. Their protein backbone is characterized by the presence of repeating sequences rich in serine, threonine, and proline residues. Many of the O-linked oligosaccharide side chains are often terminated in sialic acid, sulfonic acid, or l-fructose. As a result, mucins are negatively charged at physiological pH.

Mechanisms of polymer attachment to mucosal surfaces are not yet fully understood. However, certain theories of bioadhesion have suggested that it might occur via physical entanglement (diffusion theory) and/or chemical interactions, such as electrostatic, hydrophobic, hydrogen bonding, and van der Waals' interactions (adsorption and electronic theories). Positively charged polymers, such as chitosan, can bind to mucin via electrostatic interactions with the negatively charged sialic acid moieties. However, ionic interactions with sialic acid are merely one possible mechanism of polymer-mucin binding. In addition, it has been shown that anionic polymers usually provide better bioadhesion than cationic or uncharged polymers. Therefore, other mechanisms, including hydrophobic interactions, hydrogen bonding, and van der Waals' interactions, are also possible, which probably involve other parts of the mucin molecules. Moreover, hydrogen bonds and hydrophobic interactions are classical interactions that are desirable for mucoadhesion. Recently, covalent bonds and disulfide bonds (through disulfide exchange reactions) have also been reported to be responsible for mucoadhesion.

The bioadhesion phenomenon of the polymer is dependent on its physicochemical properties. The most important physicochemical factors of such mucoadhesive polymers are followings:

- Generally hydrophilic molecules that contain numerous hydrogen bond forming groups.
- Surface tension characteristics suitable for wetting mucus/mucosal tissue surfaces.
- The polymers are predominantly anionic in nature containing many carboxyl groups. Usually have a high molecular weight (greater than 100, 000).
- Sufficient flexibility to penetrate the mucus network or tissue crevices.

Several mechanisms of polymer/substrate interaction involvement in mucoadhesive bond formation have been suggested, namely, the electronic, adsorption, wetting, diffusion and fracture theories.

Wetting Theory

It describes the ability of a bioadhesive polymer to spread on biological surfaces. This theory is predominantly applicable to liquid bioadhesive systems. Moderately wettable polymers have been shown to exhibit optimal adhesion to human endothelial cells. The ability of the adhesive to spread spontaneously on mucin influences development of intimate contact between the mucoadhesive and mucin, and consequently influences the mucoadhesive strength. The thermodynamic phenomenon of adhesion is a function of the surface tension of the surface in contact as well as the interfacial tension. A small value of interfacial tension would mean a more intimate contact between the two surfaces.

Diffusion Theory

The basis of the diffusion theory is chain entanglement between glycoproteins of the mucus and the mucoadhesive polymer. Upon initial contact between these two polymers, diffusion of the bioadhesive polymer chain into the mucus network creates an entangled network between the two polymers. Sufficient polymer chain flexibility, adequate exposure for the surface contact of both polymers, similar chemical structures, and the diffusion coefficient of the bioadhesive polymer are among the factors which influence the inter-diffusion of the macromolecule network. The diffusion theory describes interpenetration of the mucoadhesive (polymer) and substrate (mucin) to a sufficient depth and creation of a semipermanant adhesive bond. In bioadhesion, the polymer is first brought into intimate contact with the mucus, and over time, the concentration gradient across the interface causes the diffusion of the chains of the bioadhesive into the mucus layer and also the diffusion of the glycoprotein chains of the mucus into the bioadhesive polymer. The rate of the diffusion is dependent on the chemical potential gradient and the diffusion coefficient of a macromolecule through a cross-linked network. The chains that have diffused across the interface serve as anchors to aid in securing semi-permanent adherence/localization of bioadhesive device in place. The interpenetration distance that is necessary for good bioadhesion is approximately equal to end to end distance of the macromolecular chains (Fig. 3.1).

Despite the inter-diffusion within compatible polymers as has been demonstrated by radiometric studies, the exact depth of penetration required to achieve adequate mucoadhesion is not known. However, the mean diffusional path length (S), can be derived as,

$$S = (2tD) 1/2$$

where D is the diffusion coefficient. The diffusion coefficient depends on the molecular

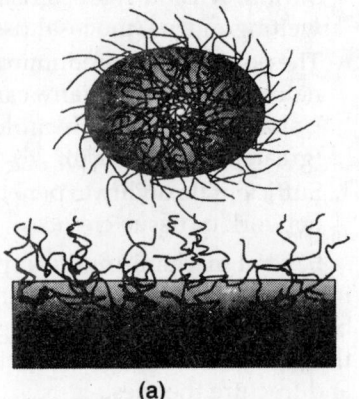
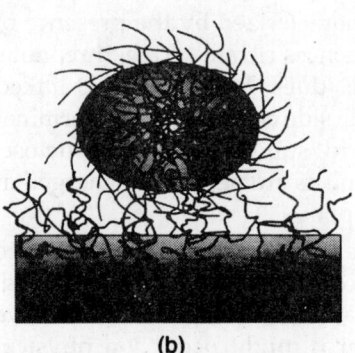

(a)   (b)

Fig. 3.1: Interpenetration of bioadhesive and mucous polymer chains

weight of the polymer strand. It decreases significantly with increasing cross-linking density, indicating that flexibility and chain segment mobility of the mucoadhesive polymer and mucous glycoprotein molecules are important parameters which control inter-chains diffusion.

Electronic Theory

Because of different electronic properties of the mucoadhesive polymer and the mucus glycoprotein, electron transfer between these two surfaces occurs. Electron transfer contributes to formation of a charged double layer at the interface of the mucus and the polymer, which results in forces of attraction in this region and interdiffusion of the two surfaces with subsequent adhesion. The mucin glyco-protein and mucoadhesive polymer possess different electronic structures, therefore electronic transfer is likely to occur when contact is established. Hence, the adhesive/ mucin interface can be treated as a capacitor, which is charged when the two surfaces are in close contact and it discharges when the surfaces are separated.

Adsorption Theory

In the adsorption theory, primary and secondary chemical bonds of the covalent and non-covalent (electrostatic and van der Waals' forces, hydrogen, and hydrophobic bonds) types are formed following the initial contact between the mucus and the mucoadhesive polymer. Most of the initial interfacials bonding forces are attributed to non-covalent forces. The formation of secondary chemical bonds greatly depends on the properties of the polymer.

The attachment of adhesive to biological tissues on the basis of group of interactions is known as 'secondary forces'. The van der Waals' forces of attraction are the sum of all attractions between uncharged molecules. These attractive forces include:

- Polar or Keesom forces developed due to orientation of permanent dipoles in two molecules
- Induction debye forces developed due to induced dipole and permanent dipole
- Dispersion or London forces developed due to the changes in the charge distribution at or around nonpolar molecules
- Hydrogen bonding developed between two non-polar groups, due to the tendency of water molecules to exclude nonpolar molecules, or between ionized carboxyl groups or surfaces.

Fracture Theory

The fracture theory relates the force required for the detachment of polymers from mucus associated through their adhesive bonds. It has been found that the work fracture is greater when the network strands are longer or the degree of cross-linking is reduced.

The most useful theory for studying bioadhesion through tensile experiments has been the fracture theory, which analyzes the forces required to separate two surfaces after adhesion. The maximum tensile strength (m) produced during detachment can be determined by dividing the maximum force of detachment, F_m, by the total surface area (A_o) involved in the adhesion interaction.

$$m = F_m / A_o \qquad (3.1)$$

In a uniform single-component system, fracture strength (f), which is equal to the maximum stress of detachment (m), is proportional to fracture energy (c), Young's modules of elasticity (E) and critical crack length (C) of the fracture site, as described in the following equation (Kammer, 1983),

$$f \times \frac{(cE / C)}{2} \qquad (3.2)$$

Fracture energy (c) can be obtained from the sum of the reversible work of adhesion, W_r, (i.e. the energy required to produce new fracture surfaces) and the irreversible work of adhesion, W_i, (i.e. the work of plastic deformation at the tip of the growing crack), where both values are expressed per unit area of the fracture surface (Af),

$$c = W_r + W_i \qquad (3.3)$$

The elastic modulus of the system (E) is related to stress (F) and strain (l) through Hooke's law,

$$E = [F/A_o/l/l_o]\, t_0 \qquad (3.4)$$

In this equation, stress is equal to the charging force (F) divided by the area (A_o), and strain is equal to the chain thickness (l) of the system divided by the original thickness (l_o). Equation (3.4) suggests that the system being investigated is of known physical dimensions and composed of a single uniform-bulk material. Considering this, equation (3.2) and (3.4) cannot be applied to analyze the fraction site of the multi-component bioadhesive bond between a polymer microsphere and either mucous or mucosal tissue. For such analysis, the equation must be expanded to accommodate dimensions and elastic module of each component. Moreover, to determine fracture properties of an adhesive union from separation experiments, failure of the adhesive bond must be assumed to occur at the bioadhesive interface. However, it has been demonstrated that fracture occurs at the interface rarely, but instead it occurs close to it. Despite these limitations, because the fracture theory deals only with analyzing the adhesive force required for separation, it does not assume or require entanglement, diffusion or interpenetration of polymer chains. Therefore, it is appropriate to use equation (3.1) to calculate fracture strength of adhesive bonds involving hard bioadhesive materials in which the polymer chain may not penetrate the mucous layer.

Mucoadhesion is considered in terms of three stages, wetting, interpenetration and interaction of substrate and polymer. The mucoadhesive must 'wet' the substrate to develop intimate contact between the interacting molecules. The hydrophilic properties of the polymer also important because mucoadhesive interaction occurs in the presence of water (mucous consists of 95% of water). A low water-polymer contact angle will encourage hydration of the polymer chains and increase segmental mobility. Spreading of the polymer over the mucous also promots an intimate contact. Then, it is important that the polymer chains are able to diffuse into the mucous network so that interdigitation between the interacting species may occur. Thus, the polymer must have a sufficient linear chain length (molecular weight consideration) to ensure interpenetration to occur. The segmental mobility of the polymer chain is of great importance to encourage entanglement between the interacting molecules. The proposed mechanism of adhesion of hydrocolloids suggested that upon hydration the synthetic polymer molecules become more freely mobile and even able to orient adhesive sites favorably with those of the substrate. As the level of the hydration increased, adhesive properties are found to be reduced since mucoadhesive properties get reduced due to mucoadhesive bonds become over-extended.

Based on estimates of the rate of a polymer rediffusion through mucous networks and the depth of penetration required for muco-adhesion, interdigitation alone could not be account for the mucoadhesive interaction because of the time dependency of the process. Therefore, it seems that the secondary bond formation (van der Waals' interactions) should play a significant role. The hydrogen bond forming capacity of the linear polymer relates to this effect, and explains the well-documented mucoadhesive properties of polymers possessing numerous carboxyl groups such as carbopol and polycarbophil. The *in vitro* mucoadhesive properties of synthesized polycarbophil hydrogels can be modified as a function of pH. At pH values above the pK_a of the polymer, the strength of the interaction tends to reduce as a greater proportion of the carboxyl groups are ionized and thus precluded from hydrogen bond formation. Also, the greater swelling of the polymer as the degree of ionization increases, leads to a reduction in mechanical strength with a concomitant reduction in mucoadhesive properties. However, another study challenges the importance of hydrogen bonding between the mucoadhesive and the glycoprotein. *In vitro* work of adhesion in separating carbopol 907 tablets from porcine gingiva was equivalent at pH 5 and 7.4. In this pH range, the number of ionized carboxyl groups (pK$_a$-4.75) increased from 9 to 96%. The results of the study conclusively suggested that the physical mechanisms of mucoadhesion (interpenetration and entanglement) are more important than secondary bond formation.

It may be thus inferred that the most efficient mucoadhesive polymers have physio-chemical properties that are closely related to those of the mucous substrate. The mucus layer is composed of an entangled, hydrated network of high molecular glycoprotein molecules. The glycoprotein generally referred to as having a bottle brush structures, which is an amino acid backbone with numerous carbohydrate side chains. The terminal groups of the side chains are sialic acid residues (pK$_a$ >3), or sulfated galactose or N-acetyl glucosamine. The linkage of the side chain to the backbone is usually through an O-glucoside bond between C1 in N-acetyl galactosamine and hydroxyl group of serine or threonine. Thus, under appropriate pH conditions (pH of saliva generally 5.8–7.4), the terminal groups confer upon the glycoprotein an overall negative charge. The structural similarities of the two polymers that is salivary glycoprotein and mucoadhesive, would suggest an existence of a small interfacial tension that upon mixing promotes interaction and the development of a mucoadhesive bond.

BIOADHESION AT EXPOSED EPITHELIAL SURFACE

Bioadhesion at an epithelial surface can occur when continuity of the mucous layer is physically interrupted due to abrasion or altered chemically by mucolytic agents. The attachment of bioadhesive polymers at epithelial surface serves the following advantages:

- Maintains continuity of the mucous layer and minimizes the exposed area
- Replaces the mucous layer and provides a protective covering for the underlying cell layers from physical and chemical stress
- Acts as a platform for drug delivery to local tissues and facilitates recovery of the damaged or diseased cell layers.

The cell membrane is viewed as a two-dimensionally oriented viscous lipid solution where proteins are free to move. The membrane is surrounded by exopolysaccharides either on or in the periphery of all cells. For animal cell membrane, the carbohydrates are bound covalently to proteins and lipids to form glycoproteins and glycolipids, which are oriented asymmetrically in the plasma membrane with the carbohydrate chains projecting to the exterior of the cell wall. All the polysaccharide-containing structures on the external surface of the cells are collectively referred to as the glycocalyx, which may be a dynamic component of the cell and is maintained, synthesized continuously by underlying cells, appears to be partly responsible for the adhesive property of the cell.

Sucralfate, a basic aluminium salt of sulfated sucrose was found to adhere selectively to ulcerous and eroded surface of epithelial cell by electrostatic attraction. Other possible mechanisms for cellular attachments of bioadhesives include charge distribution and redistribution.

NATURALLY OCCURRING BIOADHESIVES

There are some specialized macromolecules that are synthesized by cells and have potential to be used as mucoadhesives [e.g. fibronectin, lectin and several cell adhesin molecules (CAMs)]. Fibronectin is a major glycoprotein constituent of plasma and other body fluids and is present on epithelial surfaces. It is a component of extracellular matrix, and is synthesized by endothelial and glial cells. Fibronectin is an important adhesive protein that binds certain forms of collagen and glycosaminoglycans and mediates the adhesion and spreading of cells in culture. Some small bioadhesive synthetic peptides can be derived from fibronectin.

Lectins that exist on the surface of a diversity of mammalian cells are carbohydrate binding proteins and glycoproteins (e.g. limulin, carcinoscorpin, Limax flavus and achatinin) (Tables 3.1, 3.2). They possess two important properties;

- Specificity for particular sugar residues
- They are bivalent or polyvalent in nature

Lectins belong to Two Main Categories

- Integrated lectins, which are integrated with the membranes and require detergents for solubilisation. They bind glycoconjugates to the membranes at the cell interface or within vesicles, thus localize the glycoconjugates at particular membrane sites
- Soluble lectins, which move freely in the aqueous compartments intra- and extracellularly, and interact with complementary glycoconjugates on and around the cells that release them.

FACTORS AFFECTING BIOADHESION

Bioadhesive characteristics relate to both the bioadhesive polymer and the medium in which the polymer exists. A variety of factors affect the mucoadhesive properties of polymers, such as molecular weight, flexibility, hydrogen bonding capacity, cross-linking density, charge, concentration, and hydration (swelling) of a polymer, are briefly addressed here (Table 3.3).

Polymer-related Factors

In general, it has been shown that the bioadhesive strength of a polymer increases with molecular weights above 100,000. As an example, the direct correlation between the bioadhesive strength of polyoxyethylene polymers and their molecular weights, in the range of 200,000 to 7,000,000, has been shown.

Flexibility

Bioadhesion starts with the diffusion of the polymer chains in the interfacial region. Therefore, it is important that the polymer chains contain a substantial degree of flexibility in order to achieve the desired entanglement with the mucus. A recent publication demonstrated the use of tethered poly (ethylene glycol)-poly (acrylic acid) hydrogels and their copolymers with improved mucoadhesive properties. The increased chain interpenetration was attributed to the increased structural flexibility of the polymer upon incorporation of poly (ethylene glycol). In general, mobility and flexibility of polymers can be related to their viscosities and diffusion coefficients, where higher flexibility of a polymer leads to greater diffusion into the mucus network.

Table 3.1: Natural role of lectins in their origin

Origin of lectins	Functions in their origin
Plants	Defence against phytopathogens;protection against predators (insects and animals); proteins storage;symbiosis mediation.
Animals	Binding of bacteria to epithelial cells; apoptosis; endocytosis and translocation of glycoproteins; defence against microorganism; regulation of cell migration and adhesion; recognition determinants in phagocytosis
Microorganism	Attachments to host cells; recognition determinants in phagocytosis; recognition determinants in cell adhesion.

Table 3.2: Properties of some lectin-particle conjugates

Lectin general name	Sugar specificity	Carrier nature
Tomato lectin (TL)	N-acetylglucosamine	Polystyrene latex
Roman snail (HP)	N-acetyl galactosamine	Polystyrene latex
Red kidney bean (PHA)	Galactose/N-acetyl galactosamine	Polystyrene latex
Wheat germ (WGA)	Sialic acid/N-acetyl glucosamine	Polystyrene latex
Concanavalin A (Con A)	Mannose/glucose	Polystyrene latex
Lotus/Asparagus pea (AL)	L-fucose	Polystyrene latex
Furze (UEA)	L-fucose	Liposomes; vicilin nanoparticles

Table 3.3: Polymers and systems for nonspecific bioadhesion

Formulations	Polymers
Tablets	Sodium carboxy methyl cellulose, hydroxy propyl cellulose
Tablets	Chitosan and sodium hyaluronate
Polymer dispersion	Chitosan HCl and carbomer 934P
Microspheres	Poly (caprolactone) and poly (fumaric-co-sebacic anhydride) copolymer
Microspheres	Calcium alginate and poly (fumaric-co-sebacic anhydride) copolymer
Nanoparticles	Polystyrene, poly (N-isopropylacrylamide), poly (vinyl amine), poly (methacrylic acid) and poly (N-vinyl acetamide)
Pressure sensitive adhesive (PSA) matrix	2-ethylhexyl acrylate and acrylic acid copolymer
Nanoparticles	Poly (hexyl cyanoacrylate), poly (lactic acid), poly (hydroxy propyl methacrylate) and poly (ethylbutyl cyanoacrylate)

Hydrogen Bonding Capacity

Hydrogen bonding is another important factor in mucoadhesion of a polymer. Park and Robinson found that for mucoadhesion to occur, the polymers must have functional groups that are able to form hydrogen bonds. They have also confirmed that flexibility of the polymer is important to improve this hydrogen bonding potential.

Polymers such as poly (vinyl alcohol), hydroxylated methacrylate, and poly (methacrylic acid), as well as their copolymers, are the polymers with good hydrogen bonding capacity.

Cross-linking Density

The average pore size, the number average molecular weight of the cross-linked polymers, and the density of cross-linking are three important and interrelated structural parameters of a polymer network. Therefore, it seems reasonable that with increasing density of cross-linking, diffusion of water into the polymer network occurs at a lower rate which, in turn, causes insufficient swelling of the polymer and a decreased rate of interpenetration between polymer and mucin. Flory has reported a general property of polymers, in which the degree of swelling at equilibrium has an inverse relationship with the degree of cross-linking of a polymer.

Charge

Some generalizations about the charge of bioadhesive polymers have been made previously, where nonionic polymers appear to undergo a smaller/lower degree of adhesion compared to anionic polymers. Peppas and Buri have demonstrated that strong anionic charge on the polymer is one of the required characteristics for mucoadhesion. It has been shown that some cationic polymers are likely to demonstrate superior mucoadhesive properties, especially in a neutral or slightly alkaline medium. Additionally, some cationic high molecular-weight polymers, such as chitosan, and its derivatives possess good adhesive properties.

Concentration

The importance of this factor lies in the development of a strong adhesive bond with the mucus, and can be explained by the polymer chain length available for penetration into the mucus layer. When the concentration of the polymer is too low, the number of penetrating polymer chains per unit volume of the mucus is small, and the interaction between polymer and mucus is unstable. In general, the more concentrated polymer would result in a more number of longer penetrating chains and better adhesion. However, for each polymer, there is a critical concentration, above which the polymer produces an unperturbed state due to a significantly coiled structure. As a result, the accessibility of the solvent to the polymer decreases, and chain penetration of the polymer is drastically reduced. Therefore, higher concentrations of polymers do not necessarily improve on the contrary in some cases, actually diminish mucoadhesive properties. One of the studies addressing this factor demonstrated that high concentrations of flexible polymeric films based on polyvinyl-pyrrolidone or poly (vinyl alcohol) as film-forming polymers did not further enhance the mucoadhesive properties of the polymer. On the contrary, the desired strength of mucoadhesion was decreased.

Hydration (Swelling)

Hydration is required for a mucoadhesive polymer to expand and create a proper macromolecular mesh of sufficient size, and also to induce mobility in the polymer chains in order to enhance the interpenetration process between polymer and mucin. Polymer swelling permits a mechanical entanglement by exposing the bioadhesive sites for hydrogen bonding and/or electrostatic interaction between the polymer and the mucous network. However, a critical degree of hydration of the mucoadhesive polymer exists where optimum swelling and bioadhesion do occur.

Environmental Factors

The mucoadhesion of a polymer not only depends on its molecular properties, but also on the environmental factors adjacent to the polymer. Saliva, as a dissolution medium, affects the behavior of the polymer. Depending on both the saliva flow rate and method of determination, the pH of this medium has been estimated to be between 6.5 and 7.5. The pH of the microenvironment surrounding the mucoadhesive polymer can alter the ionization state and, therefore, the adhesion properties of a polymer. Mucin turnover rate is another environmental factor. The residence time of dosage forms is limited by the mucin turnover time, which has been calculated between 47 and 270 min in rats and 12–24 hours in humans. Movement of the buccal tissues while eating, drinking, and talking, is another concern which should be considered when designing a dosage form for the oral cavity. Movements within the oral cavity continue even during sleep, and can potentially lead to the detachment of the dosage form. Therefore, an optimum time span for the administration of the dosage form is necessary in order to avoid many of these interfering factors.

pH: pH influences the charge on the surface of both mucus and polymers. Mucus will have a different charge density depending on pH, because of difference in dissociation of functional groups on carbohydrate moiety and amino acids of the polypeptide backbone, which may affect adhesion.

Applied strength: To place a solid bioadhesive system, it is necessary to apply a defined pressure. Whichever may be the polymer the adhesion strength of polymers increases with the increase in the applied pressure.

Initial contact time: The initial contact time between mucoadhesive and the mucus layer determines the extent of swelling and the interpenetration of polymer chains. The mucoadhesive strength increases as the initial contact time increases.

Selection of the model substrate surface: The handling and treatment of biological substrates during the testing of mucoadhesive is an important factor, since physical and biological changes may occurs in the mucus gels or tissues under the experimental conditions.

Swelling

The swelling characteristic is related to the polymer itself, and also to its environment. Inter-penetration of chains is easier as polymer chains are disentangled and free of interactions. More is the swelling of polymeric matrix higher will be the adhesion time of polymers.

Physiological Variables

Mucin turnover and disease state of mucus layer are physiological variables, which may affect bioadhesion.

MODULATION OF MUCOADHESION

So many factors that influence the chemical and/or physical characteristics of the mucin or mucoadhesive layer will have an effect on the extent of interaction and strength of mucoadhesion. They are:

1. A number of substances interact with mucin and are known as mucous thickening or thinning agents, (e.g. tetraborate and progesterone etc.)
2. Aggregation may be caused by the formation of bridges or by reduction of electrostatic charges of the mucin molecules with a simultaneous change in conformation of the mucin network.
3. Calcium precipitates mucin, and when used to adjust media tonicity, it reduces the shear stress.

4. The degree of hydration of the mucoadhesive (e.g. polycarbophil) is decreased with a subsequent decrease in tensile stress, as result of increasing ionic strength of the media.
5. The mucin network can be altered by mucolytic agents, which may reduce the viscosity of mucous by altering the molecular composition of mucous (depolymerization of mucin molecules and breaking of mucin network) through rupture of disulfide bonds or by the proteolytic action of enzyme. Disulphide bond breaking agents act directly to split the disulfide bridges connecting different glycoprotein molecules (e.g. acetyl cysteine, carbocysteine and dithiothreitol) (Merriott, 1983). Proteolytic enzymes exert their activity only by gaining an access to protein regions, that are nonglycosylated (e.g. bacterial enzymes in normal enteric microflora).
6. Structural breakdown of the mucous can be carried out by the addition of sodium deoxycholate and lysophospatidyl choline. These substances can degrade the mucin oligosaccharide side chains extensively and more so mucin polypeptide core, however to a lesser extent.
7. Duodenogastric reflux disrupts the structure of the mucin network and leads to gastric ulcer.
8. Some diseases also disrupt the integrity of the mucin layer. For example, ulceration and inflammation of the intestine result in thinning of the mucin layer, while cystic fibrosis causes thickening of mucin layer and may lead to obstruction of bronchi.

ADHESION PROMOTERS

The use of adhesion promoters for the enhancement of mucoadhesion is recommended. The macroscopic adhesive properties of synthetic hydrogels and the impact of polymer chain diffusion (adhesion promoter diffusion) on the adhesion of gel-mucin systems have been examined. Tethering of one polymer chain to another polymer, is one of the mucoadhesion promoting approaches was proposed.

Tethered polymer chains are polymer chains with one of their ends attached on a d-dimensional surface, where $d = 1$ denotes comb polymers and $d = 2$ denotes normal, flat surfaces. Tethered chains on hydrogel surfaces as bioadhesion promoters were exploited (Fig. 3.2). Tethering of long poly (ethylene glycol) (PEG) chains on poly (acrylic acid) hydrogels and their copolymer can be achieved by grafting reactions or by copolymerization in the presence of several PEG-containing acrylates. The hydrogels exhibit mucoadhesive properties due to enhanced anchoring of the chains with the mucosa. Experimental results indicated that the chain interpenetration is a strong function of the PEG molecular weight, the polymer swelling and the mucosa composition.

Though the diffusion coefficient of tethered chains is lower than that of the free chains at interfaces due to their geometric constraints, they still have a significant ability to penetrate into the mucin network. Tethered adhesion promoters have the following advantages over free chains:

- One of their ends covalently bonded with the hydrogel, thus, it can be expected that possible adhesion strength enhancement

would be higher than that of the free loaded chains.
- The amount and length of tethered chains are easier to control.
- Tethered hydrogel surfaces can be obtained by a grafting reaction after the hydrogels have been prepared. Consequently, it is not necessary to change the bulk properties of the hydrogel, which can be designed separately.
- More importantly, promoting adhesion by tethered chains, may lead to the ability of a matrix to have units that are specifically designed to adhere to a given surface.

MUCOADHESIVE POLYMERS USED IN THE ORAL CAVITY

Desired Characteristics

The polymer-related factors have been briefly discussed in the previous section. Generally, some of the necessary structural characteristics for bioadhesive polymers include strong hydrogen bonding groups, strong anionic or cationic charges, high molecular weight, chain flexibility, and surface energy properties favoring spreading on a mucus layer.

Classification

In general, adhesive polymers can be classified as synthetic and natural, water-soluble vs. water insoluble, and charged vs. uncharged

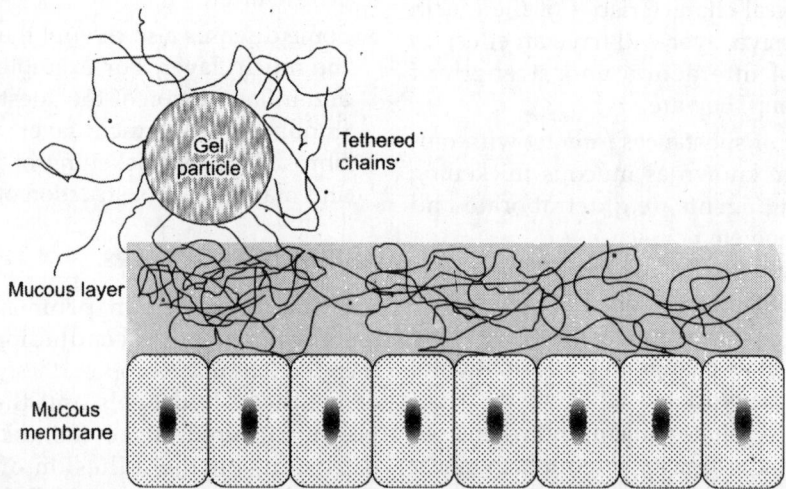

Fig. 3.2: The interpenetration between tethered chains and mucous gel layer (Huang et. al., 2000)

polymers. Natural bioadhesive macromolecules share similar structural properties with the synthetic polymers. They are generally linear polymers with high molecular weight, contain a substantial number of hydrophilic, negatively charged functional groups, and form three-dimensional expanded networks. In the class of synthetic polymers, poly (acrylic acid), cellulose ester derivatives, and poly-methacrylate derivatives are the current choices. Chitosan and various gums, such as guar and hakea (from *Hakea gibbosa*), are classified as semi-natural/natural bioadhesive polymers. Poly (acrylic acid), a linear or random polymer, and polycarbophil, a swellable polymer, represent water-soluble and water-insoluble polymers, respectively. The charged polymers are divided into cationic and anionic polymers, such as chitosan and polycarbophil, respectively, while hydroxypropylcellulose is an example of uncharged bioadhesive polymers.

New Generation of Mucoadhesive Polymers

Bioadhesive polymers are classified as first generation and second generation polymers. The older generation of mucoadhesive polymers, referred to as off-the shelf polymers; they lack specificity and targeting capability. They adhere to the mucus non-specifically, and suffer short retention times due to the turnover rate of the mucus. The chemical interactions between mucoadhesive polymers and the mucus or tissue surfaces are generally non-covalent in nature, and are classified as consisting mostly of hydrogen bonds, hydrophobic, and electrostatic interactions. However, newer polymers are capable of forming covalent bonds with the mucus and the underlying cell layers, and hence, exhibit improved chemical interactions. The new generation of mucoadhesives (with the exception of thiolated polymers) can adhere directly to the cell surface, rather than to mucus. They interact with the cell surface by means of specific receptors or covalent bonding instead of non-specific mechanisms. Examples of such polymers are the incorporation of l-cysteine into thiolated polymers and the target specific, lectin-mediated adhesive polymers. These classes of polymers hold promise for the delivery of a wide variety of new drug molecules, particularly macromolecules, and create new possibilities for more specific drug- receptor interactions and improved targeted drug delivery (Table 3.4).

The possibility of developing a bioadhesive polymer which is able to selectively create specific molecular interactions with a particular target, such as a receptor on the cell membrane of a specific tissue, seems to be an attractive strategy for targeted delivery. The potential of a specific receptor-bioadhesive polymer interaction can circumvent the

Table 3.4: Examples of different bioadhesive polymers	
Cationic polymers	Chitosan (hydrogel polymers)
Anionic polymers	Polyacrylic acid (hydrophilic soluble polymer)
	Carbopol 934P, 971P, 980 (hydrogel polymers)
	Polycarbophil (hydrogel polymers)
	Poly (methacrylic acid)
	Sodium alginate
Nonionic polymers	Methocel (HPMC) K100M, K15M, K4M
	Hydroxyethylcelullose (HEC)
	Hydroxypropylcelullose (HPC)
	Polyoxyethylene (POE)
Ion exchange resins	Cholestyramine (Duolite AP-143)
Miscellaneous	Sucralfate, gliadin

limiting factors of rapid mucus turnover and short residence time. Unlike general muco-adhesive polymers, which bind to the mucosal surface ubiquitously, a specific receptor mediated interaction with the mucosal surface could allow for direct binding to the cell surface, rather than only the mucus layer. Specific proteins or glycoproteins, such as lectins, which can bind certain sugars on the cell membrane, can increase bioadhesion as well and potentially improve drug delivery via specific binding. This type of bioadhesion should be more appropriately termed as cytoadhesion. A site-specific interaction with the receptor could potentially trigger inter-cellular signaling for internalization of the drug or the carrier system (endocytosis through cytoadhesion) into the lysosomes or into other cellular compartments.

Bacterial Adhesion

The adhesive properties of bacterial cells, as a more complicated adhesion system, have recently been investigated. The ability of bacteria to adhere to a specific target is rooted from particular cell-surface components or appendages, known as fimbriae, which facilitate adhesion to other cells or inanimate surfaces. These are extracellular, long thread-like protein polymers of bacteria that play a major role in many diseases. Bacterial fimbriae adhere to the binding moiety of specific receptors. A significant correlation has been found between the presence of fimbriae on the surface of bacteria and their pathogenicity. The attractiveness of this approach lies in the potential increase in the residence time of the drug on the mucus and its receptor-specific interaction, analogous to those of the plant lectins.

EVALUATION OF BIOADHESIVE DRUG DELIVERY SYSTEMS

In Vitro Evaluation

The morphological evaluation of the drug carrier (especially microcarriers) systems includes scanning electron microscopy (SEM), transmission electron microscopy (TEM) and fourier transform infrared spectroscopy (FTIR). *In vitro* release studies of various bioadhesive drug delivery systems are carried out by using dissolution apparatus either paddle or basket type, diffusion membrane method and simple incubation of the for-mulation in the medium. Bioadhesion is the exclusive and important property useful in the evaluation of the bioadhesive systems.

EVALUATION OF VARIOUS BIOADHESION PROPERTIES

Shear Stress Measurement

Two smooth, polished plexi glass blocks are selected one block is fixed with adhesive 'Araldite' on a glass plate, which is fixed on a leveled table. The level is adjusted with a spirit lamp. To the upper block a thread is tied and the thread is passed down through a pulley. The length of the thread from pulley to pan is approx. 12 cm. At the end of the thread a pan of weight 17g is attached to which the weights can be added.

Different polymer solutions of 3% w/v strength are prepared using water as a solvent. A fixed amount (one drop) of polymer solution is kept on the center of the first block with a pipette and then the second block is placed on the first block and pressed by applying 100 g weights such that the drop polymer spreads as a uniform film between the two blocks. After keeping it for fixed time intervals of 5, 10, 15 and 30 min, the weights are added to the pan. The weights just sufficient to pull the upper block or to make it slide down from the base block represent the adhesion strength, i.e. the shear stress required. Ishida et al., 1983, have developed one more shear tester that measures the force required to separate two polymer coated glass slides joined by a thin film of natural or synthetic mucous. The results of this technique correlate well with *in vivo* test results.

Detachment Force Measurement

This method is used to measure *in vitro* mucoadhesive capacity of different polymers. It is a modified method developed by Martti Marvola to assess the tendency of muco-adhesive to adhere to the oesophagus. The assembly consists of single organ bath, a stand, glass rod, a pan for keeping beaker and a reservoir for addition of water into beaker. Immediately after slaughter, the intestine is removed from the sheep and transported to laboratory in tyrode solution (composition: sodium chloride 8 g/L, potassium chloride 0.2 g/L, calcium chloride. $2H_2O$ 0.134 g/L, sodium bicarbonate 1.0 g/L, sodium dihydrogen phosphate 0.05 g/L and glucose H_2O 1.0 g/L). During the experiment the solution is aerated with pure oxygen and kept at 37°C and 6–7 cm long segments of intestine are cut. The lower end of the intestine segment is tied off and then tied to the aerator tube; the upper end is tied around a glass tube of diameter 15 mm. 6 mm plain tablets, tablets layered on one side with adjusted that in resting state the tablet should be at the middle of the intestinal piece. To the other end of the glass rod a pan is tied in which a beaker is placed. After inserting the tablet into intestinal segment and lightly pressing the intestinal segment with tablet by a forceps. The assembly is kept undisturbed for a fixed time interval of one hour and 30 min. Then water with a burette is added slowly drop by drop into the beaker. The amount of water required to pull out the tablet from the intestinal segment represents the force required to pull the tablet against the adhesion. The force in Newton is calculated by the equation,

$$F = 0.00981 \ W/2$$

where W = amount of water.

Following characteristics can be studied from the experiment:

- The effect of the contact time for which the product remains in intestine and the force needed to detach it.

- The strength of different mucoadhesive polymers and the effect of amount of polymer in the formulation on the force needed to detach it.

Wilhelm Plate Technique

This technique has traditionally been used for dynamic contact angle measurement and involves a microbalance or tensiometer. A glass slide is coated with the polymer of interest and then dipped into a beaker of synthetic or natural mucous. The surface tension, contact angle and adhesive force can be automatically measured using available software (Fig 3.3).

Tensile Studies on Mucoadhesive Polymer Conjugates

The lyophilized polymer conjugates (30 mg), control and unmodified polymers are compressed to flat-faced discs. Tensiometeric studies with these discs are carried out on native porcine intestinal mucosa. Test discs are therefore, attached to the mucosa with a force of 2.5 mN (Table 3.5).

Mucoadhesion Studies

In order to evaluate the binding of the mucosa as well as the cohesiveness of the tablet, an appropriate new method has been established.

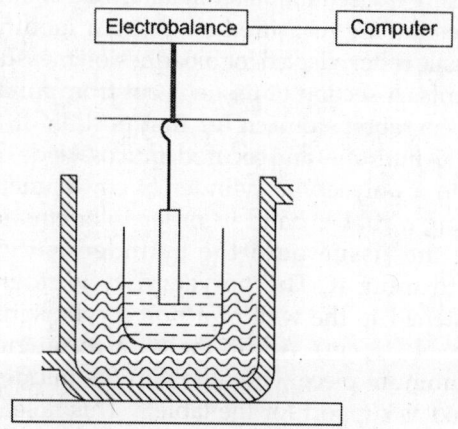

Fig. 3.3: The Wilhelmy plate method

Table 3.5: Criteria for conjugates

Particulate systems	Ligands
• Water insolubility biodegradability and immunogenicity	• Interact specificity with a marker or a receptor present at the site of immobilization
• Biodegradability and biocompatibility	• Ensure recognition of the site of interest for adhesion and anchoring of the bioadhesive system on the site surface
• Lack of toxicity and immunogenicity	
• Capacity to protect the loaded drug and to control the release	
• Availability of suitable functional groups for stable association with the chosen ligand	

The prepared tablets (flat-surface discs) are attached to freshly excise intestinal porcine mucosa, which has been spanned on a stainless steel cylinder (diameter 4.4 cm, height 5.1 cm, apparatus 4-cylinder, USP XXII). Thereafter, cylinder is placed in the dissolution apparatus according to the USP containing 100 mM TBS pH 6.8 at 37 ± 0.5°C and then fully immersed cylinder is agitated (250 rpm). The detachment, disintegration and/or erosion of test tablets are observed and recoded within a time period of 10 hours.

Measurement of Tablet Bioadhesion

The maximum adhesion force and the work of adhesion-shear to separate the tablet from freshly excised rabbit stomach tissue or small intestine are measured by using a modified tensile tester adapted for bioadhesion measurements. A section of tissue is cut from fundus of the rabbit stomach (or first portion of the small intestine) and secured, mucosal side out, onto a polyacrylic cylinder (3 cm diameter) using a rubber band in order to adequately fix the tissue onto the cylinder without deforming it. The polyacrylic cylinder is fastened to the wall of a polyacrylic square vessel (13 cm). Additionally, a rectangular aluminum piece with a hole in the middle is used as support for the tablets. This hole has a diameter of 2 mm greater than that of the tablets to allow swelling of tablet due to

absorption of medium. The experiment is carried out in a constant volume of test medium (USP simulated gastric or intestinal fluid). After 30 min, the adhesion and shear forces required to separate two parallel surfaces (tablet-tissue) are recorded as a function of time, until the tablet have crossed the tissue surface (cross head speed 1 mm/min; chart speed 20 mm/min; full scale load 1 kg). The mechanical parameters are then calculated.

Adhesion Force Measurement

The adhesion properties of bioadhesive polymer tablets can be evaluated by measuring the force required to separate the tablet from an adherent. The tablet is attached to the holder with cyanoacrylate type adhesives. Buffer solutions (2 ml; pH 2.0, 3.5 and 5.0) are gently added on the tablet to hydrate the tablet surface for 5 min at 25°C. Otherwise lyophilized porcine dermis and rabbit peritoneal membrane excised from male New Zealand white rabbits (3.0–3.5 kg) are used as adherents. The rabbits are killed by pentobarbital injection; the peritoneal membrane is extracted and stored at 10°C before the experiment and thawed at 4°C in an isotonic saline solution before it is used. The residual water on the surface is removed with the help of a filter paper. The porcine dermis of rabbit peritoneal membrane, which is cut into round shape with a diameter of 5 mm, is attached to the tip of an adapter in tensiometer with the help of a cyanoacrylate type adhesive. The adherents are then immersed in buffer solutions (pH 2.0, 3.5 and 5.0) for 5 min at 25°C before the measurement. The holder wearing the sample tablet is lifted up in contact with the adherent, which is primarily hydrated in the buffer solutions by applying a pressure of 250 g/cm^2. The tablet and the adherent are kept in contact with each other for 3 min. The tablet is then stretched from the adherent at an extension rate of 4 mm/s and the force required to detach the tablet from the adherent is recorded (Fig. 3.4).

Adhesion Studies of Hydrogels

The adhesion capacity of hydrogels is determined by applying the tensile-tester. The hydrogel is adhered to the upper support and the substrate to the lower support using a cyanoacrylate adhesive. Upon contact of hydrogel and substrate, a defined force is applied for certain time. This is followed by an extension phase at a defined rate until total separation of components is achieved.

The optimum conditions including two hydration environments influencing the adhesion are:

- An applied force of 0.5 N and a contact time of 20 min

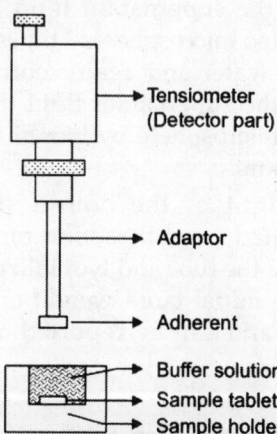

Fig: 3.4: The representation of experimental setup for determination of bioadhesive force

- **Assays where water is limited:** Studies are carried out using dry tanned leather as substrate. Water (25 ml) is homogeneously extended on the hydrogel situated on the upper support of the tension apparatus.
- **Assays where there is no water limitation:** The same assay is used with the conditions as discussed but the substrate and hydrogel are previously introduced into 25 ml of water at 37°C.

Bioadhesion Measurement of Tablets

This experiment determines the colonic bioadhesion of the tablets. The GIT of male Wister rats (200–300 g) is used as the biological substrate in these experiments. Animals are allowed free access to food and water until they are sacrificed by carbon dioxide asphyxia. Immediately after the death of the animal, the carcass is opened. The GIT is isolated and divided into 4 segments namely; stomach, proximal small intestine (PSI), distal small intestine (DSI), and the colon.

The sections are opened laterally to expose the mucosal surface, washed gently with physiological (pH 7) phosphate buffer to remove the luminal contents, flash-frozen in liquid nitrogen and stored at –18°C. The control experiments employing fresh tissue are conducted in order to confirm the validity simultaneously of the approach and utilized within 24 hours of dissection. It behaves similar to biomaterial obtained immediately after isolation from the animal.

The tissue under test is allowed to thaw to room temperature before it is fixed onto a tissue clamp so as to expose a 3.8 cm^2 circular area. The clamped tissue is then immersed in 75 ml of an isotonic solution, buffered at a predetermined pH (depending on the intestinal section tested) and kept at 37°C, where it is further allowed to stand for 5 min before each measurement. The water bath is placed on a vertically moving platform that is positioned beneath the sensor arm of the balance (GEC-Avery, UK). Using a pestle and mortar mills the polymeric materials under test is forwarded. The powdered fraction that passes through a 55 mm sieve is collected and used for the adhesion studies. Circles of 6 mm diameter are cut from double-sided adhesive film and one is attached to a 1.4 g weight. The protective film is peeled off through the free side and the weight is repeatedly placed against a sample of the test powder until its surface is completely covered with particles. The surface is cleared of loosely held particles, by exposing it to the compressed air for 2 min, and then attached to the sensor arm, which is positioned directly above the mucosal surface. The platform is raised at maximum speed until the disk and the weight are completely immersed in the buffer. The balance is tared and the platform is raised slowly until the negative reading of the balance remained constant for 5 seconds. The surfaces are allowed to interact for 2 min and then the platform is lowered at a rate of 1 mm min^{-1} until adhesive joint failure occurs. The maximum detachment force and the work of adhesion are calculated as the mean of six set of measurements. The tissue is also examined in order to identify the position at which the fracture of the adhesive joint has occurred. The apparatus for assessing bioadhesion is shown in Fig. 3.5.

Unique Flow Chamber Technique

A polymeric microsphere is placed on the surface of a natural mucous layer and fluid,

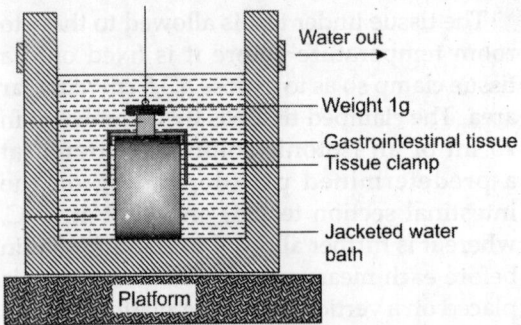

Fig 3.5: Apparatus for assessing bioadhesion (Kakoulides et al., 1998)

moving at physiological rate, is introduced into the chamber, and movement of the micosphere is monitored by videographic device. By measuring the size and speed of the microsphere, it is possible to calculate the bioadhesive force.

Everted Sac Technique

- Everted sac experiments (Fig 3.6) are performed using viable segments of rat jejunum. Unfasted rats (400 g, male) are sacrificed and intestinal tissue is excised and flushed with 10 ml of ice-cold phosphate buffered saline, pH 7.2 containing 200 mg/dl glucose (PBSG).
- Evert the segments of jejunum (6 cm) with the help of stainless steel rod and wash with the PBSG to remove the contents. Ligatures are placed at both ends of the segment and the sac is filled with 1–1.5 ml of PBSG. Tissue is maintained at 4°C prior to incubation and the sacs are introduced into a 15 ml tube containing 60 mg of bioadhesive microspheres and 5 ml of PBSG.
- The sacs are incubated at 37°C and agitated end-over-end and after 30 min, the sacs are removed and the solution of PBSG and unbound microspheres is centrifuge for 30 min.
- Discard the supernatant fluid and wash sedimented microspheres 3 times with 5 ml distilled water and again centrifuge and discard the supernatant fluid then freeze dry the microsphere by lyophilization for 24–48 hours.
- The weight of the bound spheres is determined by subtraction of the tared weight of the tube and lyophilized spheres from the initial tared weight of tube and spheres and can be reported as percent binding.

In Vivo Evaluation Methods

In vivo methods used for evaluation of mucoadhesive systems are based on the

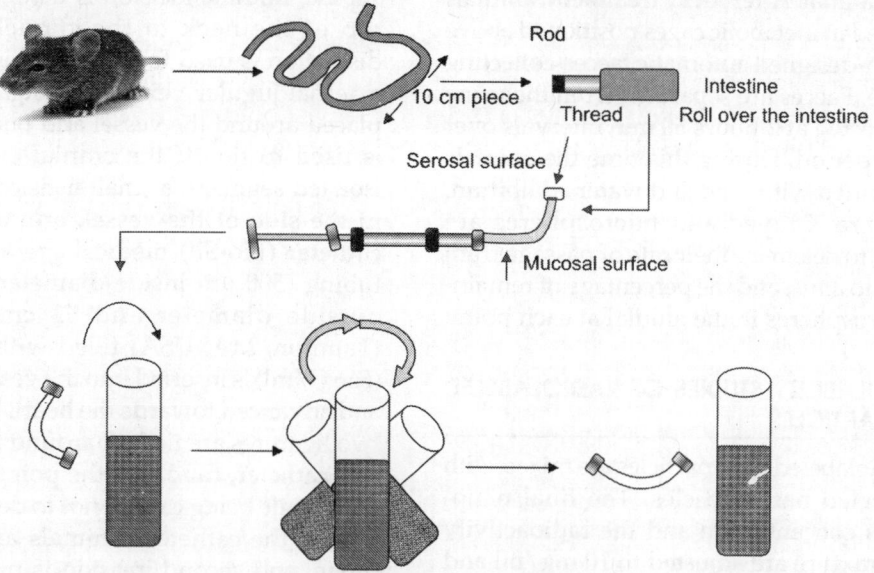

Fig. 3.6: The everted sac technique

administration of polymers to a laboratory animal and tracking their transit through the GI system. Administration methods include forced oral gavage, surgical stomach implantation and infusion through a loop placed *in situ* in the small intestine. Tracking generally followed with the help of X-ray studies, radio-opaque markers, radioactive elements and fluorescent dyes are incorporated in the device. Various animals including rats, rabbits, guinea pigs, mice and sheeps have been used for the studies.

X-RAY STUDIES FOR MONITORING GI TRANSIT

X-ray Studies on Bioadhesive Tablets

- Barium sulfate (BaSO$_4$) tablets of 8 mm diameter should be prepared in 3 different types of polymers
  - Control or plain tablets of BaSO$_4$
  - BaSO$_4$ tablets layered on one side with mucoadhesive polymer
  - BaSO$_4$ and polymer as matrix mixture in the ratio of 2:1

Ten healthy rabbits of same age and weight are taken as subjects. They are fasted overnight and the next day morning the tablets are administered to them followed by 25 ml of water. At different intervals of 1, 3, 5 and 8 hours, the rabbits are X-ray photographed and observed for the nature and position of the tablet for 8 hours after administration of the tablets. During the study, the rabbits are fed after 5 horus of tablet administration, so that the effect of food can be assessed.

X-ray GI Transit Monitoring of Radio-opaque Microspheres

Prior to administration, 200 mg of barium sulfate loaded microspheres are suspended in 1 ml of 0.9% sodium chloride. Male rats (250–300 g), fasted overnight, are anaesthetized with methoxyflurane and a silicone feeding tube (2 mm OD) is used to administer microspheres suspensions into their stomach. Following administration rats are allowed to recover from anaesthesia. Since, it is difficult to assure that 100% of the intended microspheres dose has been delivered; therefore a post-administration counting method should be used. Animals are re-anesthatized and X-rayed, thereby verifying for the presence of microspheres in lumen of the stomach. From these X-rays, it is possible to determine the number of microspheres initially administered to each animal. After X-ray treatment, animals are placed in metabolic cages positioned above a custom-designed automatic faeces-collecting machine. Faeces are separated from the urine and collected at 2 hours 50 min intervals over a 3-day period. During this time the animals are provided with food and water ad libitum. Faeces are X-rayed and microspheres are counted to determine their rate of passage from stomach to anus, and the percentage of remaining microspheres in the animal at each point.

BIOAVAILABILITY STUDIES OF RADIOLABELED NANOPARTICLES

The radiolabeled nanoparticles are mixed with non-labeled nanoparticles. The final nanoparticles concentration and the radioactivity in this mixture are adjusted to 10 mg/ml and 0.3–0.5 kBq/ml, respectively. An aqueous solution of PEG is prepared as a control. The concentration of non-labeled PEG is adjusted to 10 mg/ml and a small amount of tritiated PEG is added to this solution, to yield 0.3–0.5 kBq/ml radioactivities. The prepared dosing solution is given orally to male rats simultaneously they are kept fasted overnight (200–250 g) at a dose of 25 mg of nanoparticles in a 2.5 ml solution/kg of body weight. The aqueous solution of PEG is administered to rats under the same conditions at 5, 30 and 60 or 120 min after administration, rats are sacrificed by ether inhalation overdose and both stomach and small intestine are removed. The intestine is cut into 10 cm sections and radioactivity in each segment is measured with the gamma counter or a beta-counter (GM counter).

BIOAVAILABILITY STUDIES OF DRUG ENCAPSULATED BIOADHESIVE MICROSPHERES

Blood Sampling Set Up

- Bioavailability studies require catheters for repeated blood sampling. Male rats (200–250g) are anaesthetized with an intraperitoneal injection of sodium phenobarbital (60 g/kg). With the animals supine, midline incision is made from the top of the neck to the clavicle. Blunt dissection is used to locate and isolate the external jugular vein. Three ligatures are placed around the vessel and one ligature is used to tie off the cranial end of the isolated segment, a small incision is made in the side of the vessel, and a silicone catheter (Bio-Sil) medical grade silicone tubing (500 μm inside diameter, 940 μm outside diameter and 53 cm length) (Taunton, MA, USA) filled with heparin (666 U/ml) is inserted into the vessel lumen and advanced towards the heart. The other two ligatures are tied off around the vessel and catheter, caudal to the point of insertion, while being careful not to deform and restrict the catheter. Animals are turned prone, and second incision is made from the base of the skull to the midpoint between the scapulae. Forceps are used to tunnel subcutaneously to the opening of the ventral incision. The free end of the catheter is pulled beneath the skin to emerge from the dorsal incision at the base of the neck. The ventral incision is sutured. The free end of catheter is fed through a 30.5 cm long stainless steel spring tethered with 22-gauge swivel. The button-end of the tether is sutured to the facial covering of the muscles in the back of the neck, and a pure-string stitch is used to close the dorsal incision.

- Tall cages (Fig 3.7) are constructed for untangled movement of the tether. To produce an enclosure 33 cm high, two rat cages (36 × 30 × 16 cm) are joined; one inverted on top of the other, with 4 derlin spacers (1 cm thick) to allow adequate airflow. Additional air holes are drilled, and a derlin collar is glued into the center of the top cage. The swivel-end of the tether is passed through the top of the upper cage and secured in the collar with a setscrew.

- Three-way stopcock is attached to the swivel on the outside of the cage with a small section of silicone tubing (8 cm) to

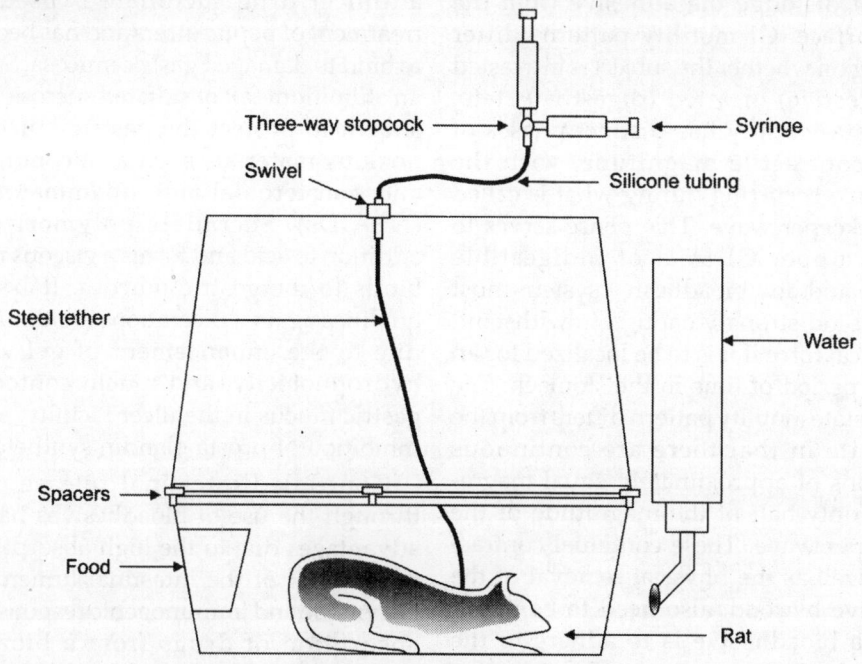

Fig. 3.7: Tall cages used for catheterized rats

facilitate syringe changes without breaking the closed-catheter system. The set up allows blood samples to be drawn from outside the cages without handling or anesthetizing the animals. Moreover, animals are seen in near normal mobility.

Applications

Along with the physicochemical characteristics of the bioadhesive and mucin-epithelium surface, physiological events in the area in which adhesion occurs must be addressed to optimize a drug delivery system. Most delivery systems utilizing bioadhesives are designed to be topically applied to a targeted tissue. Drug delivery systems using bioadhesives can be applied to many areas of the body, such as the oral cavity, gastric, intestinal, rectal, vaginal, ocular, and dermal areas. Each tissue type has its own unique properties which can be exploited for the delivery of drugs. Each biological membrane has its own permeability, enzymatic activity, and immunology, which have to be taken into

consideration if both satisfactory bioadhesion and improved bioavailability of drug are to be achieved.

A. Gastrointestinal

Most drug delivery systems are taken orally with the absorption of the drug occurring mainly in the proximal small intestine. To be effective either locally or systematically, a bioadhesive drug delivery system must be able to overcome the harsh gastric environment, motility of the gastrointestinal (GI) tract, immunogenic responses, enzymatic degradation, and dynamic changes in localization of the drug. The intestinal route is a desirable despite these conditions because of its high absorptive characteristics compared to other routes of administration, which often need permeability enhancement of the tissue to increase bioavailability of the drug. For a bioadhesive to adhere to either the stomach or intestine for an extended period of time, it must overcome the shear force associated with the motility patterns of the GI tract, which can physically dislodge the adhesive from the mucus surface. GI motility patterns differ depending on whether the subject is in a fasted (inter-digestive) or a fed (digestive) state. Fasted-state motility has distinct phases of varying contractile magnitude, with the largest force occurring during what is called the housekeeper wave. This phase serves to clear the upper GI tract of indigestible materials, and any bioadhesive system must therefore bind strongly enough to withstand this physical force if it is to be localized for an extended period of time in the stomach. The digestive state motility pattern differs from the fasted state in that there are continuous contractions of approximately equal magnitude but only half of the magnitude of the housekeeper wave. These continual contractions, as well as the physical removal of the bioadhesive by food, also need to be considered if a bioadhesive is to adhere to the mucus or underlying mucosal layer for an extended period of time. The gastric turnover of mucin in both the fasted and fed state is a significant issue for bioadhesion in case of the oral route. The relatively rapid and continual production and subsequent removal of older mucus by luminal peptic activity makes long-term (i.e., 24 to 48h) bioadhesion to the gastric mucin layer impractical. Some researchers have tried to deliver drugs to the intestine at a controlled rate using bioadhesives in the stomach but because of the mucus exchange and the motility conditions, only little can be expected in long-term gastric retention in humans. Because of the high turnover rate of gastric mucin, for a bioadhesive to remain in the stomach for an extended period of time it would therefore need to adhere to the epithelial layer instead of the mucus. This has been exploited in the use of an antiulcer drug that can adhere to damaged gastric epithelial tissue. Ulcerations are formed in the gastric and intestinal regions, where the protective mucus layer has been altered, and the underlying tissue is thus subject to proteolytic degradation by pepsins and bacteria. The antiulcer drug sucralfate is used for the treatment of peptic ulcers and has been shown to bind to damaged gastric mucosa. Sucralfate, an aluminum salt of sulfated sucrose, has been shown to protect the gastric mucosa from noxious materials such as alcohol, aspirin, and nonsteroidal anti-inflammatory drugs (NSAIDs). Sucralfate polymerizes upon addition to acid and forms a viscous mass that binds to the gastric mucosa. Its protective qualities against ulcerations are thought to be due to the enhancement of gel viscosity, hydrophobicity, and mucin content of the gastric mucus in the ulcer vicinity, as well as inhibition of prosta glandin synthetase.

Controlled intestinal release of drugs through the use of bioadhesives has certain advantages due to the high absorptivity and neutral pH of the intestinal lumen. Barring enzymatic and immunogenic responses, tissue absorption of drugs from a bioadhesive platform can be high if retained in the intestine for extended periods of time. *In situ* experiments in rats have shown increased residence time of certain cross-linked acrylic polymers in the intestine. This increased residence time in the lumen of the intestine increases the bioavailability of poorly absorbed drugs. Enzymatic and immunogenic degradation of both drug and bioadhesive must be addressed irrespective of route of administration but seems to be very important in the GI tract. Another drawback to the gastrointestinal route is that drugs that enter the general circulation are subject to first-pass metabolism as they pass through the hepatic-portal system leading to lower systemic availability.

B. Rectal

Most recently the drugs administered for either local or systemic therapy are given in the suppository form. Normally, after insertion, suppositories tend gradually to migrate and rest in the upper portion of the rectum. Drugs that are absorbed through this area into the blood stream enter the hepatic-portal system and are subjected to first-pass metabolism; which in turn degrades many susceptible drugs and leaves them ineffective. The blood flow to lower rectum, however, drains directly into the general circulation, and first-pass metabolism of a drug can be avoided if the delivery system can be maintained in the lower region. Suppositories containing bioadhesives can reduce this migration toward the upper rectum and hence improve drug bioavailability. Penetration enhancers that improve the uptake of compounds into the epithelium can also be incorporated into such a delivery system. These enhancers are often used for hydrophilic compounds (especially peptides and proteins), which show low permeability through the barrier membrane. Although penetration enhancers have obvious benefits in absorption of drugs through the epithelium, they may also cause adverse effects to the tissue as well as local or systemic side effects. Yet because of the localization of delivery systems, the concentration of enhancers can be minimized, thus reducing adverse effects. Indeed, promising results have been shown in case of penetration enhancers used in the rectum for compounds that normally show poor bioavailability. For example, insulin uptake into the bloodstream has been shown to increase when coadministered with enhaners in the rectum. Controlled release of antipyrine and theophylline using cross-linked hydroxyethyl methacrylate (HEMA) as a bioadhesive have shown sustained availability of rectally administered or applied drug in humans. The combination of permeability enhancement and localization by bioadhesives has the potential in increasing drug bioavailability significantly through rectum route.

C. Nasal

Nasal delivery systems are usually in the form of aqueous sprays in which the drug is distributed into the nasal cavity. This area provides an excellent route for drug absorption because of its large surface area and vascularity as well as a thin layer of mucus secreted from local mucosal glands. Absorption into the blood stream via the nasal route also eliminates hepatic first pass metabolism. This combination makes the nasal cavity an excellent route for localized treatment, (e.g. nasal inflammation and allergic responses) as well as for systemic drug delivery. A suitable bioadhesive could then be hydrated by the nasal mucus and form a viscous gel covering the nasal cavity. The ciliary removal of mucus must be taken into consideration when using bioadhesives in the nasal cavity.

Many researchers have taken advantage of this potential route using bioadhesives as a delivery system. Hydrophilic compounds that are normally poorly absorbed in the nasal cavity can still be utilized using penetration enhancers in conjunction with a site retentive delivery system. Using degradable starch microspheres and a penetration enhancer, the nasal absorption of gentamicin was shown to be improved. These microspheres form a gel when come in contact with the moist nasal mucosa. Using these degradable starch microspheres, nasal administration of insulin has been shown to be improved on co-administration with penetration enhancers. Insulin has also been administered in freeze-dried form with Carbopol® 934 (a cross-linked polyacrylic acid polymer) to achieve a sustained release effect (Table 3.6).

Using polyacrylic acid, other researchers have shown an increased availability of both insulin and calcitonin following nasal administration in rats. The nasal route of administration for insulin, as opposed to the daily subcutaneous injections commonly used, has obvious benefits with respect to patient compliance, although systemic levels of drug thus far attainted have been lower as compared to equivalent dose parenteral administration.

D. Vaginal

The vaginal and cervical route of administration is unique as compared with other routes in that the tissue environment is subject to many changes throughout a woman's life.

Table 3.6: Penetration enhancers used in nasal mucosal drug delivery

Name of the class	Examples
Surfactants	Laureth-9
Bile salts	Glycol-taurocholate and deoxy cholate
Chelators	EDTA and citric acid
Fatty acid salts	Oleic, caprylic, capric and lauric acid salt
Phospholipids	L-lysophosphatidylcholine (DDPC) Didecanoylphophotidylcholine
Fusidates	Sodium taurodihydofusidate (STDHF)
Glycyrrhitinic acid derivatives	Cabenoxolone, glycyrrhizinate
Cyclodextrins	α-, β-cyclodextrins ,hydroxypropyl β-cyclodextrins and dim ethyl β-cyclodextrins, randomly methylated β-cyclodextrin (RAMEB)
Polymers	Microcrystalline cellulose and chitosan
Particulate carriers	Starch microspheres and liposomes

Depending on whether the woman is pre- or postmenopausal, the tissue and mucus of the vaginal and cervical areas can be vastly different. Decreased endogenous levels of estrogen, cervical shrinkage, cell atrophy, and lower cervical mucus levels are characteristics of postmenopausal women. Thus, a vaginal bioadhesive delivery system administered to the older women would need to address these conditions to optimize drug availability. A women's menstrual cycle can also affect the vaginal environment. Vaginal mucus originates in the cervix, then migrates into the vaginal area. Monthly fluctuations in the properties of cervical mucin have been documented, showing lower viscoelasticity when estrogen is dominant and thicker, more viscoelastic mucin when progesterone dominates. Again, a bioadhesive delivery system must take these considerations into account to optimize the bioavailability of drug to the tissue. Most vaginally administered drugs have been delivered in the form of creams, foams, suppositories, gels, or tablets. The women's health care market is very large and profitable and hence Copyright © 2003 by Taylor and Francis Group, LLC a number of delivery systems utilizing bioadhesives have started to appear. The patented use of soluble hydroxypropyl cellulose (HPC) cartridge for vaginal delivery of drugs has been shown to release the drug for an extended period of time. The polymer forms a hydrated gel of high viscosity in the vaginal cavity and releases the drug directly into the vaginal area. The anticancer drugs bleomycin, carbazilquinone, and 5-fluorouracil have been administered directly into the cervix using disk- and rod-shaped dosage forms containing a combination of HPC and Carbopol®.

These dosage forms were shown to stay in the diseased area for a longer period of time than vaginal suppositories containing the same drug. Compared to suppositories, local side effects of these dosage forms were significantly reduced. Such a system has potential in the treatment of cervix carcinoma.

During a woman's reproductive years, the vaginal bacterial flora is capable of maintaining an acidic environment which can reduce vaginal infection by limiting the bacterial growth often associated with other disease states. Maintenance of this slightly acidic pH is then crucial for vaginal health, and thus drug delivery systems that address this phenomenon have obvious therapeutic benefits. A vaginal moisturizer containing the bioadhesive polycarbophil has been shown to alleviate postmenopausal vaginal dryness (Replens, Columbia Laboratories, Hollywood,

Florida). The cream has the ability to remain in the vaginal cavity for 2 to 3 days after only one administration and maintains a healthier vaginal environment through hydration of the mucosa.

E. Oral Cavity

Drug administration to the oral cavity has many advantages from both a patient and a therapeutic point of view. Both local and systemic availability can be achieved using bioadhesives in the oral cavity. Anesthetic, anti-inflammatory, and antimicrobial agents can be administered locally for increased residence time using bioadhesives. Besides the use of adhesives for retention of dentures, the dental industry has taken advantage of using bioadhesives for other localized applications. The anesthetic lidocaine, used locally for toothaches, has been shown to have an increased duration of activity when administered in a mucoadhesive tablet containing a combination of freeze-dried hydroxypropyl cellulose and Carbopol® 934. This has advantages over the usual forms of topical administrations, which show little precision in site specificity and can quickly be washed away by saliva. The analgesic lignocaine has also been studied when applied as a bioadhesive patch. Various polymeric systems have been employed to deliver fluorides to the oral cavity. Others have reported therapeutic treatment of buccal lesions, such as aphthae and lichen planus using bioadhesives. These dosage forms have the advantage over standard oral ointments of being applied directly to the lesion and achieving high drug levels because of increased duration at the site of inflammation.

Systemic delivery of drugs through mouth has gained popularity in recent years. Drugs that are susceptible to degradation due to the harshness of the gastrointestinal route can be administered intact. This avoids first-pass metabolism of susceptible compounds by the hepatic system and offers the patient a more desirable route of administration than injec-

tion. Due to the limited area of the oral cavity, the delivery system itself is restricted in size, and hence potent compounds, such as proteins and peptides, are often more suited to such delivery systems. The oral cavity can be divided into three distinct functional areas—the lining mucosa (buccal, sublingal, and soft palate), the masticatory mucosa (hard palate and gingiva), and the specialized mucosa (dorsal tongue). The thickness and keratinization of the tissue differ between these regions and hence the permeability of each is unique. The hard palate and gingiva are highly keratinized and subsequently offer limited permeability for drug delivery. The use of enhancers, however, has been shown to increase the permeability through keratinized tissues from bioadhesive delivery platforms. The majority of the work for systemic delivery of drugs using bioadhesives systems through oral cavity has been concentrated on the buccal (cheek) route of administration because of its large surface area and nonkeratinization. Bioadhesive buccal tablets or patches have been utilized as delivery systems. They are usually designed to be unidirectional in their delivery, (i.e. delivering the drug from the side of the patch attached to the buccal mucosa and not to rest of the mouth). This is often accomplished by an impermeable backing membrane facing the oral cavity. The bioadhesive of choice can then serve two purposes—as an adhesive keeping the delivery system in place and/or as a drug-containing matrix in which the compound diffuses from the matrix and permeates the mucosa to reach into the general circulation. When administered in a mucoadhesive tablet, similar to the tablet containing lidocaine above but with the addition of an oil base and the penetration enhancer glycocholate, insulin has shown an increased absorption through the oral mucosa. Insulin blood levels, however were significantly lower in comparison to systemic levels achieved by intramuscular injection. The reason for the low bioavailability could be due to poor tissue permeability, even with the enhancer. Mucoadhesive dosage forms have also been used for the treatment of cardiovascular disorders such as angina and hypertension. When administered as an adhesive delivery system, nifedipine showed plateau drug levels after 8 hours which was maintained until removal of the delivery system. Another delivery system using nitroglycerin in a bioadhesive buccal tablet has also been shown to have a sustained effect (Table 3.7).

F. Ocular

Drug delivery to the eyes is difficult due to dilution of drug in the tears and the natural mechanisms of blinking and high tear turnover rate, which protect the eye from external contaminants. Traditional aqueous, ocular delivery systems are administered dropwise, and due to the foregoing conditions, bioavailability is severely limited for either local or systemic therapy.

Although many attempts have been made to prolong drug release of ocular delivery systems, a few have proven to be successful when patient acceptance, drug bioavailability, and cost are considered. For a drug to be sustained in the eye, it must be maintained in the precorneal area and should deliver drug to this area over an extended period of time. Ocular bioadhesive delivery systems could therefore show a sustained effect if they penetrate the aqueous tear film and interact with the underlying mucin or cell layer. If firmly attached to the surface, the dosage form could remain in the preocular area for longer than conventional ocular dosage forms, and if dissolution of drug release is controlled, therapeutic utilization of water-soluble drugs can be increased significantly. Pilocarpine is a drug commonly used in glaucoma therapy to relieve intraocular pressure (IOP), which is a cause of great discomfort to the patient. Piloplex is a sustained-release product based on an emulsion system of pilocarpine bound to a polymeric carrier. Piloplex could prolong a reduction in IOP as compared to standard pilocarpine hydrochloride drops. This is attributed to its bioadhesive properties, which keep the drug in the precorneal area longer than conventional ocular dosage forms.

The release of progesterone used as a model drug in an ocular delivery system consisting of cross-linked acrylic acid has been shown to be sustained. The delivery system showed increased bioavailability 4.2 times greater than a suspension without polymer and shown excellent bioadhesion to the conjunctinal mucosa of the albino rabbit. Another system utilizing polycarbophil also showed increased bioavailability of a fluorometholone steroid suspension used for the treatment of inflammation.

CHALLENGES

Challenges and opportunities in the field of mucoadhesive polymers demand for development of novel, more adhesive polymers, as well as the discovery and utilization of further characteristics of mucoadhesive polymers, with cytoinvasive properties. Further challenges and opportunities are encountered in the use of mucoadhesive polymers for oral drug delivery where the adhesive properties are in most cases still insufficient to provide and assure a prolonged residence time in certain GI-segments. The localisation of mucoadhesive delivery systems within a certain GI-segment, ideally where the drug has its absorption window T, would lead to a tremendous improvement in the oral bioavailability of these drugs. The absorption of riboflavin, for instance, which has its absorption window T in the stomach, as well as the upper small intestine, could be strongly improved in human volunteers by oral administration of mucoadhesive microspheres. Apart from the presence of food and the high motility of this organ in the form of peristaltic waves, the main reason for insufficient mucoadhesion in the GI-tract seems to be the fact that polymers reach the mucosa already in a prehydrated state. Hence, the driving force for polymer mucus interpenetration, which provides comparatively high mucoadhesive properties, is customized.

Thus, polymers must reach the GI-mucosa in a dry form. The problem, however, cannot be solved by a simple enteric coating, as the coating material does not, even at a relatively high pH, readily dissolve. In contrast, the coating material swells slowly and creates an isolating layer between the mucoadhesive polymer and the mucus gel layer. First attempts to tackle this problem focused on mucoadhesive polymers that swell like an enteric coating material only at a higher pH. Clausen et al., for instance, developed a mucoadhesive poly (methacrylic acid)/starch composition that remains stable in gastric fluids and swells in intestinal fluids. Liposomes coated with mucoadhesive polymers, such as carbopol or chitosan, for instance, showed a significantly improved effect of orally administered calcitonin in rats. Particulate delivery systems exhibit per se a prolonged GI residence time. By diffusing into the mucus gel layer their transit time is often significantly reduced even when they are devoid of any mucoadhesive properties. Coupe et al., for instance, could show in human volunteers that 50% of an orally administered particulate formulation remains still in the small intestine, while single unit dosage forms have already left this gut segment. The potential of micro- and nanoparticles in oral drug delivery could already be demonstrated in various *in vivo* studies. Optimized combinations of both the promising strategies, i.e. the use of mucoadhesive polymers on the one hand and micro- and nanoparticulate formulations on the other hand should further improve the delivery properties of such systems. Further opportunities have found use of mucoadhesive polymers to target other mucosal membranes that have not yet been thoroughly investigated. Sakagami et al., recently demonstrated in preliminary studies the potential of mucoadhesive polymers in pulmonary delivery systems. Some of the patents related to these systems are summarized in Table 3.8.

Table 3.7: Carbopols and mucin, similar features and mechanisms of interaction

Similar features	Mechanism of interaction
Macromolecular expanded network	Electrostatic interaction
Negative charges	Hydrogen bonding
Significant hydration in aqueous media	Hydrophobic interaction
Significant number of carboxyl groups	Inter-diffusion

Table 3.8: List of some patents related to bioadhesive systems

Cited patent	Issue date	Original assignee	Title
US4915948	Apr 10, 1990	Warner–Lambert company	Tablets having improved bioadhesion to mucous membranes
US5077051	Dec 31, 1991	Warner–Lambert company	Sustained release of active agents from bioadhesive microcapsules
US5672356	Sep 30, 1997	Adir Et Compagnie	Bioadhesive pharmaceutical composition for the controlled release of active principles
US6303147	Oct 16, 2001	Janssen Pharmaceutica, N.V.	Bioadhesive solid dosage form
US4615697	Oct 7, 1986	Bio-Mimetics, Inc.	Bioadhesive compositions and methods of treatment therewith
US5314915	May 24, 1994	McNeil-PPC, Inc.	Bioadhesive pharmaceutical carrier
US5330761	Jul 19, 1994	Edward Mendell Co. Inc.	Bioadhesive tablet for nonsystemic use products

Contd.

Table 3.8: List of some patents related to bioadhesive systems *(Contd.)*

Cited patent	Issue date	Original assignee	Title
US5314915	May 24, 1994	McNeil-PPC, Inc.	Bioadhesive pharmaceutical carrier
US5330761	Jul 19, 1994	Edward Mendell Co. Inc.	Bioadhesive tablet for nonsystemic use products
US5364634	Nov 15, 1994	Southwest Research Institute	Controlled-release PH sensitive capsule and adhesive system and method
US6063404	May 16, 2000	Jenapharm GmbH & Co. KG	Bioadhesive tablet
US6248358	Jun 19, 2001	Columbia Laboratories, Inc.	Bioadhesive progressive hydration tablets and methods of making and using the same
US6284235	Sep 4, 2001	National Starch and Chemical Company Investment Holding Corporation	Bioadhesive composition
US6585997	Jul 1, 2003	Access Pharmaceuticals, Inc.	Mucoadhesive erodible drug deliver device for controlled administration of pharmaceuticals and other active compounds
US6624200	Sep 23, 2003	Columbia Laboratories, Inc.	Bioadhesive progressive hydration tablets
US7846478	Jul 10, 2012	Archimedes Development Limited	Method of managing or treating pain

SUGGESTED READINGS

1. Alpar HO, Somavarapu S, Atuah KN, Bramwell VW (2005), *Advanced Drug Delivery Reviews*. 3: 411.
2. Abdallah M, Martin W, Yuichi, T and Hirofumi, T (2011), *J. Cont. Rel.*, 149, 81–8.
3. Guo LY, Zhao YP (2006), *Journal of Adhesion Science and Technology*. 20 (12): 1281.
4. Huntsberger J.R. (1967), Treatise on adhesion and adhesives, (Ed. R Patrick), Vol. 1, New York: Marcel Dekker Inc.
5. Lee WF, Lin WJ (2001), *Journal of Polymer Research*. 9 (1): 23
6. Lenaerts V, Gurny R (1990), *Bioadhesive Drug Delivery Systems*, CRC Press. 25.
7. Luciano M, Freitas D, Osvaldo (2005), *Drug Development and Industrial Pharmacy*, 3: 293.
8. Sudhakar Y, Kuotsu K, Bandyopadhyay AK (2006), Journal of Controlled Release 1: 15.
9. Valenta C, Kast EC, Harich I, Bernkop-Schnürch A (2001), *Journal of controlled release*. 77 (3): 323–32 .
10. Hongyi Q, Wenwen C, Chunyan H, Li L, Chuming C, Wenmin L and Chunjie W (2007), *Int. J. Pharm.*, 337, 178–87.

11. Huimin Y, Lu X, Fei H, Xin C, Yang D, Min W, Jiao G, Xiaolei S and Sanming L (2008), *Int. J. Pharm.*, 364, 21–6.
12. In-Kwon H, Young BK, Hung-Sik, K, Donggeun, Sul., Woon-Won, J, Hee Jeong, C. and Yu-Kyoung, O. (2006) Methods, 38, 106–11.
13. Christian K, Karin A, Melanie, G, Christian, W, Paul, D and Andreas, B (2008), *Magnetic Resonance Imaging*, 26, 638–43.
14. Barthelmes J, Perera G, Hombach J, Dünnhaupt S and = Bernkop-Schnürch A (2011), *Int. J. Pharm.*, 416, 339–45.
15. Bernkop-Schnürch, A, Weithaler, A, Albrecht, K and Greimel A (2006), *Int. J. Pharm.*, 317, 76–81.
16. Chayed, S and Françoise MW (2007), *Eur. J. Pharm. Biopharm.*, 65, 363–70.
17. Choi HG, Oh YK, Kim CK, *Int. J.Pharm.* 165(1), 1998, 23–32.
18. NA Peppas, KB Keys, M Torres-Lugo AM Lowman, *J. Control. Release* 62 (1999) 81–7.
19. C Marriott, DRL Hughes, Mucus physiology and pathology in: R Gurny HE Junginger (Eds.), Germany, 1990, pp. 29–43.
20. Denk WJ, Strickler JP, Webb WW. Science. 1990; 248: 73–6.

21. Shang-Li T, Tze-Wen C, Yi-You H and Der-Zen, L. (2009), *Biomater.*, 30, 5862–8.

22. Jan, M. and Rainer, H. M. (2006), *Eur. J. Pharm. Biopharm.*, 62, 282–7.

23. Myung-Kwan, C, Hongkee, S and Hoo-Kyun C, (2005), *Int. J. Pharm.*, 297, 172–9.

24. Mazzarino, L, Travelet, C, Sonia, OM, Issei, O, Isabelle, P, Elenara, L and Redouane, B (2012) *J. Coll. Inter. Sci.*, 370, 58–66.

25. Sándor H, András F Hartwig W, Péter S, Szilvia V, Andrea T, Lóránd K, Kurunczi A, Gábor B, Levente K, István, E, Piroska S and Mária AD, (2009), *Eur. J. Pharm. Biopharm.*, 72, 252–9.

26. Mirkka, PS, Luis, MB, Ermei, MM, Jarno, JS, Päivi, HL, Kerttuli H, Markus BL, Jouni TH, Timo JL, Hélder AS and Anu JA (2012), *Biomater.*, 33, 3353–62.

27. Nielsen LS, Schubert L, Hansen J, *Eur J Pharm Sci.* 6(3), 1998, 231–9.

28. Bruschi ML, Jones DS, Panzeri H, Gremião MP, de Freitas O, Lara EH.Semisolid systems containing propolis for the treatment of periodontal disease: in vitro release kinetics, syringeability, rheological, textural, and mucoadhesive properties. *J Pharm Sci.* 2007; 96(8): 2074–89.

29. Schnürch AB Drug Discov Today 2(1), 2005, 83–87.

30. Takeuchi H, Thongborisute J, Matsui Y, Sugihara H, Yamamoto HH, Kamashima Y, *Adv. Drug Del. Rev.*; 57(11), 2005, 1583–94.

31. Lee JW, Park JH, Robinson JR, *J Pharm Sci.* 89(7), 2000, 850–66.

32. Neves JD, Amaral MH, Bahia MF. Vaginal Drug Delivery: In: Gad SC, editor. *Pharmaceutical Manufacturing Handbook.* Nj, Usa: John Willey and Sons Inc; 2007, 809–78.

33. RA Scott, NA Peppas, C Macromolecules 32 (1999) 6139–48.

34. RL Langer, AG Mikos, NA Peppas, DJ Trantolo, GE Wnek, MJ Yaszemski (Eds.), *Handbook of Pharmaceutical Controlled Release Technology*, Dekker, New York, 2000, pp. 47–64.

35. Y Huang, W Leobandung, A Foss, NA, *J. Control. Release* 65 (2000) 63–71.

36. V Dodane, MA Khan, JR Merwin, *Int. J. Pharm.* 182 (1999) 21–32.

37. Yamamoto T, Morita M, Hashida H, Sezaki NT, *J. Pharm.* 93 (1993) 91–9.

38. J.M. Smith, M. Dornish, E.J. Wood, Biomaterials 26 (2004) 3269–76.

39. M Fee, N Errington, K Jumel, L Illum, A Smith, SE Harding, *J. Eur. Biophys.* 32 (2003) 457–64.

40. L Illum I, *J. Pharm. Pharmacol.* 56 (2004) 3–17.

41. Wittaya-areekul S, Kruenate J and Prahsarn C (2006), *Int. J. Pharm.*, 312, 113–8.

42. Woolfson AD, Umrethia ML, Kett VL and Malcolm RK (2010), *Int. J. Pharm.*, 388, 136–43.

43. Yoshiki J, Milton H and Allan SH (2007), *Reactive and Functional Polymers*, 67, 1330–7.

44. Yoo JW, Dharmala K and Lee, CH (2006), *Int. J. Pharm.*, 309, 139–45.

4

■ Multiple Emulsions

INTRODUCTION

The emulsion can be defined as the dispersion of one immiscible liquid in another, stabilized by a third component called the emulsifying agent. Two main classes can be identified—the dispersion of water droplets in oil (W/O) and the reverse systems, the dispersion of oil droplets in water (O/W). Emulsion systems have been used in medical practices since the earliest time for the administration of oils and fats. Today they find use as drug-delivery systems, for nutritional and diagnostic applications, and as blood substitutes. Emulsion can be administered by injection by different route for variety of reasons. For example, W/O emulsions given by intramuscular (IM) injection are known for their sustained release properties and adjuvant effects in immunology. Oil in water emulsions are normally given by the intravenous route as carriers of lipid-soluble compounds including anticancer agents.

More complex types of emulsion can be produced in which the dispersed droplets themselves contain smaller dispersed droplets. These systems known as multiple emulsions are easily prepared by the re-emulsification of simple primary O/W or W/O system to provide O/W/O or W/O/W systems (Fig. 4.1). These systems can then be re-emulsified further to produce even more complicated systems.

Emulsion can be administered by injection through different route for a variety of reasons:
• Sustained released action
• Adjuvant effects in immunology

Sustained drugs release from the multiple emulsion systems can be explained on the basis of three possible mechanisms (i) diffusion of unionized drug through the oil layer, (ii) diffusion of unionized and/or ionized drug through oil-water lamellae (liquid membrane), (iii) coalescences of the internal

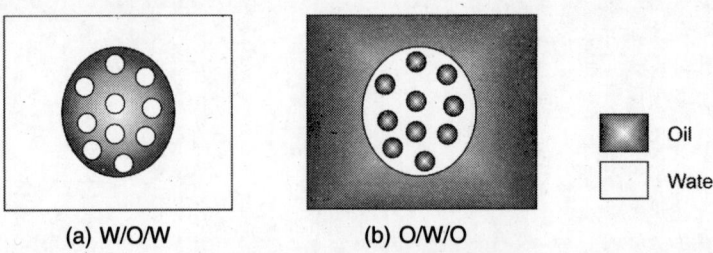

(a) W/O/W   (b) O/W/O   ■ Oil
                                      □ Water

Fig. 4.1: Multiple emulsions

82

aqueous phase and rupture of the oil droplets. A combination all three mechanisms may be possible *in vivo*.

The potential of multiple emulsions as drug delivery vehicle and drug targeting depends on successful formulation using oils and emulsifier that provide good stability characteristics and have low toxicity.

FORMULATION ASPECTS OF MULTIPLE EMULSIONS

Florence and Whitehill described three different types of multiple emulsions, which they termed A, B and C (Fig. 4.2). Type A multiple emulsions were those in which only one large internal drop was contained into the secondary emulsion droplet. In type B emulsions, there were several small internal droplets contained in the secondary emulsion droplet, and type C emulsions were those with a large number of internal droplets present. Only the type C systems have application in drug delivery and drug targeting.

Multiple emulsions can be formed purposely by re-emulsification of primary emulsion, or they can occur when an emulsion inverts from one type to another, e.g. W/O to O/W. Thus, for experimental studies multiple emulsions are best prepared by the re-emulsification of a primary emulsion employing at least two surfactants. One of which is used to stabilize the initial primary emulsion and the other to stabilize the secondary multiple emulsion. The emulsifier needs to be preferentially soluble in the dispersed phase of the emulsion type being prepared. For example, if a primary O/W emulsion is to be prepared, a lipophilic emulsifier is required, followed by a hydrophilic emulsifier for secondary emulsion (W/O). The stability of the resultant multiple emulsions will depend not only on formulation variables but also on the conditions employed in its production. The following factors are identified of importance and discussed in context to the W/O/W system:

- Emulsification equipment
- Nature of the oil phase
- Volumes of the two dispersed phase
- Nature and quantity of the emulsifying agents
- Nature of entrapped materials including the drug substances
- Added stabilizing components.

GENERAL METHODS OF PREPARATION
Two-step Emulsification (Double Emulsification)

Two-step emulsification methods involve re-emulsification of primary W/O or O/W emulsion using a suitable emulsifier agent. The first step involves, obtaining an ordinary W/O or O/W primary emulsion wherein an appropriate emulsifier system is utilized. In the second step, the freshly prepared W/O or O/W primary emulsion is re-emulsified with an excess of aqueous phase or oil phase. The finally prepared emulsion could be W/O/W or O/W/O respectively. The method is schematically illustrated in Fig. 4.3. In two-step emulsification, it was observed that on the scale of acceptability, the physicochemical characteristics of multiple emulsion systems are directly related to the ratio of the amount of Span 80 to that of a series of the hydrophilic emulsifiers existing in the entire system. It was observed that twice or less Span 80 than

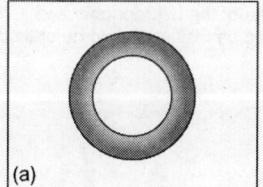 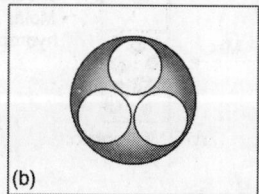 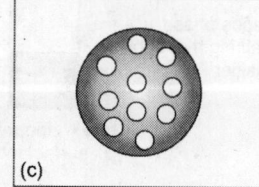

(a) (b) (c)

Fig. 4.2: Types of multiple emulsions

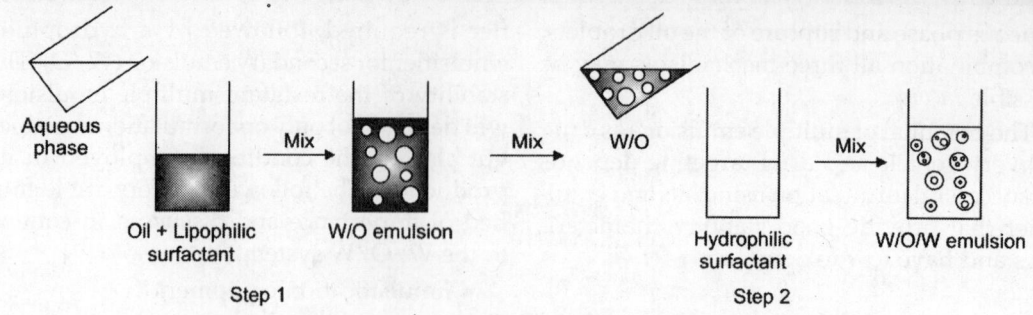

Fig. 4.3: Two-step preparation of a W/O/W multiple emulsion

Tween 80 is necessary for obtaining higher yields of O/W/O emulsions in contrast to the amount and ratio recommended for W/O/W emulsion. Recently, Okochi and Nakano, 2000 reported a modified two-step emulsification technique for the preparation of W/O/W emulsion. This method is different from the conventional two-step technique in two respects—firstly, sonication and stirring are used to obtain fine, homogenous and stable W/O emulsion. Secondly, a continuous phase is poured into a dispersed phase for preparing W/O/W emulsion (in contrast to conventional method in which a dispersed phase is poured into a continuous phase). Moreover, the composition of internal aqueous phase-oily phase-external phase is fixed at 1:4:5, which produces most stable formulation as reported for most of W/O/W emulsions.

Phase Inversion Technique (One-step Technique)

Matsumoto and coworkers first reported the development of W/O/W system during the phase inversion of the concentrated W/O emulsion. An increase in volume of dispersed phase may cause an increase in the phase volume ratio, which subsequently leads to the formation of multiple emulsions. The method typically involves the addition of an aqueous phase that contains a hydrophilic emulsifier [Tween 80/sodium dodecyl sulphate (SDS) or cetyl trimethyl ammonium salt (CTAB)] to an oil phase consisted of liquid paraffin containing a lipophilic emulsifier (Span 80). A well defined volume of oil phase is placed in a vessel of pin mixer. An aqueous solution of emulsifier is then introduced successively to the oil phase in the vessel at a rate of 5 ml/min, while the pin mixer rotates steadily at 88 rpm at room temperature. When volume fraction of the aqueous solution of hydrophilic emulsifier exceeds 0.7, the continuous oil phase is substituted by the aqueous phase containing a number of vesicular globules among the simple oil droplets, leading to phase inversion and formation of W/O/W multiple emulsion (Fig. 4.4).

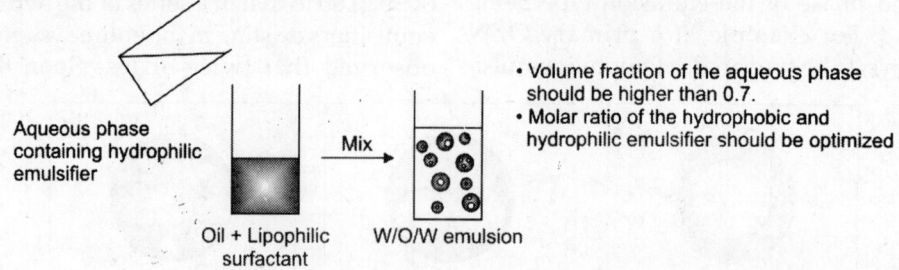

Fig. 4.4: Preparation of multiple emulsion using phase inversion technique

Membrane Emulsification Technique

In this method, a W/O emulsion (a dispersed phase) is extruded into an external aqueous phase (a continuous phase) with a constant pressure through a Porous Glass Membrane, which possess have controlled and homogenous pores. The particle size of the resulting emulsion can be controlled with proper selection of porous glass membrane as the droplet size depends upon the pore size of the membrane.

Multiple Emulsions Using Microchannel Emulsification

Monodispersed multiple emulsions are useful for both industrial applications and basic studies. Rheology, appearance, chemical reactivity, and physical properties are influenced by both the average size and size distribution, and drug-release properties of multiple emulsions depend on the size of the dispersed phase.

Monodispersed emulsions can be obtained by fractionation of polydispersed emulsion, but repeated operations are required. Several research groups are investigating how to produce quasimonodisperse W/O/W emulsions. Membrane emulsification, in which the pressurized dispersed phase permeates through a microporous membrane and forms emulsion droplets, enables us to produce monodispersed emulsions with a coefficient of variation of approximately 10%. This technique has been applied for the preparation of W/O/W emulsions. However, it is not clear how internal water droplets penetrate through the membrane pore. Recently, novel microfabricated channel emulsification method has been developed for making monodisperse emulsion droplets. This emulsification technique is called microchannel (MC) emulsification. Oil-in-water emulsions with a coefficient of variation of less than 5% and a droplet size of 3 to 100 mm have been successfully prepared using this technique. MC emulsification exploits the interfacial tension, the dominating

force on a micrometer scale, and the driving force for droplet formation. During the droplet formation, the distorted dispersed phase is spontaneously transformed into spherical droplets by interfacial tension. The dispersed phase is forced into a distorted (elongated) disk-like shape in the MC. This distorted disk-like shape is the essential point for spontaneous transformation since the disk-like shape has a higher interface area than a spherical shape, resulting in instability from the viewpoint of interface free energy. The dispersed phase with disk-like shape spontaneously transforms into spherical droplets.

Therefore, the droplets are formed without shear by continuous phase flow, and the required energy input is very low compared with conventional emulsification techniques. The mechanism is similar to the breakup of cylindrical flow at the point where transformation is caused by interfacial tension. The droplet size is controlled by MC geometry. An advantage of this technique is direct observation of emulsification through a microscope. Microchannel (MC) emulsification can be applied to prepare several types of oil-in-water emulsions, water-in-oil emulsions, lipid microparticles, and polymer microparticles. A disadvantage is its low production rate. Usually, less than 1 ml/h of dispersed phase can be emulsified.

Characterization of Multiple Emulsions

Average Globule Size, Size Distribution and Yield of Multiple Emulsions

The optical microscopy method using calibrated ocular and stage micrometer can be used for size determinations of globule both multiple emulsion droplets and droplets of internal dispersed phase as well as yield. Florence and Whitehill (1982) used inverted phase contrast microscope and a high-speed camera. With the help of this technique, they classified multiple emulsions as coarse (>3 μm diameter), fine (1–3 μm diameter) and micro-multiple emulsion (<1 μm diameter).

droplet size distribution of freshly prepared emulsion can be measured by light scattering using a Malvern Mastersizer and surface mean droplet diameter and the specific surface area (or SSA—area per unit mass of emulsion) can also be derived. Brightfield micrographs equipped with differential interference contrast optics have been used to characterize the internal droplet of multiple emulsions. Various other techniques used to characterize colloidal carriers like Coulter counter, freeze-fracture electron microscopy and scanning electron microscopy are also used to determine average globule size and size distribution of multiple emulsions.

Area of Interfaces

The average globules diameter determined can be used in the calculation of the total area of interface using the formula:

$$S = 6/D$$

where, S = Total area of interface (sq. cm)

D = Diameter of globules (cm)

Number of Globules

Number of globules per cubic mm can be measured by using the hemocytometer cell. The emulsion is appropriately diluted; a countable number of globules are observed in each small square of the cell and counted. The globules in five groups of 16 small squares (total 80 small squares) are counted and the total number of globules in per cubic mm is calculated using the formula:

$$\text{No. of globules/mm}^3 = \frac{\text{No. of globules} \times \text{Dilution} \times 400}{\text{No. of small squares}}$$

Rheological Evaluation

The rheology of multiple emulsion is an important parameter as it relates to emulsion stability and clinical performance. The viscosity and interfacial elasticity are two major parameters, which relate to product rheology. The viscosity of the multiple emulsions can be measured by Brookfield rotational viscometer. Samples are sheared for one minute at 100 rpm, using an appropriate spindle and readings are taken. Oil phase viscosity can be measured by stress viscometry using a Bohlin controlled rheometer. Three different geometries stant (5 µL) were used according to the viscosity of the samples— double gap DG 40/50, cone-plate 4/40, and concentric cylinder C25. The shear rates were varied between 0.5 and 200 s^{-1} depending on viscosity of the sample and geometry of the measuring head. The resulting viscosity was taken as the mean viscosity over the shear rate range. Interfacial film strength can be evaluated by interfacial rheology measurements, i.e. elasticity of (W/O) and (O/W) components of (W/O/W) multiple emulsions and these data may relate to emulsion stability. Interfacial rheology, (i.e. interfacial elasticity at the oil-aqueous interface) can be investigated at the mineral oil/water interface using an oscillatory surface rheometer. The effect of adding hydrophilic surfactant, Tween and Spans on interfacial elasticity can also be investigated and this may provide an insight on interfacial interactions that occur at the secondary O/W interface.

Zeta Potential

The zeta potential measurements are pivotal in the designing of surface modified or ligand anchored multiple emulsion systems. The zeta potential and surface charge can be calculated using Smoluchowski's equation from the mobility and electrophoretic velocity of dispersed globules using the zeta-potentiometer. A cylindrically bored microelectrophoresis cell equipped with platinum-iridium electrodes is used to measure the electrophoretic mobility of the diluted W/O/W emulsion and using the following equation, zeta potential is calculated.

$$\zeta = \frac{4\pi\eta m}{\varepsilon E} \times 10^3$$

where,

ζ = Zeta potential (mV)

η = Viscosity of the dispersion medium (poise)

m = Migration velocity (cm/s)

ε = Dielectric constant of the dispersion medium

E = Potential gradient (voltage applied/Distance between electrodes)

Percent Drug Entrapment

Percent entrapment of drug or active moiety in the multiple emulsion is generally determined using dialysis, centrifugation, filtration and conductivity measurements. However, recently an internal tracer/marker is used to evaluate the entrapment of an impermeable marker molecule contained in the inner aqueous phase of W/O/W emulsion. The unentrapped marker is determined and the amount entrapped can be thus calculated by deducting unentrapped amount from the initially added amount. The % drug entrapment in the inner aqueous phase of W/O/W emulsion can be determined by using the dialysis method. The % entrapment can be calculated using the following equation:

$$C = \frac{100}{[1 - n_1 V^* / n_{10} - n_1) V_1]}$$

$$V = V^* + \frac{V_d(V_1 + V_2 + V_0)}{V_s}$$

where,

n_{10} = Initial concentration of drug in inner aqueous phase

n_1 = Concentration of drug in dialysate

V_1, V_2 and V_0 represent the volume of inner and outer aqueous and middle oil phase respectively, while V_s and V_d represent volume of dialyzing media and dialyzed emulsion respectively.

In Vitro Drug Release

The drug released from the aqueous inner phase of a W/O/W emulsion can be estimated using the conventional dialysis technique. The release of drug from W/O/W emulsion is measured employing the dialysis method using cellophane tubing (Fig. 4.5). The W/O/W emulsion may be placed in the dialysis bag and dialyzed against 200 ml of phosphate saline buffer (PBS, pH 7.4) at 37±1°C and a sink condition is maintained while sink contents are stirred continuously using a magnetic stirrer. Aliquots are withdrawn at different time intervals and estimated using standard procedure and the data are used to calculate cumulative drug release profile.

In Vitro Stability Studies

Emulsion stability is determined by phase separation on storage of W/O/W emulsions. Freshly prepared multiple emulsion is allowed to stand for 1 week at room temperature and the volume of aqueous phase separated (V_{sep}) is measured at suitable time intervals and percent phase separation is calculated using following formula:

$$B(\%) = 100 \, (V_{sep}/20)/[(V_1 + V_2)/V_1 + V_2 + V_0]$$

where, V_1, V_2 and V_3 are the volumes of internal, external aqueous phase and middle oil phase respectively. Photomicrography, difference in release of model drug and analysis of mean droplet diameters of the multiple emulsion systems as a function of time could be followed and used to study the stability of W/O/W emulsions. However, to test flocculation in multiple emulsions, 5 and

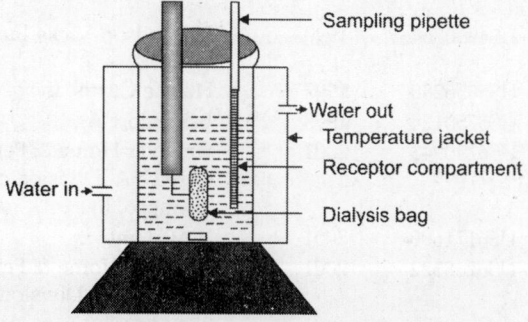

Fig. 4.5: Assembly used for *in vitro* drug release assay

---

*Indicates that no drug was detected in oil phase.

100 drops of SDS (10%) are added immediately after the measurement and the emulsion is stirred gently. Then the droplet size distribution measurement is repeated and the degree of flocculation is microscopically assessed. Change in the stability of multiple emulsions can be assessed measuring by the number and size of multiple droplets over a period of time or by studying changes in rheological properties.

APPLICATIONS

Over last 25 years, multiple emulsions had been investigated intensively with resultant revolution in emulsion technology. This system had been explored for several potential applications in cosmetics, separation sciences, pharmaceuticals, food technology, and several industrial processes and as drug delivery systems. The pharmaceutical applications include bioavailability enhancement, taste masking, drug targeting, prolonged delivery of drugs, immobilization of enzymes etc. Some of the patents related to multiple emulsion are listed in Table 4.1.

Cosmetics

Emulsions are one of the most useful systems in cosmetics and toiletries preparations because most preparations are based either on oil-in-water or water in-oil emulsions. W/O/W multiple emulsions. They provide advantage of having the external aqueous phase where any W/O type emulsion can be incorporated in water, thereby overcoming the shortcomings of conventional W/O emulsions. Multiple emulsions have preference over simple emulsions in personal care products because of the slow and controlled release of drugs. Multiple emulsion based formulations can be used for different purposes like nutritive, moisturizing and protective in cosmetics. Long-term stable multiple emulsion can overcome the stability related problems of emulsions for cosmetic use.

For increasing stability of multiple emulsions in personal cleansing system, synergistic interaction between the low HLB emulsifier and the high HLB surfactant has been investigated by many researchers. These systems produced long-term stability in multiple

	Table 4.1: List of some of the patents related to multiple emulsion		
Cited patent	Issue date	Original assignee	Title
US4650690	1987	Thomas J. Lipton Inc.	Edible water-in-oil-in-water emulsion
US4714566	1987	Meiji Milk Products Company Limited	Process for producing W/O/W type multiple emusion
US4804495	1989	Societe Anonyme Elf France	Reduced viscosity heavy hydrocarbon composition in form of multiple emulsion and its production
US4960764	1990	Richardson-Vicks Inc.	Oil-in-water-in-silicone emulsion compositions
US5656280	1997	Helene Curtis, Inc	Water-in-oil-in-water compositions
US5750124	1998	Beiersdorf Ag	W/O/W emulsions
US6290943	2001	Unilever Home & Personal Care USA, Division of Conopco, Inc.	Stable multiple emulsion composition
US6171600	2001	IFAC GmbH	Stable multiple X/O/Y-emulsion
US6268322	2001	Unilever Home & Personal Care USA, a Division of Conopco, Inc.	Dual chamber cleansing system, comprising multiple emulsion
US6022547	2000	Helene Curtis, Inc.	Rinse-off water-in-oil-in-water compositions

emulsion because of very low interfacial tension at the oil/water interface. Recently, a multiple emulsion formulation was developed for the treatment of acne vulgaris. This formulation contained tea tree oil, as an active ingredient, which is a popular antimicrobial agent for the pilosebaceous applications. Vitamin C (ascorbic acid), a moisturizing and anti-aging active ingredient are widely used in skin care products. Delivery of these agents through multiple emulsion prevents its degradation against oxidation and also provides better and prolonged release. Slow release characteristic is an additional advantage of multiple emulsion systems which are developed and meant for the cosmetic purposes.

Separation Sciences

Multiple emulsions have been explored for engineering sciences and chemistry for the separation of heavy metals (Cr, Cu, Zi, and Ni), hydrocarbons and different compounds. These have been utilized for the separation of contaminant from the waste water of industries. These have also shown potential in separation of the biological materials (nucleoside, lactic acid).

Pharmaceuticals

In pharmaceuticals the basic pathway for absorption of drug from multiple emulsion system was hypothesized to be through intestinal lymphatic system in the form of chylomicron and lipoproteins. The system either can be absorbed directly through intestinal macrophage or through microfold cells of Peyer's patch or from mesenteric lymph duct in the form of chylomicron and lipoproteins. Due to intestinal lymphatic absorption of oils present in multiple emulsions, it had also been utilized for modulating drug absorption kinetics, i.e prolonged or sustained delivery. Pharmaceutical potential of multiple emulsions has been extensively realized in areas such as bioavailability enhancement, drug targeting and prolonged

release delivery—(i) multiple emulsions (W/O/W) have been investigated for controlling the release of different categories of drugs specially those having short half-lives. Partitioning of drugs from water-to-oil phase and then to external aqueous phase for release in W/O/W multiple emulsions leads to the prolonged delivery of the drug, (ii) *Increasing bioavailability of drugs having high first pass metabolism*—multiple emulsion increases bioavailability of drugs either by protecting them in physiological, ionic/enzymatic environment in the GIT where otherwise these may get degraded especially proteins, peptides or they may bypass the hepatic first pass metabolism, (iii) *targeting drugs to lymphatics*—multiple emulsion has shown great potential in the targeting the cytotoxic drugs (highly toxic drugs) to different kinds of tumors. They have been used as lymphotropic carriers drug targeting to several organs (Liver, brain etc.) because of their selective uptake by reticuloendothelial system.

Gene Library

The use of multiples emulsion has been described for compartmentalization and selection of large gene libraries. The aqueous droplets of the w/o emulsion functions as a cell-like compartment in each of which a single gene is transcribed and translated to give multiple copies of the protein (e.g. an enzyme). While compartmentalization ensures that the gene and the protein it encodes, and the products of the activity of this protein remain linked, it does not directly offer a way of selecting for the desired activity.

Oxygen Substitute

Multiple emulsions had been tried out as a substitute to blood where hemoglobin has been incorporated in the inner phase of emulsion. A stable hemoglobin (Hb) in oil-in-water (Hb/O/W) multiple emulsion simulating red blood cell properties has been reported earlier in which gases (O_2 and CO_2) are exchanged with hemoglobin. However, for last one decade there is no report on multiple emulsion investigated for this purpose. Challenges in this area include artificiality, immune response and the questionable *in vivo* compatibility of chemicals.

Taste Masking

Taste masking of bitter drugs like chloroquine has already been investigated as one of major pharmaceutical applications of multiple emulsions. Multiple emulsions of chloroquine, an antimalarial agent has been successfully prepared and found to mask the bitter taste efficiently. Taste masking can be achieved by incorporating drugs in inner aqueous phase of W/O/W multiple emulsion which is surrounded by oil layer that masks the taste. Taste masking of chlorpromazine, an anti-psychotic drug has also been reported by multiple emulsions.

Enzyme Immobilization

Enzyme immobilization technique involves the entrapment of enzymes, which catalyze several reactions. Reports of using multiple emulsions for enzyme immobilization go back to 1972 where hydrocarbon based multiple emulsions were used to entrap urease enzyme for kidney diseases and subsequently immobilized enzymes and whole cell from *M. denitrificans* for waste water treatment. Presently, this technique has been established as a tool for immobilization of various enzymes, proteins, amino acids etc., in bio-technology. Immobilized alcohol dehydro-genase is utilized for the conversion of alcohol to acetaldehyde for industrial use.

Drug Overdosage Treatment/Detoxification

Liquid membrane system had been efficaci-ously used for the drug overdosage treatment as early as 1978. This system could be utilized for the overdosage treatment by utilizing the difference in the pH in different compartments of multiple emulsions, which affects the ionization behavior of the drug. These have been utilized for acidic drug overdosage treatment like barbiturates. In these emul-sions, the inner aqueous phase of emulsion has the basic buffer and when emulsion is taken orally, acidic pH of the stomach acts as an external aqueous phase. In the acidic phase barbiturate remains mainly in unionized form which transfers through oil membrane into inner aqueous phase and gets ionized. Ionized drug has less affinity to cross the oil membrane thereby getting entrapped. Thus, entrapping excess drug in multiple emulsions cures over dosage. Likewise, quinine sulfate overdosage treatment has been reported. Detoxifications of blood by multiple emulsions have also been reported.

Topical Applications

Multiple emulsions slowly release their contents in comparison to solutions because of the three-phase system, therefore they are of immense use in topical applications. A three-phase emulsion containing model compounds testosterone, caffeine and tritiated water for topical use is reported. The effect of Fomblin® on percutaneous absorption was investigated. Fomblin® did not affect flux of caffeine while decreased the percutaneous absorption of testosterone but increased water permeation. A successful W/O/W multiple emulsion preparation containing lactic acid in the internal aqueous phase, octadecylamine in oily phase and benzalkonium chloride in the external aqueous phase is effective for vaginal application against three microbial strains (*Escherichia coli, Staphylococcus aureus* and *Candida albicans*).

Technique for Microsphere/Microcapsule Preparation

Multiple emulsion solvent evaporation method is now one of the well-established methods used for the preparation of micro-spheres, nanospheres, nanoparticles, micro-capsules etc. In this method, multiple emulsion formation is an intermediate step which finally gives rise to the final product. A novel technique is to develop water-in-oil-in-water double emulsion solvent diffusion for encapsulation of hydrophilic drugs. Microencapsulation of different categories of drugs like enzymes, hormones, peptides, synthetic drugs has also been reported. Different polymers (ethylcellulose, eudragit, polylactic acid, polyglycolic acid, etc.) have been employed on the basis of the nature of drug and intended properties of microcapsules. Multiple emulsions have been used to prepare three kinds of hepatitis B surface antigen (HBsAg) loaded poly (d, l) lactic-co-glycolic acid (PLGA) microspheres. These microspheres showed greater antibody response in mice in comparison to the conventional aluminum-adjuvant vaccine and thus hold promise for controlled delivery of a vaccine. Likewise, tetanus toxoid loaded polylactic acid particles have also been prepared by double emulsion technique.

Vaccine/Vaccine Adjuvant

The use of w/o/w multiple emulsion as a new form of adjuvant for antigen was first reported by Herbert. These emulsions elicited better immune response than antigen alone. A multiple emulsion vaccine against *Pasteurella multocida* infection in cattle is reported. This vaccine contributed both humoral as well as cell-mediated immune responses in protection against the infection. Recently, multiple water-in-oil-in-water (W/O/W) emulsion formulations, containing influenza virus surface antigen hemagglutinin were found to be effective in antigen presentation as adjuvant. They have advantage over conventional preparation and can be effectively used as one of the vaccine delivery system with adjuvant properties.

SUGGESTED READINGS

1. Baker RW and Lonsdale HK (1974), Controlled release of biologically active agents (Tonquary, AO and Lceoy, RE, Eds.), Plenum Press, New York, pp. 15.

2. Benichou A, Aserin A, Garti N (2007), Colloids and Surfaces A: Physicochem. *Eng. Aspects* 294, 20.

3. Bhatnagar S, Nakhare S and Vyas SP (1995), *J. Microencap.*, 12, 13.

4. Boyd JV, Krog N and Sherman P (1976), The theory and practice of emulsion technology, Smith, AL., Ed., Academic Press, London,123.

5. Florence AT and Whitehill D (1985), *Macro and Micro-Emulsions: Theory and Application*, ACS Symposium Series, (Shar, D.O., Ed.), vol. 272, 1985, pp. 359.

6. Goldberg EP (1983), *Targeted drugs*, John Wiley, New York, pp. 296.

7. Hashida M, Muranishi S and Sezaki H (1977), *J. Pharmacokinetics and Biopharmaceutics*, 5, 241.

8. Nakhare S, Vyas SP and Jain NK (1994), *The Eastern Pharmacist*, 65.

9. Shinoda K and Friberge S (1986), *Emulsion and solubilization*, John Wiley and Sons, New York, pp. 33.

10. Tomlinson E, Burger JJ, Mevie JG and Hoefnagel, K (1984), *Recent advances in drug delivery systems* (Anderson JH and Kim JW, Eds.), Plenum Press, New York, pp. 199.

11. Wisse E and De Leeuw AM (1984), Microspheres and drug therapy: Pharmaceutical, immunological and medical aspects (Davis SS, Illum L, Mevie, JG and Tomlinson E, Eds.), Elsevier, Amsterdam, pp. 1.

12. RH Engel SJ Riggi, MJ Fahrenbach Nature (London), 219 (1968), pp. 850–7.

13. SG Frank, AF Brodin, D Kavaliunas Acta Pharm. Suecica, 13 (1976), pp. 41 (Supplement) ES Matulevicius, NN Li Separ. Purif. Methods, 4 (1976), pp. 73

14. S Matsumoto, Y Kita, D Yonezawa, *J. Colloid Interface Sci.*, 57 (1976), p. 353.

15. DD Eley, MJ Hey, JD Symonds, JHM Willison, *J. Colloid Interface Sci.*, 54 (1976), pp. 462–466

16. H Moor, K Muhleihale, *J. Cell Biol.*, 17 (1963), pp. 609

17. WJ Herbert Lancet, II (1965), pp. 771

18. F Brodin, SG Frank, DR Kavaliunas Acta Pharm. Suec., 15 (1978), pp. 1–12.

19. T Yoshioka, K Ikeuchi, M Hashida, S Muranishi, H. Sezaki, *Chem. Pharm. Bull.*, 30 (1982), pp. 1408–15.

20. S Fukushima, K Juni, M Nakano, *Chem. Pharm. Bull.*, 31 (1983), pp. 4048–56.

21. CJ Benoy, LA Elson, R Schneider, *J. Pharmacol.*, 45 (1972), pp. 135P

22. AJ Collings, R Schneider, *J. Pharmacol.*, 38 (1970), pp. 469.

5

Colon-Specific Drug Delivery Systems

INTRODUCTION

The colon-specific drug delivery has a number of important implications in the field of pharmacotherapy. Various diseases including inflammatory bowel diseases (IBD) can be effectively treated by the local delivery of various drugs to the large intestine. Especially, the treatment of IBD with anti-inflammatory drugs was further improved by local delivery of the agents to the bowel. By this technique, absorption of the drugs from the stomach and small intestine can be minimized until the drug reaches the large intestine. Several drug delivery systems which work on the basis of various mechanisms are developed to deliver the drugs quantitatively to the large bowel and

subsequently to trigger the release of active drug. The treatment of large intestine disorders, such as Crohn's disease, irritable bowel syndrome, colitis, colon cancer and local infectious diseases where a high concentration of active drug is needed, can be improved by colon-specific drug delivery employing various mechanism of drug release (Table 5.1). Moreover, the introduction of several peptide-based drugs requires special drug delivery systems for their delivery.

The site-specific delivery of the drugs to the target receptor sites possesses the potential to reduce the side effects and to improve the pharmacological response. However, for successful colonic drug delivery, many

Table 5.1: Colon-targeting diseases, drugs and sites		
Target sites	*Diseases and conditions*	*Drugs and active agents*
Topical action	Inflammatory bowel disease, irritable bowel disease, and Crohn's disease.	Hydrocortisone, budenoside, prednisolone, sulfasalazine, olsalazine, mesalazine and balsalazide.
Local action	Chronic pancreatitis, pancreatactomy and cystic fibrosis. Colorectal cancer	Digestive enzyme supplements 5-Fluorouracil
Systemic action	To prevent gastric irritation	NSAIDs
	To prevent first pass metabolism of orally ingested drugs	Steroids
	Oral delivery of peptides	Insulin
	Oral delivery of vaccines	Typhoid

physiological barriers must be overcome, the major one being absorption or degradation of the active drug in the upper part of the GI tract. The disease state also can potentially alter the delivery and absorption characteristics of drug from the colon. The drug targeting to colon is also exploited for systemic administration of active drugs. Most of the peptide and protein drugs are unstable in the stomach and upper part of intestine, which contains proteases. Apart from stability problems, peptides are not well absorbed from the lumen of the GIT due to their larger molecular size and high brush border peptidase activity. Comparatively, proteolytic activity of colon mucosa is much less than that observed in the small intestine. Colon-specific drug delivery systems are protecting peptide drugs from hydrolysis and enzymatic degradation in the duodenum and jejunum, and eventually releasing drugs in the ileum or colon, which leads to greater systemic bioavailability. This specific release in the colon also gives a time delay between administration and onset of action, which can be useful for diseases with varied degrees of severity, such as asthma and arthritis (Friend, 1991).

Various colon-specific drug delivery systems have been developed, which exploit advantage of the luminal pH in the ileum and the microbial enzymes in the colon, such as pectinase, amylase, dextranase, glycosidase and azoreductase in the favor of therapeutic benefits. This chapter focuses on various concepts and approaches used in the development of colon-specific drug delivery systems.

ANATOMIC AND PHYSIOLOGICAL CONSIDERATIONS

The therapy desired for local (colonic) or systemic delivery of drug, the development and aim of the drug delivery to colon, however remain to be the same. Firstly, the drug must not absorb from other regions of the GIT; also it should only suffer negligible degradation in the lumen of small intestine. Secondly, the release of the drug in the colon should be at quantitatively-controlled rate and the released drug should be absorbed from the lumen of the larg intestine without any appreciable degradation in the lumen. In order to meet these objectives, a thorough knowledge of the anatomy and physiology of gastrointestinal tract (GIT) is required (Fig. 5.1). Table 5.2

Table 5.2: Properties of human GIT and metabolic and enzymatic reactions by GIT microflora

Properties of GIT	Measured values	Microbial metabolic and enzymatic reactions in human GIT
Surface area		Hydrolysis of glucuronides, hydrolysis of glycosides, hydrolysis of –CO–NH– compounds (amides, glycine conjugates and N-acetyl compounds), hydrolysis of esters, hydrolysis of sulfamates, dehydroxylation (C-dehydroxylation and N-dehydroxylation), demethylation, dealkylation (O-demethylation, N-demethylation and other), dehalogenation, heterocyclic ring fusion, reduction of double bonds, reduction of nitro groups, reduction of azo groups, reduction of aldehydes, reduction of ketones, reduction of alcohols, reduction of N-oxides, reduction of arsenic acids, aromatization, nitrosamine formation, acetylation and esterification.
Total GIT	$2-10^6$ cm^2	
Resting volume		
Stomach	25–50 ml	
Length		
Total GIT	500–700 cm	
Duodenum	20–30 cm	
Jejunum	150–250 cm	
Ileum	200–350 cm	
Colon	90–150 cm	
pH		
Stomach	1–3.5	
Duodenum	5–7	
Jejunum	6–7	
Ileum	7	
Colon	5.5–7	
Rectum	7	

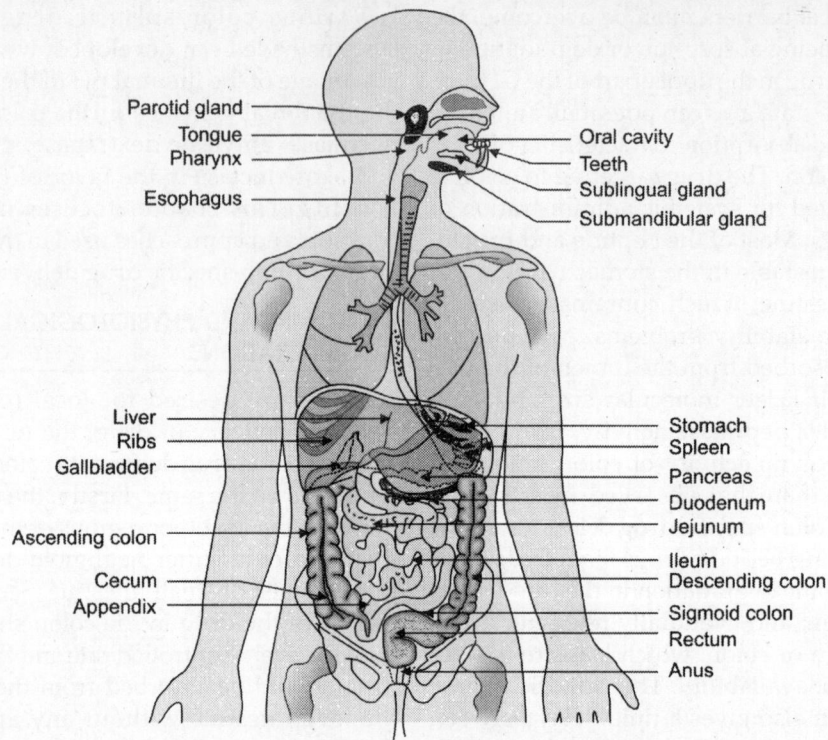

Fig. 5.1: Schematic representation of human GIT

categorically presents some important properties of human GIT. In gastrointestinal tract, large intestine starts from the ileocecal junction to the anus with a length about 1.5 m (adults) and is divided into three parts—(i) colon, (ii) rectum and (iii) anal canal. The colon consists of cecum, colon ascendens, colon transvesale, colon descendens and sigmoid colon. Colon is made up of four layers, serosa, muscularis externa, submucosa and mucosa (Samuel et al., 1968). The serosa is the exterior coat of the large intestine and consists of areolar tissue that is covered by a single layer of squamous mesothelial cells. The muscularis externa is composed of the major muscular coat of inner circular layer of fibres that surrounds the bowel and an outer longitudinal layer. Colonic longitudinal muscle fibres are composed of three flat long bands called taenia coli, which is shorter than other coats of the colon and hence results in wall contractions and formation of haustra. The submucosa is the layer of connective tissue that lies immediately below the mucosa. Lining the lumen of the colon, the mucosa is divided into epithelium, lamina propria and muscularis mucosae. The mucosa is consisted of a layer of smooth muscles and separates the submucosa from the lamina propria, which supports the epithelium. The blood capillaries and lymphatic vessels supply biofluids to lamina propria.

The adult colon is lined by at least 8 distinct epithelial cell types—(1) columnar or absorptive cells, (2) deep crypt secretory cells, (3) vacuolated cells, (4) microfold or 'M' cells, (5) undifferentiated crypt cells, (6) multivesicular or caveolated cells, (7) goblet cells and, (8) variety of enteroendocrine cells. They constitute a structural and functional barrier protecting the internal milieu from direct contact with iumenal components such as the indigenous bacterial flora or exogenously introduced antigens or viruses (Colony, 1996). The pilae semilunares (folded mucosa) and the villi of the columnar cells contribute to the larger surface area of the colon (Hamilton, 1984). Apart from stomach, the GIT has normal bacterial flora, which inhibits the growth of other organisms (Binder et al., 1987). Some species of normal microflora produce short chain fatty acids or antibiotics such as 'clostin', which prevent the growth of pathogens by competing with them for nutrients. The mucus lining of GIT forms a barrier against bacterial invasion of the gut wall. Antibodies IgA and IgG enhance the phagocytosis of GI bacteria.

FACTORS GOVERNING THE COLON DRUG DELIVERY

Physiological Factors

Gastrointestinal Transit

The drug delivery systems are first entering to stomach and small intestine through mouth and then reach colon. The nature and pH of gastric secretions and gastric mucosa influence the drug release and absorption. If the drug delivery systems successfully reach colon in an intact form, they should surpass the physiological barriers of the stomach and small intestine. In fasted state, the motility takes place in 4 phases through stomach and small intestine in 2–3 hours. Phase I is a quiescent period of 40–60 min and phase II consists of intermittent contractions for a period of 40–60 min. Phase III is a period of intense contractions sweeping material out of the stomach and down the small intestine followed by phase IV with contractions dissipating (Code and Marlett, 1987; Rubinstein and Friend, 1994). The feeding state, however affects the normal pattern by irregular contractile activity.

Small Intestinal Transit

Normally, the small intestinal transit is not influenced by the physical state, size of the dosage form and the presence of food in the stomach (Malagelada et al., 1984; Coupe et al., 1991). The mean transit time of the dosage form is about 3–4 hours to reach the ileocecal junction further the time period remains consistent. The dosage form is exposed to enzymes such as esterase, lipase, amylase, protease, nuclease and brush border enzymes (glucosidases, disaccharidases and peptidases) present in the small intestine (Hofmann et al., 1983). The release of drugs from the prodrug based systems and stability of peptides can be affected by the bacterial contents in the ileum.

Colonic Transit

The bioavailability of drugs, released from the dosage forms can be highly influenced by the colonic transit time. Unlike small intestine, colonic transit time shows a considerable variability (Schang et al., 1985; Chaussade et al., 1986). Various factors like gender and size of the dosage form, and physiological conditions such as stress, presence of food and disease state may influence the colonic transit time (Proano et al., 1991; Enck et al., 1989; Holdstock et al., 1970; Cann et al., 1983). Small particles and solutions generally pass slowly through the proximal colon and, particularly in human beings, males show shorter transit time compared to women. Small variation in dietary fibre and age do not alter the transit time significantly. The colonic transit time of a capsule in adults is 20–35 hours, the transit rate is independent of capsule density and volume. The improved residence time with the longer transit time and prolonged contact of dosage form with the microflora in the colon may govern the release and absorption of drug from the dosage form.

Gastric Emptying

Generally, in fasted state, gastric emptying is fastest and most consistent. Emptying is completed from 5–10 min. up to 2 hours, depending on phase of the stomach at the time of drug administration (Gruber et al., 1987; Davis et al., 1984; Christensen et al., 1985). Gastric emptying can be considerably slowed in case of fed state. For drug delivery to the systemic vasculature, small transit time in stomach to reduce random distribution of particulate drug in intestine is preferable for colon drug delivery. The residence time in the stomach is important for single unit sustained release system like matrix or OROS type tablets, which are designed to deliver the drugs in large intestine. Such systems may release the drug at a distant locus from the colon in case gastric emptying is retarded due to some reasons.

Stomach and Intestinal pH

Generally, the release and absorption of orally administered drugs are influenced by the gastrointestinal pH. The pH gradient in the GIT is not in increasing order, in stomach the pH is 1.5–2 and 2–6 in fasted and fed conditions, respectively (Fordtran and Locklear, 1996). The acidic pH is responsible for the degradation of various pH sensitive drugs and enteric coating may prevent it. In small intestine, the pH increases slightly from 6.6–7.5 and decreases to 6.4 in right colon. The pH of mid colon and left colon is 6.6 and 7.0, respectively (Meldrum et al., 1972; Evans et al., 1988). Since the variation in the pH from ileum to colon is minimum, the pH-dependent polymers based drug delivery may not be much selective. However, the possible exploitation of pH variation in GIT leads to successful development of various colon-specific drug delivery systems.

Colonic Microflora and Enzymes

The human alimentary canal is highly populated with bacteria and other microflora at both the ends specifically the oral cavity and the colon or rectum. Microorganisms of the oral cavity, normally do not affect the oral drug delivery, however, gut microflora of the colon have a number of effects and implications in health and the treatment of diseases such as IBD (Gorbach, 1971). The concentration of gut microflora rises considerably in the terminal ileum and reaches extraordinarily

higher levels (10–11 to 10–12 CFU/ml) in the colon. The colon microflora is predominantly consisted of bacterides, *Bifidobacterium, Eubacterium, Peptococcus, Peptostreptococcus, Ruminococcus, Propionibacterium, Veillonella* and *Clostridium,* including important facultative bacteria *Escherichia coli* and Lactobacillus (Draser and Hill, 1974; Simon and Gorbach, 1983).

The metabolic reactions are carried out by the enzymes and secretary products released from the microflora can be used to deliver drugs selectively to colon. The oxidation-reduction potential in colon is about –200mV (Gorbach, 1971). Azoreductase produced by the colonic microflora plays an important role in development of a number of delivery systems, particularly in catalyzing the release of 5-aminosalicylic acid (5-ASA) from a variety of prodrugs. The reduction of azobonds is typically an O_2-sensitive reaction mediated by low molecular weight carriers with $E_o = -200$ to -350 mV (Brown, 1981). Another class of enzymes used to trigger the release of drugs in the colon includes glycosidases and glucuronidases produced by lactobacilli, bacteroides and bifidobacteria. The activity of enzymes is associated with the population density of bacteria in particular region. The composition and population of the intestinal microflora remain unaltered and intact under normal conditions, however may vary with disease conditions (Hill, 1981). The metabolic activity of microflora is also dependent on fermentation of dietary residues. In some cases, the metabolic products of the microflora can inactivate drugs or may potentiate their side effects (Peppercorn and Goldman, 1976).

Colonic Absorption

The surface area of the colon is much less than that of small intestine, and hence not ideally favorable for absorption. Despite this problem, the colon is considered for drug delivery because the environment is devoid of endogenous digestive enzymes other than from microbial origin and the residence time of colon can be as long as 10–24 hours. Little mixing in the colon makes it possible to create local environments with optimal absorption. The higher viscosity of colonic contents delays the diffusion of drug from the lumen to mucosa. The absorption is therefore, influenced by the transport of water, electrolytes and ammonia across the mucosa. The absorption is more in the proximal colon than the distal colon. The absorption properties of colon are being studied by using *in vitro* monolayers of colon carcinoma cell lines (caco-2, T-84 and HT-29), everted sac (Tomilta et al., 1988) and colonoscopy (Gleiter et al., 1985). The mucus layer at the epithelial surface can impose a formidable physical barrier and may result in either drug-mucus binding or drug-mucus repulsion (Mirsny, 1992). The lipid bilayer of the individual epithelial colonocyte and the occluding junction complex between the colonocyte may constitute a physical barrier which may impede colonic drug absorption.

Drug molecules pass from the apical to basolateral surface of the epithelial cells by two paths (Fig. 5.2):

1. By passing through colonocytes (transcellular transport).

2. By passing between adjacent colonocytes (paracellular transport).

Small fraction of low molecular weight amphipathic drugs may surpass this barrier through transcellular transport. However, transit through the cell cytoplasm may result in its extensive enzymatic extraction and degradation. Paracellular transport may be the most promising means of general drug absorption in colon. Since the membrane fluidity of proximal colonocytes is higher than distal colonocytes, drugs can easily pass via a passive absorption process in the proximal colon. Additionally, carrier mediated uptake of drugs in the colon does not extensively operate. It usually relates to the metabolic events of the resident bacteria. Receptor-mediated endocytosis and pinocytosis could, however lead to transcellular transport of drug.

The colonic epithelial permeability of many drugs can be modified by the use of absorption enhancers (Table 5.3) effective absorption and prevention through various mechanisms (Muranishi et al., 1979; Murakami et al., 1986; Fix, 1987), are as follows:

1. Disruption of the intracellular occluding junction complex function to open paracellular route

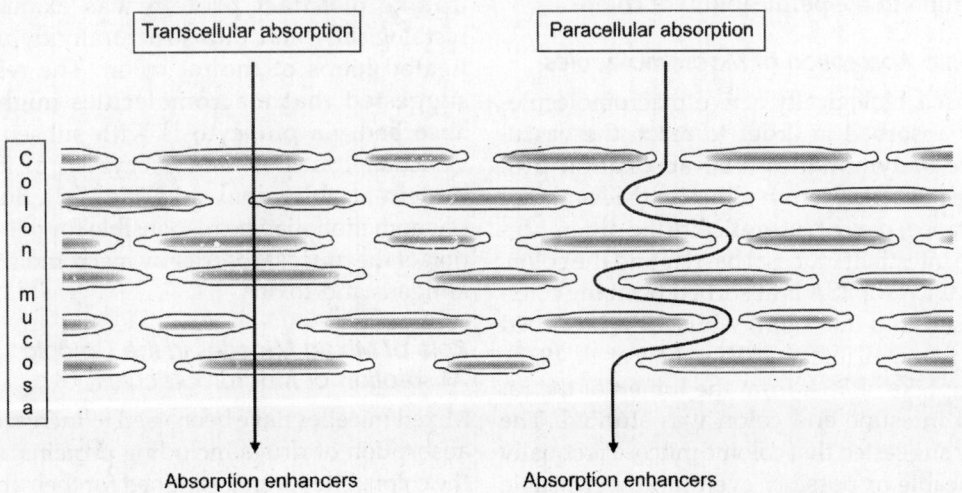

Fig. 5.2: Absorption of drugs from colon and mechanism of absorption enhancers

Table 5.3: Factors affecting colon absorption and absorption enhancers used in colon-specific drug delivery

Factors affecting colon absorption	Absorption enhancers used in colon-specific drug delivery	
• Physical properties of drug such as pK_a and degree of ionization	Class of drugs: NSAIDs	Examples: Indomethacin and Na salicylate
• Colonic residence time as commanded by GIT motility	Ca^{++} ion chelators Surfactants	EDTA and trisodium citrate Sodium lauryl sulfate
• Degradation by bacterial enzymes and metabolic products	Fatty acids	Sodium oleate and laurate
• Local physiological action of drug	Mixed micelles	Hydrogenated castor oil
• Selective and non-selective binding to mucous	Miscellaneous	Acetyl choline and phenothiazines
• Disease state		

2. Modification of epithelial permeability by denaturing membrane proteins
3. Modification of lipid protein interactions and disruption of the integrity of lipid barrier by colonic enterocytes.

Several absorption enhancers are conventionally used to enhance the absorption of polar drugs. Similarly, protease inhibitors such as aprotinin and bacitracin enhance the absorption of peptides and proteins, by preventing their destruction from aminopeptidase activity (Muranishi, 1987). The use of absorption enhancers in pharmaceutical formulations is limited since they are nonspecific in action, produce local irritation and promote irreversible alteration in the permeability of colon.

Colonic Absorption of Macromolecules

Released biologically active macromolecules must absorbed in order to reach the vasculature or lymphatics. The absorption properties of bovin serum albumin (BSA-marker substance) present categorically the differences in the intestinal mucosal barrier and the colon. Only 0.13% of BSA is absorbed from the colon (infused into the colon) while 1.7% absorbed from the small intestine (Warshaw et al., 1977). The uptake of BSA from the lumen of the rat small intestine and colon was studied. The study suggested that colonic mucosa is equally permeable or possibly even more permeable than small intestinal mucosa. In this case, the

differences in absorptive surface area between the colon and small intestine are not considered. Insulin and growth hormone were found to be absorbed intact from the lumen of colon in rats (Touitou and Rubinstein, 1986). In another study, 1.3–3.3% of a dose of 131I-labeled human serum albumin (HSA) (administered as an enema) was absorbed from the colon of dogs whilst absorption of 131I-BSA in humans was found to be negligible (Isley et al., 1959).

Horseradish peroxidase has been used to examine the permeability of biological membranes including colon epithelium (Worthington and Enwonwu, 1975). The uptake of intact protein was examined histologically and ultrastructurally by using ligated loops of the rat colon. The results suggested that macromolecules might be absorbed via pinocytosis with subsequent vesicular transport and exocytosis of intact protein at abluminal side (Fig. 5.3). Such a phenomenon may be responsible for penetration of the mucosal barrier by macromolecular antigens and toxins.

Role of Mixed Micelles in the Colonic Absorption of Macromolecules

Mixed micelles have been used to increase the absorption of drugs including proteins, from the colon. They were examined for their ability to increase absorption of interferon (IFN) from

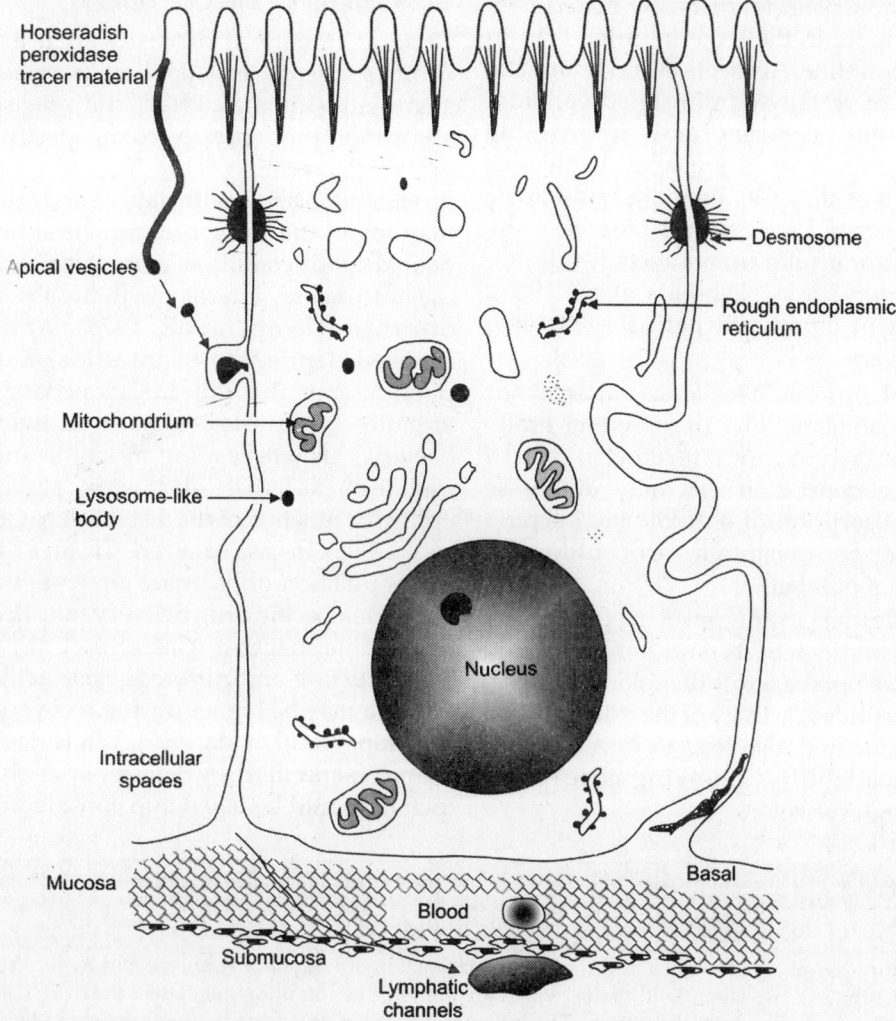

Fig.5.3: Diagrammatic representation of a surface absorptive cell from the rat colon showing progress of exogenous horseradish peroxidase tracer material from the intestinal lumen into apical vesicles, subsequent movement into intracellular spaces via vesicular exocytosis and eventual presence in blood vessels and lymphatic channels

rat's large intestine (Yoshikawa et al., 1984). Absorption of human fibroplast IFN (HuIFN-) was undetectable in serum or lymph from a saline solution or when linoleic acid and a surfactant were used as permeation enhancers. However, delivery into lymphatics was greatly enhanced when linoleic acid/surfactant mixed micelles were used. The extent of absorption of water soluble peptides with mixed micelles is dependent on the molecular weight and molecular shape (Yoshikawa et al., 1982). The use of mixed micelles as absorption enhancers is relatively nontoxic to colonic epithelia as observed microscopically. The effects appear to be reversible in that it takes only about 15 min for permeability to return normal.

The absorption of heparin was evaluated by using lipid surfactant mixed micelles in the rats (Taniguchi et al., 1980). The promoting effect of monoolein-taurocholate mixed micelles was more in the large intestine than in the small intestine. Absorption and lymphatic transport of rectally administered colloidal particles, has been reportedly improvable by using mixed lipid surfactant micelles (Muranishi et al., 1979). Enamine, a nontoxic surfactant could significantly increase the absorption of insulin from a rectally administered suppository (Nishihata et al., 1985). Problems in colonic targeting of macromolecules are:

1. Whether mixed micelles as enhancers or other adjuants, find use in either orally or rectally administered drugs will largely depend on selectivity; otherwise the absorption of enterotoxin, bacteria and opportunistic viruses could cause serious problems.

2. In addition to the problem of luminal proteolytic activity and generally low rates of uptake across the colonic mucosa, the peptidase activity of the colonic brush border could also lead to lower overall bioavailability following absorption through the colon.

Gastrointestinal Disease State

General intestinal diseases such as IBD, Crohn's disease, constipation, diarrhea and gastroenteritis may affect the release and absorption properties of colon-specific drug delivery systems (Table 5.4). Most of the diseases associated with nausea and vomiting may expel the drug content. In antibiotic-related colitic condition, plaque formation on the mucosa may interfere with the absorption of drugs (George et al., 1978). Antibiotic induced depression of intestinal motility, particularly the muscaris mucosa, may enhance antibiotic-resistant allowing for bacterial growth leading to colitis and also initiate or exacerbate diarrhea by altering the epithelial function of the distal colon (Goldhill et al., 1996). In case of severe Crohn's disease, the population of bacterial enzymes utilized for colon-specific drug delivery may decrease or become inactive (Carrette et al., 1995). Azoreductase and nitroreductase activity of bacteria may be higher during recovery from pouchitis (Raffi et al., 1997). While designing the colon-specific drug delivery systems, these factors should be taken into consideration.

Table 5.4: GIT diseases which affect the performance of colon-specific drug delivery systems

Disease	Effects on colonic absorption of drugs
Inflammatory bowel diseases (Crohn's disease and ulcerative colitis)	Diarrhea, fever, anemia, obstruction of lymphatic drainage and hyperplasia of lymphoid tissue, which are seen in this condition may affect the drug release and absorption. The inflammatory response extends from mucosa to cerosa through intestinal wall. Impairment of lymphatic drainage causes malabsorption of fats and highly lipophilic drugs. Thickening of mucosa and submucosa may reduce surface area and obstruct diffusion.
Diarrhea	Hypermotility and frequent passage of hypertonic liquid feces significantly affect drug absorption and release.
Antibiotic associated colitis	Overgrowth of *Clostridium difficile* and its toxin production that alters mucosal surface area may reduce drug absorption.
Constipation	Decreased peristaltic movement of bowel decreases diffusion and availability of drug at absorption sites. Severe constipation reduces bowel movement once or twice a week and interferes with the movement of formulations.
Gastroenteritis	Diarrhea due to increased mucosal secretion may affect the performance of formulations.
GIT infections	Diarrhea due to colonic protozoal and bacterial infections causes extremely low transit time and increased mucus production, interferes with localization of drug and absorption. Toxins produced may obstruct diffusion process.

Pharmaceutical Factors

Drug Candidates

Drugs which show poor absorption from the stomach or intestine including peptide drugs are most suitable for colon-specific drug delivery systems. The drugs used in the treatment of IBD, ulcerative colitis, diarrhea and colon cancer, are ideal candidates for the systems designed to specific drug colon delivery. Salfasalazine and 5-ASA are widely used drugs for the treatment of IBD and others include dexamethasone, prednisolone, hydrocortisone and budenoside. Various non-peptide and peptide drug candidates are listed in the Table 5.5.

Drug Carriers

The selection of carrier for particular drug candidate depends on the physiochemical nature of the drug as well as the disease for which the system is to be used. The factors such as chemical nature, stability and partition coefficient of the drug and the type of absorption enhancer chosen influence the carrier selection. Moreover, the choice of drug carrier depends on the functional groups of the drug molecule (Friend, 1991). For example, aniline or nitro groups on a drug may be used to link to another benzene group through an azo bond. The carriers, which contain additives like polymers (may be used as matrices and hydrogels or coating agents) may influence the release properties and efficacy of the systems.

TARGETING APPROACHES TO COLON

Polymer-based Approaches

Biodegradable Matrix and Hydrogel Systems

The inability to digest certain plant poly-saccharides by GIT enzymes is taken as an advantage to develop colon-specific drug delivery systems. The drug is embedded in the matrix core of the biodegradable polymer by compressing the blend of active drug, a degradable polymer and additives. Various polysaccharides such as pectin, guargum, chondroitine, etc. are being used for the purpose of colon targeting. The bacterial enzymes of colon degrade the carrier polymer

Table 5.5: Criteria for selection of drugs for colon-specific drug delivery system and various peptide and nonpeptide drugs (Antonin et al., 1992; Fara, 1989; Mackay and Tomlinson, 1993)

Criteria	Pharmacological class	Drug candidates	
		Nonpeptide drugs	Peptide drugs
1. Drugs used for local effects in colon against GIT diseases	Anti-inflammatory drugs	Oxyprenolol, metoprolol, nifedipine, diclofenac sodium, Ibuprofen, Isosorbides, theophylline, pseudoephedrine, bromophenaramine, 5-flourouracil, doxorubicin, nimustine, bleomycin, nicotine, dexamethasone, prednisolone, hydrocorti-sone, 5-aminosalicylic acid	Amylin, antisense oligo-nucleotide, calcitonin, cyclosporin, desmopressin. Epoetin, glucagon, gonadoreline, insulin, interferons, leuprolide, filgrastin, molgramoatim, protinelin, sermorelin, saloatonin, somatropin, urotoilitin, vasopressin
2. Drug poorly absorbed from upper GIT	Antihypertensive and antianginal drugs		
3. Drugs for colon cancer	Antineoplastic drugs		
4. Drug degrade in stomach and small intestine	Peptides and proteins		
5. Drugs undergo extensive first pass metabolism	Nitroglycerin and corticos-teroids		
6. Drugs need targeting	Antiarthritic and antiasthmatic drugs		

in a defined way to release the contents for localized colonic delivery or systemic absorption through colon (Hovgaard and Brondsted, 1996).

The gelling properties of pectin offer several advantages, including formation of viscous diffusional barriers and fermentability in the large intestine, which are collectively useful attributes in colon-specific drug delivery systems (Fig. 5.4) (Sriamornsak et al., 1997). Calcium pectinate is a lower water-soluble pectin salt used in colonic delivery systems. Calcium pectinate-indomethacin compressed tablets reportedly degraded by enzymes of aspergillus and colonic bacteria. Bacteroides ovatus (Rubinstein et al., 1993). Similarly, compression coated tablets comprised of natural pectin could protect the bio-susceptible core during GI transit (Ashford et al., 1993a, 1994).

Drug carriers consisted of natural and modified polysaccharide hydrogels swell following their hydration. The degree of swelling is an important property of the hydrogels. Initially, the·swollen hydrated polymer creates a diffusional barrier on the surface and eventually, allows the penetration of colonic enzymes, causing the degradation of polymer (Rubinstein and Gliko-Kabir, 1995). The swelling property therefore, limits the use of hydrogels for poorly water-soluble drugs and in case of highly water-soluble drugs, an addition of compressed polymer layer may be used to delay the diffusion of drug for longer time (Rubinstein and Radai, 1995).

Amidated pectins are more tolerant to pH variations and fluctuations in calcium levels yet remain susceptible for enzymatic degradation (Figs 5.5 and 5.6) (Wakerly et al., 1996).

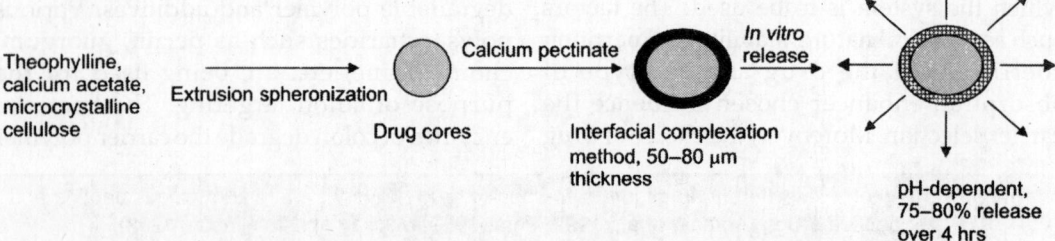

Fig. 5.4: pH dependent theophylline release from pectin based biodegradable matrix system

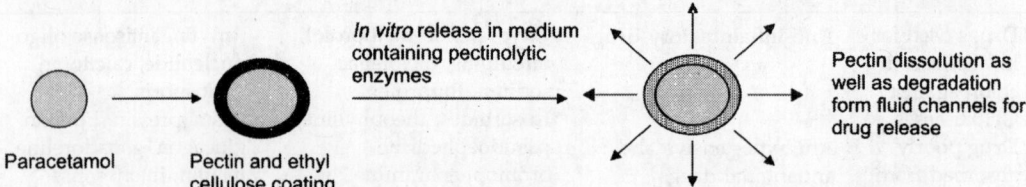

Fig. 5.5: Working principle of system based on pectin-ethyl cellulose combination

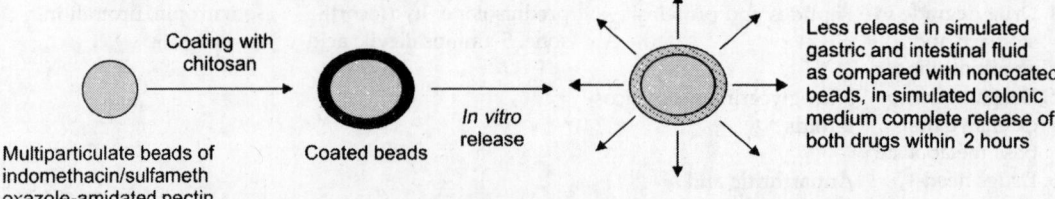

Fig. 5.6: Working principle of multiparticulate system based on amidated pectin

Inclusion of calcium as a cross-linking agent increases the viscosity of amidated pectin gels while the amidation of pectin affects the drug release rate due to matrix erosion.

Chondroitin sulfate is a soluble mucopolysaccharide (Fig. 5.7), generally used as a substrate for bacteria (Bacteroides and *B. ovatus*) in large intestine (Salyers, 1979). Chondroitin breakdown occurs by the enzyme chondroitin sulfate lyase. Natural chondroitin sulfate is cross-linked, because its higher water solubility. The hydrophilicity may be, however altered by varying the degree of cross-linking (Rubinstein et al., 1992).

Hydrogels with azo-aromatic cross-linking agents are developed to deliver drugs to the colon (Fig. 5.8) (Shanta et al., 1995). The swelling of hydrogels is increasing with increasing pH in alimentary tract initially, and swollen extensively in large intestine (alkaline pH), where the bacterial azoreductases degrade polymer. Various polymers such as cellobiose-derived monomers, carbopol 974P and copolymerized methacrylates have been explored and used for colon delivery of

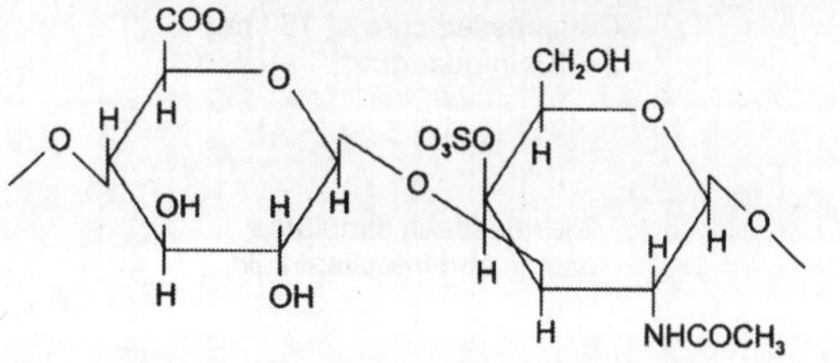

Fig. 5.7: Chemical structure of chondroitin sulfate

Mesalamine and 5-fluorouracil (Sintov et al., 1993).

Biodegradable hydrogels containing both acidic comonomers and enzymatically degradable azoaromatic cross-links were synthesized and evaluated (Fig. 5.9) for site-specific delivery of peptides, (e.g. insulin) into colon (Kopecek et al., 1992). In stomach (low pH), the gels demonstrate a low equilibrium degree of swelling and the entrapped drugs remain protected against digestion by enzymes. The degree of swelling moreover increases as the hydrogel passes down the GIT due to increased pH (Fig. 5.10). In colon, the hydrogels reach a degree of swelling that makes the cross-links accessible to azoreductase and

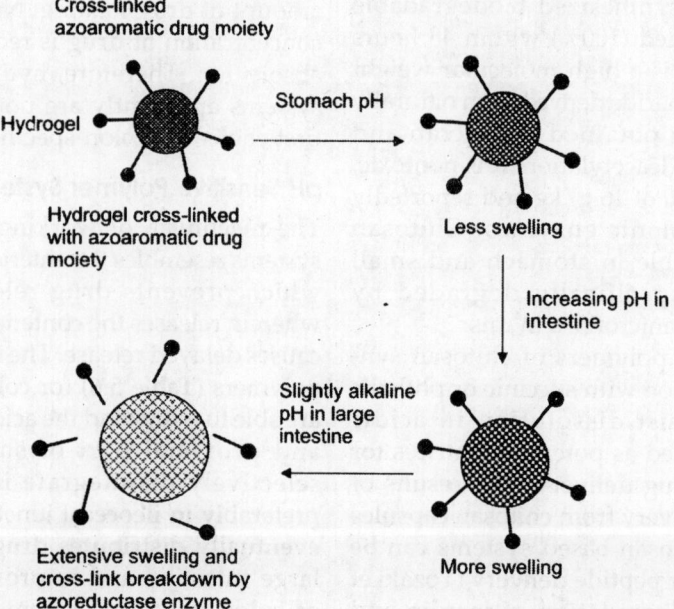

Cross-linked azoaromatic drug moiety

Hydrogel

Stomach pH

Hydrogel cross-linked with azoaromatic drug moiety

Less swelling

Increasing pH in intestine

Slightly alkaline pH in large intestine

Extensive swelling and cross-link breakdown by azoreductase enzyme

More swelling

Fig. 5.8: Working principle of system based on hydrogel-azoaromatic cross-linking

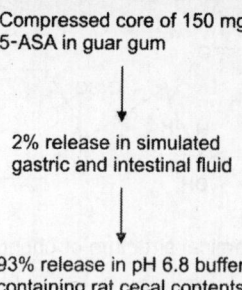

Compressed core of 150 mg
5-ASA in guar gum

↓

2% release in simulated
gastric and intestinal fluid

↓

93% release in pH 6.8 buffer
containing rat cecal contents

Fig.5.9: Schematic representation of biodegradable guar gum matrix system

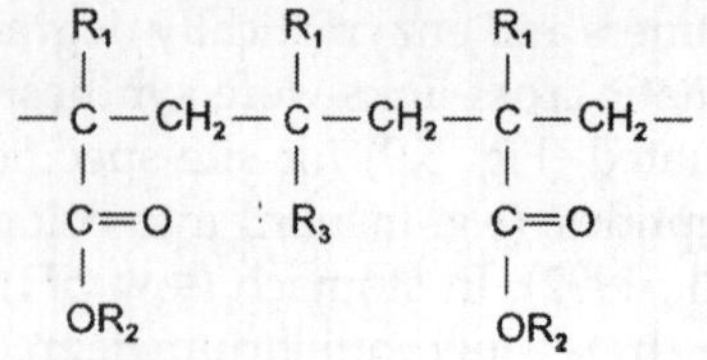

$$-\overset{\underset{\displaystyle |}{R_1}}{C}-CH_2-\overset{\underset{\displaystyle |}{R_1}}{C}-CH_2-\overset{\underset{\displaystyle |}{R_1}}{C}-CH_2-$$

$$\begin{matrix} C=O & \vdots & R_3 & & C=O \\ | & & & & | \\ OR_2 & & & & OR_2 \end{matrix}$$

R_1=CH$_3$; H
R_2=CH$_3$, CH$_3$CH$_2$–
R_3=COOH (Eudragit® L and S)
R_3=COOCH$_2$CH$_2$N+(CH$_2$)$_3$ Cl– (Eudragit® RL and RS)

Fig. 5.10: Structure of various Eudragit® polymers

other mediators. The rate of degradation essentially depends on the structure of hydrogels. The synthesized biodegradable hydrogels degraded (100%) within 48 hours *in vivo*. Chitosan is a high molecular weight cationic polysaccharide derived from naturally occurring chitin obtained from crab and shrimp shells by deacetylation. It is nontoxic, with an oral LD50 of 16 g/kg and reportedly degraded by colonic enzymes. Chitosan capsules are stable in stomach and small intestine, but specifically degraded by enzymes of cecal microflora in rats.

Semisynthetic polymers of chitosan synthesised by reaction with succinic or phthalic anhydrides, resist dissolution in acidic condition and used as potential matrices for colon-specific drug delivery. The results of insulin colon delivery from chitosan capsules suggest that chitosan based systems can be useful carriers for peptide delivery (Tozaki et al., 1997). The degradation of insulin and calcitonin in suspension of rat cecal contents

was compared. Calcitonin degraded faster than insulin; furthermore the insulin degradation was maximum at pH 6.8. Protease inhibitors like camestat and aprotinin found in large bowel prevent the degradation of insulin and calcitonin. This can improve the stability of peptides in large intestine as well as systemic absorption (Tozaki et al., 1997).

Directly compressed matrix tablets comprised of guar gum were developed (Fig. 5.12). Scintigraphic studies of guar gum matrix tablets containing tracer molecules, in human models showed that tracer on the surface of the tablet released in stomach and small intestine, and bulk of the tracer molecules released in colon. The tablets reached the colon in 2–4 hours (Krishnaiah et al., 1998).

Bacterial adherence retards the diffusion rate of salicylic acid through ethyl cellulose films and may interfere with drug release from biodegradable pectin films (Rubinstein et al., 1997). Hence, successful functioning of biodegradable systems depends on agitation and surface friction encounter in the lumen of colon. The major limitation of hydrogel based colon drug delivery system is the limited amount of drug loading. Nevertheless, more concentration of drug is required for colonic absorption. Therefore, hydrogel and matrix systems apparently are not the materials of first choice for colon-specific drug delivery.

pH Sensitive Polymer Systems

The mechnism of working of pH sensitive systems resembles the enteric coating of drugs, which prevents drug release in stomach wherein releases the contents in intestine thus causes delayed release. The ideal pH sensitive polymers (Table 5.6) for colon drug delivery are able to withstand the acidic pH of stomach and proximal part of small bowel, and selectively disintegrate in intestinal pH, preferably in ileocecal junction. This process eventually distributes drug throughout the large intestine and improves the potential of colon delivery systems. However, this approach is limited by the unpredictable

Table 5.6: Some properties of pH sensitive and biodegradable polysaccharides

pH sensitive polymers		Biodegradable polysaccharides	
Polymer	Threshold pH	Polysaccharide and its general use	Bacterial species that degrade polysaccharide
HPMC* phthalate	4.6–4.8	Amylose (tablet expient)	Bacteroides, Bifidobacterium
PVA** phthalate	6.0	Arabinogalactose (thickening agent)	Bifidobacteria
HPMC phthalate 50	5.2	Chitosan (absorption enhancing agent)	Bacteroides
HPMC phthalate 55	6.4	Cyclodextrins (solubilizing and	Bacteroides
Eudragit L-100	6.6	absorption enhancing agent)	Bacteroides
Aquateric	5.8	Chondroitin sulfate	Bacteroides
CA*** phthalate	6.0	Pectin (thickening agent)	Bacteroides, Bifidobacterium,
Eudragit L	6.0		Eubacterium
Eudragit S	6.8	Dextran (plasma expander)	Bacteroides
Shellac	7.2	Guar gum (thickening agent)	Bacteroides, Ruminococcus
CA Trimellitate	4.8	Xylan (plant hemicellulose)	Bacteroides, Bifidobacterium

*Hydroxy propyl methyl cellulose, **Polyvinyl acetate, ***Cellulose acetate

disintegration site due to gut motility. Moreover, small variations in pH caused by residues of bile acids, short chain fatty acids, carbon dioxide and fermentation products of colonic microflora affect the release properties of the system (Rubinstein, 1990). Therefore, pH-dependent polymers are not suitable for colon targeting because of poor site specificity.

Eudragit polymers (Fig. 5.10) are generally used for the development of colon-specific drug delivery systems. Eudragit-L and Eudragit-S are soluble at pH 6 and 7, respectively, hence they are used to make acid resistant film coating.

These polymers were used to develop systems containing drugs such as salsalzine, prednisolone, insulin and quinolones (Azad Khan et al., 1977; Thomas et al., 1985; Touitou and Rubinstein, 1986). Eudragit-S coated systems showed optimal delivery of insulin in ileum at pH 7 and could successfully deliver more than 60% of salfapyridine in colon (Dew et al., 1982). Partially methylated Eudragit-S soluble in slightly higher pH aqueous media, can be useful and effective for colon drug delivery (Peeters and Kinget, 1993).

Biodegradable Polymer Systems

The degrading ability of enzymes of microflora of the colon, particularly azoreductase activity is taken as an advantage for developing bacteria-biodegradable polymer (Table 5.6) coated drug delivery systems. These systems deliver drugs to the colon without releasing drug in small intestine. This is probably due to a minimum azoreductase activity found in small intestine to which these systems are susceptible. This approach totally depends on the metabolic activity of bacteria in colon, which is influenced by dietary fermentation precursors, coadministration of chemotherapeutic agents and type of food consumed (Scheline, 1973). The copolymers of styrene and hydroxy ethyl methacrylate, cross-linked with divinyl benzene and N, N'-bis- (styrene sulfonyl)-4, 4' diaminoazobenzene were used to coat insulin and vasopressin for oral delivery to rat colon (Saffran et al., 1991; Cheng et al., 1994). Glassy amylose and suspension of natural polygalactomannose in polymethacrylate are used to form biodegradable coating. The systems based on such coatings, selectively deliver drugs in large intestine following enzymatic degradation of swellable polymer layer. Polymethacrylate copolymers were used to strengthen the film forming properties of polygalactomannans.

Biodegradable azopolymers (Figs 5.11 and 5.12) (Kinget et al., 1998) with high hydrophilicity exhibit superior colon degradation

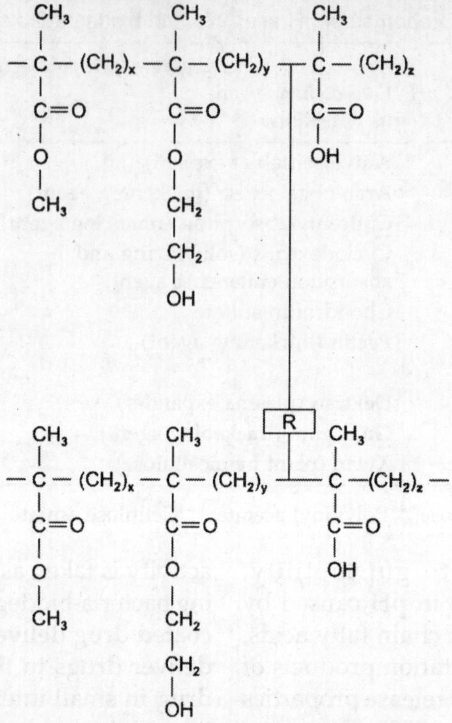

$$
\begin{array}{ccccc}
CH_3 & & CH_3 & & CH_3 \\
| & & | & & | \\
-C-(CH_2)_x- & C-(CH_2)_y- & C-(CH_2)_z \\
| & & | & & | \\
C=O & & C=O & & C=O \\
| & & | & & | \\
O & & O & & OH \\
| & & | & & \\
CH_3 & & CH_2 & & \\
& & | & & \\
& & CH_2 & & \\
& & | & & \\
& & OH & &
\end{array}
$$

$$\boxed{R}$$

$$
\begin{array}{ccccc}
CH_3 & & CH_3 & & CH_3 \\
| & & | & & | \\
-C-(CH_2)_x- & C-(CH_2)_y- & C-(CH_2)_z- \\
| & & | & & | \\
C=O & & C=O & & C=O \\
| & & | & & | \\
O & & O & & OH \\
| & & | & & \\
CH_3 & & CH_2 & & \\
& & | & & \\
& & CH_2 & & \\
& & | & & \\
& & OH & &
\end{array}
$$

Fig. 5.11: Chemical structure of biodegradable azopolymers, R-divinylbenzene, N.N'-bis-(methacryloylamino-azobenzene or N,N'-bis-(methacryloyloxyethyl)oxy(carbonylamino) azobenzene

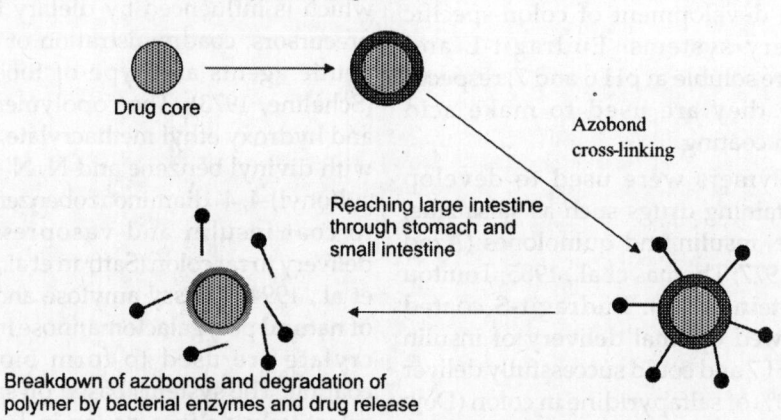

Methacrylate coating

Drug core

Azobond cross-linking

Reaching large intestine through stomach and small intestine

Breakdown of azobonds and degradation of polymer by bacterial enzymes and drug release

Fig. 5.12: Working principle of biodegradable azopolymer system

properties are used to coat capsules (Van den Mooter et al., 1992). The azopolymer-coated systems of theophylline and ibuprofen were studied in rats. The study concluded that the degree of hydrophilicity required is limited. Higher degree of hydrophilicity may cause the drug release from the system even before it reaches the colon.

Apart from azopolymers, galactomannan, which is degraded by glycolytic activity of colonic bacteria also implemented for colon drug delivery (Sarlikiotis and Bauer, 1992). Water insoluble film developed by the block polymer polyurethane with ethylated or acetylated galactomannan segments could effectively modulate the release of drugs in presence of human and pig colonic bacteria. The azopolymeric systems are not suitable for delivery of peptides, hormones and other drugs with a narrow therapeutic index, however, they are suitable for the local delivery of drugs to the colon. *In vitro* release of glutaraldehyde cross-linked dextran capsules was found to be 35% of administered drug after 24 hours (Brondsted et al., 1998). However, in simulated dextranase solution, capsules broke and as a result dose dumping occurred. Ester based dextran was also used to develop colon drug delivery systems. Mechanistic aspect of its working is depicted in Fig. 5.13. Film coating of ethyl cellulose and pectin showed that the release of drug depends on ethyl cellulose to pectin ratio. Eudragit® film coated insulin systems showed the degradation of insulin by bacteria in a degradation medium of fecal origin.

Bioadhesive Polymer Systems

When a system is coated with a bioadhesive polymer, it adheres to the wall of GIT and increases the residence time of the system, thereby improving the absorption possibilities. Despite the limited knowledge in anatomy and physiology of GIT, and attachment

site for bioadhesive systems, epithelial and mucosal adhesions are preferred as target sites (Veillard, 1989). The mucus layer is continuous on the surface as well as inside the lumen. Bioadhesive systems made up of various polymers such as polycarbophils, polyurethanes and polyethylene oxide-polypropylene oxide copolymers showed better adhesion in *in vitro* and to some extent *in vivo*.

Bioadhesive systems based on receptor mediated mechanisms, constitute another approach that essentially involve lectin. Sugar groups in mucus or on glycocalyx specifically interact and bind with plant lectins (Woodley and Naisbett, 1989). Apart from lectin, some bioadhesive microorganisms, which colonize in GIT are also exploited for the colon drug delivery. *E. coli* is able to adhere to small intestine by producing a protein (fimbriae) on the surface of organism. Fimbriae attached or coated on the surface of drug-loaded microspheres, allow it to adhere to mucus or cell wall of intestine and interact specifically with sugar groups in the mucus. The specific bioadhesive region of the fimbrial structure of *E. coli* was identified as film-H, which is characteristically polyvalent (Caston et al., 1990).

Systems Based on Particulate Ion Linking

High local concentrations of antiprotozoal drugs are required for protozoal infections of large intestine. A silica-nitroimidazole preparation which contained covalently bound drug on silica particles (5–10) was developed. The system in an experimental set up was

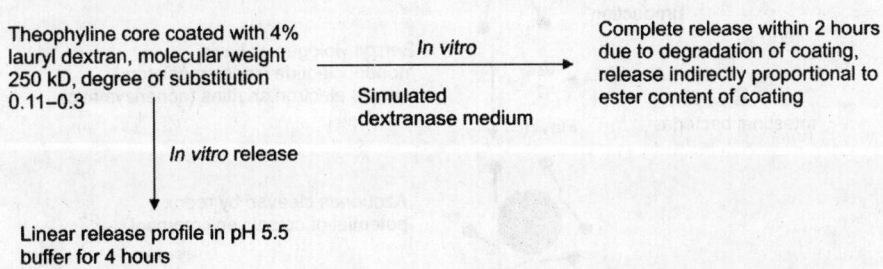

Theophyline core coated with 4% lauryl dextran, molecular weight 250 kD, degree of substitution 0.11–0.3 → *In vitro* Simulated dextranase medium → Complete release within 2 hours due to degradation of coating, release indirectly proportional to ester content of coating

In vitro release ↓

Linear release profile in pH 5.5 buffer for 4 hours

Fig. 5.13: Schematic representation of biodegradable ester based dextran system

phagocytosed and subsequently led to rapid cell death (Mirelman et al., 1989). The use of particulate carriers for colon-specific drug delivery is yet to be established. The colonic delivery using receptor-mediated cellular uptake may be explored for delivery of drug to or through specialized colonic cells.

Redox-sensitive Polymeric Systems

Novel polymers, which are hydrolyzed non-enzymatically by enzymatically produced flavins, are being used for colon targeting. The hydrolysis proceeds analogous to azobond cleavage by intestinal enzymes. Benzyl viologen and flavin mononucleotide (redox mediators) act as electron shuttles between the intracellular enzyme and extracellular substrate (Fig. 5.14) (Grim and Kopecek, 1991). Redox potential is an expression of total metabolic and bacterial activity in the colon and intestine that is determined by dietary changes. This microflora-induced change in redox potential can be used as a highly specific mechanism to target the colon. Based on the redox mechanism, systems bearing peptides coated with polymers cross-linked through azoaromatic groups were developed (Haste-Well et al., 1991). Insulin and vasopressin were incorporated in such systems, which could protect the drugs in stomach and large intestine and release them after the reduction of azobond, by the microflora present in large intestine.

Apart from azobonds, disulfide bonds can also be cleaved by redox potential of colon (Larsen et al., 1983). Various systems comprised of disulfide linkage in drug cysteine conjugates, noncross-linked redox sensitive polymers containing azo/disulfide linkage and novel polyurethane with azobonds (as coated preparation) were developed for colon-specific drug delivery (Kimura et al., 1992).

Prodrug-based Approaches

A prodrug is a pharmacologically inactive derivative of a parent compound that requires spontaneous or enzymatic conversion within the body in order to release active drug with improved release properties over the parent compound. Specific properties such as pH variation or activity of enzymes of particular sites are taken into consideration which could effect the prodrug conversion into drug. Prodrugs can be designed to release drugs systematically in specific organs and tissues such as kidneys, brain, eyes, breast and skin.

Numerous enzymes such as azoreductase, glycosidase and cyclodextrinase produced by bacterial flora have been studied and exploited for site-specific colon targeting with prodrugs. The choice of carrier is determined by the functional groups available on the drugs. For example, aniline groups on a drug (5-ASA) may be used to link another benzene ring group via an azobond. Thus, amino group on 5-ASA is diazotized to benzene-containing

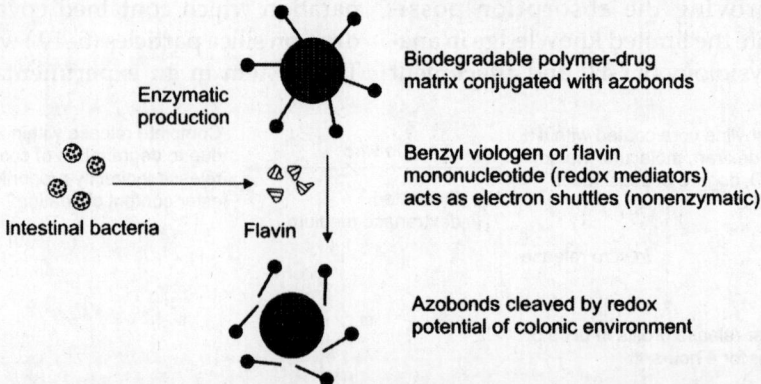

Fig. 5.14: Release mechanism of system based on redox-sensitive polymers

compounds. This approach is limited to only aniline group containing drugs. Drugs like corticosteroids, which normally possess hydroxyl groups, can be derivatized to glycoside compounds; are suitable candidates for colon-specific delivery. Carboxylic groups can be linked to dextran using carbodiimide (Friend, 1991).

Azobond Prodrugs

Low Molecular Weight Azobond Prodrugs

Salfasalazine is composed of sulfapyridine, which has antibacterial activity while 5-ASA, possesses anti-inflammatory activity, both linked through an azo bond (Azad Khan, 1982). In this case, salfasalazine is 'prodrug', salfapyridine is an intestinal 'carrier' to release active drug 5-ASA at the site of action (Fig. 5.15). In another approach, olsalazine (1 mole), which is a dimer of 5-ASA linked via an azo bond, reaches large intestine, cleaves to release 5-ASA (2 moles) (Fig. 5.16). The absorption of intact prodrugs in GIT is very limited. Clinical

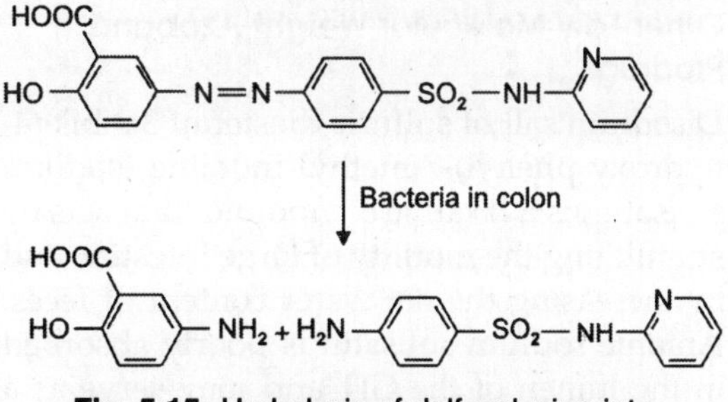

Fig. 5.15: Hydrolysis of dalfasalazine into 5-aminosalicylic acid and salfapyridine

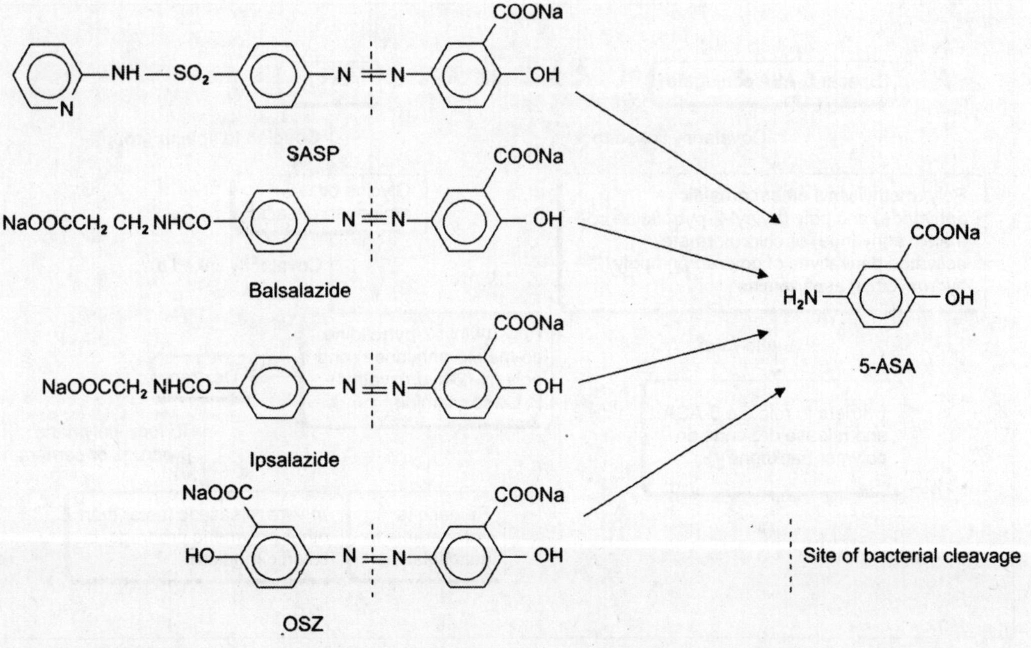

studies showed that an intact GIT and a normal microflora are required for the effective bio-cleavage or splitting of olsalazine, moreover, watery diarrhea is the major side effect as recorded in about 15% of patients (Rao et al., 1987). A second azo bond prodrug is balsalazide, in which 5-ASA is azolinked to 4-aminobenzoyl-alanine. This carrier prodrug is less toxic and poorly absorbed in upper part of GIT till it reaches colon, where it is reduced to release 5-ASA. Ipsalazide is an another prodrug carrier for 5-ASA (McIntyre et al., 1988).

Fig. 5.16: Chemical structures of sodium salfasalazine (SASP), balsalazide, ipsalazide and olzalazine (OSZ) showing the site of bacterial cleavage leading to liberation of active agent 5-ASA

Other Low Molecular Weight Azobond Prodrugs

Disodium salt of sulfuric diester of 3,3-bis-(4-hydroxy phenyl)-7-methyl indoline (sodium sulisatin) is a laxative compound, that acts by stimulating the motility of large intestine and by increasing the net water content of feces. Anionic sodium sulisatin is poorly absorbed in the lumen of the GIT and may serve as a prodrug. It passes through stomach, small intestine and eventually on reaching large intestine, it hydrolyzes by bacterial aryl sulfate sulfohydrolase to form DHMI. DHMI is a diphenolic derivative and also an active agent, which was confirmed by experiments carried out in rats (Moreto et al., 1979).

Polymer-based Azobond Prodrugs

Instead of using low molecular weight promoities, macromolecular carriers are used to deliver 5-ASA to colon. The large molecular size of polymers limit the absorption in upper GIT, moreover, polymeric carriers can accommodate large dose of drugs for local as well as systemic drug delivery.

Polymer based prodrugs have been developed by using a spacer coupling with 5-ASA via 5-amino functional group by an azobond. The synthesis and release of some prodrug are schematically presented in Fig. 5.17.

The relatively slow release of these prodrugs can be compensated by some bioadhesive polymeric prodrug systems. 5-ASA bioadhesive polymeric prodrugs containing fucosylamine (Fig. 5.18) were developed on the basis of glucose and fucose-specific adhesion mechanism of bacteria to the colon cells of guinea pigs (Rihova, 1995; Kopeckova and Kopecek, 1990). Increase rate of reduction of azobonds by the addition of redox mediator (benzyl viologen) leads to zero order release of 5-ASA however, the rate of reduction remains comparable with low molecular weight compounds. Hydrophilic binding of aromatic side chain in the polymeric backbone and delivery to colon mucosa may have a greater

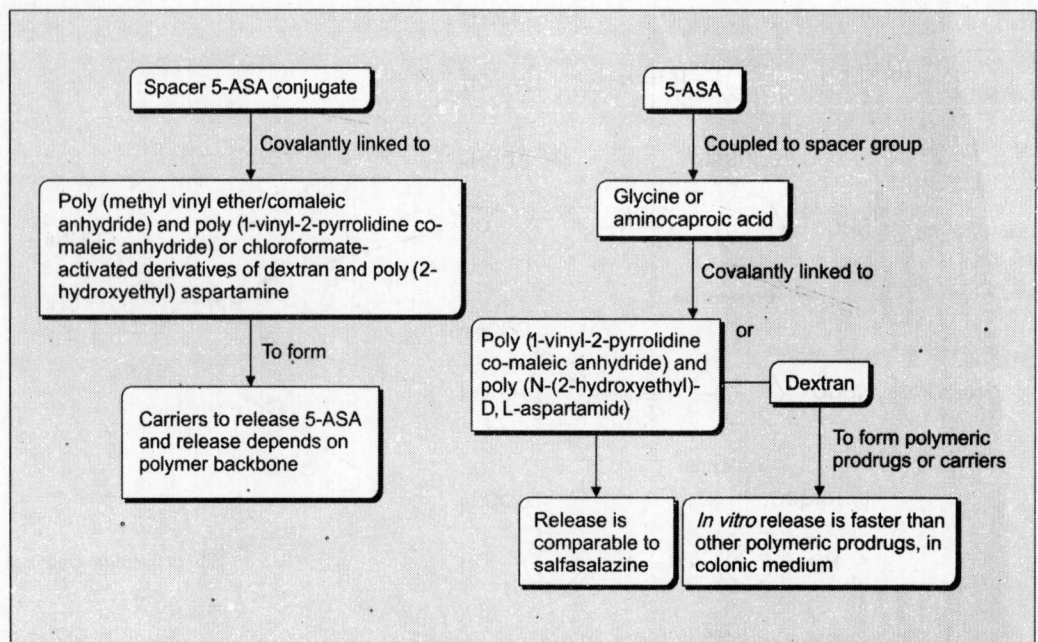

Fig. 5.17: Schematic representation of preparation and properties of 5-ASA polymeric prodrugs (Schacht et al., 1991, 1996)

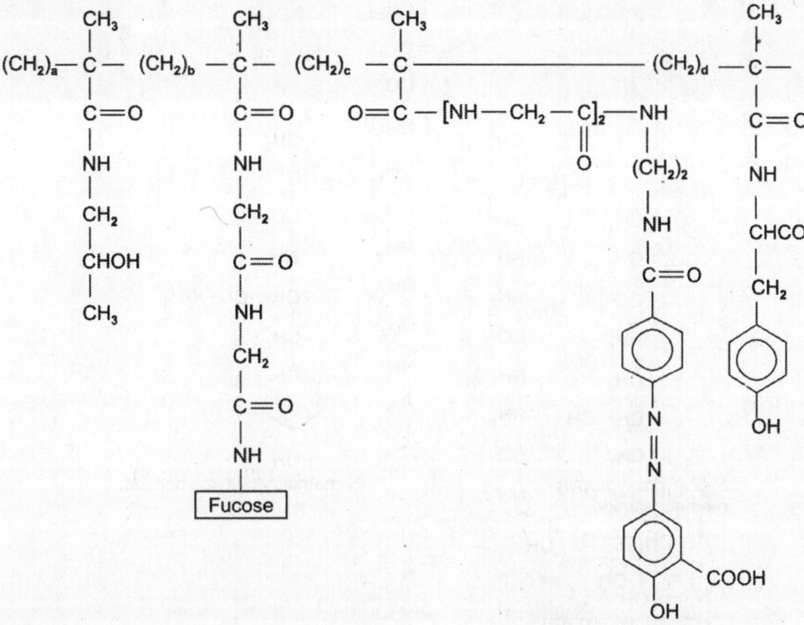

Fig. 5.18: Chemical structure of 5 -ASA polymeric prodrug of N-(2-hydroxypropyl) methacrylamide containing fucosylamine

effect than the specific recognition of native fucosylamine groups. Major limitation of polymer based azobond prodrug is the coupling of drug to polymer requires a large amount of drug. Therefore, drugs with large dose volume are not ideal candidates for these systems.

Newer acrylic type polymeric systems comprised of degradable ester or amide bonds linked to 5-ASA, have been developed for colon drug delivery (Davaran et al., 1999). The hydrolytic behavior of polymers mainly depends on their degree of swelling, type of comonomer used and the nature of hydrolyzable bond. A water-soluble polymer (polyasa) consisted of salicylate residues azo-linked at the fifth position to the polymeric backbone and polysulfonamide ethylene, is used to develop some colon-specific drug delivery systems.

Kopeckova et al., (1994) evaluated N-(2-hydroxypropyl) methacrylamide (HPMA) copolymers as colon-specific drug carriers (Fig. 5.19). These carriers designed for site-specific (5-ASA) release of the drug following enzymatic degradation or fragmentation of carrier polymer by the microbial azoreductase

of the colon. They synthesized a new 5-ASA containing monomer and incorporated into the comonomer together with the fucosylamine (bioadhesive moiety). The synthesis was conducted using free radical copolymerization. The in vitro release rate of 5-ASA from HPMA copolymers following azoreductase activity in guinea pig cecum was approximately 2.5 times slower compared to a low molecular weight analog. Both *in vitro* and *in vivo*, HPMA copolymer containing side chains terminated in fucosylamine, showed a higher degree of adherence to guinea pig colon when compared to HPMA copolymer without fucosylamine moieties. The incorporation of 5-ASA containing aromatic side chains into HPMA polymers further increased their bioadherence probably by combination of nonspecific hydrophobic binding with specific recognition.

Glycoside Conjugated Prodrugs

The glycosidases produced by human microflora are D-galactosidase, L-arabinofuranosidase, D-xylopyranosidase and D-glucosidase.

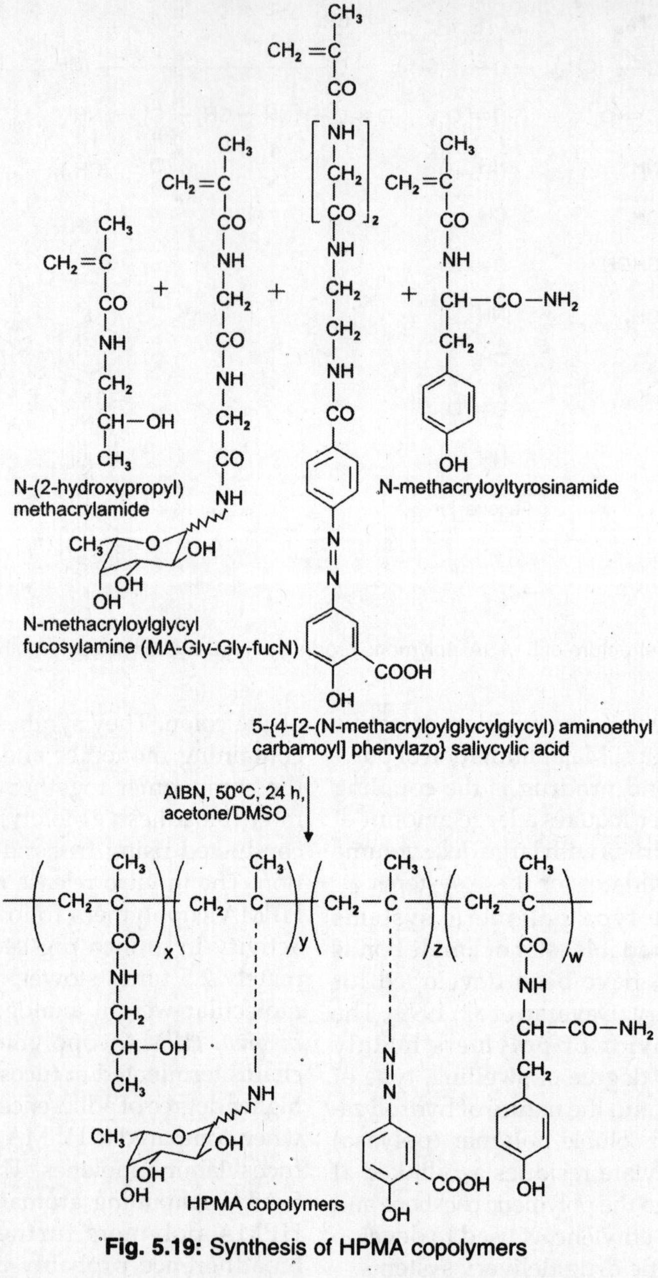

Fig. 5.19: Synthesis of HPMA copolymers

These are found in human feces (Friend, 1992). Particularly, glucosidase and glucuronidase activity is extensive in human microflora. These enzymes are located at the brush border and relatively accessible to the substrate. Various plant drugs are glycosides, upon oral administration, they reach colon through stomach and intestine. In colon, they are cleaved by glycosidases of microflora, to liberate aglycon, the active constituent that acts on colon. Plant drug glycosides are highly hydrophilic and poorly absorbed from stomach and small intestine and eventually reach colon, where they are cleaved by glycosidases. On the basis of this mechanism, numerous prodrugs of dexamethasone, prednisolone and hydrocortisone with D-galactosides and D-glucosides were synthesized (Friend and Chang, 1984).

Dexamethasone-glucoside conjugate is one of the examples for these prodrugs (Table 5.7). Tozer and coworkers (1991) studied the distribution and recovery of dexamethasone glucoside following oral administration to guinea pigs and some results are shown in Fig. 5.20.

Glucuronide Conjugated Prodrugs

Glucuronide conjugation is one of the major metabolic pathways of drugs (e.g. inactivation of naloxone by forming drug-glucuronide conjugate) glucuronidase secreted from large intestine, deglucuronidate many drugs. This concept can be used to develop colon-specific drug delivery systems. Prodrugs such as dexamethasone-D-glucuronide, naloxone and nalmefene glucuronide conjugates were developed and evaluated for colon delivery (Fujimoto, 1970). The conjugates are deglucuronidated by glucuronidase in large intestine and as a result active drug is released for local action or systemic reabsorption. Budenoside and dexamethasone conjugates of glucuronic acid and dextran prodrugs were synthesized for the treatment of ulcerative colitis (McLead et al., 1994). These prodrugs release drugs in large intestine, thereby reducing systemic toxicity (adrenal suppression) of corticosteroids. The problems associated with D-glucuronidase activity are (Danovitch et al., 1972):

1. D-glucuronidase activity is located in intracellular compartment (lysozyme) that is inaccessible to its substrates.
2. The hydrolysis of D-glucuronides in the luminal contents by mammalian D-glucuronidase is insignificant.

Dextran Conjugated Prodrugs

Most of the prodrugs of dextran synthesized with NSAIDs, are directly coupled to dextran by using carboxylic groups present in the drugs. *In vitro* release of naproxen from dextran prodrug is 17-fold higher in cecum and colon homogenate of the pig than the homogenate of small intestine (Larsen et al., 1989). Dextran prodrugs of methyl prednisolone and dexamethasone were synthesized and evaluated. They reached large intestine and colon, where dextranases and esterases liberate the active drug (Mcleod et al., 1993). The compounds which do not possess carboxylic groups such as anti-inflammatory corticosteroids, are chemically derived to glucocorticoid carbonates, benzyl alcohol carbonates and metronidazole hemisters (Mcleod et al., 1994). Succinic acid is generally used as a spacer molecule to synthesize corticosteroid-dextran conjugate or prodrug.

Cyclodextrin Conjugated Prodrugs

Cyclodextrins are cyclic oligosaccharides consisted of 6–8 dextrose units (cyclodextrins)

Table 5.7: Pharmacokinetic parameter values (mean S.D.) of dexamethasone conjugated D-glucoside and plain dexamethasone (Del Soldato et al., 1985; Gallone et al., 1980)

Intravenous administration Animal : Guinea pigs						Oral administration
Terminal half-life (h)	Mean residence time (h)	Volume of distribution (L/kg) Terminal phase	Steady state	Clearance (L/h/kg) unchanged	Fraction excreted	Bioavailability
Dexamethasone conjugated D-glucosidase						
0.26 ± 0.02	0.27 ± 0.02	0.76 ± 0.40	0.57 ± 0.25	2.00 ± 0.91	0.97 ± 0.11	<0.01
Dexamethasone						
1.82 ± 0.18	2.58 ± 0.28	1.43 ± 0.33	1.43 ± 0.32	0.55 ± 0.13	0.20	1.12

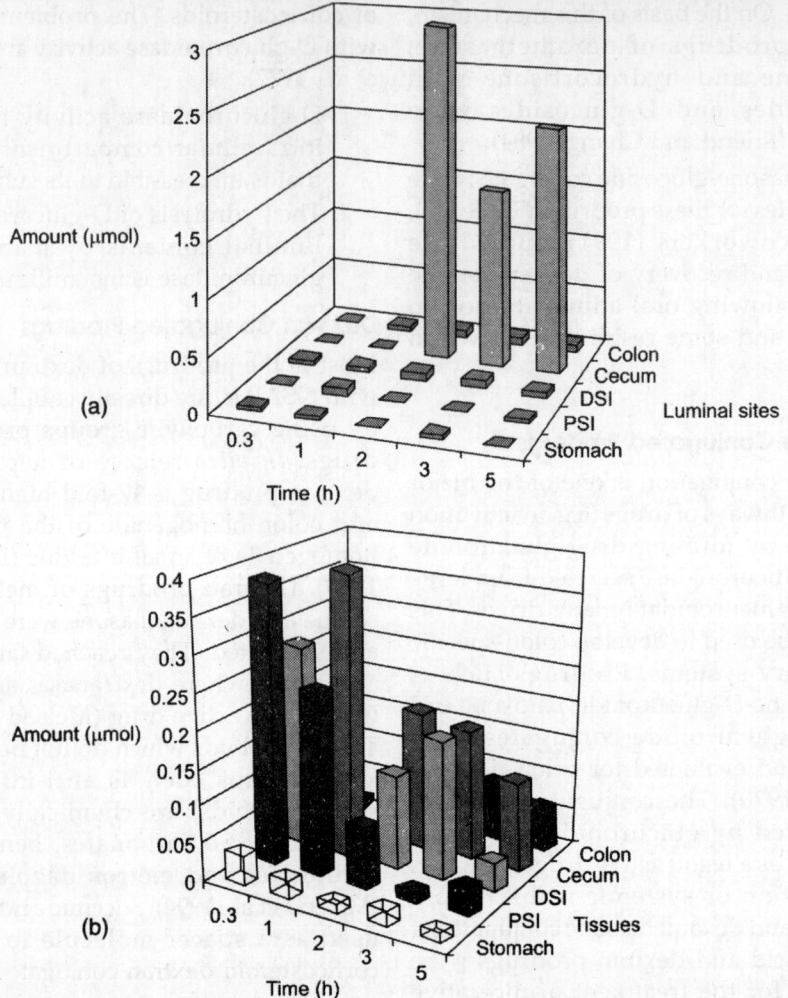

Fig. 5.20: Amount (μmol) formed and remaining in the luminal contents (a) and tissues (b) of the GIT of fasted guinea pig at various times after gastric incubation of 54.1 μmol/kg of dexamethasone-D-glucoside. Dexamethasone appears in the lumen of the large intestine by 2 hours. The drug appears in the tissues of both the large and small intestine, a result of high hydrolytic activity in the contents of cecum and colon and perhaps the high glucosidase activity of the small intestine brush border (Tozer et al., 1991)

linked through 1–4 bonds (Fig. 5.21) (Irie and Uekama, 1997) (Table 5.8). They are well-accepted pharmaceutical carriers as they are stable against nonenzymatic and enzymatic degradation in body fluids and tissue homogenates. Moreover, they possess appreciable biocompatibility ensuring *in vivo* safety. Cyclodextrins readily form inclusion complexes with many drugs since the interior of the molecules is relatively lipophilic and exterior is hydrophilic. The complexes are in equilibrium with aqueous medium. The cyclodextrin absorption from GIT is relatively less due to its bulky and hydrophilic nature. They are used as drug carriers for some drugs, which are released in aqueous fluid and remain in GIT. The cyclodextrins are more resistant to gastric, salivary and pancreatic

Table 5.8: Physiochemical properties of cyclodextrins (Reddy et al., 1999)

Property	α-cyclodextrin	β-cyclodextrin	γ-cyclodextrin
Molecular weight	973	1135	1297
Glucose residues	6	7	8
Aqueous solubility (g/100 ml)	14.5	1.85	23.2
Melting point (°C)	276	280	275
pK_a	12.3	12.2	12.1
Enzymatic hydrolysis (by bacterial-amylase)	Negligible	Slow	Rapid
Half-life of ring opening (h) in 1N HCl at 60°C	6.2	6.4	3.0

enzymes as well as gastric pH than cyclo-dextrin, which is slowly digested in small intestine, but completely degraded by colonic microflora.

Hydrophilic cyclodextrins are used to formulate controlled release preparations of many water-soluble drugs including peptides and proteins (Hirayama et al., 1996). Synthesis, properties and *in vitro* evaluation of bip-

henylyl acetic acid (an anti-inflammatory drug) cyclodextrin conjugated prodrug, are given schematically in Fig. 5.21.

Various esters and amide-linked biphenylyl acetic acid α or β or γ cyclodextrin conjugates demonstrated potential to deliver drugs to colon and may also be used to develop delayed release systems (Fig. 5.22). Chemical derivatization of cyclodextrins (xenobiotics,

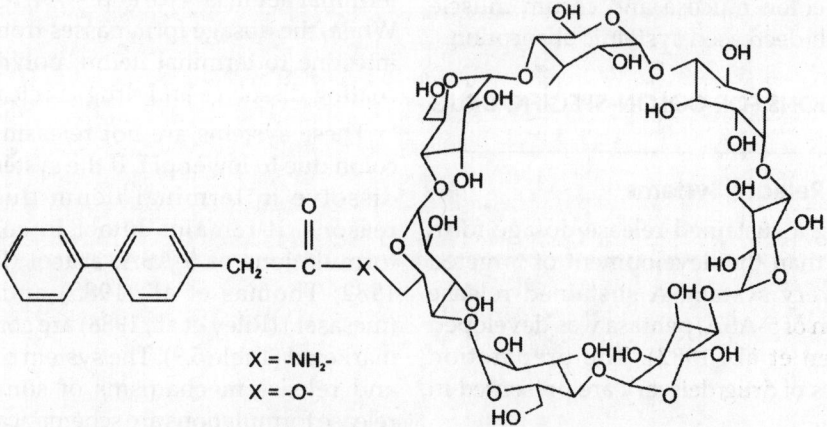

X = -NH₂-
X = -O-

Fig. 5.21: Structure of biphenyl acetic acid-cyclodextrin conjugates

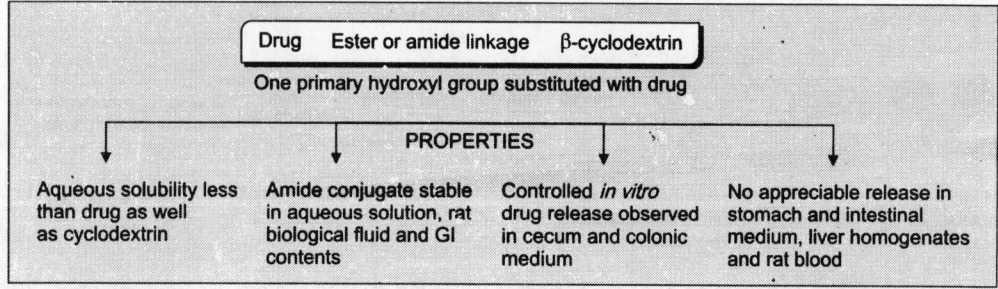

Fig. 5.22: Properties of ester or amide-type drug conjugate of β-cyclodextrin (Hirayama et al., 1996)

e.g. epichlorhydrin-DM-cyclodextrin and HP-cyclodextrin-drug conjugates) are more resistant to intestinal hydrolases, hence absorption is very low and it is almost completely excreted in the faeces.

Polypeptide Conjugated Prodrugs

Some enzymes of gut microflora are able to cleave certain peptide and ester bonds. Despite the systemic side effects, glucocorticoids are used in the treatment of severe inflammatory bowl diseases (IBD). Prodrug approach can deliver glucocorticoids in colon and may reduce the required dose of drug as well as its side effects. Poly (L-aspartic acid) conjugate of dexamethasone was synthesized and evaluated for the selective release in large intestine (Leopold and Friend, 1995). The study concluded that significantly higher localized concentration of drug is attained in cecum, colon mucosa and cecum muscle tissues with decreased systemic absorption.

FORMULATIONS FOR COLON-SPECIFIC DRUG DELIVERY

Sustained Release Systems

Developing a sustained release dosage form is simpler than the development of targeted drug delivery system. A sustained release formulation of 5-ASA, pentasa was developed (Rasmussen et al., 1982). The preparation and process of drug delivery are presented in Fig. 5.23.

Pentasa shows little localization in colon, but enough amount of drug is released in colon, which enables effective treatment of IBD. The drawbacks of Pentasa are;

1. Under normal transit conditions drug release is 100%, but accelerated transit conditions during IBD drug release reduced to 88%.

2. 5-ASA is unstable in gastric juice and fastly absorbed from small intestine. The absorbed drug is not available for the local action. So, 5-ASA delivery by azobond drugs is superior to the sustained release dosage forms.

Delayed and Timed Release Dosage Forms

Various delayed release dosage forms of 5-ASA have been developed based on the pH gradient of GIT. Eudragit-S polymer, soluble in pH above 7 is used to develop such systems. The pH of proximal small intestine and terminal ileum is ≈ 6.6 and ≈ 7.4, respectively. While, the dosage form passes from proximal intestine to terminal ileum, polymer enteric coating dissolves and drug is released.

These systems are not releasing drugs to colon due to lower pH. If the system does not dissolve in terminal ileum due to some reasons, it remains intact in colon. Some formulations of 5-ASA, asacol (Dew et al., 1982; Thomas et al., 1985) and claversal (mesasal) (Riley et al., 1988) are commercially marketed (Table 5.9). The system components and release mechanisms of some delayed release formulations are schematically presented in Fig. 5.24. Osmet, a miniature osmotic pump releases drugs over 8 hours in colon

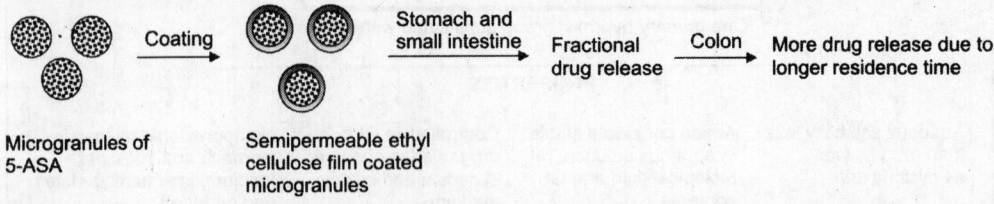

Fig. 5.23: Preparation and working principle of pentasa delayed release system (Rasmussen et al., 1982)

Table 5.9: Marketed colon-specific drug delivery systems for the treatment of ulcerative colitis and Crohn's disease (Hawkey et al., 1992; Dipirio et al., 1989)

Drugs	Dose	Formulation	Trade name	Presentation
Sulfasalazine	Either 1–2 or 2–4 g daily	5-ASA linked to sulfapyridine	Azulfidine and salazopyrin	500 mg tablets
Olsalazine	1 g/day	5-ASA dimer	Dipentum	250 mg capsules and 500 mg tablets
Mesalazine	1.5–4 g daily	Controlled release ethyl cellulose coated pellets. Eudragit-S coated tablets	Pentaza	250 mg tablets
		Eudragit-L coated tablets Eudragit-L 100 coated tablets	Asacol	400 mg tablets
			Salotalic Claversal and Mesasal	250 mg tablets Tablets (250 and 400 mg)
Budenoside	9 mg/day	Controlled-release capsules	Entocort	3 mg capsules

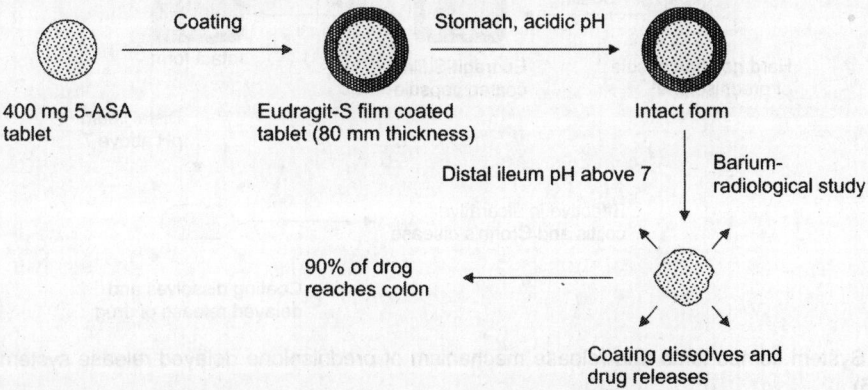

Fig. 5.24: Preparation and working principle of asacol delayed release system (Dew et al., 1982; Riley et al., 1988)

after passing through stomach and small intestine in intact form.

Numerous timed-release release systems such as pulsincap (Fig. 5.25), time clock (Fig. 5.26) and time-controlled explosion (Fig. 5.27), ethyl cellulose system (Fig. 5.28), two-layer system (Fig. 5.29), and multiple-coated system (Fig. 5.30) are discussed in the literature. The components and working principles of these systems are presented in Figs 5.31 to 5.33.

A multiparticulate system ordansetron and budenoside loaded cellulose acetate butyrate

(CAB) microspheres coated with Eudragit-S, were prepared (Rodriguez et al., 1998). The variation in hydrophobic CAB polymer concentration (6 and 8%) influenced the drug release rate. The microspheres remained intact in stomach while reaching small intestine, the enteric coat dissolved releasing the drug.

Clinical Evaluation of Colon-specific Drug Delivery Systems

Colonic drug delivery systems are developed for the treatment of various diseases such as ulcerative colitis, colonic cancer and Crohn's

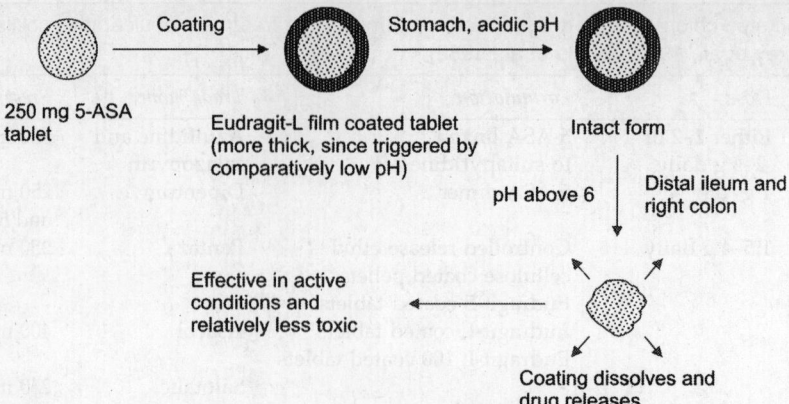

Fig. 5.25: Preparation and working principle of claversal delayed release system (Rutgeerts, 1989; Rachmilewitz, 1988)

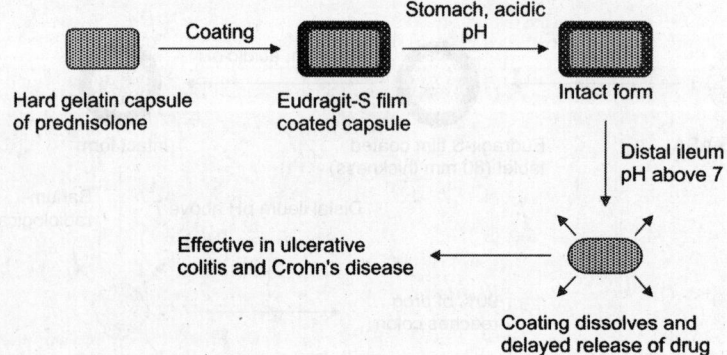

Fig. 5.26: System components and release mechanism of prednisolone delayed release system (Thomas et al., 1985)

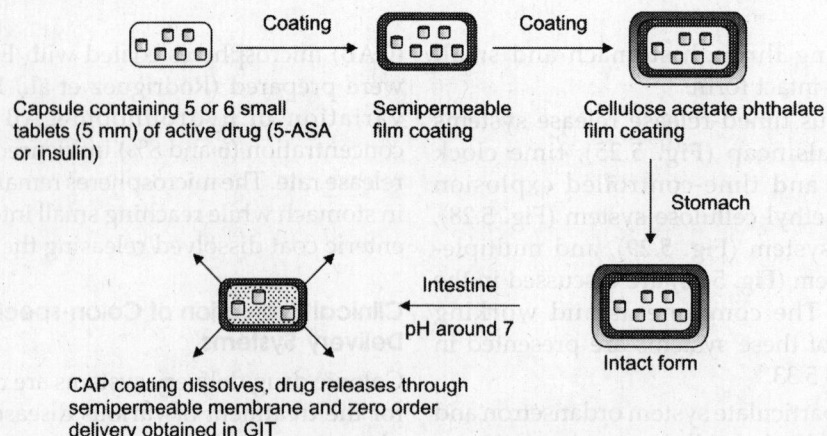

Fig. 5.27: Preparation and release mechanism of Oros-CT delayed release system (Theeuwes et al., 1991)

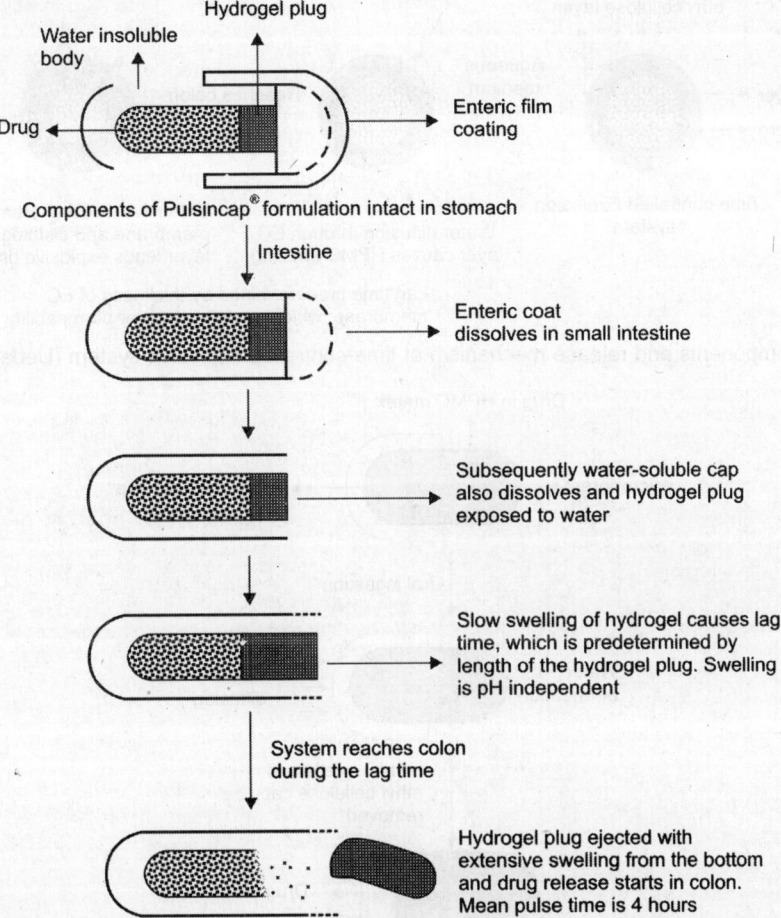

Fig. 5.28: Components and working principle of Pulsincap® time-dependent release system (MacNeil et al., WO 9009168)

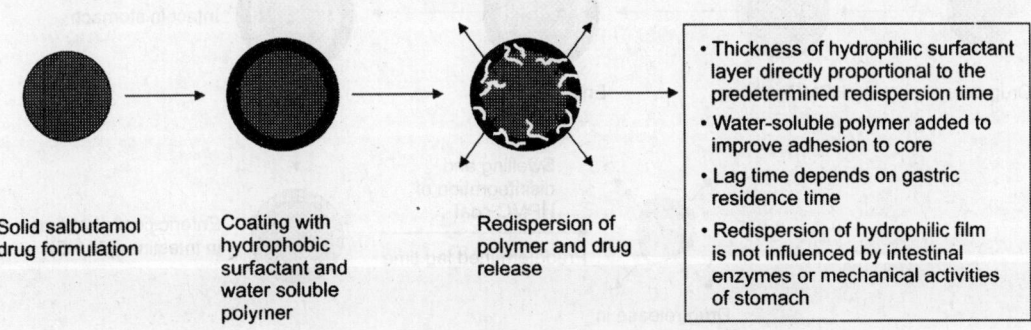

Fig. 5.29: Components and working principle of time clock (Pozzi et al., 1994)

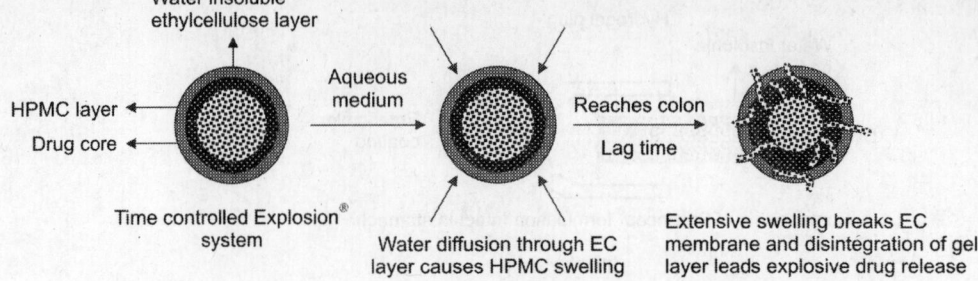

Fig. 5.30: Components and release mechanism of time-controlled explosive system (Ueda et al., 1994)

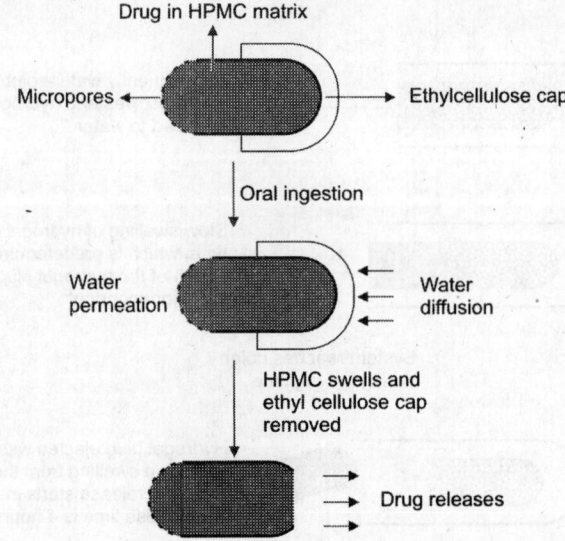

Fig. 5.31: Components and working principle of ethylcellulose capsule system (Niwa et al., 1995)

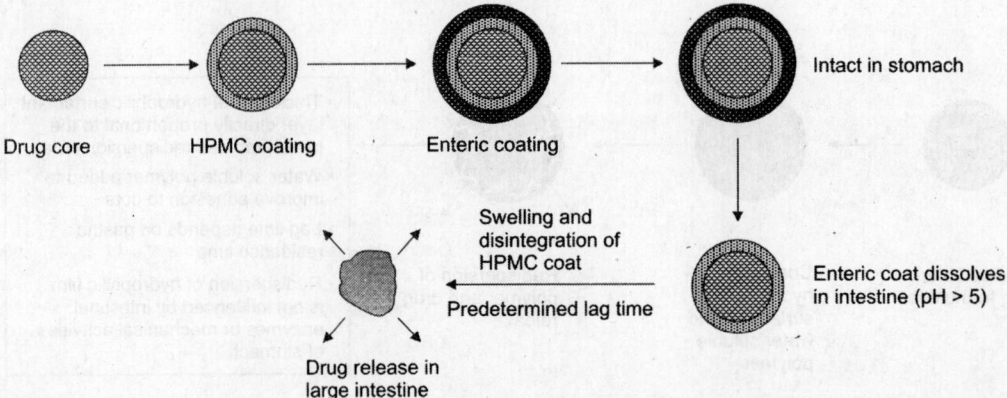

Fig. 5.32: Components and release mechanism of two-layered polymer system (Gazzaniga et al., 1994)

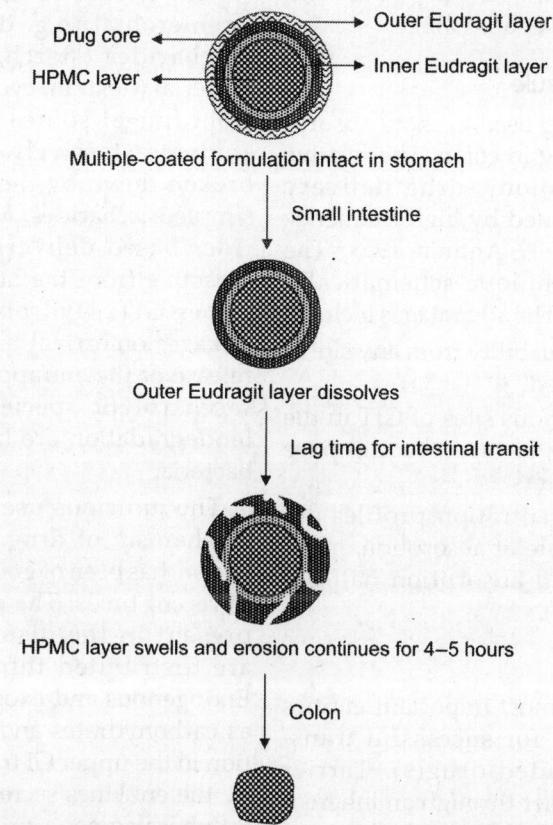

Drug core

HPMC layer

Outer Eudragit layer

Inner Eudragit layer

Multiple-coated formulation intact in stomach

Small intestine

Outer Eudragit layer dissolves

Lag time for intestinal transit

HPMC layer swells and erosion continues for 4–5 hours

Colon

Inner Eudragit layer dissolves (pH around 7) and drug releases

Fig. 5.33: Components and release mechanism of delayed-release multiple coated tablet formulation (Reddy et al., 1999)

disease as well as to increase the systemic uptake of peptides and hydrophilic drugs. The absorption of drugs from these systems is monitored by colonoscopy and intubation. The pharmacokinetic data obtained from systems can be used to evaluate absorption properties indirectly (Lee, 1992). Currently, scintigraphy and high frequency capsules are the most preferred techniques employed to evaluate colon drug delivery systems.

γ-Scintigraphy

By using scintigraphic technique, the transit of dosage form through the GIT can be monitored. The formulations are additionally comprised of emitting radionuclides coentrapped with drugs and the images of distributed radiotracer within the body, are captured by camera. The radiations emerge from the subject is collimated and detected by a crystal. The energy is transformed to light scintillation and amplified to give digitalized results (Ashford et al., 1993a, 1993b). This technique is noninvasive and even low level radiation in patients can be measured and monitored. The gastric emptying of dosage forms and transit of food also can be precisely followed. Visualization of the drug delivery process also possible with this technique (Ishibashi et al., 1998). Study conducted using scintigraphy showed that out of 36 tablets administered orally to 6 human subjects, 50% of capsules reached colon in 5 hours, 72% in 8 hours and 89% in 12 hours (Dew et al., 1982).

High-frequency Capsule

This technique is being used to check absorption properties of drug in colon. The relative bioavailability of colonic-drug delivery systems can be evaluated by high-frequency capsule (Staib et al., 1989; Antinin, 1993). The principle of this technique schematically presented in Fig. 5.34. The advantages include:

1. The relative bioavailability from any site of GIT can be evaluated.
2. Drug release at various sites of GIT in the same subject may be used to compare absorption parameters.
3. Plasma-drug concentration profiles are used to calculate rate of absorption, mean residence time and absorption half-life (Harder et al., 1990).

Carrier Systems

Carrier is one of the most important entities essentially required for successful transportation of the loaded drug(s). Carrier systems can do so either through an inherent characteristics or acquired (through structural modification), to interact selectively with biological targets, or otherwise they are engineered to release the drug in the proximity of target cells in need of an optimal pharmacological action.

Biodegradable Polysaccharide Carriers

The polysaccharides naturally occurring in plant (e.g. pectin, guar gum, inulin, locust bean gum, glucomannan, Khaya and Albizia gums), animal (e.g. chitosan, chondroitin sulfate, hyaluronic acid), algae (e.g. alginates), or microbial (e.g. dextran), starch polysaccharides (starch, amylase, cellulose), bacterial (dextran, cyclodextrin, curdlan) and from fungal source (sceleroglucan), were studied extensively previously. These are broken down by the colonic microflora to simple saccharides. Most of the polysaccharides based delivery systems protect the bioactive from the hostile conditions of the upper GIT. Hydrolysis of the glycosidic linkages on arrival in the colon, triggers the release of the entrapped bioactive. The main saccharolytic species responsible for this biodegradation are bacteroides and bifidobacteria.

The judicious use of GI microflora as a mechanism of drug release in the colonic region, has been of great interest to researchers in recent times. The majority of bacteria are present in the distal gut, although they are distributed throughout the GI tract. Endogenous and exogenous substrates, such as carbohydrates and proteins escape digestion in the upper GI tract, but are metabolized by the enzymes secreted by colonic bacteria. Sulphasalazine, a prodrug consisting of the active ingredient mesalazine, was the first bacteria-sensitive delivery system designed to deliver the drug to the colon. The use of polysaccharides offers an alternative substrate for the bacterial enzymes present in the colon. Most of the polymers are used in pharmaceutical compositions and regarded as safe (GRAS) excipients. Pectin alone and in combination with other polymers has been studied for colon-specific drug delivery. Pectin, when used alone, is needed in large

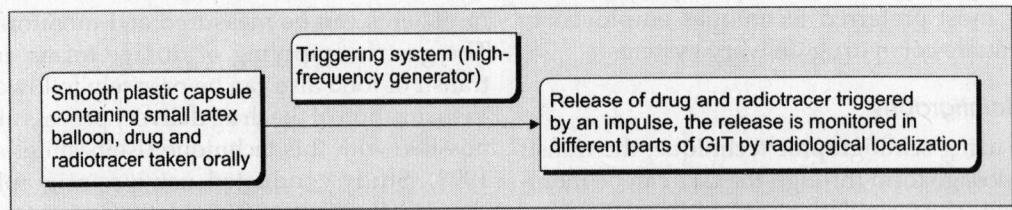

Fig. 5.34: Schematic representation of high-frequency capsule method

quantities to control the release of the drug through the core. A coating composition of a mixture of pectin, chitosan and hydroxypropyl methylcellulose has been proven to be an efficient as the tablets coated with this composition could pass intact through the stomach and small intestine and eventually disintegrated.

Microspheres-based Systems

In the treatment of inflammatory bowel disease (IBD), sustained release devices like pellets, capsules or tablets have limited effect due to diarrhea, a symptom of IBD that enhances their elimination and reduces the total time available for drug release. It has been shown that drug carrier systems with a size larger than 200 μm would be subjected to speedy bowel evacuation due to diarrhea, resulting in a decreased GI transit time and decreased efficiency. Therefore, a multiparticulates system in the micron size range could be a useful option in the design of a suitable dosage form for IBD. The Eudragit P-4135 F, a new pH-sensitive polymer was used to prepare microparticles of tacrolimus, an immunosuppressant drug, for colonic delivery. In a previous study by the same authors, the use of Eudragit P-4135 F in the microencapsulation of 5-fluorouracil for the

treatment of colorectal cancer has also been reported. Eudragit P-4135 F belongs to the pH-sensitive polymer group of polyacrylates and possesses a dissolution threshold pH slightly above 7.2. This is very useful, ulcerative colitis mainly affects the distal parts of the colon and an early drug loss towards the noninflamed tissue would be undesirable. Most of the currently employed pH-responsive colonic-drug delivery systems utilize Eudragit S and L, which dissolve in the pH range of 6–7 and therefore liberate the drug at the terminal ileum, which may lower the efficiency and risk of adverse effects. Eudragit P-4135 F might prove a useful alternative for systems intended for targeting to the distal colon (Fig. 5.35).

Microspheres in the Delivery of Peptides

The colon has always attracted attention as a potential site for the systemic absorption of peptides on account of low proteolytic enzyme activity. In this context, several research groups have attempted to develop oral delivery systems for insulin. An azo-polymer based system which depends on cleavage by colonic microflora has also been reported for the delivery of insulin. The insulin-containing polyanhydride microspheres were developed and shown to adhere to the walls of the small

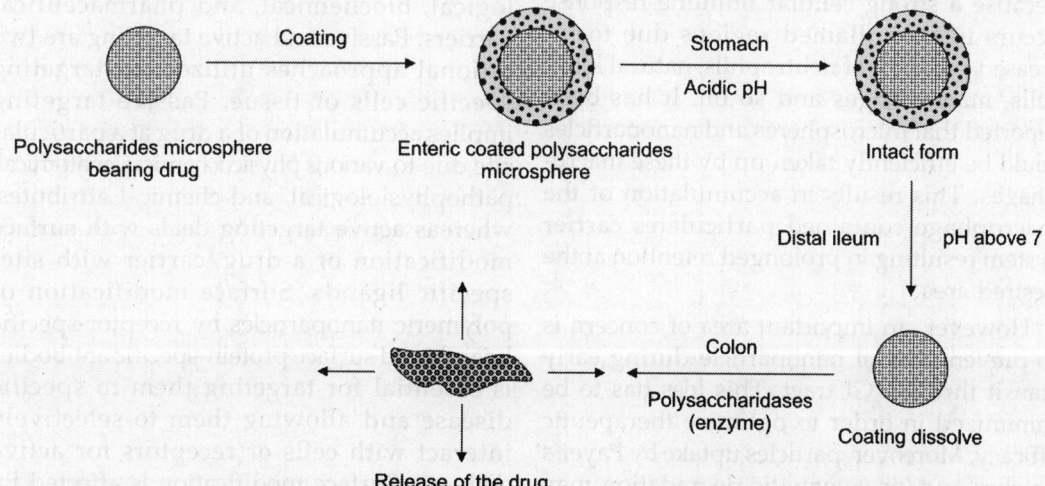

Fig. 5.35: Schematic representation of polysaccharide-based colon-specific microspheres

intestine and release the insulin upon degradation of the polymeric carrier. In a study, pH responsive poly (methacrylic-g-ethylene glycol) hydrogels were investigated as oral delivery vehicles for insulin. Insulin was loaded in polymeric microspheres and administered orally to healthy and diabetic Wistar rats. The gel particles did not swell in the acidic environment of the stomach thereby protecting insulin from proteolytic degradation, however, when they come in contact of basic and neutral environment of the small intestine, the gels rapidly swelled and released the entrapped insulin. This resulted into strong hypoglycemic effects in both healthy and diabetic rats within 2 hours of its administration.

Nanoparticle-based Systems

Nano-sized colloidal carriers consisted of natural or synthetic polymers have also been investigated for colon targeting. Orally administered nanoparticles serve as carriers for different types of drugs and have been shown to enhance their solubility, permeability and bioavailability characteristics. Nanoparticles have also been investigated for the delivery of protein and peptide drugs. For colonic pathologies, it was shown that nanoparticles tend to accumulate at the site of inflammation especially in IBD. This is because a strong cellular immune response occurs in the inflamed regions due to increased presence of neutrophils, natural killer cells, macrophages and so on. It has been reported that microspheres and nanoparticles could be efficiently taken up by these macrophages. This results in accumulation of the macrophage contained particulates carrier system resulting in prolonged retention at the desired area.

However, an important area of concern is to prevent loss of nanoparticle during early transit through GI tract. This loss has to be minimized in order to optimize therapeutic efficacy. Moreover, particles uptake by Payer's patches and/or enzymatic degradation may result in the release of entrapped drug leading to systemic drug absorption and side effects. In order to overcome this problem, drug loaded nanoparticles were entrapped into pH sensitive microspheres, which serve to deliver the incorporated nanoparticles to their site of action, thereby preventing an early drug leakage.

The use of Eudragit P-4135F prevents drug release in the upper GI tract during intestinal passage and permits selective drug delivery to or in the colon.

Furthermore, the use of nanoparticles as bioadhesive carriers has also been investigated. Nanoparticles have a large specific surface, which is indicative of high interactive potential with biological surfaces. Since the interaction is of nonspecific nature, bioadhesion can be induced by binding nanoparticles with different molecules. However, for covalent attachment, the nanoparticle surface should possess free functional groups, such as carboxylic or amine residues.

Ligand-anchored Functional Polymeric Nanoparticles

Targeting of drugs at molecular and cellular levels has emerged as a paradigm with immense potential in therapeutics and diagnosis. However, such targeting poses enormous challenges and needs to overcome physiological, biochemical, and pharmaceutical barriers. Passive and active targeting are two rational approaches utilized for targeting specific cells or tissue. Passive targeting implies accumulation of a drug at a particular site due to various physicochemical, anatomical, pathophysiological, and chemical attributes, whereas active targeting deals with surface modification of a drug/carrier with site-specific ligands. Surface modification of polymeric nanoparticles by receptor-specific ligands and surface protein-specific antibodies is essential for targeting them to specific disease and allowing them to selectively interact with cells or receptors for active delivery. Surface modification is affected by coupling these site-specific moieties by various physical and chemical means. Physical means mainly include adsorption of ligand and antibodies to the surfaces of nanoparticles by hydrophobic and ionic interaction, whereas chemical means are comprised of covalently or noncovalently conjugated target-specific ligands on to the surfaces of nanoparticle. Coupling of receptor-specific ligands and antibodies to the nanoparticles surface is known to increase their probability of interaction with corresponding targets, resulting in high therapeutic efficiency. Surface functionalization of nanoparticles for active delivery is either based on direct coupling or coupling of the ligands on stealth particles. This modulates spatial placement of nanoparticles to specifically defined targets. The incorporation of various site-directing ligands on colloidal carriers enables site specificity towards receptors associated with target sites. Such a functional system represents for future-generation active-drug delivery systems. Ligand-anchored nanoparticles represent an active mode of drug delivery. The ligand-mediated carrier system can be used to deliver anticancer drug(s) to colorectal cancer (Fig. 5.36).

Enteric-coated Systems

Enteric-coated systems are designed to provide protection to tablets and other version of novel drug delivery systems in the stomach. Application of a thicker coat causes a delay in drug release in the small intestine and slows down drug release rate, which is both pH and time controlled. This time-controlled drug release may be retarded by 3–4 hours. This ensures drug delivery to the colon. For the preparation of such tailor-made formulations, the selection of a polymer with a suitable coat level is crucial. Most of the commercially available systems for colon-specific drug delivery utilize Eudragit® (L-100/S-100) or cellulose acetate phthalate (CAP). Other coating polymers such as shellac (SH) and ethyl cellulose (EC) may be used as alternative polymers for the development of these systems. Eudragit S-100 (ES) is a methacrylic acid methylmethacrylate copolymer, which is soluble at a pH of 7. Cellulose acetate phthalate is also an effective enteric film coating material, as it dissolves at a pH of 6.0. As an enteric coating polymer, it is used at a concentration at or above 0.5–0.9%.

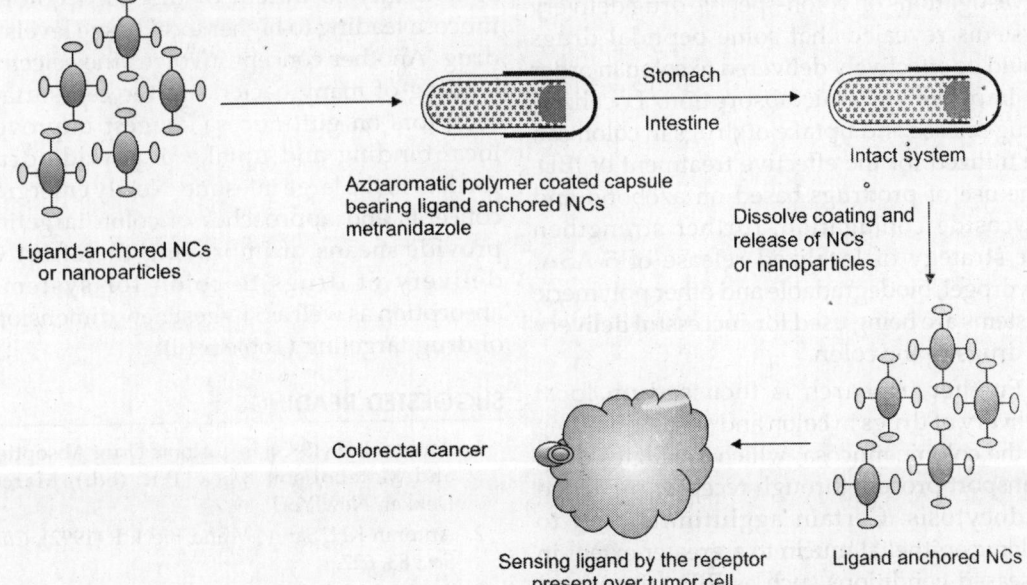

Ligand-anchored NCs or nanoparticles

Azoaromatic polymer coated capsule bearing ligand anchored NCs metranidazole

Stomach

Intestine

Intact system

Dissolve coating and release of NCs or nanoparticles

Colorectal cancer

Sensing ligand by the receptor present over tumor cell

Ligand anchored NCs

Fig. 5.36: Schematic representation of colon-specific ligand anchored nanoparticles for colorectal cancer

Table 5.10: Patents on colon drug delivery

Patent	Year	Original assignee	Title
Us4863744	1989	Alza Corporation	Intestine drug delivery
Us4968508	1990	Eli Lilly and Company	Sustained release matrix
Us5525634	1996	Perio Products, Ltd. Jerusalem	Colonic-drug delivery system
Us5656290	1997	The Procter and Gamble Company	Bisacodyl dosage form with multiple enteric polymer coatings for colonic delivery
Us5656294	1997	Cibus Pharmaceutical Inc.	Colonic delivery of drugs
Us5866619	1999	Perio Products Ltd, Jerusalem	Colonic drug delivery system
Us6506407	2003	Yamanouchi Pharma. Co. Ltd	Colon-specific drug release system
Us6972132	2005	Mochida Pharma. Co. Ltd	System for release in lower digestive tract
Us7196059	2007	Biocon Limited	Pharmaceutical compositions of insulin drug-oligomer conjugates and methods of treating diseases therewith
Us7384653	2008	Purdue Pharma LP	Oral dosage form comprising a therapeutic agent and an adverse-effect agent
Us7670624	2010	Astella Pharma Inc.	Gastrointestinal-specific multiple drug release system
Us7842308	2010	Smithkline Beecham	Limited Pharmaceutical formulation
Us 2011/0117154a1	2011	Activbiotics Pharma, LLC	Use of rifalazil to treat colonic disorder
Us 2011/0171275a1	2011	Team Academy of Pharmaceutical Science	Gastroretentive drug delivery system, preparation method and use thereof
Us 2011/0271357a1	2011	Celera Corporation	Colon disease targets and uses thereof

CONCLUSION

Investigations on colon-specific drug delivery systems revealed that some peptidal drugs could be effectively delivered to colon in order to improve systemic absorption. Localized drug release and uptake of drugs in colon can be utilized for the effective treatment of IBD. The use of prodrugs based on azobond and glycoside conjugation, further strengthen the strategy of localized release of 5-ASA. Hydrogel, biodegradable and other polymeric systems are being used for successful delivery of drugs to the colon.

Further, research is focussed on local delivery of drugs in colon and specific binding to the colonic mucosa, which facilitates drug transport process through receptor-mediated endocytosis. Certain agglutinins bind to colonic epithelial mucin to a greater extent in diseased conditions such as IBD, cancer and adenomatous mucin. Coupling a drug to agglutinins via a bioreversible linkage, bind specifically to mucin of diseased colonic mucosa leading to higher local tissue levels of drug. Another concept involves the selective binding of many bacteria to the cell surface receptors on gut mucosa suggest improved local binding and uptake of peptide drug carriers in the large intestine. Newly emerging concepts and approaches of colon targeting provide means of improving the effective delivery of drugs to colon for systemic absorption as well as suggest new dimensions of drug targeting (Table 5.10).

SUGGESTED READINGS

1. Antinin KH (1993), In: Colonic Drug Absoption and Matabolism, Bieck, P.R. (ed.), Marcel Dekker, New York, 89.
2. Antonin KH, Sanno V and Bieck P (1992), *Clin. Sci.*, 83, 627.
3. Ashford M, Fell J, Attwoods D, Sharma H and Woodhead P (1993b), *J. Control. Rel.*, 26, 213.

4. Ashford M, Fell J, Attwoods D, Sharma H and Woodhead P (1994), *J. Control. Rel.*, 30, 225.

5. Ashford M, Fell JT, Attwood D, Sharma H and Woodhead PJ (1993a), *Int. J. Pharm.*, 95, 193.

6. Azad Khan AK, Truelove SC and Aronson JK (1982), *Br. J. Clin. Pharmacol.*, 13, 523.

7. Anil K Philip and Betty Philip. Oman Med J. (2010) 25(2): 79–87.

8. Asghar LF, Chandran S, (2006), *J Pharm Pharm Sci.* 9(3): 327–38.

9. Azad Khan KA, Piris J and Truelove SC (1997), Lancet, 2, 892.

10. Binder HJ, Foster ES, Budinger ME and Hayslett JP (1987), *Gastroenterology*, 93, 449.

11. Brockmeier D (1993), In: Colonic Drug Absoption and Matabolism, Bieck, P.R. (ed.), Marcel Dekker, New York, 109.

12. Bauer KH and Kesselhut JF (1995), *STP Pharm. Sci.*, 5, 54.

13. Brondsted H and Kopeckova P (1991), *Biomaterials*, 12, 584.

14. Brondsted H, Anderson C and Hovgaard L (1998), *J. Control. Rel.*, 53, 7.

15. Brondsted H, Hovgaard L and Simonsen L (1995), *STP Pharm. Sci.* 5, 60.

16. Basit A, *Bloor J Pharmtech* 2003, 185.

17. Basit AW. Drugs. (2005) 65(14): 1991–2007.

18. Brown JP (1981), *Appl. Environ. Microbiol.*, 41, 1283.

19. Chourasia MK, Jain SK. *J Pharm Pharm Sci.* 2003. 6(1): 33–66.

20. Cann PA, Read NW, Brown C, Hobson N and Holdsworth, CD (1983) Gut., 24, 405.

21. Carrette, O., Favier, C. and Mizon, C. (1995) Dig. Dis. Sci., 42, 133.

22. Caston AJ, Davis SS and Williams P (1990), In: Proceedings of the 16th International Symposium on Controlled Release Bioactive Materials, Lee, V.H.L. (ed.), CRC Press, 313.

23. Chassuade S, Roche H, Khyari A, Couturier D and Guerre J (1986), *Gastroenterol. Clin. Biol.*, 10, 385.

24. Cheng CL, Gehrke, SH and Ritschel WA (1994), *Methods Find Exp. Clin. Pharmacol.*, 16, 271.

25. Christensen FN, Davis SS, Hardy JG, Taylor MJ, Whalley DR and Wilson CG (1985), *J. Pharm. Pharmacol.*, 37, 91.

26. Code CF and Marlett JM (1975) *J. Physiol., (Lond)* 246, 289.

27. Colony PC (1996), *Dig. Dis. Sci.*, 41, 88.

28. Coupe AJ, Davis SS and Wilding IR (1991), *Pharm. Res.*, 8, 360.

29. Danovitch SH, Gallucci A and Shora W (1972), *Am. J. Dig. Dis.*, 17, 977.

30. Davaran S, Hanaee J and Khosravi A (1999), *J. Control. Rel.*, 58, 279.

31. Davis SS, Hardy JG, Taylor MJ, Whalley DR and Wilson CG (1984), *Int. J. Pharm.*, 21, 331.

32. Del Soldato P, Fosch D, Varin L and Daniotti (1985), *Agents Actions* 6, 393.

33. Dew MJ, Hughes PJ, Lee, MG, Evans BK and Rhodes, J. (1982), *Br. J. Clin. Pharmacol.*, 14, 405.

34. Dipirio JT, Posey LM and Bowden TA (1989), *In: Pharmaco-therapy, A Pathophysiologic Approach, Dipirio*, J.T. et al. (eds.), Elsevier: New York, 444.

35. Draser BS and Hill, MJ (eds.) (1974), Human Intestinal Flora, Acadamic Press, London.

36. Simon GL and Gobach SL (1983), In: Colon, Structure and Function. Bustos-Fernandez, L. (ed.), Plenum, New York, 103.

37. Dressman JB and Yamada K (1991), *In: Pharmaceutical Bioequivalance* (Vol. 48) Welling, P.G., Tse, F.L.S. and Dighe, S.V. (eds.), Marcel Dekker, New York, 727.

38. Enck P, Merlin V, Erckenbrecht JF and Weinbeck, M. (1989), *Gut.*, 30, 455.

39. Evans DF, Pye G, Bramley R, Clark AG, Dyson, TJ and Hardcastle JD (1988), *Gut.*, 29, 1035.

40. Fara JW (1989), *In: Novel Drug Delivery and its Therapeutic Application*, Presscot, LF and Nimmo, WS (eds.), Wiley, Chichester, 103.

41. Fix, J.A. (1987), *J. Control. Rel.*, 6, 151.

42. Fordtran JS and Locklear TW (1966), *Am. J. Dig. Dis.*, 11, 503.

43. Friend DR (1991), *Adv. Drug Del. Rev.*, 7, 149.

44. Friend DR (1992), In: *Oral-Colon Specific Drug Delivery, Friend*, DR (ed.), CRC Press, Boca Raton, 153.

45. Friend DR and Chang, GW (1984), *J. Med. Chem.*, 27, 261.

46. Fujimoto JM (1970), *Proc. Soc. Exp. Biol. Med.*, 133, 317.

47. Gallone L, Olmi L and Marchetti V (1980), *World J. Surg.*, 4, 609.

48. Gazzaniga A, Maroni A, Sangalli ME, Zema L. Expert Opin Drug Deliv. 2006. 3(5): 583–97.

49. Gardner N, Haresign W and Spiller R (1996), *J. Pharm. Pharmacol.*, 48, 689.

50. Gazzaniga A, Iamartino P, Maffione G and Sangalli, ME (1994), *Int. J. Pharm.*, 108, 77.

51. George WL, Sutter VL and Finegold SM (1978), *Curr. Microbiol.*, 1, 55.

52. Gleiter CH, Antonin KH and Bieck P (1985), *Gastrointest. Endosc.*, 31, 71.

53. Goldhill JM, Rose K and Percy WH (1996), *J. Pharm. Pharmacol.*, 48, 651.

54. Gorbach SL (1971), *Gastroenterol.*, 60, 1110.

55. Gorbach SL (1971), *Gastroenterol.*, 86, 174.

56. Grim Y and Kopecek J (1991), *New Polymer Mater.* 3, 49.

57. Gruber P, Longer MA and Robinson JR (1987), *Adv. Drug Del. Rev.*, 1, 1.

58. Hamilton SR, (1984), *Scand. J. Gastroenterol.* 19 (Suppl. 93), 13.

59. Harder S, Fuhr U, Beerman D and Staib AH (1990), *Br. J. Clin. Pharmacol.*, 30, 35.

60. Hastewell J, Phillips J, Lloyd AW, Martin GP, Marriott C and Williams M (1991), *J. Pharm. Pharmacol.*, 43 (Suppl.), pp. 62.

61. Hawkey CJ, Mahida YR and Hawthorne AB (1992), *Agents Actions Spec* No: C22-6.

62. Hawksworth G, Draser BS and Hill MJ (1971) *J. Med. Microbiol.*, 4, 451.

63. Hill MJ (1981), *Cancer Res.*, 41, 3778.

64. Hirayama F, Minami K and Uekama K (1996), *J. Pharma. Pharmacol.*, 48, 27.

65. Hirsch S, Binder V, Kolter K, Kesselhut JF and Bauer KH (1997), *Proc. Int. Symp. Control. Rel. Bioact. Mater.*, 24, 379.

66. Hofmann AF, Pressamn JH, Code CF and Witztum KF (1983), *Drug Dev. Ind. Pharm.*, 9, 1077.

67. Holdstock DJ, Misiewicz JJ, Smith T and Rowlands EN (1970), *Gut.*, 11, 91.

68. Holtenius K and Bjornhag G (1985), *Comp. Biochem. Physiol.*, 82A, 537.

69. Hovgaard L and Brondsted H (1996), *Crit. Rev. Ther. Drug Carr. Syst.*, 13, 185.

70. Irie T and Uekama K (1997), *J. Pharm., Sci.* 86, 147.

71. Ishibashi T, Pitcairn GR, Yoshino H, Mizobe M and Wilding IR (1998), *J. Pharm. Sci.*, 87, 531.

72. Isley JK, Sanders AP, Sharpe KW, Reeves RJ and Baylin GJ (1959), *Am. J. Roentgenol. Rad. Ther. Nuc. Med.*, 81, 89.

73. Jain SK, Jain A. Expert Opin Drug Deliv. (2008), 5(5): 483–98.

74. Jung Y, Kim YM. Expert Opin Drug Deliv. (2010) Feb; 7(2): 245–58.

75. KV Vinay Kumar, T Sivakumar, T Tamizh mani, *Int J Pharm Biomed Sci* (2011), 2(1), 11–19.

76. Kim H. *Curr Drug Deliv.* 2012 Mar 1; 9(2): 132–47.

77. Kothawade PD, Gangurde HH, Surawase RK, Wagh MA, Tamizharasi S. e-JST. 2011. (2)6, 33–56.

78. Kumar P, Mishra B. Curr Drug Deliv. 2008. 5(3): 186–98.

79. McConnell EL, Liu F, Basit AW. *J Drug Target.* (2009). 17(5): 335–63.

80. Patel M, Shah T, Amin A. Crit Rev Ther Drug Carrier Syst. (2007). 24(2): 147–202.

81. Patel MM. Expert Opin Drug Deliv. (2011). 8(10): 1247–58.

82. Roldo M, Barbu E, Brown JF, Laight DW, Smart JD.

83. Kararli TT (1995), *Biopharm. Drug Dispos.*, 16, 351.

84. Kimura Y, Makita Y and Kumagai, T. (1992) Polymer, 33, 5294.

85. Kinget R, Kalala W, Vervoort L and Van den Mooter G (1998), *J. Drug Target.*, 6, 129.

86. Kopecek J (1990), *J. Control. Rel.*, 11, 279.

87. Kopecek J, Kopeckova P, Brondsted H, Rathi R, Rihova B, Yeh PY and Ikesue K (1992), *J. Control. Rel* 19, 121.

88. Kopeckova P and Kopecek J (1990), *Macromol. Chem.*, 191, 2037.

89. Kopeckova P, Ikesue K, Fornusek L and Kopecek J (1990), *Proc. Int. Symp. Control. Rel. Bioact. Mater.*, 17, 130.

90. Kopeckova P, Rathi R, Takada S, Rihova B, Berenson MM and Kopecek J (1994), *J. Control. Rel.* 28, 211.

91. Krishnaiah YS, Satyanarayana S and Rama Prasad YV (1999), *Drug Dev. Ind. Pharm.*, 25, 651.

92. Krishnaiah YS, Satyanarayana S, Rama Prasad YV and Narasimha Rao S (1998), *J. Control. Rel.*, 55, 245.

93. Larsen C, Harboe E, Johenson, M. and Olesen, H.P. (1989) Pharm. Res., 6, 1989.

94. Larsen, G.L., Larson, J.P. and Gustafsson, J.A. (1983) Xenobiotica, 13, 687.

95. Lee, V.H.L. (1992) Biopharm., 5, 39.

96. Leopold CS and Friend DR (1995), *J. Pharmacokinet. Biopharm.*, 23, 397.

97. Levy G (1964), *Arch. Int. Pharmacodyn. Ther.*, 152, 59.

98. Mackey M and Tomlinson E (1993) In: Colonic Drug Absorption and Metabolism Bieck P (ed.), Marcel Dekker, New York, 159.

99. MacNeil ME, Rashid A and Stevens HNE, WO 9009168.

100. Malagelada JR, Robertson JS and Brown ML (1984), *Gastroenterol.*, 87, 1255.

101. McIntyre PB, Rodrigues CA and Lennard-Jones, JE (1988), *Aliment. Pharmacol. Ther.*, 2, 237.

102. McLead AD, Feclorak RN, Friend DR, Tozer, TN and Cui N (1994), *Gastroenterol.*, 108, 1688.

103. McLeod AD and Tozer TN (1992), In: Oral Colon-Specfic Drug Selivery, Friend, DR (ed.) CRC Press, Boca Raton., 85.

104. McLeod AD, Friend DR and Tozer TN (1993), *Int. J. Pharm.*, 92, 105.

105. Meldrum SJ, Watson BW, Riddle HC, Bown RL and Sladen GE (1972), *Br. Med. J.*, 2, 104.

106. Mirelman D, De Meester F, Stolarsky T, Burchard GD, Ernst-Cabrera K and Wilcheck M (1989), *J. Infect. Dis.*, 159, 303.

107. Mirsny RJ (1992), *J. Control. Rel.*, 22, 15.

108. Molly K, Vande Woestyne M and Verstraete W (1993), *Appl. Microbiol. Biotechnol.*, 39, 254.

109. Moreto M, Gonalons E, Mylonakis N, Girldez, A and Torralba A (1979), *Arzneim-Forsch/Drug Res.*, 29, 1561.

110. Munjeri O, Collet JH and Fell JT (1997), *J. Control. Rel.*, 46, 273.

111. Murakami M, Yoshikawa H, Takada K and Muranishi S (1986), *Pharm. Res.*, 3, 35.

112. Muranishi S (1987), *Proc. Int. FIP Satell. Symp.*, L18.

113. Muranishi S, Muranishi N and Sezaki H, (1979), *Int. J. Pharm.*, 2, 101.

114. Niwa K, Takaya T, Morimoto T and Takada K (1995), *J. Drug Target.*, 3, 83.

115. Nishihata T, Okamura Y, Kamada A, Highuchi T, Yagi T, Kawamori R and Shichiri M (1985), *J. Pharm. Pharmacol.*, 37, 22.

116. Nord CE Heimdahl A, (1986), *J. Antimicrob. Chemother.*, 18 (Suppl. C), 159.

117. Peeters R and Kinget R (1993), *Int. J. Pharm.*, 94, 125.

118. Pettersson G, Ahlman H and Kewenter J (1976), *Acta. Chir. Scand.*, 142, 537.

119. Peppercorn MA and Goldman P (1976), *Rev. Drug Metab. Drug Interact.*, 2, 75.

120. Pozzi F, Furlani P, Gazzaniga A, Davis SS and Wilding IR (1994), *J. Control. Rel.*, 31, 99.

121. Proano M, Camilleri M, Philips SF, Thomforde, GM, Brown ML and Tucker RL (1991), *Am. J. Physiol.*, 260, G13.

122. Rachmilewitz D (1988), *Br. Med. J*, 298, 82.

123. Ruseler-Van Embden, JGH and Asad YF (1997), *Dig. Dis. Sci.*, 42, 133.

124. Rao SSC, Read NW and Holdsworth CD (1987), *Gut.*, 28, 1474.

125. Rasmussen SN, Bondeson S, Hvidberg EF, Honore Honsen S, Binder V, Halskoz S and Flachs H (1982), *Gastroenterol.*, 83, 1062.

126. Reddy MS, Sinha RV and Reddy DS (1999), *Drugs of Today*, 35(7), 537.

127. Renwick AG (1982), In: Clinical Pharmacology and Therapeutics (Vol. 1), George, CF, Shand, G and Renwick AG (eds.), Butterworth, London, 3.

128. Rihova B (1995), *Adv. Exp. Med. Biol.*, 371B, 1491.

129. Riley SA, Tavares IA, Bennet A and Mani V (1988), *Br. J. Clin. Pharmacol.*, 26, 173.

130. Rodriguez, M., Vila-Jato, J.L. and Torres, D. (1998), *J. Control. Rel.*, 55, 67.

131. Rubinstein A (1990), *Biopharm. Drug Dispos.*, 11, 465.

132. Rubinstein A and Friend DR (1994), In: Polymer Site-Specific Pharmacotherapy, Domb, A.J. (ed.) John Wiley and Sons, Sussex, 267.

133. Rubinstein A and Gliko-Kabir I (1995), *STP Pharm. Sci.*, 5, 41.

134. Rubinstein A and Radai R (1995), *Eur. J. Pharm. Biopharm.*, 41, 291.

135. Rubinstein A and Sintov A (1992), *In: Oral Colon-Specfic Drug Selivery*, Friend, D.R. (ed.) CRC Press, Boca Raton, 233.

136. Rubinstein A, Naker D and Sintov A (1992), *Pharm. Res.*, 9, 276.

137. Rubinstein A, Radai R, Ezra M, Pathak S and Rokem JS (1993), *Pharm. Res.*, 10, 258.

138. Rubinstein A, Radai R, Friedman M, Fischer P and Rokem JS (1997), *Pharm. Res.*, 14, 503.

139. Ruckbusch Y and Buene L (1976), *Br. J. Nutr.*, 35, 397.

140. Rutgeerts P (1989), *Aliment. Pharmacol. Ther.*, 3, 183.

141. Saffran M, Field JB, Pena J, Jones RH and Okuda Y (1991), *J. Endocrinol.*, 131, 267.

142. Salyers AA (1979), *Am. J. Clin. Nutr.*, 32, 158.

143. Samuel PG, Sypol GM, Meilman E, Mosbach EH and Chafizadeh M (1968), *J. Clin. Invest.*, 42, 2070.

144. Sarlikiotis AW and Bauer KH (1992), *Pharm. Ind.*, 54, 873.

145. Schacht E, Callant D and Verstraete W (1991), *Proc. Int. Symp. Control. Rel. Bioact. Mater.*, 18, 686.

146. Schacht E, Gevaert A and Kenawy ER (1996), *J. Control. Rel.*, 39, 327.

147. Schang JC, De Vroede G, Duguay C, Hemonds, M and Hebert M (1985), *Gastroenterol. Clin. Biol.*, 9, 480.

148. Scheline RR (1973), *Pharmacol. Rev.*, 25, 451.

149. Shanta KL, Ravichandran P and Rao KP (1995), *Biomaterials*, 16, 1313.

150. Simon GL and Gorbach SL (1884), *Gastroenterol.*, 86, 174.

151. Sintov A, Ankol S, Levy, DP and Rubinstein, A. (1993), *Biomaterials*, 14, 483.

152. Sriamornsak P, Prakongpan, S, Puttipipatkhochorn, S and Kennedy, RA (1997), *J. Control. Rel.*, 47, 221.

153. Staib AH, Woodcock BG, Loew D and Schuster, O (1989), *In: Novel Drug Delivery and its Therapeutic Application*, Prescott, LF and Nimmo, WS (eds.), Wiley, Chichester, 79.

154. Shah N, Shah T, Amin A. Expert Opin Drug Deliv. 2011.8(6): 779–96.

155. Shareef MA, Khar RK, Ahuja A, Ahmad FJ, Raghava S, *AAPS Pharm. Sci.* 2003. 5(2): E17.

156. Szente V, Zelkó R. Acta Pharm Hung. (2007). 77 (3): 185–9.

157. Tsibouklis J. Expert Opin Drug Deliv. 2007. 4(5): 547–60.

158. Taniguchi K, Muranishi S and Sezaki H (1980), *J. Pharm. Dyn.*, 5, 69.

159. Theeuwes F, Yum SI, Haak R and Wong P (1991), In: Temporal Control of Drug Delivery, Hrushesky, WJM, Langer R and Theeuwes, F. (eds.), *NY Acad. Sci.*, New York.

160. Thomas P, Richards D and Richards A (1985), *Int. J. Pharm.*, 4, 219.

161. Tomita M, Hayashi M, Horie T, Ishizawa T and Awazu S (1988), *Pharm. Res.*, 5, 786.

162. Touitou E and Rubinstein A (1986), *Int. J. Pharm.*, 30, 95.

163. Tozaki H, Emi Y, Horisaka, E, Fujita, T., Yamamoto A, and Muranishi S (1997), *J. Pharm. Pharmacol.*, 49, 164.

164. Tozer TN, Rigod J, McLeod AD, Gungon R, Hoag MK and Friend DR (1991), *Pharm. Res.* 8, 445.

165. Ueda S, Iibuki R and Kawamuza A (1994), *J. Drug Target.*, 2, 133.

166. Van den Mooter G Expert Opin Drug Deliv. 2006. 3(1): 111–25.

167. Van den Mooter G, Samyn C and Kinget R (1992), *Int. J. Pharm.*, 87, 37.

168. Van den Mooter G, Samyn C and Kinget R. (1995), *Pharm. Res.*, 12, 244.

169. Veillard M (1989) In: Bioadhesion-Possibilities and Future Trends, Gurny, R. and Juginger, H.E. (eds.), Wissenschaftliche Verlag, Stuttgart, 124.

170. Bioactive Materials, Pearlman R and Miller JA (eds.), CRC Press, 58.

171. Worthington BS and Enwonwu C (1975), *Dig. Dis.*, 20, 750.

172. Yoshikawa H, Takada K, Muranishi S, Satou YI, and Naruse N (1984), *J. Pharm. Dyn.*, 7, 59.

173. Yoshikawa, H., Muranishi, S. and Sezaki, H. (1982), *J. Pharm. Dyn.*, 5, 69.

6

■ Transdermal Drug Delivery Systems

INTRODUCTION

In contemporary therapeutics, the oral route has been the most preferred route of drug administration. The rise to prominence of modern therapeutics is based on so many existing medicinal agents. The drugs of future; due to their poor oral availability generated a need of focusing the attention on nonoral route for routine and effective drug administration. The nonoral routes, which include nasal rectal buccal, vaginal, and transdermal are considered, as due to first pass metabolism drug availability is poor or administered drug

moles are poorly permeable across gastro-intestinal barrier. Due to frequent pricking, need of constant medical supervision and lack in patient compliance, the transdermal route has been introduced as an alternative to bolus system. Transdermal drug delivery systems (TDDS) are specifically designed to obtain systemic blood levels. Schematic representation of drug levels in blood from transdermal routes of administration are shown in Fig. 6.1. A TDDS is designed to release the drugs at a predetermined rate continuously, avoiding unnecessarily high peaks and subtherapeutic

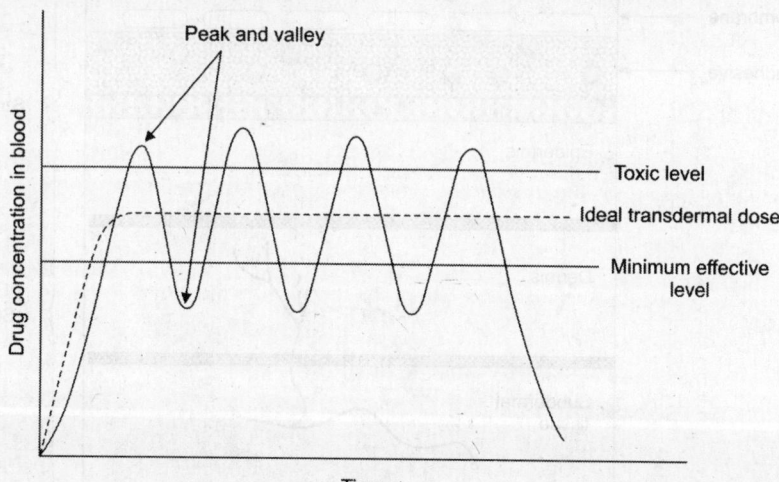

Fig. 6.1. Hypothetical blood level pattern from a conventional multiple dosing schedule and the idealised pattern from TDDS

troughs in plasma drug levels. Transdermal permeation, or percutaneous absorption, can be defined as the passage of a drug substance, from the outside of the skin through its various layers into the bloodstream (Fig. 6.2).

Advantages

The positive features of delivering drugs across the skin to achieve systemic effect are summarised as follows:

1. Avoidance of significant presystemic metabolism (degradation in the gastrointestinal tract or by the liver), and, therefore, resulting to a lower daily dose.
2. Reduced inter- and intra-patient variability, this is particularly true for those situations in which drug release from the transdermal patch is slower than drug diffusion or flux across the stratum corneum.
3. Drug levels can be maintained in the systemic circulation, within the therapeutic window, (i.e. above the minimum effective concentration, but below the level at which

side-effects become apparent), for prolonged periods of time.
4. Thus, the duration of drug action following a single administration of the drug can be extended, and the frequency of dosing is reduced.
5. Improved patient compliance and acceptability of the drug therapy.
6. Drug input can be terminated simply by removal of the patch.

Disadvantages

The limitations of transdermal drug delivery are essentially associated with the barrier function of skin, which severely constrain the absolute amount of a drug that is absorbed across a reasonable area of skin during a dosing period. Thus, the major disadvantage of the method is that its limitation to potent drug molecules, typically those requiring a daily dose of the order of 10 mg or less. Usually, this suits the best for drugs with effective plasma concentrations in the ng/mL

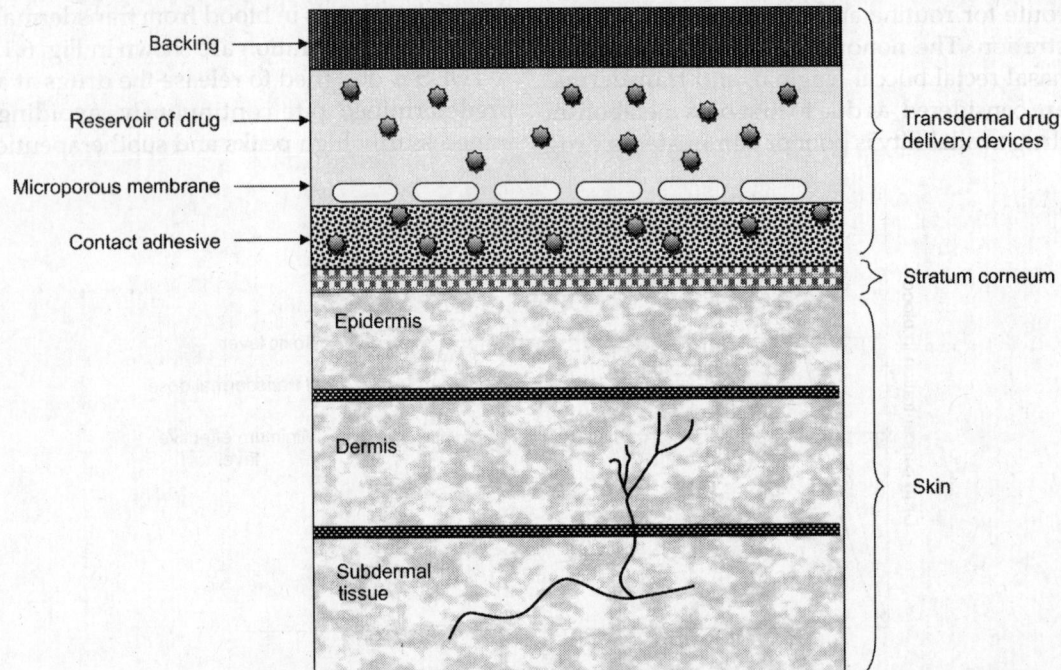

Fig. 6.2: Scheme of transdermal drug delivery system

(or lower) range. Even if the drug is sufficiently potent, it must yet satisfy other criteria to be considered as a viable candidate for transdermal delivery. First, its physicochemical properties must allow it to be absorbed percutaneously. This means that its molecular weight should be appropriate (see above), and that it should have adequate solubility in both lipophilic and aqueous environments, to reach the dermal microcirculation and gain an access to the systemic circulation.

The molecule must cross the stratum corneum (a lipoidal barrier) and then traverse through the much more aqueous-in-nature viable epidermis and upper dermis. Absence of either oil or water solubility will preclude desirable permeation. Second, the pharmacokinetic and pharmacodynamic characteristics of the drug must be such that relatively sustained and slow input is required from transdermal delivery to produce desirable therapeutic effect. Tolerance-inducing compounds are not proper candidates for this mode of administration unless an appropriate 'wash-out' period is programmed in between the dosing regimen. Drugs with short biological half-lives are subject to major first-pass metabolism, necessitating inconvenient frequent oral or parenteral dosing (with the concomitant problems of side-effects and poor compliance), are good candidates. On the other hand, drugs that can be given orally once a day, with reproducible bioavailability, and well tolerated by the patient, do not really need a transdermal formulation. Third, the drug must not be locally irritating or sensitising, since provocation of significant skin reactions beneath a transdermal delivery system will most likely prevent its regulatory approval.

SKIN: A BIOLOGICAL BARRIER TO DRUG TRANSPORT

The skin is consisted of the epidermis, the dermis, and the subcutis or subcutaneous tissues, which anchor the skin to underlying tissues. Each layer is physically and functionally distinct with appendages, including hair follicles, sweat ducts and sebaceous glands, bridging between the layers and the skin surface. The barrier function of skin is due to, entirely and quite remarkably, by the outermost few microns of the skin, i.e. the stratum corneum (SC), a compositionally and morphologically unique biomembrane. This extremely thin (approximately one-hundredth of a mm), least permeable of skin layers is the ultimate stage in the epidermal differentiation process, forming a laminate of compressed keratin filled corneocytes (terminally differentiated keratinocytes) anchored in a lipophilic matrix. The lipids of this extracellular matrix are distinctive in many respects: (1) they provide a continuous phase (and diffusion pathway) from the skin surface to the base of the SC; (2) the composition (ceramides, free fatty acids and cholesterol) is unique among biomembranes and particularly noteworthy is the absence of phospholipids; (3) despite of this deficit of polar bilayer-forming lipids, the SC lipids exist as multilamellar sheets; and (4) the predominantly saturated, long-chain hydrocarbon tails facilitate a highly ordered, interdigitated configuration and the formation of gel-phase membrane domains, as opposed to the more usual (and more fluid and permeable) liquid crystalline membrane systems (Fig. 6.3).

Any superior problem-solving or solution-creating approach must be goal-oriented, and the goal must take the form of the 'ideal system'. Some of the characteristics of an ideal

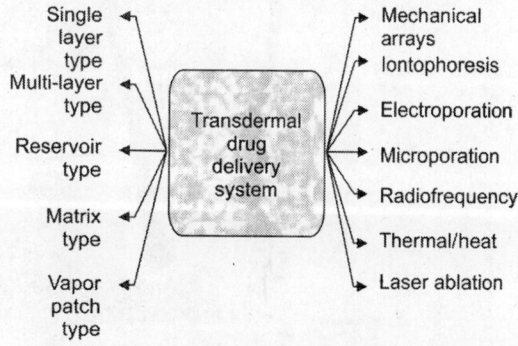

Fig. 6.3: Transdermal drug delivery systems

transdermal drug delivery system (Table 6.1) are specified below:

1. *Agent independent:* The ideal drug delivery system (IDDS) should be capable of delivering any drug, regardless of size or structure, at the specified rate of delivery.
2. *Selected delivery profile:* Drug as per quantity-time profile specified, is delivered by the IDDS.
3. *Multiple drugs:* The IDDS should also be capable of delivering more than one therapeutic agents at a time.
4. *Flexibility:* The IDDS should have the capability for changing or adjusting the rate or timing of delivery, or the quantity to be delivered.
5. *Sensoring/monitoring and decision-making:* The system will sense patient needs, determine appropriate action, and deliver the necessary quantities in accordance with a calculated quantity-time delivery profile. Such system is referred to as 'smart' delivery system.
6. *Targeting:* The IDDS has the (optional) capability of focusing drug transport towards target sites (minimum drug losses to other-than-target sites).

7. *Capacity:* The system should be capable of making repeated deliveries between bioreplacements.
8. *Absence of problems:* The IDDS raises or causes no new problems or concerns.
9. *Reliability:* The IDDS consists of few parts and has reliability in keeping with other (competitive) delivery systems.
10. *Marketplace value:* The IDDS should offer high value by featuring maximum functionality at minimum system complexity and cost.

MECHANISTIC ASPECTS OF DRUG DELIVERY IN TDDS

Designing of transdermal delivery systems, requires an understanding of the permeation behavior of drug through the skin. The amount of active agent accumulated in different strata of the skin, the flux through the skin into systemic circulation and an additional aspect to consider the mechanism of penetration, i.e. the fractional contribution of bulk strata versus the appendageal pathway to total absorption are some of the factors responsible for drug transdermal permeability. Figure 6.4 shows different possible pathways which may allow penetration via

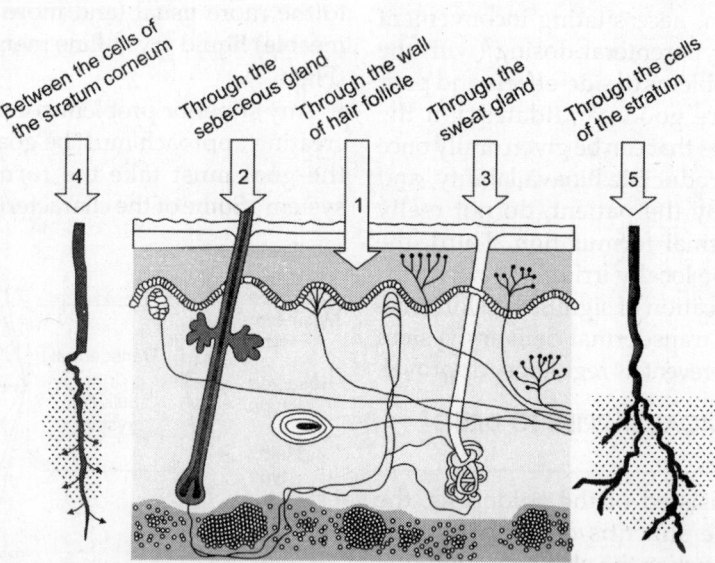

Fig. 6.4: Different pathways of penetration into and through the unbroken viable skin

Table 6.1: Ideal properties of drug for TDDS

Parameter	Properties
Dose deliverable	>10 mg day^{-1}
Half-life (hr)	Should be 10 or less
Molecular weight	<500 Da
Partition coefficient	(octanol-water)
Log P	between –1 and 3
Skin permeability coefficient	Less than 0.5×10^{-3} cm/hr
pH	5–9
Dose deliverable	<10 mg/day
Aqueous solubility	>1 mg ml^{-1}
Lipophilicity	$10 < K_{w/o} < 1000$
Melting point	<200°C
Oral bioavailability	Should be low
Therapeutic index	Should be low

intact viable skin. The transfollicular pathway, in which the drug travels through cells and across them, is the shortest way that most likely provides relatively large area for diffusion of a molecule. The intracellular pathway avoids the cell contents. It is an aqueous pathway, which is considerably more tortuous. The transfollicular pathway involves passage or diffusion of drug molecule through the hair-shaft openings, which are presumably filled with sebum. This route offers substantially lower diffusional resistance to the most of the drugs, that are generally not permeated fairly through other routes. However, the path length is relatively long, while the density of hair follicles in human skin quite low (Table 6.2). Scheuplein (1967) using a mathematical model for diffusion through the skin, concluded that the major pathway for penetration of small polar molecules is likely to be transcellular and through the stratum corneum. Although the skin appendages offer less diffusional resistance, they occupy and

represent for only 0.1% of the surface area of the skin surface, therefore contribute relatively little to the total flux. After the attainment of the steady state flux, most of the molecules penetrate the skin via shunt pathways. In the case of molecules with very small diffusion coefficient in stratrum corneum, such as the polar steriods, a significant proportion of the drug even after steady state is absorbed through appendages and glands. The intercellular route seems an unlikely avenue because of its volume and long path length (Blank et al., 1967).

The principle mechanism for drug delivery using transdermal drug delivery system is 'a slow process of diffusion dependent on the drug gradient between the high concentration in the delivery system and the zero concentration prevailing in the skin'. The transdermal permeation of most neutral molecules is primarily a process of passive diffusion across the intact stratum corneum and through the transfollicular region (Fig. 6.5). The rate of skin permeation (dQ/dt) can be expressed mathematically by the following relationship:

$$\frac{dQ}{dt} = P_S (C_P - C_R) \qquad (6.1)$$

where C_P and C_R are, respectively, the concentrations of a penetrant in the donar compartment, e.g. on the surface of the stratum corneum, and in the receptor compartment, e.g. in the body P_S is the skin permeability coefficient, defined as follows:

$$P_S = \frac{K_S D_{SS}}{H_S} \qquad (6.2)$$

where K_S is the partition coefficient of the penetrant at the interface between the delivery system and the skin tissues, D_{SS} is the diffusion coefficient for the diffusion of a

Table 6.2: Pathways through the human skin

Route	Relative surface area (%)	Diffusional path length (m)	Relative viscosity of stratum corneum (%)
Transcellular	99.0	25	90–99
Intercellular	0.7	350	1–10
Transfollicular	0.1	200	0.1

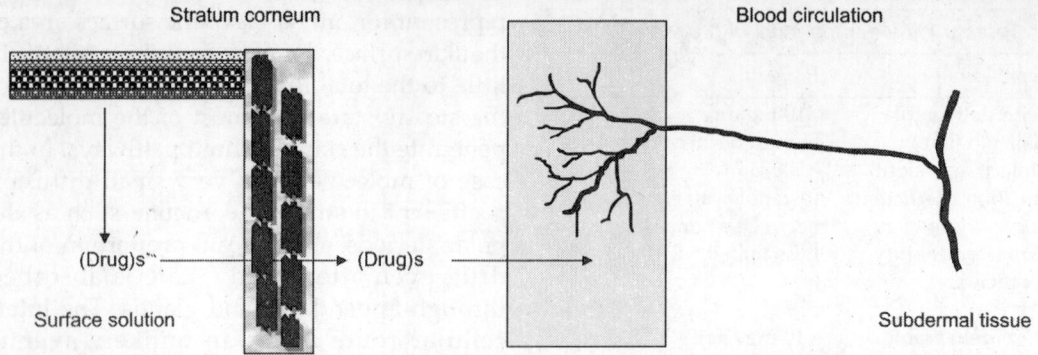

Fig. 6.5: Diagrammatic representation of the transdermal drug permeation and drug uptake by the skin

penetrant through the skin tissues at steady state, and H_S is the thickness of the skin tissues. The skin permeability coefficient (P_S) is a constant, since the other terms in equation 6.2 (K_S, D_{SS} and H_S) will be constant under constant conditions.

FACTORS AFFECTING PERCUTANEOUS ABSORPTION

The passive diffusion is the principal transport mechanism that operates in mammalian skin by following which drug molecules are transported via the transepidermal route at steady state or transappendageal route at non-steady state. The factors, which control the percutaneous absorption can be physico-chemical properties of penetrants, physico-chemical properties of the drug delivery systems and the physiological and patho-logical conditions of the skin.

Physicochemical Properties of Penetrant

The route through which permeation occurs is largely dependent on the physicochemical characteristics of the penetrant, the most important being the relative ability to partition into each skin phase. Each phase of the membrane can be characterized in terms of diffusional resistance (R), which usually is a function of thickness.

$$R = \frac{H_S}{D_{SS}K_S} \tag{6.3}$$

$$P_S = \frac{K_S D_{SS}}{H_S} \tag{6.3a}$$

(H_S) of the phase, the permeant diffusion coefficient (D_{SS}) within the phase, and the partition coefficient (K_S) between the membrane phase and external phase are expressed as equations 6.2–6.5, where P_S is permeability coefficient as earlier discussed in equation 6.2. The permeability coefficient is related to membrane flux (J), as given by relationship (Eq. 6.4)

$$J = A_{PS} (C_P - C_R) \tag{6.4}$$

in which $C_P - C_R$ is the difference in permeant concentration across the membrane, and A is the area of application. Combining the (Eqs 6.2 and 6.4), we get Eq. 6.5, as follows:

$$\frac{J}{A} = \frac{D_{SS}K_S(C_P - C_R)}{H_S} \tag{6.5}$$

From Eq. 6.5, it is evident that three major variables account for difference in the rate, at which drugs permeate the skin; the concentration of the drug in the vehicle, the partition coefficient of the drug between the stratum corneum and the vehicle, and the diffusivity of the drug through the stratum corneum.

Drugs with partition coefficients indicating an ability to dissolve in both lipid and water are favorably absorbed through the skin and would be the ideal candidates for transdermal delivery. Transdermal permeability has linear relationship with partition coefficient. A lipid/water partition of one or greater is generally required for transdermal permea-bility. The mobility of a permeating molecule within a specific membrane phase can numeri-cally be described by a diffusion coefficient.

This parameter, D_{SS}, depends, to a large extent, on degree of interaction between the diffusant and the surrounding medium, and tends to decrease with an increase in permeant molecular volume (V):

$$D_{SS} \infty \, V^{-1/3} \qquad (6.6)$$

This relationship suggests that only a slight variation in diffusivity occurs with an increase in molecular size. However, any factor that tends to promote interaction between the permeant and the membrane will hinder the diffusion. As the drug transport is a passive diffusion process, the concentration of penetrant molecule on the surface layer of the skin, increases with an increase in the concentration of penetrant delivered from the delivery system.

The release of a therapeutic agent from a formulation applied to the skin surface and its transport to the systemic circulation is a multistep process, which involves (a) dissolution within and release from the formulation, (b) partitioning into the skin's outermost layer, the stratum corneum (SC), (c) diffusion through the SC, principally via a lipidic intercellular pathway, (i.e. the rate-limiting step for most compounds), (d) partitioning from the SC into the aqueous viable epidermis, (e) diffusion through the viable epidermis and into the upper dermis, and (f) uptake into the local capillary network and eventually the systemic circulation (Fig. 6.6).

Basic Components of Transdermal Device(s)

The components of a transdermal device include (1) the polymer matrix or matrices that regulate the release of drug, (ii) the drug absorption/permeation enhancer, (iii) excipients, and (iv) adhesives.

Polymer Matrix

The polymer that is used in the preparation of various components of transdermal drug delivery systems, should fulfill the following requirements:

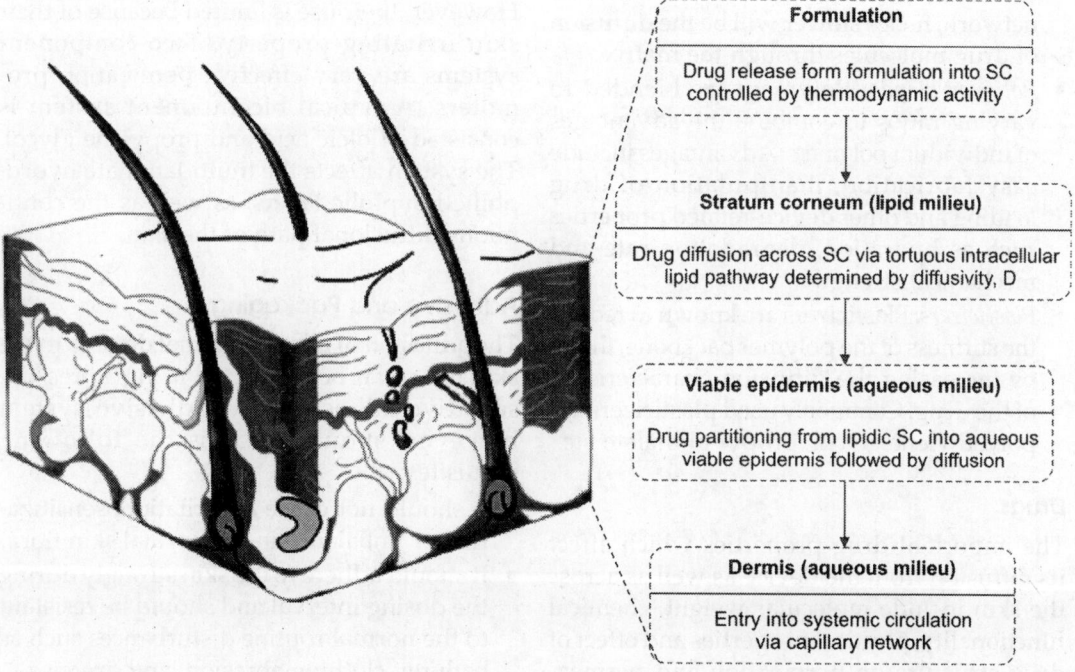

Fig. 6.6: Schematic representation of the drug transport processes involved after the release of the drug from the formulation

- Molecular weight, physical characteristics and chemical functionality of the polymer, must allow the diffusion of the drug substances.
- The nature of the polymer should be chemically nonreactive.
- The polymer and its degradation products must be nontoxic.
- The polymer must not decompose on storage or during the life of the device.
- The polymer must be easy to manufacture and fabricate into the desired product. It should allow incorporation of large amounts of active agent.
- The cost of the polymer should not be excessively high. Various techniques, which are frequently employed to modify the polymer properties and thus drug release rates are as follows:

Techniques Relating to Matrix Preparation

- *Cross-linked polymers:* Higher the degree of cross linking, the more dense is the polymer network, hence slower will be the diffusion of drug molecules through the matrix.
- *Polymer blends:* Polymers are blended in varying ratios to combine the advantages of individual polymers. Advantages include easy fabrication, manipulation of drug loading and other device-related properties such as hydration, degradation rate and mechanical strength.
- *Plasticizers:* Plasticizers are known to reduce the stiffness of the polymer backbone, thereby increasing the diffusion characteristics of the drug. Commonly used plasticizers are polyethylene glycol, propyl phthalate etc.

Drugs

The important drug properties which affect its diffusion from the device as well as across the skin include molecular weight, chemical functionality, physical properties and effect of drug structure on permeation and permeability. The diffusion of drug in an adequate amount to produce a satisfactory therapeutic effect is of paramount importance. Other parameters such as skin irritation and clinical need should also be considered before a drug is selected as a candidate for transdermal delivery. The drug should be nonirritating and nonallergic to the human skin.

Penetration Enhancers and Excipients

Skin permeability enhancers and other excipients which promote skin permeation are considered as an integral part of the most of transdermal formulations because of the barrier properties of the stratum corneum. The penetration enhancers have been classified into three categories, i.e. lipophilic solvents, surface-active agents, and two-component systems. Lipophilic solvents have been found to increase permeation of lipophilic drugs. Dimethyl sulfoxide increases the permeation of lipophilic drugs, possibly by affecting the continuous lipophilic pathway of the skin. Surface-active agents also enhance the skin permeation especially of hydrophilic drugs. However, their use is limited because of their skin irritating property. Two-component systems are very effective permeation promoters. A typical bicomponent system is consisted of oleic acid and propylene glycol. The system affects the multi-laminate hydrophilic lipophilic layers, as well as the continuous diffusional path of the skin.

Adhesive and Packaging

The adhesion of all transdermal devices to the skin has so far been affected using a pressure sensitive adhesive. The adhesive system however, should possess the following requisites:

- It should not cause an irritation, sensitization or imbalance in the normal skin flora.
- It should adhere to the skin strongly during the dosing interval and should be resistant to the normal routine disturbances such as bathing, clothing abrasion, and exercise.
- It should easily be removable without leaving any unwashable remains.

- It should have an intimate contact with the skin at the both macroscopic and microscopic levels.

Pressure-sensitive Adhesive

A pressure-sensitive adhesive is generally defined as a material that adheres to a substrate when a light pressure is applied and leaves no residue when removed. In transdermal drug delivery systems, a pressure sensitive adhesive requires to maintain an intimate contact of TDD systems with the skin surface. In TDD systems adhesive should be nonirritant to skin, physically and chemically compatible with drug, and should be moisture resistant. The pressure-sensitive adhesive currently used in transdermal delivery devices may one of the three different categories—butyl rubbers and polyisobutylenes, acrylics, and silicones.

The pressure sensitive adhesive can be positioned on the face of the delivery (face adhesion systems). The devices have to fulfill the additional requirements, which include

- It should be physically compatible with the drug and other dosage form excipients.
- It should not interfere with the permeation characteristics of the drug.
- It should allow the delivery of simple or blended percutaneous absorption enhancers.
- The adhesive properties should not deteriorate on ageing or on storage of delivery system or release of drug.

Butyl Rubber and Polyisobutylenes

Widely used pressure-sensitive adhesives both as primary elastomers, and as tackifiers and modifiers are elastomeric polymers. Butyl rubber is a copolymer of isobutylene with trace levels of isoprene (less than 3%) while polyisobutylene is a homopolymer. Butyl rubber is fairly inert and stable because the C-H backbone is fairly large (containing 40,000 –60,000 units) with only few double bonds and other reactive sites. Small and regularly spaced side groups of polymer chain impart low permeability to gas, air, and moisture. Butyl rubbers are mainly differentiated on the basis of the number of isoprene units per 100 monomer units in the chain as well as molecular weight. In butyl rubbers, stabilizers like zinc dibutyl dithiocarbamate, BHT, are added.

The polyisobutylenes are very similar to butylrubbers, but differ in terminal unsaturation and have a wide molecular weight range. The crosslinking of polymer makes the internal structure completely amorphous and gives them flexibility, tack, internal mobility, and similar desirable properties. The low molecular weight poly-isobutylenes are permanently tacky, clear to white yellow semiliquids containing no stabilisers. They are primarily used as tackifiers. Such polymers provide tackiness, softness, and flexibility and assist in improving the adhesion.

Acrylic Adhesives

The pressure-sensitive acrylic adhesives derive their pressure sensitivity from acrylic esters, which are found in polymers of low glass transition temperature (T_g) and can be copolymerized with acrylic acid and many other functional monomers. The suitable monomers include alkyl acrylate and methyl methacrylates with 4 to 17 carbon atoms and these are excellent pressure sensitive adhesives. 2-ethylhexyl acrylate, butyl acrylate and acrylic acid are commonly used monomers. The polymer properties can be varied by copolymerization with other monomers. Normally, the T_g is used to predict the pressure-sensitive adhesive application of a polymer and the effect of a comonomer on the copolymer properties. Pressure-sensitive properties, such as peel adhesion, may be correlated with T_g. A polymer that is too soft and fails cohesively, when peeled can be improved by copolymerization using a monomer that increases its T_g. Similarly, a hard polymer that fails in peel because of stick-slip manner, may be improved by incorporation of a low T_g causing monomer. The homopolymer must have a low T_g to give good tack. 2-ethylhexyl acrylate ($T_g = -54°C$) and n-butyl acrylate ($T_g = -54°C$), have good tack. They are good pressure sensitive adhesives.

Silicone Adhesives

Silicone pressure-sensitive adhesives exhibit the flexible characteristics of silicone rubber and the temperature resistance of the silicone resins. Moreover, they are nonreacting and are stably functional between extremely low and high temperatures, giving them versatility. Such adhesives are based on two components, a gum and a resin. The resin functions as a tackifier for optimizing the physical properties of the pressure-sensitive adhesives. A broad range of tack and peel adhesion properties are achieved in combination by varying the gum/resin ratio. There are two different types of silicone gum, i.e. methyl and phenyl.

Methylated silicone-based pressure-sensitive adhesives exhibit a wide range of viscosities (100–90,000 cp) and, typically contain approximately, 50% solids. Increases with the addition of a dry-type adhesive. A dry type of methyl-based adhesive having peel strength of 1110 g/cm, may be blended with a tacky adhesive in order to increase its peel strength from 400 g/cm to about 800 g/cm (about 30% dry type and 70% tacky type). These methyl types of adhesives are universal. The phenyl-based adhesives are also available in two viscosity ranges—6,000 to 25,000 cp and 50,000 to 100,000 cp. Phenyl adhesives have good tack and peel strength and high viscosity.

Based on the components used for the preparations of these delivery systems, they could essentially be classified as:
1. Membrane moderated
2. Adhesion diffusion controlled
3. Matrix dispersion type
4. Microreservoir type

Membrane moderated TDDS (reservoir type device)

In membrane moderated systems, the drug reservoir is encapsulated in a shallow compartment molded from a drug impermeable metallic plastic lamination, whilst the drug delivery side is covered by a rate-controlling polymeric membrane. The drug molecules are released only through the release rate-controlling membrane. In the drug reservoir compartment, the drug solids are dispersed in a solid polymer matrix or suspended in an unleachable viscous fluid that forms a paste like suspension. On the external surface, a thin layer of drug compatible adhesive polymer may be applied for an intimate skin contact. The rate of drug release from this type of transdermal drug delivery system can be tailored by varying the polymer composition permeability coefficient and thickness of the rate-limiting membrane. Several transdermal therapeutic systems have been successfully developed using this technology, i.e. Transderm Scop® for 3-day protection of motion sickness and Transderm nitro® for once a day medication of angina pectoris. This approach has also been used for the development of transdermal therapeutic system for the controlled percutaneous absorption of estradiol, clonidine, and prostaglandin (Fig. 6.7).

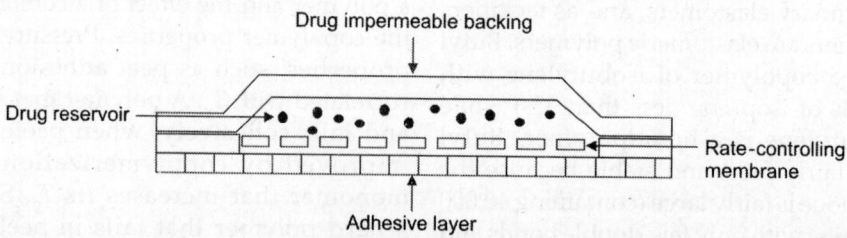

Fig. 6.7: Cross-sectional view of membrane moderated transdermal drug delivery system

Adhesion diffusion controlled TDDS

This type of delivery system, is a simplified form of the membrane moderated drug delivery system. Instead of completely encapsulating the drug reservoir in a compartment, the drug reservoir is prepared by directly dispensing the drug in an adhesive polymer and then spreading the medicated adhesive by solvent film-casting method over a flat sheet of drug impermeable metallic-plastic backing membrane to form a thin drug

reservoir layer. The drug reservoir layer is covered by a nonmedicated rate-controlling adhesive polymer of constant thickness to produce an adhesive diffusion-controlled drug delivery system (Fig. 6.8).

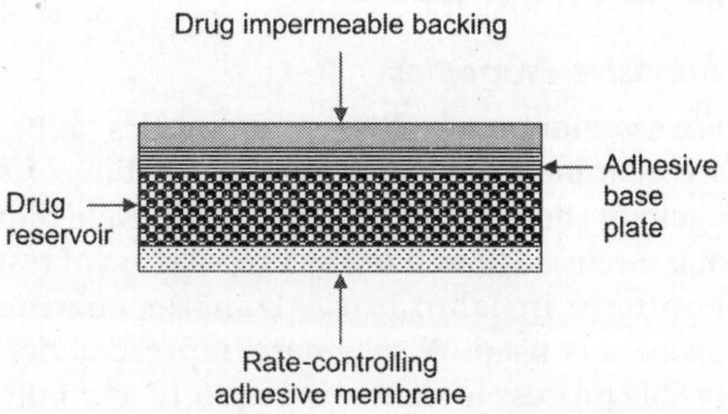

A transdermal patch or skin patch is a medicated adhesive patch that is placed on the skin to deliver a specific dose of medication through the skin and into the bloodstream. The first commercially available prescription patch was approved by the United States Food and Drug Administration in December 1979, which successfully administered scopolamine for motion sickness [Figs 6.9 (a), (b) and (c)].

Fig. 6.8: Cross-sectional view of adhesion diffusion type transdermal drug delivery system

Matrix dispersion type TDDS

The matrix dispersion type transdermal systems are formed by homogeneously dispersing the drug in a hydrophilic lipophilic mix polymeric matrix and the polymer matrix, is then molded into a form of a medicated disc of defined surface area and thickness. The drug reservoir containing polymer disc is then

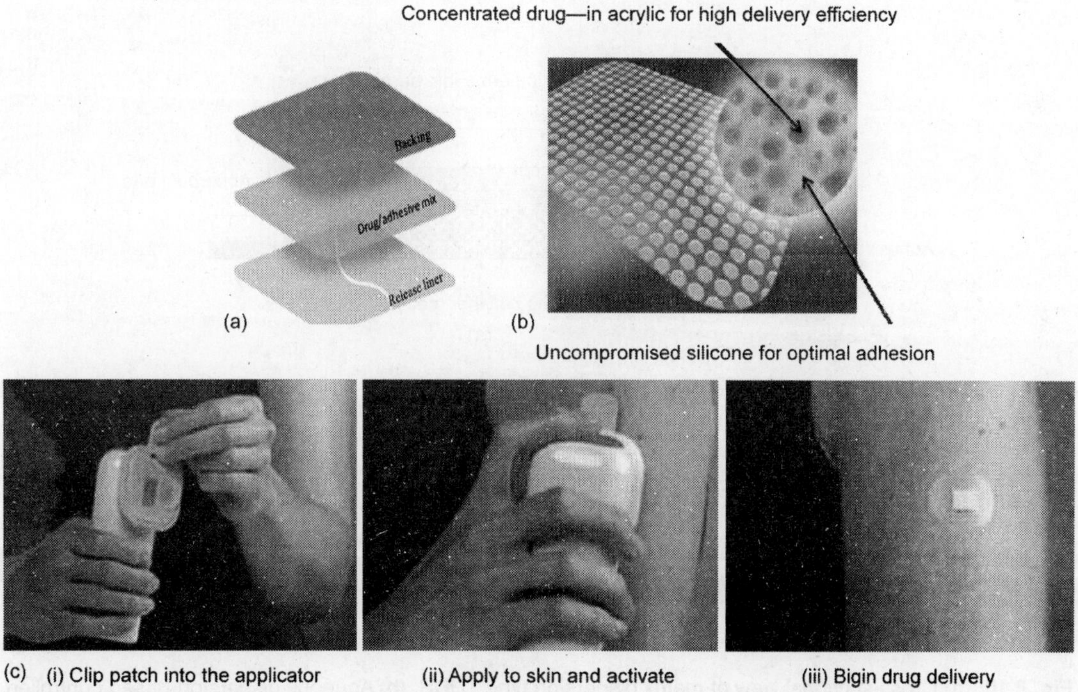

Fig. 6.9: (a) Drug in adhesive patch, (b) DOT matrix® patch, (c) applying the passport system to the skin

glued over an occlusive base plate consisted of a compartment fabricated using an impermeable plastic backing. Instead of spreading the adhesive polymer on to the surface of the medicated disc, the polymer is applied along the circumference to form an adhesive rim around the medicated disc. This type of polymeric device is exemplified by Nitro Dur® system, which is used for once a day medication of angina pectoris. The delivery system can also be used for transdermal administration of estradiol diacetate and verapamil [Figs 6.10 (a) and (b)].

Microreservoir type TDDS

This type of delivery systems have some of the essential features of both, i.e. reservoir and matrix dispersion type drug delivery systems. In this approach, the drug reservoir is formed by suspending the drug as solid in an aqueous solution of water-soluble liquid dispersion, by high shear mechanical agitation to form thousands of unleachable microspheres of the drug. This thermodynamically unstable

dispersion is stabilized by immediate cross-linking of the polymer chains in-situ. This technology has been utilized in the development of Nitro Dur® for one day treatment of angina pectoris (Fig. 6.11).

CHARACTERIZATION OF TRANSDERMAL DRUG DELIVERY SYSTEMS

Evaluation of Pressure-sensitive Adhesives

The pressure-sensitive adhesives are evaluated for general adhesive properties as well as for dermal toxicity.

Adhesive Properties

For evaluation of adhesive properties, adhesive laminates are prepared, consisting of a backing sheet or membrane, an adhesive film and a release liner. For the preparation of test laminate in laboratory, transfer coating process is used. A schematic representation of this process is shown in Figs 6.12 and 6.13. Pressure-sensitive adhesive can be evaluated on the basis of their three basic properties— peel adhesion, tack, and shear strength.

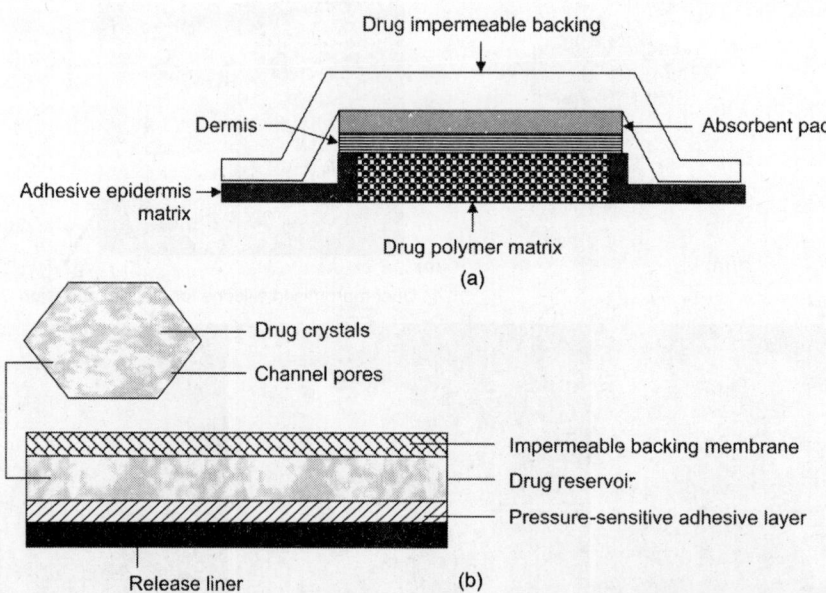

Fig. 6.10: (a) Cross-sectional view of matrix dispersion type TDDS. (b) Aqueous dispersion-based controlled transdermal monolithic system

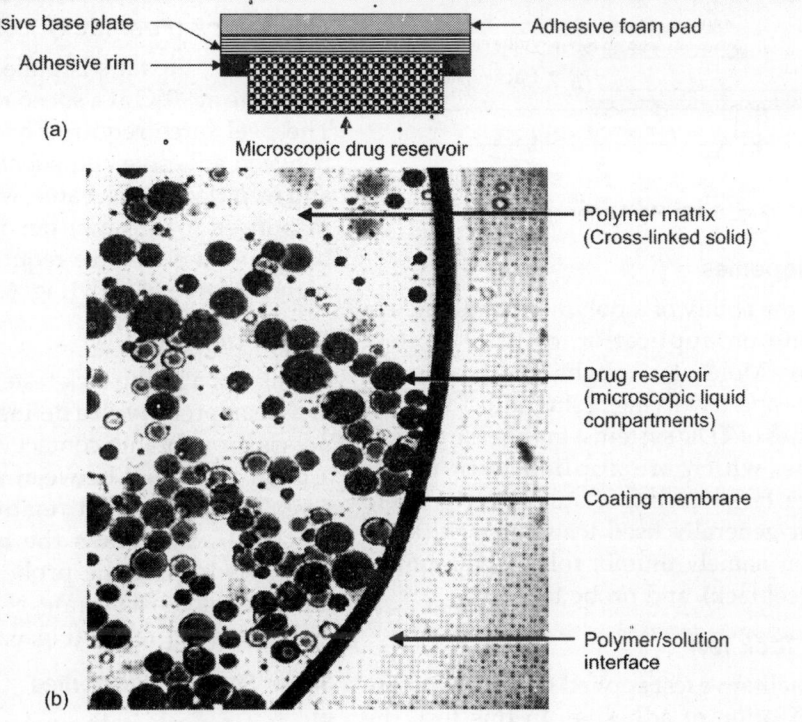

Occlusive base plate
Adhesive rim
Adhesive foam pad
(a)
Microscopic drug reservoir

Polymer matrix
(Cross-linked solid)

Drug reservoir
(microscopic liquid
compartments)

Coating membrane

Polymer/solution
interface

(b)

Fig. 6.11: (a) Cross-sectional view of matrix dispersion type TDDS. (b) Microreservoir drug delivery system showing the microscopic structure of system

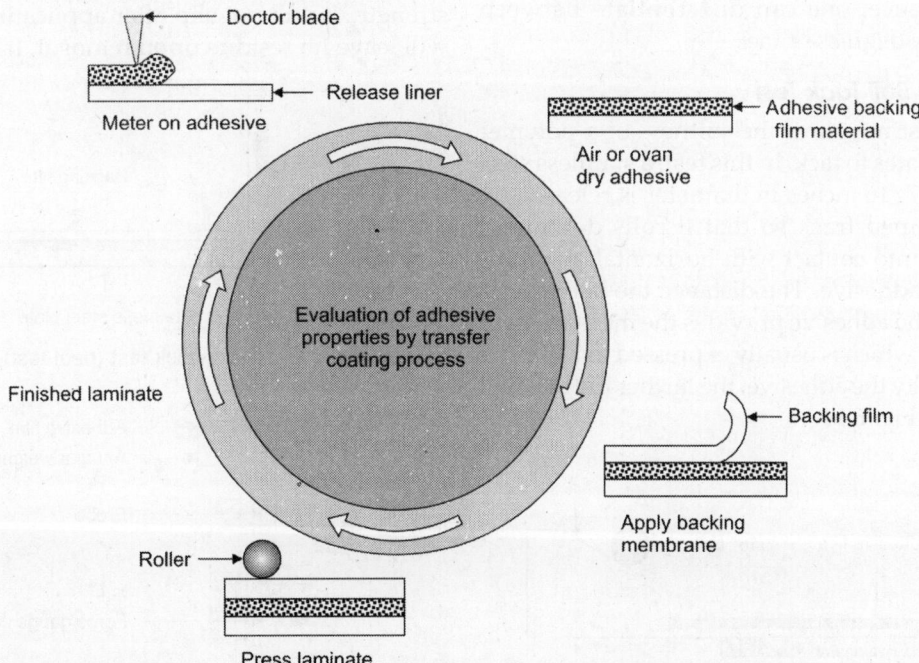

Doctor blade

Release liner

Meter on adhesive

Adhesive backing
film material

Air or ovan
dry adhesive

Evaluation of adhesive
properties by transfer
coating process

Finished laminate

Backing film

Apply backing
membrane

Roller

Press laminate

Fig. 6.12: Schematic representation of preparation of test laminates by transfer coating process

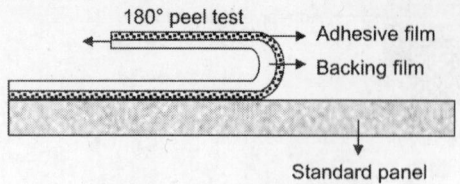

Fig. 6.13: Peel adhesion text

Tack Properties

Tack is the ability of a polymer to adhere to a substrate on application of little contact pressure. Molecular weight, composition of polymer and tackifying resins, affect the tack properties of TDD systems. In the case of TDD systems, which are applied with finger pressure, tack is an important property. There are four generally used tests for tack determination namely thumb, rolling ball, quick-stick (peel-tack), and probe tack test.

Thumb Tack Test

It is a qualitative test applied for tack property determination of adhesive. In this test, the thumb is simply pressed on the adhesive and the relative tack property is detected. By experience, one can differentiate between relative degrees of tack.

Rolling Ball Tack Test

This test measures the softness of a polymer that relates to tack. In this test, a stainless steel ball of 7/16 inches in diameter is released on an inclined track so that it rolls down and comes into contact with horizontal, upward-facing adhesive. The distance the ball travels along the adhesive provides the measurement of tack, which is usually expressed in inch. The less tacky the adhesive, the farther the ball will travel (Fig. 6.14).

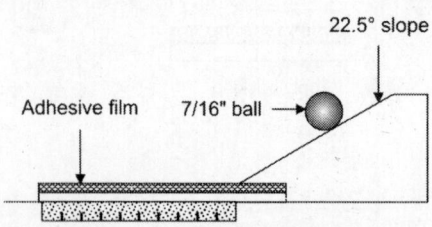

Fig. 6.14: Rolling ball tack test

Quick-stick (Peel-tack) Test

In this test, the tape is pulled away from the substrate at 90°C at a speed of 12 inches/min. The peel force required breaking the bond between adhesive and substrate is measured and recorded as tack value, which is expressed in ounces (or grams) per inch width. The higher values of force required indicates the higher degree of tack (Fig. 6.15).

Probe Tack Test

In this test a probe tack tester is used. The tip of a clean probe with a defined surface roughness is brought into contact with an adhesive; a bond is formed between probe and adhesive. The subsequent removal of the probe mechanically breaks the bond. The force required to pull the probe away from the adhesive at constant rate, is recorded as tack (expressed in grams) (Fig. 6.16).

Shear Strength Properties

Shear strength is the measurement of the cohesive strength of an adhesive polymer. If transdermal device has adequate cohesive strength, it will not slip after application and will leave no residue upon removal. It can be

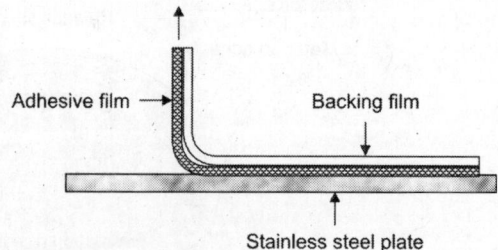

Fig. 6.15: Quick-stick test (peel test)

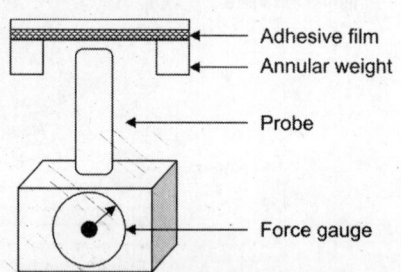

Fig. 6.16: Probe tack tester

influenced by the molecular weight, the degree of cross-linking and the composition of polymer, as well as by the type and the amount of tackifier added. In this particular test, adhesive-coated tape is applied onto a stainless steel plate. A specified weight is hung from the tape, for its pulling in a direction parallel to the plate. Shear strength is determined by measuring the time it takes to pull the tape off the plate. The longer the time taken for removal, greater is the shear strength.

In Vitro Release Kinetics

Controlled-release kinetics of drug from technologically different transdermal therapeutic systems, can be evaluated and compared by using Franz diffusion cell assembly. For example, in the case of nitroglycerine TDD systems, the release of nitroglycerine from Transderm Nitro (a membrane-moderated transdermal system) and Deponit (an adhesive diffusion-controlled system) can be compared by plotting the data for cumulative amount of drug released from these systems as a function of time (Qv/st).

In Vitro Skin Permeation Kinetics
Animal Model and Human Cadaver

In vitro permeation kinetics studies can be performed on hairless mouse skin or human cadaver skin by using either Franz diffusion cell or two-reservoir diffusion cell (Valia-Chien permeation cell). In two-reservoir diffusion cells, sink conditions can be maintained. The permeation of nitroglycerine across human cadaver and hairless mouse skin from different TDD therapeutic systems, was compared for their kinetics. It was noted that the rates of skin permeation generated from the excised skins of hairless mouse, agree fairly with the data obtained from human cadaver skin, suggesting that hairless mouse skin could be an acceptable animal model as an option for human skin permeation kinetics studies.

Transdermal Delivery—New Approaches

Several new techniques have recently been developed, which reduce the barrier properties of the stratum corneum and as a result significantly enhance the skin permeation of drugs. Potential approaches used in overcoming the skin barrier properties are as follows. Over the last two decades, many more transdermal products have been approved for sales in market (Table 6.3).

Physical approaches (Fig. 6.17)

1. Iontophoresis
2. Ultrasound

Table 6.3: Marketed transdermal drug delivery products			
Product name	*Drug*	*Manufacturer*	*Indication*
Androderm®	Testosterone	TheraTech/Glaxo Smith Kline	Hypogonadism (males)
Nitro-dur®	Nitroglycerin	Key Pharmaceuticals	Angina pectoris
Nitrodisc®	Nitroglycerin	Roberts Pharmaceutical	Angina pectoris
Minitran®	Nitroglycerin	3M Pharmaceuticals	Angina pectoris
Deponit®	Nitroglycerin	Schwarz-Pharma	Angina pectoris
Climaderm®	Estradiol	Ethical Holdings/ Wyeth-Ayerest	Postmenstrual syndrom
Estraderm®	Estradiol	Alza/Norvatis	Postmenstrual syndrome
FemPatch®	Estradiol	Parke-Davis	Postmenstrual syndrome
Alora®	Estradiol	TheraTech/Proctol and Gamble	Postmenstrual syndrome
Prostep®	Nicotine	Elan Corp./Lederle Labs	Smoking cessation

Contd.

Table 6.3: Marketed transdermal drug delivery products *(Contd.)*

Product name	Drug	Manufacturer	Indication
Nicoderm®	Nicotine	Alza/Glaxo Smith Kline	Smoking cessation
Habitraol®	Nicotine	Novartis	Smoking cessation
Nuvelle TS	Estrogen/Progesterone	Ethical Holdings/Schering	Hormone replacement therapy
CombiPatch®	Estradiol/Norethindrone	Noven Inc./Aventis	Hormone replacement therapy
Ortho-Evra®	Norelgestromin/Estradiol	Ortho-McNeil Pharmaceuticals	Birth control
Duragesic®	Fentanyl	Alza/Janssen Pharmaceutic	Moderate/severe pain
Catapres-TTS	Clonidine	Alza/Boehinger Ingelheim	Hypertension

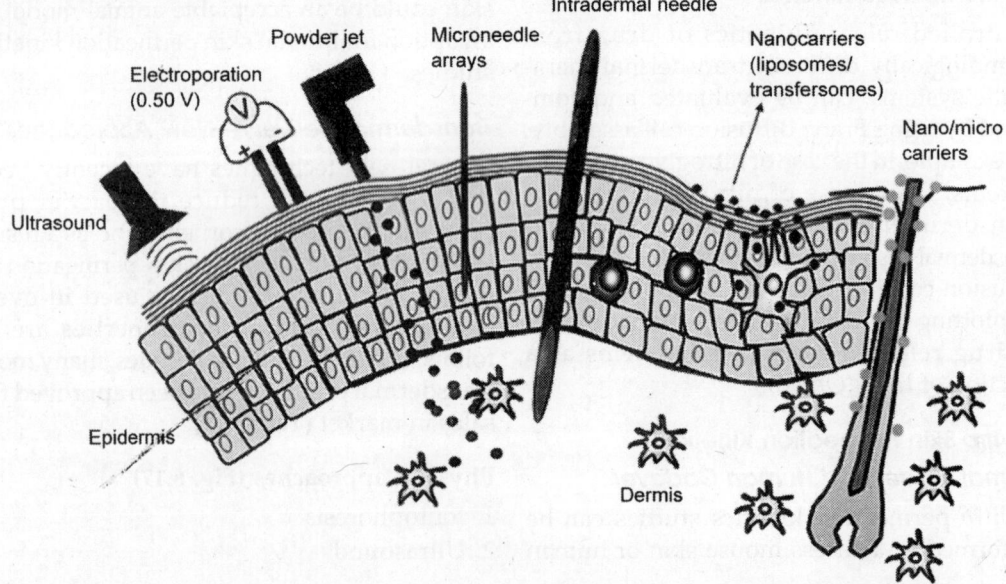

Fig. 6.17: Schematic illustration of physical approaches and devices developed for TDDS

3. Thermal energy
4. Stripping of stratum corneum
5. Hydration of stratum corneum

Chemical approaches

1. Delipidization of stratum corneum
2. Synthesis of lipophilic analogs
3. Coadministration of cutaneous enzyme inhibitor

Biochemical approach

1. Synthesis of bioconvertible prodrugs
2. Coadministration of cutaneous enzyme inhibitors

Advanced Penetration Enhancement Techniques

a. **Iontophoresis:** One of the most evolved of these technologies is iontophoresis that uses a small electrical current (usually, 500 micro-amperes cm^{-2}) to facilitate the transfer of drugs across the skin (Fig. 6.18). Charged species are repelled into and through the skin as a result of an electrical potential across the membrane; the efficiency of this process is dependent on the polarity, valency, and ionic mobility of the permeant as well as on the composition of the delivery formulation and the current profile.

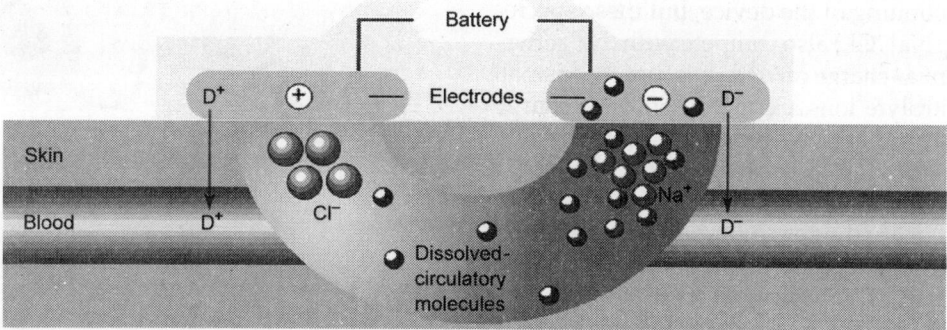

Fig. 6.18: Schematic of an iontophoretic device

Typically, two electrolyte chambers containing electrodes (one of which contains the ionized therapeutic molecule of similar polarity, i.e. cationic drug in anodal chamber) are placed on the skin surface and driven by a constant current source. The magnitude of current determines the amount of charge generated in the circuit and, in turn, the number of ions transported across the skin; this ensures a controlled and efficient method of drug delivery because the amount of compound delivered is directly proportional to the quantity of charge passed. The anodal delivery of small cationic drugs is generally favored because the skin carries a net negative charge at physiological pH, which renders it permselective to the positively charged species under the imposition of an electrical field. As a corollary, the preferential transport of small cations (e.g. buffer salts, Na^+) induces a net solvent flow in the direction of cation movement (anode to cathode) as these ions collide with solvent molecules in their path. The resulting electro osmotic flow consequently enables the transport of neutral (as well as positively charged) species that can now literally be ferried from the anode to the cathode. In fact, for cationic drugs, the relative contribution of electro osmosis (compared with the classical electro repulsive effect) becomes increasingly significant with increasing molecular weight, such that it is probably the predominant mechanism for the iontophoretic transport of peptides and small proteins. It should be noted that a unidirectional solvent flow is the consequence of a permselective membrane; a positively charged membrane will be permselective to anions and will therefore induce a net solvent flow in the sense of anion movement (cathode to anode). Conversely, an uncharged membrane that is equally favorable to anions and cations will not give rise to a bulk solvent flow. This means that modification of the skin's charge (through changes in formulation pH) has the potential to change the balance of electroosmotic and electrorepulsive contributions to iontophoretic transport, and this has now been convincingly demonstrated in *in vitro* systems. The formulation pH, in fact, plays a crucial role in the efficiency of the iontophoretic delivery process in that, it influences not only the skin's permselectivity, but also the ionization state of the permeant, which in turn determines its electrical mobility. The fine tuning of such formulation parameters is critical to the optimization of an iontophoretic device, which is required to deliver therapeutic levels of medicament swiftly (in order to minimize the period of current passage) across a relatively small surface area. For instance, the inclusion of an electrolyte is obviously essential for the electrochemical functioning of the device, but these species (e.g. Na^+, Cl^-) also compete with the 'active' agent as charge carriers; because these small electrolyte ions are highly efficient charge carriers themselves, they are preferentially transported across the skin, and their incorporation in the device must therefore be carefully regulated. Although, the pharmaceutical industry still awaits the approval of iontophoretic patch-like devices that contain both the medicament and the microelectronic processing device in a small portable unit, iontophoresis has been shown to be an effective method to administer ionized drugs in dermatological, physiotherapeutic and diagnostic applications within the clinic. Small battery-operated power supplies coupled to 'fillable' electrodes are now widely available to the physician for routine use in the clinic. A long-standing diagnostic test for cystic fibrosis consists of assaying chloride levels in sweat, the secretion of which is stimulated by the cutaneous iontophoresis of a cholinergic (and cationic) drug, pilocarpine. First FDA approved pre-filled active anesthetic patch LidoSite® (lidocaine HCl/epinephrine topical iontophoretic patch) 10%/0.1% – Vyteris (Fig. 6.19), a revolutionary active patch provides fast, effective analgesia prior to blood is drawn; by venipunctures, and other superficial dermatological procedures. More recently, IONSYS™ (Fig. 6.20) is indicated in the short-term management of acute postoperative pain in adult patients requiring opioid analgesia during hospitalization.

b. **Ultrasound (phonophoresis, sonophoresis):** The application of ultrasound to deliver therapeutic compounds through the skin is generally referred to as sonophoresis (also known as phonophoresis), and dates back to the 1950s. Ultrasound is defined as sound having a frequency above 18 kHz. Most modern ultrasound devices are based on

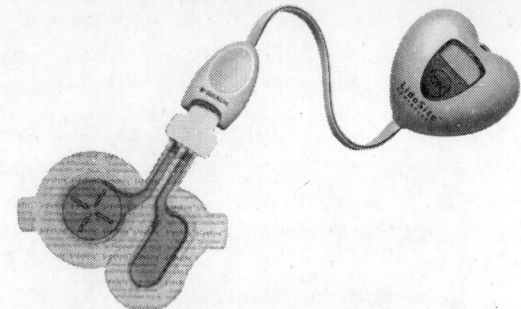

Fig. 6.19: Vyteris' LidoSite®

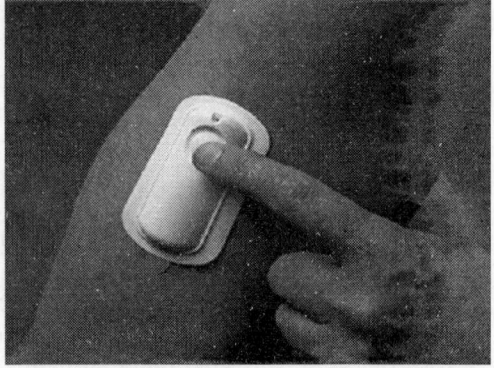

Fig. 6.20: IONSYS™

the piezoelectric effect. This is achieved by applying pressure to quartz crystals and some polycrystalline materials, such as lead zirconate-titanium or barium titanate, causing electric charges to develop on the outer surface of the material. Thus, application of a rapidly alternating potential across the opposite faces of a piezoelectric crystal will induce corresponding alternating, dimensional changes, thereby converting electrical energy into vibrational (sound) energy (Fig. 6.21).

The ultrasound wave is longitudinal in nature (i.e. the direction of propagation is the same as the direction of oscillation). Longitudinal sound waves cause compression and expansion of the medium at a distance of half a wavelength, leading to pressure variations in the medium. The resistance of the medium to the propagation of sound wave is dependent on the acoustic impedance (Z),

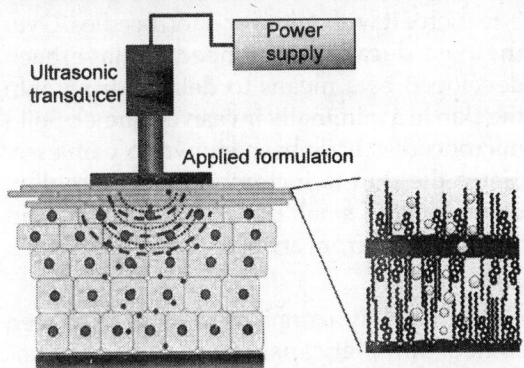

Fig. 6.21: Basic principle of phonophoresis

which is related to the mass density of the medium (ρ) and the speed of propagation (C), according to Eq. 1:

$$Z = \rho \times C \tag{1}$$

The specific acoustic impedances for skin, bone, and air are 1.6×10^6, 6.3×10^6 and 400.0 kg/(m²s), respectively.

As ultrasound energy penetrates the body tissues, biological effects are generally expected to occur, especially if the tissues absorb the energy. The absorption coefficient (a) is used as a measure of the absorption in various tissues. For ultrasound consisting of longitudinal waves with perpendicular incidence on homogeneous tissues, Eq. 2 applies:

$$I(x) = I_0 \times e^{-ax} \tag{2}$$

where $I(x)$ is the intensity at depth x, I_0 is the intensity at the surface and a is the absorption coefficient.

To transfer ultrasound energy to the body, it is necessary to use a contact medium because of the high impedance of air. Many types of contact media are currently available for ultrasound transmission; they can be broadly classified as oils, water-oil emulsions, aqueous gels and ointments. There are three distinct sets of ultrasound conditions based on frequency range and applications:

- High-frequency or diagnostic ultrasound in clinical imaging (3–10 MHz).
- Medium-frequency or therapeutic ultrasound in physical therapy (0.7–3.0 MHz).
- Low-frequency or power ultrasound for lithotripsy, cataract emulsification, liposuction, cancer therapy, dental descaling and ultrasonic scalpels (18–100 kHz).

Mechanism

The mechanism of improved transdermal transport by ultrasound has been studied for over past 20 years. In spite of the large number of studies that have been published, the mechanism is still not well understood or characterized. A possible mechanism of improved percutaneous transport by ultrasound suggested that ultrasound might interact with the structural lipids located in the intercellular channels of the stratum corneum. This is similar to the postulated effects of some chemical transdermal enhancers that act by disordering lipids. Tachibana and Simonin postulated that the energy of ultrasonic vibrations enhances the transdermal permeability through the transfollicular and transepidermal routes, suggesting that microscopic bubbles (cavitation) produced at the surface of the skin by ultrasonic vibration might generate a rapid liquid flow, thereby increasing skin permeability. Mitragotri et al., evaluated the role played by various ultrasound-related phenomena, including cavitation, thermal effects, generation of convective velocities and mechanical effects. It is hypothesized that transdermal transport during low-frequency ultrasound application, occurs across the keratinocytes rather than the hair follicles and suggested that cavitation causes the disorder of the stratum corneum lipids, resulting in significant water penetration into the disordered lipid region. This might cause the formation of aqueous channels through the intercellular lipids of the stratum corneum through which permeants could move. All recent studies indicate that cavitation plays an important role in the enhancing skin penetration mechanism. Several attempts have been made to establish a suitable mathematical model to describe the trans-skin permeation enhancement phenomenon and predict the enhancement ratio for different drugs. A unique design for a transducer system intended to be utilized in an active transdermal drug delivery system, powered by ultrasound was developed as encapsulation systems. The system postulated that a small, light-weight battery powered ultrasonic transducer could be attached to a transdermal patch and used to enlarge the sweat and hair follicle pores of the skin.

Electroporation

Electroporation or electropermeabilization is the transitory structural perturbation of lipid bilayer membranes on application of high voltage pulses. Electrical exposures typically involve electric field pulses that generate transmembrane potentials of 0.5–1.0V voltage for a short period of $10\mu s$ to $100\mu s$. This phenomenon occurs in different kinds of lipid bilayer membranes—artificial (liposomes), cellular (bacteria, yeast, plant, mammalian cell) or in a more complex structure (stratum corneum). Reversible electrical breakdown and high molecular transport are observed, resulting from structural rearrangements of the cell membrane (Fig. 6.22).

Microneedles

A conceptually straightforward way to selectively permeabilize the stratum corneum is to pierce it with micro or nano needles. Over the past decade, microneedles have been developed as a means to deliver drugs into the skin in a minimally invasive manner. Solid microneedles have been shown to painlessly pierce the skin to increase skin permeability to a variety of small molecules, proteins and nanoparticles from an extended-release patch (Fig. 6.23).

Alternatively, drug formulations have been coated on or encapsulated within microneedles for rapid or controlled release of peptides and vaccines in the skin. Hollow microneedles have been used to deliver insulin and vaccines by infusion. In general, microneedles (i) increase skin permeability by creating micron-scale pathways into the skin, (ii) can actively drive drugs into the skin either as coated or encapsulated cargo introduced during microneedle insertion or via convective flow through hollow microneedles and (iii) target their effects to the stratum corneum, although microneedles typically pierce across the epidermis and into the superficial dermis too. Several recent advances in microneedle design and development are worthy of note. Original fabrication methods involving sterile preparation of silicon-based structures have moved to low-cost manufacturing methods to make microneedles out of metals and

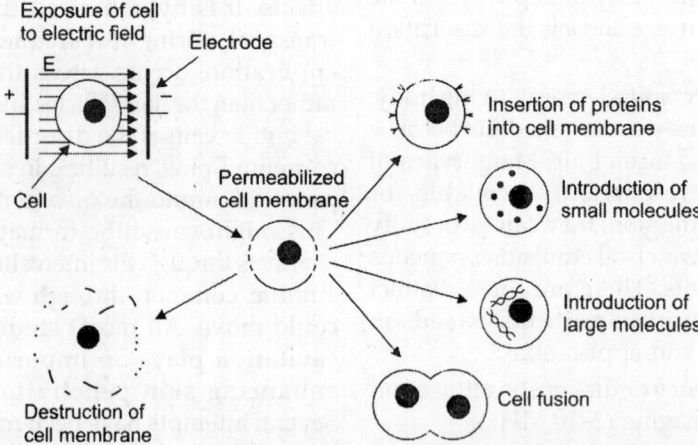

Fig. 6.22: Schematic representation of delivery of bioactives via electroporation technique

Zosano's drug-coated patch   Magnified section of drug-coated microprojections

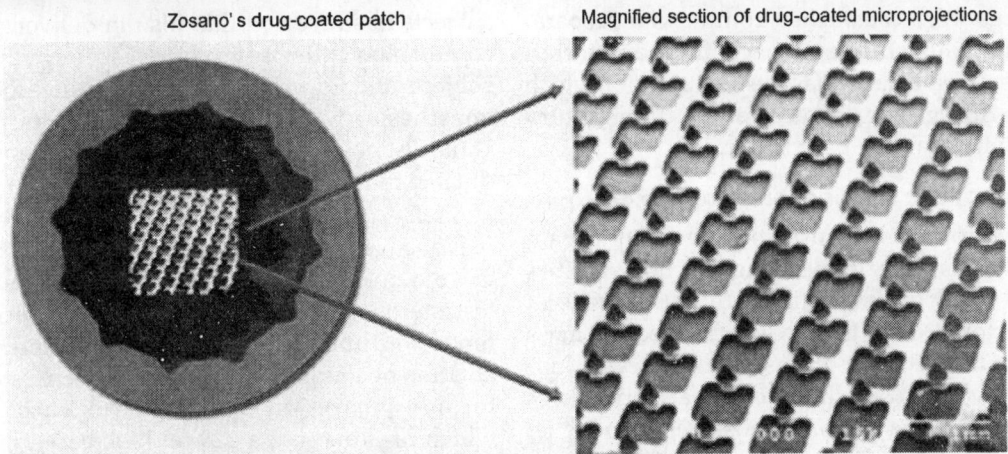

Fig. 6.23: Cross-sectional view of microneedle-based TDDS

polymers commonly found in FDA-approved devices and parenteral formulations. Micro-needles are dip coated with a variety of compounds, including small molecules, proteins, DNA, and virus particles. Micro-needles have also been made of water-soluble polymers that encapsulate various compounds within the needle matrix. These microneedles dissolve in the skin over a timescale of minutes and thereby leave no sharp medical waste after use. Advances have also been made in the delivery to humans using microneedles. In a recent study, naltrexone was administered to healthy volunteers, whose skin was pretreated with microneedles. After applying a naltrexone patch, blood levels of naltrexone reached the therapeutic range. Transdermal delivery without microneedle pretreatment yielded naltrexone levels below detection level. Microneedle treatment was reported to be painless by the volunteers and was generally well tolerated. Other unpublished human studies have demonstrated delivery of parathyroid hormone from coated microneedles, which have advanced from animal studies through clinical trials. Vaccine delivery using microneedles has also been a focus for research. Animal studies have demonstrated delivery of live attenuated virus, inactivated virus, protein subunit, and DNA vaccines against influenza, hepatitis B, Japanese encephalitis and anthrax using solid and hollow microneedles. Human studies have demonstrated the reliability of hollow microneedles to achieve intradermal injection without special training. Administration of influenza vaccine using these microneedles has recently progressed through completion of clinical trials.

Prodrug Approach for Transdermal Delivery

The prodrug approach has been investigated to enhance dermal and transdermal delivery of drugs with unfavorable partition coefficients. The prodrug design strategy generally involves addition of a promoiety to increase partition coefficient and hence solubility and transport of the parent drug in the stratum corneum. Upon reaching the viable epidermis, esterases release, the parent drug following hydrolysis thereby optimising solubility in the aqueous epidermis. The intrinsic poor permeability of the very polar 6-mercaptopurine was increased up to 240 times using S6-acyloxymethyl and 9-dialkylaminomethyl promoieties. The skin permeability of 5-fluorouracil, a polar drug with was increased up to 25 times by forming N-acyl derivatives. The prodrug approach has also been investigated for increasing skin permeability of nonsteroidal anti-inflammatory drugs, naltrexone, nalbuphine, buprenorphine, β-blockers and other drugs. Well-established commercial preparations using this approach include steroid esters (e.g. betamethasone-17-valerate), which provide greater topical anti-inflammatory activity than the parent steroids.

Therapeutic Applications (Table 6.4)

New approach focuses on minimizing pain and bruising by minimizing injection volumes and depth of penetration. Multi use nozzle jet injectors (MUNJIs), have been used for mass immunization programs for diseases including measles, smallpox, cholera, hepatitis B, influenza and polio. Disposable cartridge jet injectors (DCJIs), have been used for delivery of several proteins. Most work has been done on delivery of insulin and growth hormones, while erythropoietin and interferon have also been delivered using this approach. Insulin administration by jet injectors led to a faster delivery into systemic circulation, possibly due to better drug dispersion at the injection site.

Microneedles have been studied *in vitro,* in animals and in humans for a variety of applications. Microneedle piercing has been shown to increase skin permeability by orders of magnitude to a variety of compounds ranging from low molecular weight tracers to proteins, DNA and even nanoparticles. A recent study reported on delivery of naltrexone, which is used to treat alcohol and opioid addiction, at therapeutic levels in normal human subjects using this approach. Solid microneedles have also been coated with a number of different compounds, including low molecular weight drugs, proteins, DNA, virus particles and microparticles. Dissolving polymeric microneedles have been developed which encapsulate various compounds, including erythropoietin and enzymes. The bio-actives have shown to retain activity after encapsulation and even after at least two months of storage at room temperature. Hollow microneedles have been shown to deliver insulin to rodent models and modulate blood glucose levels. Recent work on human

subjects has revealed that insulin delivery to control blood glucose levels in diabetic human subjects and lidocaine delivery to induce local anesthesia in normal human subjects are clinically possible in a therapeutically reproducible manner.

ViaDerm™ has been tested extensively *in vitro* for delivery across porcine skin and in in vivo on pigs and Sprague-Dawley rats of testosterone, granisetron hydrochloride, diclofenac sodium and plasmid DNA. Thermal ablation by Passport system™ has been tested for administration of adenovirus vaccine, which resulted into a 120-fold increase in reporter gene expression in various mice strains (Bramson, Dayball et al., 2003). Recently, delivery of interferon-γ has been shown to be successful using passive and iontophoretic patch in rat model. The device has also been tested for delivery of influenza antigens, tetanus antigen, erythropoietin and fentanyl citrate in preclinical studies.

Levonorgestrel, a potent contraceptive agent, formulated as transdermal protransferosome gel can provide enhanced, prolonged and controlled delivery and overcome GI disturbances, weight gain, irregular bleeding, headache etc., associated with oral dosing. Ester prodrug of ketorolac provides enhanced permeation, whereas nanostructured lipid carrier serves as controlled-release system therby avoiding gastric ulceration and renal failure associated with frequent long-term oral dosing.

Drugs used for long-term dosing in chronic diseases like captopril, verapamil, terbutaline sulfate, pinacidil, propranolol have short biological half-life, considerable first pass metabolism, therefore can be formulated as TDDS to achieve prolonged steady state plasma concentration.

Rising Interest in Transdermal Vaccines

Transdermal delivery offers convincing opportunities to improve vaccine administration. Although vaccines are typically macromolecules, viral particles, or other large supramolecular constructs, their small (microgram) doses may facilitate the possibility of transdermal delivery. Vaccine delivery via the skin is even more attractive therapeutically, because it targets the potent epidermal Langerhans and dermal dendritic cells that may generate a strong

Table 6.4: List of patents on transdermal drug delivery

Patent	Year	Original assignee	Title
US4405616	1983	Nelson Research & Development Company	Penetration enhancers for transdermal drug delivery of systemic agents
US4626539	1986	Alza Corporation	Skin permeation enhancer compositions
US4626539	1986	E. I. DuPont de Nemours	Transdermal delivery of opioids and company
US4706676	1987	The United States of America	Dermal substance collection device as represented by the secretary of the army
US4746515	1988	ALZA Corporation	Skin permeation enhancer compositions using glycerol monolaurate
US4764379	1988	Alza Corporation	Transdermal drug delivery device with dual permeation enhancers
US4801586	1989	Nelson Research and Development Co.	Penetration enhancers for transdermal delivery of systemic agents
US4888360	1989	American Home Products Corporation	Carvone in enhancement of transdermal drug delivery
US4888362	1989	American Home Products Corp.	Eugenol in enhancement of transdermal drug delivery
US4906475	1990	Paco Pharmaceutical Services	Estradiol transdermal delivery system
US4927687	1990	Biotek Inc.	Sustained release transdermal drug delivery composition
US4931283	1990	American Home Products Corp. (Del)	Menthol in enhancement of transdermal drug delivery
US5023252	1991	Conrex Pharmaceutical Corporation	Transdermal and transmembrane delivery of drugs
US5142044	1992	Whitby Research Inc.	Penetration enhancers for transdermal delivery of systemic agents
US5196410	1993	Pfizer Inc.	Transdermal flux enhancing compositions
US5196416	1993	Eli Lilly and Company	Transdermal flux-enhancing pharmaceutical compositions comprising azone, ethanol and water
US5221254	1993	Alza Corporation	Method for reducing sensation in iontophoretic drug delivery
US5391548	1995	Pfizer Inc.	Transdermal flux enhancing compositions to treat hypertension, diabetes and angina pectoris
US5500222	1996	Alza Corporation	Transdermal administration of oxybutynin
US5662925	1997	TheraTech, Inc.	Transdermal delivery system with adhesive overlay and peel seal disc
US7470433	2008	Antares Pharma IPL AG	Formulations for transdermal or transmucosal application
US7879344	2011	Kimberly-Clark Worldwide Inc.	Transdermal delivery of oleocanthal for relief of inflammation

immune response at much lower doses than deeper injection. The most successful vaccine of all time the smallpox vaccine, which have eradicated the disease worldwide was administered via the skin with the aid of a small needle device used to breach the stratum corneum barrier. Although, it was effective, however this approach does not provide good control over delivery, which has motivated development of new delivery methods. Elimination of the need for hypodermic needles further motivates transdermal vaccine development. In the situations, where needle reuse kills at least 1.3 million people per year from hepatitis B and AIDS, needle-free, patch-based vaccination could have large utility and relevance. In addition, the possibility of administering vaccine patches by minimally trained personnel or patients themselves could not only facilitate compliance with routine, seasonal and pandemic vaccination, but could also expedite vaccination campaigns in developing countries, where medical personnel are limited in terms of availability.

SUGGESTED READINGS

1. Aggarwal G, Dhawan SA, Pharmainfo. net. 2009; 7(5).
2. Chein YW and Valia KH (1985), *Drug Dev. Ind. Pharm.* 11, 1195.
3. Altea Therapeutics, www.alteatherapeutics.com.
4. Aarti Naik, Yogeshvar N Kalia and Richard H Guy, *PSTT* Vol. 3, No. 9, 2000.
5. Akomeah FK (2010), *Curr. Drug Deliv.* 7(4), 283–96.
6. Aslani, P. and Kennedy, R.A., J. Contr. Rel., 1996, 42, 75–82.
7. Baichwal MR. MSR Foundation; 1985, 136–47.
8. BW Barry, *Euro J Pharma Sci*, 14 (2001), 101–114.
9. BB Michniak-Kohn, Transdermal Delivery Systems, 2001.
10. Blank IH, Scheuplein J and MacFarlane DJ, (1967), *J. Invest. Dermatol.*, 49, 582.
11. Bodor N and Loftsson T, US Patent 4,885, 174, 5 Dec 1989.
12. Bodor N and Loftsson T, US Patent 4, 983, 396, 8 Jan 1991.
13. Bal SM, Ding Z Van, RE, Jiskoot W, Bouwstra, JA (2010), *J. Control. Rel.* 148(3), 266–82.
14. Batheja P, Thakur R, Michniak B. (2006), *Exp. Opin. Drug Deliv.*, 3(1), 127–38.
15. Chein YW and Lambert HJ (1976b), US Patent, 3, 992, 518.
16. Chein YW and Lambert HJ (1977), US Patent, 3, 953, 580.
17. Chein YW and Lambert HJ, (1976a) US Patent, 3, 946, 106.
18. Chein YW, (1978), JR Robinson (Ed.), Marcel Dekkar, 8, 223.
19. Degim IT, Burgess DJ, Papa dimitra kopoulos, F. (2010), *J. Microencapsul.*, 27(8), 669–81.
20. Dixit N, Bali V, Baboota S, Ahuja A, Ali J (2007), *Curr. Drug Deliv.* 4(1), 1–10.
21. Durand, C., Alhammad, A., Willett, K.C. (2012), *Am. J. Health Syst. Pharm.*, 69(2), 116–24.
22. Foldvari, M. J. (2010) Biomed. Nanotechnol. 6(5), 543–57.
23. Fawzi MB, Iyer UR and Mahjour M, U.S. Patent 4, 783, 450, 8 Nov 1988.
24. Francoeur ML and Potts RO, US Patent 5, 023, 085, 11 Jun 1991.
25. Foco A, Hadziabdic J and Becic F (2004), *Med. Arch.*, 58, 230–34.
26. FDA Advisory Committee for Pharma Sci and Clinical , Pharmacol, 2009.
27. Guy RH (1996), *Pharm Res.* 13, 1765.
28. Guo R, Du X, Zhang R, Deng L, Dong A, Zhang J (2011) *Eur. J. Pharm. Biopharm.* 79(3), 574–83.
29. Heather AE Benson, *Current Drug Delivery,* 2005, 2, 23–33.
30. Ito Y, Hasegawa R, Fukushima K, Sugioka N, Takada K (2010), *Biol. Pharm. Bull.*, 33(4), 683–90.
31. Ilana Lavon and Joseph Kost, DDT Vol. 9, No. 15, 2004.
32. Keshary PR and Chein YW (1994), *Drug Dev. Ind. Pharm.* 10, 883.
33. Lvovich VF, Matthews E, Riga AT, Kaza L (2010), *J. Control. Rel.* 145(2), 134–40.
34. Misra N and Rao VU (1996), *Ind. J. Expt. Bio.* 34(2), 171.
35. Mundada AS and Avari JG (2011), *Curr. Drug Deliv.* 2011, 8(5), 517–25.
36. Mark R Prausnitz and Robert Langer, Nat Biotechnol. 2008; 26(11): 1261–8.
37. Okabe H, Suzuki E, Saitoh T, Takayama K and Nagai T (1994), *J. Control Rel.* 32, 243.
38. Patil S, Singh P, Szolar-Platzer C and Maibach H (1996), *J. Pharm. Sci.* 85(3), 249.
39. Pierre MB, Miranda DS and Costa I (2011), *Arch. Dermatol. Res.*, 303(9): 607–621.

40. Robinson JR and Lee, VHL (1987), *Controlled Drug Delivery: Fundamentals and Applications*, Marcel Dekker, New York, 523.

41. Shah HS, Genier S, Yu CD and Patel B (1993), US Patent 5,219,877.

42. Sharata HH and Burnette RR (1988), *J. Pharm. Sci.*, 77(1), 27.

43. Stinchcomb AL, Swaan PW, Ekabo O, Harris KK, Browe J, Hammell DC, Cooperman TA, Pearsall M J. *Pharm. Sci.*, 2002, 91, 2571–8.

44. Sung KC, Fang JY; Wang JJ, Hu OY Eur. *J. Pharm. Sci.*, 2003, 18, 63–70.

45. Sung KC, Fang JY, Hu, OY, *J. Control Rel.*, 2000, 67, 1–8.

46. Samad A, Ullah Z, Alam MI, Wais M, Shams MS (2009), *Recent Pat. Drug Deliv. Formul.* 3(2), 143–52.

47. Swain S, Beg S, Singh A, Patro ChN, Rao ME (2011), *Curr. Drug Deliv.* 8(4), 456–73.

48. Schroeter A, Engelbrecht T, Neubert RH, Goebel, AS (2010), *J. Biomed. Nanotechnol.* 6(5), 511–28.

49. Scheuplein J, (1965), *J. Invest. Dermatol.*, 48, 334.

50. ScheupleinJ, (1967a), *J. Invest. Dermatol.*, 48, 79.

51. Scheuplein J, (1967b), *J. Invest. Dermatol.*, 45, 334.

52. Scheuplein J, Blank IH, Burner GJ, Mac Farlane DJ (1965), *J. Invest. Derma*, 52, 63.

53. Tamura G, Ichinose M, Fukuchi Y, Miyamoto, T (2012), *Allergol. Int.* 25.

54. Walters KA and Olejink O (1983), *J. Pharm. Pharmacol.*, 35, 79P.

55. Wert PW and Downing, DT (1982), *Science* 217, 1261.

56. Walters KA, Walker M and Olejink O (1988), *J. Pharm. Pharmacol.* 40, 525–9.

57. Wurster DE and Kramer SF (1961), *J. Pharm. Sci.*, 50, 288–93.

58. Shaw JE and Mitchell C (1984), *J. Toxi. Cutene. and Ocul. Toxi.*, 2, 249–66.

59. Thorsteinsson T, Masson M, Loftsson T, Haraldsson GG, Stefansson E. Pharmazie, 1999, 54, 831–6.

60. Prausnitz MR, Gill, HS; Park, JH. Modified Release Drug Delivery. In: Rathbone, MJ; Hadgraft, J.; Roberts, MS.; Lane, ME., editors. New York: Informa Healthcare; 2008.

61. Sivamani RK, Liepmann D, Maibach HI. *Expert Opin Drug Deliv* 2007; 4:19–25.

62. Denet AR, Vanbever R, Preat V. *Adv Drug Deliv Rev* 2004; 56: 659–74.

63. Machet L, Boucaud A. *Int J Pharm* 2002; 243: 1–15.

64. Guy RH; Hadgraft J, editors. New York: Marcel Dekker; 2003.

65. Williams, A. London: Pharmaceutical Press; 2003.

66. Prausnitz MR, Mitragotri S, Langer R, *Nat Rev Drug Discov* 2004; 3: 115–24.

67. PC Mills, SE Cross/. *The Veterinary Journal* 172 (2006) 218–33.

68. Talukdar AH, Calhoun ML, Stinson AW (1972), *Amer J. Vet Res*, 33, 2365–90.

69. Cowen T, Trigg P, Eady RA (1979), *Distribution of mast cells in human dermis: development of a mapping technique. British J Dermat*, 100, 635–40.

70. Cross SE, Anderson C, Roberts, MS (1998), *British J ClinPharma*, 46, 29–35.

71. Pharmatutor-Art-1235, www.Pharmatutor forum. com.

72. Elias PM, *J. Invest. Dermatol.* 80,44–9, 1983.

73. Lampe MA et al. *J. Lipid Res.* 24, 120–30, 1983.

74. Bouwstra JA, Gooris GS, Dubbelaar FE, Ponec M, *J. Lipid Res.* 42, 1759–70.

75. Fartasch M, Bassukas ID, *Dipegen TL Br. J. Dermatol.* 128, 1–9, 1993.

76. Pellet M, Raghavan SL, Hadgraft J, Davis A. In: Guy RH, Hadgraft J (Eds.) Transdermal Drug Delivery. 2nd Edition, Marcel Dekker, New York, 2003, pp. 305-326.

77. Barry BW, *Eur. J. Pharm. Sci.* 14, 101–114, 2001.

78. Cross SE, Roberts MS, 1, 81–92, 2004.

79. Preat V, Vanbever R. In: Guy RH, Hadgraft J (Eds.) Transdermal Drug Delivery. 2nd Edition, Marcel Dekker, New York, 2003, pp. 227–54.

80. Down JA, Harvey NG. In: Guy RH, Hadgraft J (Eds.) Transdermal Drug Delivery. 2nd Edition, Marcel Dekker, New York, 2003, pp. 327–59.

81. Daniels R. Issue 25, http://www.scf-online. com/english/25_e/galenic_25_e.htm.

82. Cevc G. Eur Pat Appl 1992; A 61 k 9/50.

83. Cevc G, In Gregoriadis G (Ed.) Liposome Technology. 2nd Edition, CRC Press, Boca Raton, 1992, pp. 1–36.

84. Schmalfuss U, Neubert R, Wohlrab WJ, *Control. Release* 46, 279–85, 1997.

85. Specht C, Stoye I, Mueller-Goymann CC. *Eur. J. Pharm. Biopharm.* 46, 273–8, 1998.

86. Pittermann W, Jackwerth B, Schmitt M. Toxic. in Vitro 10, 17–21, 1997.

87. Gaur PK, Mishra S, Purohit S, Dave K. Asian *J Pharma Clinical Res.* 2009; 2: 14–20.

88. MR Prausnitz, S Mitragotri, R Langer. *Nature Reviews, Drug Discovery*, 2004, 3: 115–24.

89. Front Line Strategic Consulting Inc. 2002.

90. Loyd V. Allen Jr, Nicholas G. Popovich, Howard C. Ansel, 8th Edition., Wolter Kluwer Publishers, New Delhi, 2005 pp. 298–9.

91. Lvovich VF, Matthews E, Riga AT, Kaza L (2010), *J. Control. Rel.* 145(2), 134–40.

92. Hadgraft J, Guy R, In; Marcel Dekker, Inc., New York, and Basel, Vol. 35, 296.

93. Keleb E, Sharma RK, *Int J. Adv Pharma Sci.* 2010; 1: 201–11.

94. Lee WR, Shen SC, Lai HH, Hu CH, Fang JY. *J Control Rel.* 2001; 75:155–66.

95. Lec ST, Yac SH, Kim SW and Berner B. *Int. J Pharm.* 1991; 77: 231–7.

96. Rhaghuram Reddy K, Muttalik S, *AAPS Pharm. Sci. Tech.* 2003; 4:4.

97. Shaila L, Pandey S and Udupa N. *Ind J Pharm. Sci.* 2006; 68: 179–84.

98. Patani GA, Chien YW, In; Swerbrick, J. Eds., *Encyclopedia of Pharmaceutical Technology*, Vol. 18, Marcel Dekker Inc., New York, 1999, 317–20, 329.

99. Jayaswal SB and Sood, R, *The Eastern Pharmacist*, 1987, 30(357), 47–50.

100. Finnin BC and Morgan TM (1999), *J. Pharm. Sci.*, 88(10), 955.

101. Sun YM, Huang JJ, Lin, FC and Lac, JY, *Biomat.*, 1997, 18, 527–33.

102. Transdermal Delivery of Drugs, Kydonieus, Berner, CRC.

103. Press 1987.

104. www.ionsys.net

105. www.vyteris.com

106. www.noven.com

107. www.macroflux.com

108. www.dermisonics.com

109. www.zars.com

110. www.transpharma-medical.com

111. Tsai JC, Guy RH, Thornfeldt CR, *Jour. Pharm. Sci.*, 1998; 85: 643–8.

112. Berner B and John VA Jour. Clinical pharmacokinetics 1994; 26(2): 121–34.

113. Baker W and Heller J, Eds. Marcel Dekker, Inc., New York 1989 pp. 293–311.

114. Wiechers J. Acta Pharm. 1992: 4: 123.

115. Singh J, Tripathi KT and Sakia TR (1993), *Drug Dev. Ind. Pharm.* 19: 1623–8.

116. Wade A, Weller PJ Handbook of pharmaceutical Excipients. Washington, DC:American Pharmaceutical Publishing Association; 1994: 362–6.

117. Willams AC, Barry BW (2004), *Adv Drug Del Rev.* 56:603–18.

118. Vyas SP and Khar RK Targetted and controlled Drug Delivery Novel carrier system 1st Ed., CBS Publishers and distributors, New Delhi, 2002; 411–47.

119. Williams AC, Barry BW 9; 305–53, 1992.

120. Yogeshvar N Kalia, Richard H Guy, *Adv Drug Deliv Rev*, 48 (2001) 159–72.

121. Yadav KS, Malviya, RK and Sharma P (2011), *Curr. Drug Therapy*, 6(8), 223–30.

7 ■ Spherical Crystallization

INTRODUCTION

Spherical crystallization is a particle designing technique, by which crystallization and agglomeration can be carried out simultaneously in one step. The spherical crystallization technique also involves the use of a bridging liquid that improves compressibility by acting as granulating fluid. Thus, spherical crystallization (Fig. 7.1) is a method that helps achieve good flow ability and compressibility. Spherical crystallization can be achieved by various methods such as simple spherical crystallization, emulsion solvent diffusion, ammonia diffusion, and neutralization. The principal steps involved in the process of spherical crystallization are flocculation zone, zero growth zone, fast growth zone, and constant size zone. Factors controlling the process of agglomeration are solubility profile, mode and intensity of agitation, temperature of the system and residence time. Spherical crystallization is having wide applications in pharmaceuticals like improvement of flow ability and compressibility of poorly compressible drugs, masking bitter taste of drugs and improving the solubility and dissolution rate of poorly soluble drug. In the pharmaceutical industry, the crystal size growth and the formation of the spherical crystal agglomerates are very important for preparing the solid dosage forms (e.g. capsules, tablets,

etc.). The particle size of the agglomerates produced by the spherical crystallization techniques is 300–500 mm in diameter and their shape is more or less spherical. The agglomerates have very good flow property, high bulk density, and compressibility values. They can be used directly for capsule-filling (without excipients) and direct tablet making (without granulation, drying, etc.). The drug materials produced by the spherical crystallization technique are economical in the development of the solid dosage forms. The typical spherical crystallization technique employs three solvents—one is the substance dissolution medium, another is a medium, which partially dissolves the substance, and third is the wetting solvent for the substance. The traditional crystallization processes (salting-out precipitation, cooling crystallization, crystallization from the melting, etc.) can also be used to produce spherical crystal agglomerates. It may be called a nontypical spherical crystallization process.

METHODS OF SPHERICAL CRYSTALLIZATION

The methods of spherical crystallization are categorized as:

- Quasi emulsion solvent diffusion method (QESD)
- Ammonia diffusion method (AD)
- Solvent change method (SC)
- Salting-out method (SO)

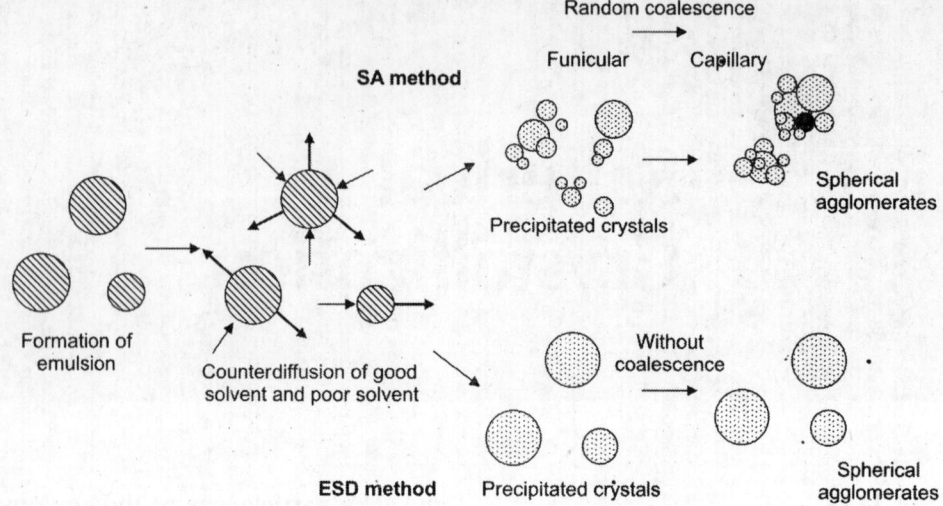

Fig.7.1: Mechanism of spherical crystallization

Quasi Emulsion Solvent Diffusion (QESD)

In the emulsion solvent diffusion, the affinity between the drug and the good solvent is stronger than that between the good solvent and the poor solvent. The drug is dissolved in the good solvent, and the solution is dispersed into the poor solvent, producing emulsion (quasi) droplets, even though the pure solvents are miscible. The good solvent diffuses gradually, out of the emulsion droplets into the surrounding poor solvent phase, and the poor solvent diffuses into the droplets resulting into drug crystallization within the droplets. The method is considered to be simple than the SA method, but it can be difficult to find a suitable additive to keep the system emulsified and to improve the diffusion of the poor solute into the dispersed phase.

Ammonia Diffusion (AD) Method

In this method, the mixture of three partially immiscible solvent, i.e. acetone, ammonia water, and dichloromethane was used as a crystallization system. In this system ammonia water acted as bridging liquid as well as a good solvent. Acetone was the water miscible however, it acts as a poor solvent, thus drug precipitated out by solvent change without forming ammonium salt. Water immiscible solvents include hydrocarbons or halogenated hydrocarbons, e.g. dichloromethane induced liberation of ammonia water.

Principle Steps Involved in the Process of Spherical Crystallization

Bermer and Zuider Wag proposed that four steps are involved in the growth of agglomeration.

I. Flocculation zone

In this zone, the bridging liquid displaces the liquid from the surface of the crystals and these crystals are brought in close proximity by agitation; the adsorbed bridging liquid links the particles by forming a lens bridge between them. In these zones, loose open flocs of particles are formed by pendular bridges.

II. Zero growth zone

Loose floccules get transferred into tightly packed pellets, during which the entrapped fluid is squeezed-out followed by squeezing of the bridging liquid onto the surface of small flocs causing poor space in the pellet to be completely filled with the bridging liquid. The driving force for the transformation is provided by agitation of the slurry causing liquid turbulence, pellet-pellet and pellet-stirrer collision.

III. Fast growth zone

The fast growth of the agglomerates takes place, when sufficient bridging liquid is squeezed-out of the surface on the small agglomerates. This formation of large particles following random collision of well-formed nucleus is known as coalescence. Successful collision occurs, only if the nucleus has a slight excess of surface moisture. This imparts plasticity to nucleus and enhances particle deformations and subsequent coalescence. Another reason for the growth of agglomerates is attributed to growth mechanisms that describe the successive addition of material on already formed nuclei.

IV. Constant size zone

In this zone agglomerates cease to grow or even show marginal decrease in size. Here, the frequency of coalescence is balanced by the breakage frequency of agglomeration. The size reduction may result due to attrition, breakage and shatter. The rate-determining step in agglomerates growth that occurs in zero growth zones, when bridging liquid is squeezed-out of the pores as the initial floccules are transformed into small agglomerates. The rate determining step is the collision of particles with the bridging liquid droplets prior to the formation of liquid bridges. The rate is also governed by the speed of agitation. The strength of the agglomerates is determined by interfacial tension between the bridging liquid and the continuous liquid phase, contact angle and the ratio of the volumes of the bridging liquid to solid particles.

Solvent Change (SC) Method

The solution of the drug in a good solvent is poured in a poor solvent under controlled condition of temperature and speed to obtain fine crystals. These crystals are agglomerated in the presence of bridging liquid. The poor solvent has miscibility with good solvent, but low solubility with solvent mixture, so during agitation of the solvent system the crystals formed. The drawback of this system is that it provides low yield because the drug shows significant solubility in the crystallization solvent due to cosolvency effect. This method is not applicable for water insoluble drugs.

Salting-out (SO) Method

This method involves the addition of suitable salt that relatively makes good solvent to be poor solvent, thus drug tends to crystallize out in the presence of bridging liquid.

Crystallization Mechanism of Nanomaterials

The controllable synthesis of new nano-structures has an enormous impact on the fabrication and application of nanomaterials and continues to be a central challenge in nanoscience and nanotechnology. In order to explore the growth kinetics of the crystallization of nanomaterials, endeavors have been made to a large extent to the parallel experiments, in situ observations, and theoretical modelings. Despite some exciting results, essential factors, which can modify and effect the thermodynamics and kinetics are still ambiguous. Understanding of colloidal nanocrystal growth mechanism is essential for the preparation of nanocrystals with desirable chemical/physical properties. Recent in situ experiment has suggested that colloidal nanoparticles can grow either by monomer attachment from solution or by particle coalescence. However, atomic-scale in situ observations are still beyond our scope.

Composition-controlled Crystallization of Nanomaterials

In addition to structural controlled synthesis, composition-controlled crystallization appears especially important for nanomaterials. Doping can enhance the performances of semiconductors by providing a powerful method to control their optical, electronic, transport, and spintronic properties. Furthermore, introducing specific dopants could also lead to dramatic changes in morphology except altering the atomic composition and structure of the nanocrystals. Doping models of nanomaterials are summarized in Table 7.1. Models proposed at present are aimed at the host crystal, whose structure remains unchanged during the whole doping process, and doping models that take into account the structural transition are thus needed. Moreover, recent study indicates that the influence of shape parameter on doping content and doping state can provide an alternative approach to adjust the doping degrees of doping materials. Ion exchange reaction has been demonstrated to be another effective approach to increase the compositions of inorganic functional materials in various solution-based chemistry approaches. Such crystallization process is associated with localized chemical conversions of the host structure, which can serve as a solid state precursor (Table 7.2).

Spherical Agglomeration (SA)

A near saturated solution of the drug in a good solvent is poured into a poor solvent. Provided that the poor and good solvents are freely miscible and the affinity between the solvents is stronger than the affinity between the drug and the good solvent, crystals will precipitate immediately. In the spherical agglomeration method also a third solvent called the bridging liquid is added in a smaller amount to promote the formation of agglomerates. Under agitation, the bridging liquid (the wetting agent) is added. The bridging liquid should not be miscible with the poor solvent and should preferentially wet the precipitated crystals. As a result of interfacial tension and capillary forces, the bridging liquid acts to adhere the crystals to one another. The spherical agglomeration method has been applied to several drugs, and it has been found that the product properties are quite sensitive to the amount of the bridging liquid. Less than the optimum amount of bridging liquid produces plenty of fines, while more than optimum amount produces very coarse particles. Also the choice of bridging liquid, the stirring speed and the concentration of solids (or of the

Table 7.1: Nanocrystal doping models		
Doping model	*Model description*	*Characteristics*
Statistical model	Dopant solubility remains the same as in the bulk crystal, and nanocrystals tend to be pure simply, since they contain so few atoms owing to their smaller volume.	Decreasing size
Trapped-dopant model	The impurity adsorbs on the surface of nanocrystal and then incorporates into nanocrystal. Doping is thus relative easy for the nanocrystal exposed surface favorable for impurity binding	Growth and incorporation
Self-purification model	Nanocrystals are difficult to dope due to thermodynamic limitations and dopants are therefore expelled from bulk.	Dopant bulk diffusion
Novel models for the doping process accompanied by structural transformation		Structural transformation

Table 7.2: Different crystallization models of nanoparticles

Crystallization model	Model description	Characteristics
Classical nucleation theory (CNT)	Surface energy and chemical potential (related to monomer supersaturation) codetermine the nucleation of nanoparticles.	It fails to provide information about the size and distribution. Only Gibbs-Wulff morphology can be simulated.
First-order reaction-diffusion model	By combining Fick's first law and first-order reaction rate, particle radius with time can be obtained.	Size distribution and its role in the nanoparticle growth process is still beyond the scope of this model.
Combination of CNT and reaction-diffusion growth equations	It can simulate the growth state of nanocrystals.	The assumed initial seeding distribution curve has an intensive relation with final results.
Rate-equation-based growth model	Evolution of the entire size distribution with time can be described	It requires solving rate equations skillfully. No information about growth morphology can be provided. Growth approach should be initially assumed.
Surface area limited model	It combines surface diffusion, step-growth rate and surface site availability to describe an isotropic coarsening of faceted nanoparticles.	The effective number of sites available for monomers adsorbtion determine nanoparticle shape evolution.
Chemical bonding theory of single crystal growth	Chemical-bonding processes play a critical role in crystallization.	Morphological evolution during crystallization process can be successfully simulated.

solute) are of importance. In case of lactose, the agglomerate size distribution was affected by both the size of raw particles and the amount of bridging liquid used. On increasing stirring rate the agglomeration was reduced because of increasing disruptive forces. Higher stirring rate produces agglomerates that are less porous and more resistant to mechanical stress, while the porosity decreases. The viscosity of the continuous phase has an effect on the size distribution of the agglomerates. The choice of bridging liquid exhibits an influence on the rate of agglomeration and also on the strength of the agglomerates.

Factors Controlling the Process of Agglomeration

Solubility

The selection of solvent is dictated by solubility characteristics of drug. A mutually immiscible three solvent system, consisting of a poor solvent (suspending liquid), good solvent and bridging liquid are necessary. Physical forms of product, i.e. microagglomerates or irregular macroagglomerates or paste of drug substance can be controlled by selection of proper solvent proportion. The proportion of solvent to be used is determined by carrying out solubility studies and constructing triangular phase diagram to define the region of mutual immiscibility by using ternary diagram.

Agitation

High speed agitation is necessary to disperse the bridging liquid throughout the system. Any change in agitation pattern or fluid flow would be reflected as a change in force acting on agglomerate, which ultimately affects the shape of agglomerate. The extent of mechanical agitation in conjuction with the amount of bridging liquid determines the rate of formation of agglomerate and their final size.

Temperature

Study revealed that the temperature has a significant influence on the shape, size and texture of the agglomerates. The effect of temperature on spherical crystallization is probably due to the effect of temperature on the solubility of a drug substance in the ternary system.

Residence Time

The time for which agglomerates remain suspended in reaction mixture affects their strength.

Advantages of Spherical Crystallization

1. Spherical crystallization technique has been successfully utilized for improving flowability and compressibility of drug powder.
2. This technique could enable subsequent processes such as separation, filtration, drying, etc. to be carried-out more efficiently.
3. By using this technique, physicochemical properties of pharmaceutical crystals are dramatically improved for pharmaceutical process, i.e. milling, mixing, and tabletting because of their excellent flowability and packagability.
4. This technique may enable crystalline forms of a drug to be converted into different polymorphic forms having better bioavailability.
5. For masking of the bitter taste of drug.
6. Preparation of microsponge, microspheres and nanospheres, microbaloons, nanoparticles and micropellets as novel particulates drug delivery system.

Amphiphilic Microenvironments Conducive to Crystallization

The first report of successful membrane protein crystallizations constituted a paradigm for membrane protein crystallization; transfer membrane proteins from their native environment into particulate detergent micelles in order to purify and to crystallize them in the same way as soluble proteins. It was reasoned that homogenous, lipid-free protein detergent micelles of uniform size would be most suitable for crystallization processes. The choice of the detergent for crystallization purposes is based on three factors—(i) stabilization of the native conformation of the membrane protein in monodisperse form, (ii) enabling protein-protein contacts in the packed crystal and, (iii) preventing detrimental phase separations during crystal growth. This line of thinking was expanded in the recent years, particularly with respect to lipids being recognized as beneficial and sometimes crucial crystallization components. Most detergents belong to one of the following categories—ionic, nonionic or Zwitterionic. Their characteristic behavior depends on their shape, stereochemistry of the head group and tail. According to the 'intrinsic curvature hypothesis' they form supramolecular structures in water due to the hydrophobic effect and their shape. At sufficiently high concentrations, i.e. above the critical micellar concentration (CMC), detergents form micelles. These form roughly spherical objects in which detergent molecules are primarily packed with their orienting alkyl chains towards the center and their head groups towards the surface. Detergent molecules in micelles are flexible and exhibit a high degree of mobility, allowing for dramatic fluctuations in overall micellar shape including deformations, fusion, and fission Amphiphiles generally display a rich phase behavior commonly described with help of phase diagrams. Detergents typically have consolute boundaries, separating a single-phase micellar region from a dual micellar phase, wherein the latter of which consists of a detergent rich and a detergent depleted phase. At the cloud point a clear homogenous detergent solution turns to be turbid upon heating. Importantly, the addition of salt, variations of pH, etc. and in particular the introduction of additional components may have profound, but essentially unpredictable effects on amphiphile phase behavior. The fact that a 'simple' ternary system consisting of oil, water and block copolymer amphiphile may form nine different isothermal phases spectacularly illustrates this polymorphism, which is a typical feature of amphiphiles. Lipid polymorph phases include fluid isotropic phases, planar, positively and negatively curved bilayer phases, rod-shaped hexagonal phases, micellar phases and bicontinuous cubic phases and they occur, among other shapes, as a function of composition, hydration, pressure, and temperature. Some integral membrane proteins may be introduced into detergent micelles following there refolding. Indeed, since β-barrel proteins can be expressed in *Escherichia coli* as inclusion bodies, membrane proteins such as OmpA or NspA can be purified in unfolded form and crystallized without any exposure or contact with lipids, thus ensuring that once reconstituted into detergent micelles they would form true detergent-protein micelles. In most of the cases, however, membrane proteins are extracted concomitantly with associated lipids from their native environment, i.e cellular membranes. Such mixed systems, consisting of detergent, lipids and membrane proteins form the so-called, protein detergent complexes (PDCs). The phase behavior of PDCs is expectedly complex and only in some selects cases portions of phase diagrams have been mapped-out. It is this state; however, that is usually employed in membrane protein crystallization trials and in many cases detergents as well as lipids are present in membrane protein crystals. Two-methodological advances have substantially aided many membrane protein crystallizations based on PDCs—(i) the introduction of small amphiphiles such as 1,2,3-heptanetriol to modify micelle dynamics and size and, (ii) the increase of the size of the hydrophilic portion by complexing with monoclonal antibodies or fragments thereof. The range of alternative amphiphilic vehicles for membrane proteins useful for crystallization purposes has increased in the recent years. Besides protein-detergent micelles and PDCs, membrane protein crystallizations were started from membraneous structures. The latter may be obtained by adding lipids to create structures that are small in size and planar such as bicelles or that are large such as in extended planar membranes or those that exhibit positive, or negative curvature. Curved bilayers membrane proteins include proteoliposomes or bicontinuous lipidic cubic phases. Furthermore, the quantity and type of lipid added to PDCs determine the nature of the resulting amphiphile phase. For some membrane proteins, it is very difficult to identify detergent-based conditions that could preserve their native conformation. This predicament has inspired several research groups to expand the range of solubilization strategies by designing new amphiphiles and to investigate the richness of their phase behavior for the purpose of membrane protein crystallization. Among these, amphiphiles are peptitergents, lipopeptide detergents, amphiphiles and new detergents with reduced alkyl chain mobility such as tripod amphiphiles. They all are self-assembled into small micelles, can be used to disperse lipid membranes. They are gentle, nondenaturing amphiphiles, which preserve the native structure of the test protein such as bacteriorhodopsin and other membrane proteins in solution for an extended periods of time.

Amphiphilic Microenvironment Inside Membrane Protein Crystals

Membrane protein crystals consist of three major molecular species—water, amphiphile, and membrane protein. Water and dissolved solutes form a fluid phase within the rigidly packed protein network, while amphiphiles may tightly bind to the protein surface and/or form a disordered state. The morphology and the strength of intermolecular contacts in protein crystals were investigated by Matsuura and Chernov (2003). It was found that soluble proteins form crystal contacts frequently involving water molecules, which form specific intermolecular hydrogen bonds on top of nonspecific attractive electrostatic interactions. Similar contacts are present between hydrophilic protein surfaces of membrane proteins in crystals. In some cases amphiphiles form interactions that are crucial to crystal packing. The structures that amphiphiles form within membrane protein crystals, are remarkably diverse and go beyond the simple two-types of classification introduced. According to these categories, type I crystals are consisted of stacked membraneous layers. They stick together via hydrophobic interactions in the plane of the layers, resembling 2D crystals, and polar contacts mediated interlayer interactions. Conversely, type II crystals possess contacts involving the polar regions of membrane proteins only. The hydrophobic perimeter is embedded in a torus of detergent molecules. Typical type I crystals have been found in all cases, where membrane proteins were crystallized with the cubic phase method. Bacteriorhopsin packs in a unidirectional way 'head to tail', while halorhodopsin packs in layers, where heads interact with heads and tails with tails, and sensory rhodopsin II packs in layers with mixed up-down arrangements. Bacteriorhodopsin crystals were shown by mass spectrometry to contain native lipids that were copurified, namely 2,3-di-O-phytanyl derivatives of phosphatidylglycerol, phosphatidylglycerol sulfate, phosphatidylglycerol phosphate methylester, triglycosyldiether, sulfated triglycoside lipid and sulfated tetraglycosyldiphytanylglycerol, when crystallized from lipidic cubic phases and they contained similar lipids, when crystallized as PDCs. Amphiphile phase transitions occur during crystallization. The crystallization process consists of two steps, nucleation, and crystal growth. Nucleation is a critical phenomenon and hardly anything is known specifically for membrane protein crystallizations. Soluble protein crystallization growth is mainly initiated and driven by modification of the water structure, creating conditions that allow and favor the defined association of proteins. Similar conditions need to be created for the hydrophilic sections of membrane proteins, i.e. screening of repulsive electrostatic surface charges by ions and providing conditions, where the protein is at supersaturation. The latter effect was investigated by Rosenow et al. (2003), who concluded from biochemical studies that membrane protein crystallization is favored by those amphiphiles that optimize the solubility of integral membrane proteins. At the same time, conditions are needed to be provided for the hydrophobic sections to maintain or to rearrangement into the suprastructures. Crystallizations involve phase transitions, an initial homogenous medium separates into a depleted phase and rich in amphiphile and membrane protein, the crystal. The association of protein/detergent micelles or PDCs into a type II packed crystal can easily be understood within the framework of present crystallization theory. The mechanism for PDC crystallization was studied and investigated by Marone et al. (1998), for photosynthetic reaction centers. These were shown to exist predominantly in the monomeric form throughout the entire crystallization process. Comparable experiments were used to characterize the effects of crystallization additives on the shape of pure detergent micelles (Littrell et al., 2000). It was found that micelles were elongated and rod-shaped and that their size grew on increasing the ionic strength whilst decrease when glycerol or PEG was added. In order to form continuous structures such as layered type I crystals or crystals with a continuous network of amphiphile phase, PDCs need to fuse and allow detergent and lipid molecules to rearrange into the supramolecular architecture as described above. Snijder et al. (2003) pointed out that the continuous detergent network in their crystals and the hydrophobic crystal contacts suggest that OmplA molecules approach each other closely and coalesce their detergent belts. The formation of the polar contacts might actually drive crystallization and induce the merging of micelles. They hypothesized that micelle fusion and the stabilization of a continuous network is mediated by the organic solvent and the amphiphile 2-methyl-2,4-pentanediol. Indeed, many of the putative type III crystal yielding conditions include the use of rather high concentrations of organic solvents or small molecule amphiphiles such as 1,2,3-heptanetriol. The picture emerges that this crystallization process may be driven partly or possibly be dominated by amphiphiles undergoing a phase transition prompted by an increase in system complexity.

Characterization of the Spherical Crystals

The spherical agglomerated crystals show significant effect on the formulation and manufacturing of pharmaceutical dosage forms, therefore, it is necessary to evaluate them by using different parameters.

Particle Size, Size Distribution and Particle Roundness

For the determination of the particle size (length, breadth, and roundness) light microscope fitted with image processing and analysis system is used. Size of the particles and their distributions can also be determined by simple sieve analysis. Now, with the help of Ro-Tap sieve shaker, particle size analysis can be performed. In advance technology, image-analyzer is used to determine the size and volume of the particle.

Roundness is a shape-related factor that provides information about the circularity of particles. It is calculated by using software according to the following formula:

Roundness = (Perimeter)^2/4 area *1.064

The perimeter is calculated from the horizontal and vertical projections, with an allowance for the number of corners. An adjustment factor of 1.064 corrected the

perimeter for the effect of the corners produced by digitization of the image. When roundness value is close to one, the particles are near to spherical in shape.

Particle Shape/Surface Topography

Following methods are used:

Optical Microscopy

The shape of the spherical crystals is studied by observing them under an optical microscope. The observations are made using 10X, 45X, 60X magnification (Fig. 7.2).

Scanning Electron Microscopy

The surface topography, type of crystals, polymorphism, and crystal habit of the spherical crystals are analyzed by using scanning electron microscopy.

X-ray Powder Diffraction

This is an important technique for establishing batch-to-batch reproducibility of a crystalline form. The form of crystal in agglomerates can be determined by using X-ray diffraction techniques. An amorphous form does not produce a pattern. The X-ray scatters in a reproducible pattern of peak intensities at distinct angle (2θ) relative to the incident beam. Each diffraction pattern is a characteristics of a specific crystalline lattice of a compound.

Flow Property

Flow property of the material largely depends on the force that is developed between the particles, particle size, particle-size distribution, particle shape, surface texture or roughness and surface area. Flowability of the agglomerates is much improved as the agglomerate exhibits lower angle of repose than that of single crystals. The improvement in the flowability of agglomerates could be attributed to the significant reduction in inter-particles friction, due to their spherical shape and relatively a low-static electric charge.

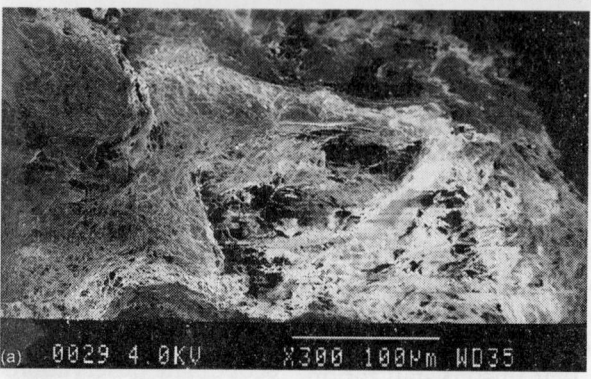

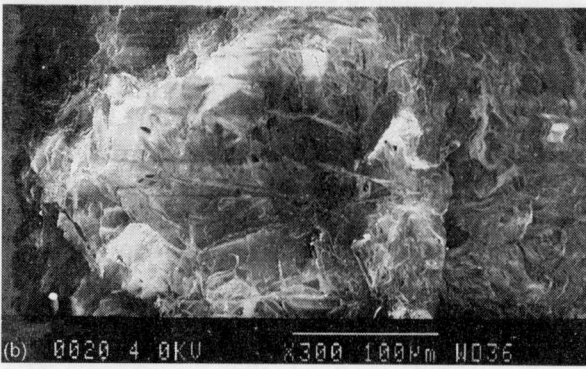

Fig. 7.2: Scanning electron photomicrographs of spherical crystal agglomerates—(a) reference sample, (b) agglomerates of ibuprofen—Eudragit®

Following are the methods used to determine of flow property:

Angle of Repose

This is a common method used to determine the flow property. The angle of repose is the angle between the horizontal plane and the slope of the heap or cone of solid dropped from some elevation. Values for angle of repose 30° usually indicate free flowing material and angle 40° suggest for a poor flowing material. The angle of repose can be obtained using following equation:

$$\tan \theta = h/0.5\, d$$

where, h—height of the cone and d—diameter of the cone

Compressibility or Carr Index

A simple indication of an ease with which a material can be induced to flow is given by application of compressibility index

$$I = (1 - V/V_o) * 100$$

where, V = the volume occupied by a sample of powder after being subjected to a standardized tapping procedure and V_o = the volume before tapping. The value below 15%, indicates good flow characteristics and value above 25% indicates poor flowability.

Hausner Ratio

It is calculated from bulk density and tapped density.

Hausner ratio = Tapped density/Bulk density

Values less than 1.25, indicate good flow (20% Carr Index) and a value greater than 1.25 indicates poor flow (33% Carr index).

Density

Density of the spherical crystals is the mass per unit volume.

$$\text{Density} = M/V$$

Porosity

Porosity of granules affects the compressibility. Porosities are of two types namely intragranular and intergranular and these are measured with the help of true and granular densities.

Intragranular = 1–granular density/true porosity   density.

Intergranular = 1–bulk density/granular porosity   density

Total porosity = 1–bulk density/true density

Packability

Improved packability has been reported for agglomerates prepared by spherical crystallization. The angle of friction, shear cohesive stress and shear index are lower than that of single crystals, which can improve the packability of the agglomerates.

The packability of agglomerates is improved as compared to those recorded for the original crystals and that the agglomerated crystals are adaptable to direct tabletting. The packability assessed by analysis of the tapping process with the Kawakita (I) and Kuno (II) method and using the parameters $a, b, 1/b, k$ in the equation

$$N/C = 1/(ab) + N/a \qquad (i)$$
$$C = (V_o - V_n)/V_o,$$
$$a = (V_o - V_h)/V_o$$
$$r_f - r_n = (r_f - r_o) \exp(-kn) \qquad (ii)$$

where: N = Number of tapping
C = Difference in volume (degree of volume reduction) and a, b are constants.

Compression Behavior Analysis

Good compactibility and compressibility are essential properties of directly compressible crystals. The compaction behavior of agglomerated crystals and single crystals is obtained by plotting the relative volume against the compression pressure. Spherical agglomerates possess superior strength characteristics in comparison to conventional crystals. It is suggested that the surfaces are freshly created fractures during compression

of agglomerates, which enhances the plastic-interparticle bonding, resulting in a lower compression force required for compressing the agglomerates under plastic deformation compared to that of single crystals.

Compaction behavior of agglomerated crystals is evaluated by using following parameters:

Heckel Analysis

The following Heckel's equation is used to analyze the compression process of agglomerated crystals and assessed their comapactibility.

$$In[1/(1-D)] = KP + A$$

where:

A—constant to represent particle rearrangement.

D—relative density of the tablets under compression pressure

K—slope of the straight portion of the Heckel plot

The reciprocal of K is the mean yield pressure (P_y).

The following equation gives the intercept obtained by extrapolating the straight portion of the plots

$$A = In[1/(1-D_0)] + B$$

where:

B is constant to represent particle rearrangement.

D_0 is the relative density of the powder bed when $P = 0$.

The following equation gives the relative densities corresponding to A and B.

$$D_A = 1 - e - A$$
$$D_B = D_A - D_0$$

Stress Relaxation Test

A specific quantity of spherical agglomerated crystals sample is placed in a die of a specific diameter, i.e. the surface of which is coated with magnesium stearate in advance, then used the universal tensile compression tester to compress the sample at a constant pressure. After the certain limit of pressure applied or attained, the upper punch held in the same position for 20 minutes, during which the time for the reduction of the stress applied on the upper punch is measured. The result is corrected by subtracting the relaxation measured without powder in the die from the measured force under the same conditions.

The following equation establishes the relationship between relaxation ratio $Y(t)$ and time t, calculated parameters A_s and B_s, and also the assessed relaxation behavior.

$$t/Y(t) = 1/A_s B_s - t/A_s$$
$$Y(t) = (P_0 - P_t)/P_0$$

where, P_0 is the maximum compression pressure, and P_t is the pressure at time t.

Mechanical strength

Spherical crystals should possess good mechanical strength as directly reflected from the mechanical strength of compact or tablet. It is determined by using the following two methods.

Tensile strength

Tensile strength of spherical crystals is measured by applying maximum load required to crush the spherical crystal. This method is a direct method of tensile strength measurment of spherical crystals.

Crushing strength

It is measured by using 50 ml glass hypodermic syringe. The modification includes the removal of the tip of the syringe barrel and the top end of the plunger. The barrel is then used as hallow support and the guide tube with close fitting tolerances to the plunger. The hallow plunger with open end served as load cell in which mercury could be added. A window is cut into the barrel to facilitate placement of granule on the base platen. The plunger acts as a movable plates and sets directly on the granules positioned on the lower platen, as the rate of loading may affect crushing load (gm). Mercury is introduced from reservoir into the upper chamber at the rate of 10 gm/sec until the single granule crushed; loading time should be <3 minutes. The total weight of the plunger and the mercury required to fracture a granule is measured as the crushing load.

Friability Test

The friability of the spherical crystals is the combination of the attrition and sieving process of a single operation. Granules along with the plastic balls are placed on a test screen. The sieve is then subjected to the usual motion of a test sieve shaker to impart the necessary attrition motion to the granules. The weight of powder passing through the sieve is recorded as a function of time. The friability index is determined from the slop of the plot between % weights of granules remaining on the sieve as a function of time of shaking. Friability of agglomerates is determined by using following formula:

$$\text{Friability}(X) = [1 - W/W_0]/100$$

where:

W_0 = Initial weight of the crystalline agglomerates placed in sieve;

W = Weight of the material, which does not pass through sieve after 5 min.

Moisture Uptake Study

The study indicates the uptake of moisture by drug and the prepared spherical crystals, which affects the stability. The weighed quantity of drug and spherical crystals is placed in a crucible at accelerated condition of temperature and humidity, 40 C ± 10C and 75% ± 3% respectively. The gain in weight of drug and spherical crystals is measured.

Drug Loading Efficiency

The drug loading efficiency of crystals are determined by dissolving 100 mg of crystals in 100 ml of appropriate solvent, followed by measuring the absorbance of appropriately diluted solution by using spectrophotometer, other appropriate analysis procedure may be used.

Solubility Studies

A quantity of crystals (about 100 mg) is shacked with an appropriate solvent in a shaking water bath (100 agitations per min) for 24 hours at room temperature. The solution is then passed through a 0.45 mm membrane filter and the amount of the drug dissolved is analyzed spectrophotometerically.

APPLICATIONS OF SPHERICAL CRYSTALLIZATION IN PHARMACEUTICALS

To Improve the Flowability and Compressibility

Today the tablet is the most popular dosage form of all pharmaceutical preparations manufactured. From the manufacturing point of view, tablets can be produced at much higher rate than any other dosage form. Tablet is the most stable readily ingestable and conveniently consumed dosage form. The formulation of tablet is optimized to achieve the goals. The focus today in the business is not only a better drug delivery concept, but also the preparation of the simple standard formulations as economical as possible. One of the most economical solutions is to find directly compressible drug materials and this is especially of interest in case of large volume products. There have been renewed interests in examining the potential of direct compressibility for tabletting over recent years. Since in comparison to traditional granulation process, such manufacturing of the tablets involves simple mixing and compression of powders, which give benefits like time and cost saving. An interesting alternative is to manufacture larger particles in situ by agglomeration of the small crystals during the crystallization. In addition, it has been revealed that agglomerates have properties that make them suitable for direct compression or tabletting. Crystals could be generated employing any of the available techniques like sublimation, solvent evaporation, vapor diffusion, thermal treatment and crystallization from melt precipitation by change in pH, growth in presence of additives or the grindings. Thus, the novel agglomeration techniques that transform crystals directly into a compact spherical form during crystallization process are desired. The use of spherical crystallization as a technique, thus appears to be an efficient alternative for obtaining suitable particles for direct compression. Due to different crystal habit(s), many drugs show inconvenient flowability and compressibility. These problems can be solved by converting them into agglomerated crystals by changing the crystal habit and spheronization, so as to increase both the flowability and compressibility. Patents on spherical crystallization are shown in Table 7.3.

Table 7.3: Patents on spherical crystallization			
Patent	Year	Original assignee/inventor	Title
US 4675339	1987	Nippon Kayaku Kabushiki	Spherical amino acid preparation Kaisha
US 5817173	1998	Josuke Nakata	Method for making spherical crystals
US 6150364	2000	Roche Vitamins Inc.	Purification and crystallization of riboflavin
US 6825218	2004	Aventis Pharma S.A.	Spherical agglomerates of telithromycin, their preparation process and their use in the preparation of pharmaceutical forms
US2006/ 0275219A1	2006	Taisho pharmaceutical co. Ltd.	Radial spherical crystallization product, process for producing the same, and dry powder preparation containing the crystallization product
US 7427413	2008	Skendi Finance Ltd.	Stable shaped particles of crystalline organic compounds
US2009/ 0176096A1	2009	Council of scientific & industrial research, New Delhi, IN	Free flowing 100–500 micrometer size spherical crystals of common salt and process for preparation thereof
US2011/ 0033707A1	2011	National institute for materials science, Ibaraki JP	Spherical boron nitride nanoparticles and synthetic method thereof

For Masking Bitter Taste of Drug

Microcapsules are prepared to mask the bitter taste of the drug. They are suitable for coating granules, since spherical material can be uniformly coated with a relatively small amount of polymer.

For Increasing Solubility and Dissolution Rate of Poorly Soluble Drug

Spherical crystallization has been described as an effective technique in improving the dissolution behavior of some drugs, which possess low water solubility and a slow dissolution profile.

SUGGESTED READINGS

1. Wells JI (1988), *Pharmaceutical preformulation, in: M.M. Rubinstein* (Ed.), The physicochemical Properties of Drug Substances, Ellis Horwood Limited, Chinchester, UK, pp. 209.

2. Kawashima Y. New processes-application of spherical crystallization to particulate design of pharmaceuticals for direct tabletting and coating and new drug delivery systems. *In: Powder Technology and Pharmaceutical* Processes. Handbook of Powder Technology, 1994; 9: 493–512.

3. Shangraw RF. Compressed tablets by direct compression. In: Lieberman HA, Lachman L, Schwartz JB. Pharmaceutical Dosage Forms: Tablets, vol. 1. Marcel Dekker, New York, 1989; 195–246.

4. Heckel RW (1961), *Trans. Metall. Soc.*, AIME 221, 671.

5. Kawakita K and Ludde KH (1971), *Powder Technol.*, 4 61.

6. Guillory JK. Polymorphism in pharmaceutical solids. Marcel Dekker, New York (1989), 183–226.

7. Schacher FH, Elbert J, Patra SK, Yusoff SF, Winnik MA, Manners I (2012), *Chem.*, 18(2), 517–25.

8. Iacovella CR, Keys AS, Glotzer SC (2011), *Proc. Natl. Acad. Sci.*, 108(52), 20935–40.

9. Pawar AP, Paradkar AR, Kadam SS, Mahadik KR (2004), *AAPS Pharm Sci Tech.*, 5(3), e44.

10. Maghsoodi M (2011), *Pharm. Dev. Technol.*, 16(5), 474–82.

11. Maghsoodi M and Tajalli Bakhsh AS (2011), *Pharm. Dev. Technol.*, 16(3), 243–9.

12. Nokhodchi A, Maghsoodi M (2008), *AAPS Pharm. Sci. Tech.*, 9(1), 54–9.

13. Katta J and Rasmuson AC (2008), *Int. J. Pharm.*, 348(1–2), 61–9.

14. Usha AN, Mutalik S, Reddy MS, Ranjith AK, Kushtagi P, Udupa N (2008), *Eur. J. Pharm Biopharm.* 70(2), 674–83.

15. Thati J and Rasmuson AC (2012), *Eur. J. Pharm. Sci.*, 45(5), 657–67.

16. Varshosaz J, Tavakoli N and Salamat FA (2011), *Pharm. Dev. Technol.*, 16(5), 529–35.

17. Michel H, General and practical aspects of membrane protein crystallization. 1991.

18. Crystallization of membrane proteins. CRC Press Inc., Boca Raton, FL, pp. 73–88.

19. Michel H (1983). Crystalization of membrane proteins. *Trends Biochem. Sci.* 8, 56–9.

20. Michel H, Oesterhelt D (1980), *Three-dimensional crystals of membrane proteins: bacteriorhodopsin.* PNAS 77 (3), 1283–5.

21. Nollert P (2002), *J. Appl. Cryst.* 35, 637–640.

22. Nollert P, Qiu H, Caffrey M, Rosenbusch JP, Landau EM (2001), *FEBS Lett.* 504, 179–86.

23. Pebay-Peyroula E, Garavito RM, Rosenbusch JP, Zulauf M, Timmins PA (1995), *Structure* 3(10), 1051–1059.

24. Piazza R, Pierno M, Vignati E, Venturoli G, Francia F, Mallardi A, Palazzo G, (2002).

25. Pautsch A, Schulz GE (1998), *Nat. Struct. Biol.* 5, 1013–1017.

26. Popot, et al., (2003), *Cell Mol. Life Sci.* 60, 1–16.

27. Rosen (1978). Surfactants and Interfaceial Phenomena. Wiley, New York.

28. Rosenow MA, Brune D, Allen JP (2000), *Acta Crystallogr.* D 59, 1422–8.

29. Royant A, Nollert P, Edman K, Neutze R, Landau, EM, Pebay-Peyroula E, Navarro J (2001), *Proc. Natl. Acad. Sci. USA* 98, 10131–6.

30. Santarsiero BD, Yegian DT, Lee CC, Spraggon G, Gu J, Scheibe D, Uber DC, Cornell EW, Nordmeyer RA, Kolbe WF, Jin J, Jones AL, Jaklevic JM, Schultz PG, Stevens RC (2002), *J. Appl. Cryst.* 35, 278–81.

31. Schafmeister CE, Miercke LJW, Stroud RM (1993), *Science* 262, 734–8.

32. Sennoga C, Heron A, Seddon JM, Templer RH, Hankamer B (2003), *Acta Crystallogr.* D 59, 239–46.

33. Snijder HJ, Timmins PA, Kalk KH, Dijkstra BW, (2003), *A. J. Struct. Biol.* 141, 122–31.

34. Takeda K, Sato H, Hino T, Kono M, Fukuda K, Sakurai I, Okada T, Kouyama T (1998), *J. Mol. Biol.* 283(2), 463–74.

35. Tanford C (1973), The Hydrophobic Effect-Formation of Micelles and Biological Membranes. Wiley Interscience, New York.

36. Tanford C (1980), The Hydrophobic Effect. Wiley, New York. Tanaka S, Ataka M, Onuma K, Kubota T, (2003), Rationalization of membrane protein crystallization with polyethylene glycol using a simple depletion model. *Biophys. J.* 84 (5), 3299–306.

37. Tielemann DP, van der Spoel D, Berendsen, HJC, (2000), *J. Phys. Chem.* B, 104, 6380–8.

38. Tribet, C., Audebert, R., Popot, J.-L., 1996. Proc. Natl. Acad. Sci. USA 93, 15047–50.

39. Weber PC (1991). *Advances in Protein Chemistry*, 41.

40. Wennerstroem H, Lindman B, (1979), *Phys. Reports* 52, 1–86.

41. Wiener MC, (2001), *Curr. Opin. Coll. Int. Sci.* 6, 412–9.

42. Wiener MC, Snook F, (2001), *J. Cryst. Growth* 232, 426–31.

43. Faham S, Bowie JU (2002), *J. Mol. Biol.* 316, 1–6.

44. Fromme P (2003). Crystallization of Photosystem I. In: Iwata, S. (Ed.), Methods and Results in Membrane Protein Crystallization. University Line, La Jolla, CA.

45. Fromme P, Witt HT (1998), *Biochim. Biophys. Acta* 1365, 175–84.

46. Garavito RM, Ferguson-Miller S (2001), *J. Biol. Chem.* 276 (35), 32403–406.

47. Garavito RM, Rosenbusch JP (1980), *J. Cell. Biol.* 86 (1), 327–9.

48. Garavito RM, Picot D (1990). The art of crystallizing membrane proteins. Method: A Companion to Methods Enzymology 1, 57–69.

49. Grabe M, Neu J, Oster G, Nollert P (2003), *J. Biophys.* 84, 854–68.

50. Gruner SM (1985), *Proc. Natl. Acad. Sci.* USA 82, 3665–9.

51. Henderson R, Shotton D (1980), *J. Mol. Biol.* 139, 99–109.

52. Hino T, Kanamori E, Shen JR Kouyama T (2004), *Acta Crystallogr. D* 60 (5), 803–809.

53. Hitscherich Jr C, Aseyev V, Wiencek J, Loll PJ, (2001), *Acta Crystallogr. D* 57, 1020–1029.

54. Hunte C, Michel H (2002), *Curr. Opin. Struct. Biol.* 12, 503–508.

55. Hunte CC, von Jagow G, Schagger H (2003), Membrane Protein Purification and Crystallization: A Practical Guide. Academic Press, San Diego.

56. Iwata S (2003), *Methods and Results in Crystallization of Membrane Proteins*. In: Iwata, S, (Ed.), International University Line, Biotechnology Series.

57. Iwata S, Ostermeier C, Ludwig B, Michel H (1995), Structure at 2.8A? resolution of cytochrome c oxidase from Paracoccus denitrificans. Nature 376, 660–69.

58. Kam Z, Shore HB, Feher G (1978). On the Crystallization of Proteins. *J. Mol. Biol.* 123, 539–55.

59. Katona G, Andreasson U, Landau EM, Andreasson LE, Neutze R (2003), *J. Mol. Biol.* 331 (3), 681–92.

60. Kolbe M, Besir H, Essen LO, Oesterhelt D (2000), *Science* 288 (5470), 1390–96.

61. Landau EM, Rosenbusch JP (1996), *Proc. Natl. Acad. Sci.* USA 93, 14532–5.

62. Lemieux MJ, Reithmeier RAF, Wang, DN (2002), *J. Struct. Biol.* 137, 322–32.

63. Liu Z, Yan H, Wang K, Kuang T, Zhang J, Gui L, An X, Chang W (2004), *Nature* 428 (6980), 287–92.

64. Littrell K, Urban V, Tiede D, Thiyagarajan P (2000), *J. Appl. Cryst.* 33, 577–81.

65. Marheineke K, Gruenewald S, Christie W, Reilaender H (1998), *FEBS Lett.* 441, 49–52.

66. Marone PA, Thiyagarajan P, Wagner AM, Tiede, DM (1998), *J. Cryst. Growth* 191, 811–9.

67. McGregor CL, Chen L, Pomroy NC, Hwang P, Go S, Chakrabatty A, Prive GG (2003), *Nat. Biotechnol.* 21 (2), 171–6.

68. Matsuura Y, Chernov AA (2003), *Acta Crystallogr. D* 59, 1347–56.

8 ■ Microemulsion

INTRODUCTION

Microemulsion can be defined in general as thermodynamically stable isotropically clear dispersion of two immiscible liquids, consisting of microdomains of one or more liquids stabilized by interfacial films of surface active molecules. Schulman and coworkers (1959) introduced the term microemulsion to describe the clear, fluid system obtained by titration to the point of clarity of an ordinary milky emulsion (macroemulsion) by the addition of a medium chain alcohol, such as pentanol or hexanol. Thus, over the year the terms thermodynamically stable emulsions, transparent emulsion, micellar emulsions, swollen micelles and reverse micelles have been used in the literature to describe precisely the same systems that were called microemulsion by Schulman. Microemulsions are thermodynamically stable, transparent (or translucent) dispersions of oil and water that are stabilized by an interfacial film of surfactant molecules. The surfactant may be pure or a mixture, or combined with a cosurfactant such as a medium-chain alcohol (e.g. butanol, pentanol). These homogeneous systems, which can be prepared over a wide range of surfactant concentrations and oil-to-water ratios (20–80%), are all fluids of low viscosity. The term microemulsion, which implies a close relationship to ordinary emulsions, is seemingly misleading because the microemulsion state includes a number of different microstructures, most of which are little in common with ordinary emulsions. Although, microemulsions may be composed of dispersed droplets of either oil or water, it is now accepted that they are essentially stable, single phase swollen micellar solutions rather than unstable two-phase dispersions. Microemulsions are readily distinguished from normal emulsions by their transparency, their low viscosity, and more fundamentally their thermodynamic stability and ability to undergo the process of spontaneous formation. The dividing line, however, between the size of a swollen micelle (10–140 nm) and a fine emulsion droplet (100–600 nm) is not well defined, although microemulsions are very labile systems and a microemulsion droplet may disappear within a fraction of a second whilst another droplet forms spontaneously elsewhere in the system. In contrast, ordinary emulsion droplets, though small in size yet exist as discrete entities until coalescence or Ostwald ripening occurs (Table 8.1).

METHODS OF PREPARATION

Phase Titration Method

Microemulsions are prepared by the spontaneous emulsification method (phase titration method) and can be depicted with the help of

Table 8.1: Comparison of microemulsion with conventional emulsion

Property	Microemulsion	Conventional emulsion
Appearance	Transparent (or translucent)	Cloudy
Preparation	Facile preparation, relatively lower cost for commercial	Require a large input of energy, higher cost production
Viscosity	Low viscosity with Newtonian behavior	Higher viscosity
Optical isotropy	Isotropic	Anisotropic
Interfacial tension	Ultra-low	High
Microstructure	Dynamic (interface is continuously and spontaneously fluctuating)	Static
Droplet size	20–200 nm	>500 nm
Stability	Thermodynamic stability, long shelflife	Thermodynamic unstability (kinetic stable) will eventually phase separate
Phases	Monophasic	Biphasic

phase diagrams. Construction of phase diagram is a useful approach to study the complex series of interactions that can occur when different components are mixed. Microemulsions are formed along with various other association structures (including emulsion, micelles, lamellar, hexagonal, cubic, and various gels and oily dispersion) depending on the chemical composition and concentration of each component. The understanding of their phase equilibria and demarcation of the phase boundaries are essential aspects of the study. As quaternary phase diagram (four component system) is time consuming and difficult to interpret, pseudoternary phase diagram is often constructed to find the different zones including microemulsion zone, in which each corner of the diagram represents 100% of a particular component. The region can be separated into W/O or O/W microemulsion by simply considering the composition, whether it is oil rich or water rich. Observations should be made carefully so that the metastable systems are not included.

Phase Inversion Method

Phase inversion of microemulsions occurs upon addition of excess of the dispersed phase or in response to temperature. During phase inversion drastic physical changes occur including changes in particle size that can affect drug release both *in vivo* and *in vitro*. These methods make use of changing the spontaneous curvature of the surfactant. For nonionic surfactants, this can be achieved by changing the temperature of the system, forcing a transition from an O/W microemulsion at low temperatures to a W/O microemulsion at higher temperatures (transitional phase inversion).

During cooling, the system crosses a point of zero spontaneous curvature and minimal surface tension, promoting the formation of finely dispersed oil droplets. This method is referred to as phase inversion temperature (PIT) method. Instead of the temperature, other parameters such as salt concentration or pH value may be considered as well instead of the temperature alone. Additionally, a transition in the spontaneous radius of curvature can be obtained by changing the water volume fraction. By successively adding water into oil, initially water droplets are formed in a continuous oil phase. Increasing the water volume fraction changes the spontaneous curvature of the surfactant from initially stabilized a W/O microemulsion to an O/W microemulsion at the inversion locus. Short-chain surfactants form flexible monolayers at the O/W interface resulting in a bicontinuous microemulsion at the inversion point.

STRUCTURE OF MICROEMULSION

Microemulsions can be classified into three types—water-in-oil (water/oil), bicontinuous, and oil-in-water (oil/water) (Fig. 8.1).

Two types of phases are thus shown to be associated with microemulsions:

- Droplet phases
- Bicontinuous phases

Droplet Phases

At higher water concentration microemulsion is consisted of small oil droplets dispersed in water, i.e. O/W microemulsion, whereas at lower water concentration the situation is reversed and the system tends to be consisted of water droplets dispersed in oil, i.e. W/O microemulsion (Fig. 8.2). In each phase, the oil and water are separated by a surfactant rich film. The oil droplets in O/W microemulsions are surrounded by the electrical double layers, which can extend into the external phase up to a considerable distance (up to 100 nm), depending on the electrolyte concentration. Thus, the hard sphere volume of the droplet is considerably greater than the oil core volume, which creates a strong osmotic (repulsive) force at relatively low disperse

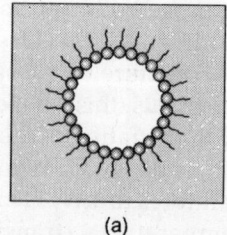 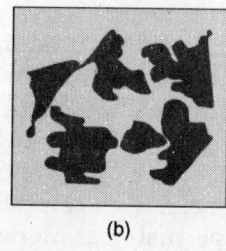 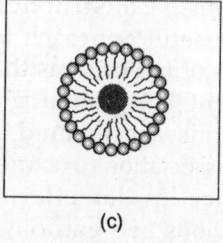

(a)   (b)   (c)

Fig. 8.1: Schematic representation of different types of microemulsion systems—(a) W/O microemulsion, (b) bicontinous microemulsion, (c) O/W microemulsion

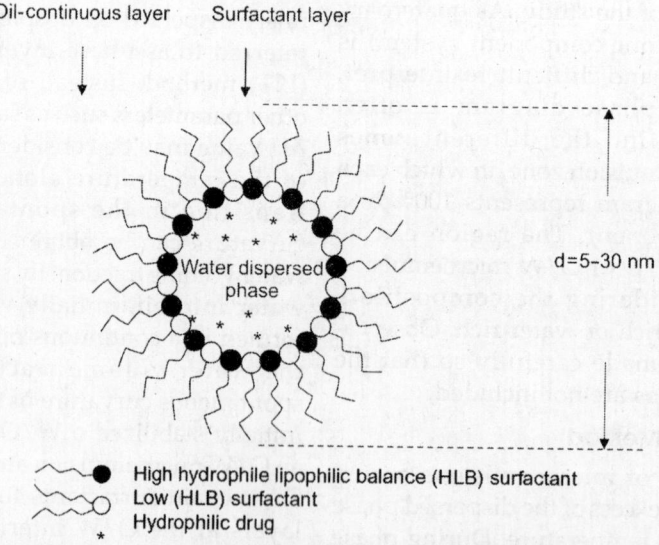

Fig. 8.2: Representative example of W/O emulsion

phase concentrations. In contrast, W/O systems are stabilized primarily by steric interactions between the absorbed films in such a way that the hard sphere volume of the droplets is only slightly greater than that of the water pools. The droplet interaction can take place at relatively short distances of separation, where the tail of the hydrocarbon chains can interpenetrate with each other. This allows a great increase in droplet number concentration before a strong osmotic force is felt.

Bicontinuous Phases or Middle Phase Microemulsions

In many cases, it is possible to affect a gradual transition from O/W to W/O microemulsion simply by changing the volume fraction of oil and water. The intermediate region, which contains approximately equal volumes of oil and water is composed of lamellar or bicontinuous structures. In this region both the oil and the water domains extend over macroscopic distances and the surfactant forms an interface of rapidly fluctuating curvature, but the net curvature is near zero.

Theoretical Basis of Microemulsification

When oil, water, and surfactants are mixed, microemulsions are only one of a number of association structures (including ordinary emulsions, micellar, and mesomorphic phases of various constructions such as lamellar hexagonal cubic and various gels and oily dispersions) that can form depending on the chemical nature and concentration of each of the components, as well as prevailing temperature and pressure.

When a surfactant is added to a mixture containing equal amounts of oil and water, either W/O or O/W emulsion will form depending on the molecular interaction of the surfactant with both the oil and water. Different interaction strengths on both sides of the surfactant film induce a tension gradient across the surfactant membrane and consequently produce curvature. A geometrical model has been proposed to describe

quantitatively, the correlation between the structure of surfactant aggregates and the geometric packing of surfactants at the interface. It is a packing ratio or critical packing parameter (CPP). CPP defined as the ratio of cross-sectional area of hydrocarbon chain to that of the polar head of the surfactant molecule at the interface, i.e.

$$V/a_0 lc$$

where, V = volume of the hydrocarbon chain of surfactant; a_0 = optimal cross-sectional area per polar head in a planar interface; lc = approximately 80–90% of the fully extended length of the surfactant chain.

A greater cross-sectional area of the tail than that of the head ($V/a_0 lc > 1$) would favor the formation of W/O droplets, whereas a smaller cross area of the tail than that of the head ($V/a_0 lc < 1$) would favor the formation of O/W droplets. A planer interface dictates $V/a_0 lc = 1$, leading to the formation of lamellar structure. Many approaches have been used to explore the mechanisms of microemulsion formation and stability. Some emphasise on the formation of an interfacial film and the production of ultra-low interfacial tensions (mixed film theories); other emphasise the monophasic nature of many microemulsions (solubilization theories). Thermodynamic theories consider the free energy of formation of microemulsions and the bending elasticity of the film. No one approach alone covers all aspects of microemulsion structure. The stability and all structures have a place in the overall understanding of microemulsions.

FORMULATION OF MICROEMULSION

In the microemulsification, the film curvature and interfacial tension are crucial factors which determine the formation of microemulsions. Thus, the key to microemulsion preparation lies in decreasing the interfacial tension and increasing the free energy of the newly created surfaces. In this respect, a relatively large amount of surfactant along with cosurfactant, such as a short chain alcohol is required to lower the interfacial tension in formulating conventional microemulsion. Thus, the formulation of microemulsion usually involves a combination of three to five components viz., an oil phase, an aqueous phase, a primary surfactant and in many case secondary surfactants (cosurfactant), and sometimes an electrolyte. The formation of microemulsion is highly specific process involving spontaneous interactions among the constituent molecules. The type of association structure formed from these components at a particular temperature depends not only on the chemical nature of each component, but also on their relative concentrations. Thus, it is essential for a systematic study of micro-emulsion composition to establish phase diagrams for the system under investigation (Fig. 8.3).

Oil

In the microemulsion formulations, usually aliphatic and aromatic oils are employed together with synthetic or natural amphiphiles to homogenize water forming isotropic transparent and stable dispersion of either water-in-oil or oil-in-water for various industrial purposes. The solubilization of single-chain oil (ethyl ester of fatty acid oil) is easier than the three-chain (triglycerides) oil and within the same series of oil; the oil with shorter alkyl chain length is solubilized to greater extent than the longer chain length oils. Thus, as expected, the structure and in part the molecular volume of the oils used influenced the amount of oil incorporated within the microemulsion. Within the triglyceride series of oils, tributyrin, the smallest molecular volume oil could be incorporated up to 3% w/w at a surfactant concentration of 35% w/w, while the larger molecular volume oils could only be solubilized to 2 and 1 % w/w at approximately 30% w/w and 10–35% w/w surfactant for miglycol 812 and soyabean oil respectively. Similarly, for the ethyl esters, the smallest molecular volume, ethyl butyrate was solubilized to the greatest extent, i.e. 16% w/w using a surfactant concentration of 30% w/w, whereas the larger molecular volume oils, ethyl caprylate and ethyl oleate were incorporate at levels of 7% and 3% w/w respectively, at surfactant concentration

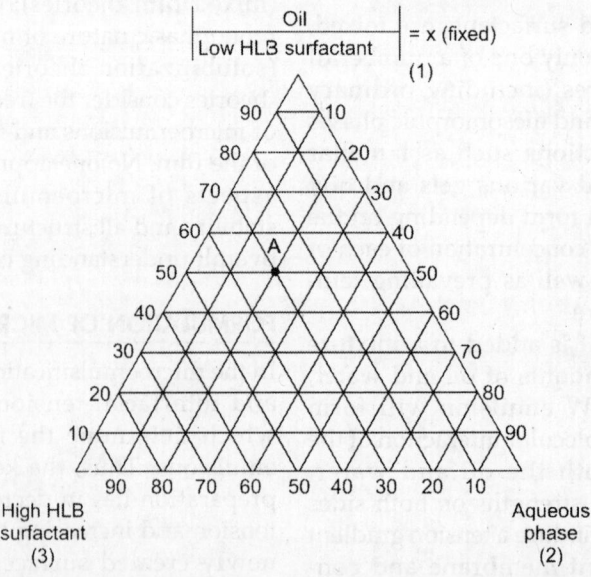

Fig. 8.3: A pseudoternary phase diagram reading. Point A stands for a mixture 50% oil containing the low HLB surfactant at a fixed ratio x (w/w), 20% aqueous phase and 30% high HLB surfactant

of 25% w/w. Surprisingly, this trend was reversed in O/W microemulsions produced using a longer unsaturated alkyl chain surfactant, where the largest molecular volume were solubilized to the greatest extent.

Surfactants

In the preparation of microemulsion, a crucial step is in the choice of surfactant (if necessary) and cosurfactant for particular oil. The chosen surfactant must:

- Lower the interfacial tension to a very small value to aid to the dispersion processes during the preparation of the micro-emulsion.
- Provide a flexible film that can readily deform around small droplets.
- Be of an appropriate hydrophilic lipophilic character to provide the correct curvature at the interfacial region for the desired microemulsion type, O/W, W/O, or biconti-nuous. Preparation of microemulsion is shown in Fig. 8.4.

These conditions could be achieved in several ways. For example, by using a combination of an anionic or cationic surfactant of high hydrophile–lipophilic balance (HLB) with a cosurfactant of lower HLB; a double-chained surfactant of the appropriate molecular composition; or a single-chained nonionic surfactant of the polyethylene glycol alkyl ether type at appropriate temperature. In order to reduce the interfacial tension, it is necessary to maximize the interfacial adsorption of surfactant. A surfactant with a balanced hydrophilic and lipophilic property is desirable, meaning that a surfactant with equal solubility in both water and oil is preferentially adsorbed at the oil-water interface. The relative sizes of the hydrophilic and hydrophobic groups of the surfactant molecules, that is, their HLB must be correctly balanced for a given oil and aqueous solution to produce a microemulsion. The HLB scheme, though originally defined for oil and water emulsions stabilized by nonionic surfactants, can be extended to microemulsion formulation and many ionic emulsifiers. Figure 8.5, represents hypothetical ternary phase diagram and schematic representation of the dispersed phase structure of micelles, reverse micelles, O/W microemulsions, and W/O microemulsions. Recently, much attention has been paid to the use and application of the phospholipids in formulating pharma-ceutically acceptable microemulsions. Their nontoxic nature makes them an ideal choice. Attempts to use lecithin as an amphiphile for the preparation of efficient microemulsions, must be taken into consideration the characteristic solution properties of lecithin, which are as follows:

- Very strong hydrophobicity due to two long hydrocarbon chains
- A strong hydrophilicity due to the zwitter-ionic polar head groups, which have dipole moments and are strongly hydrated.

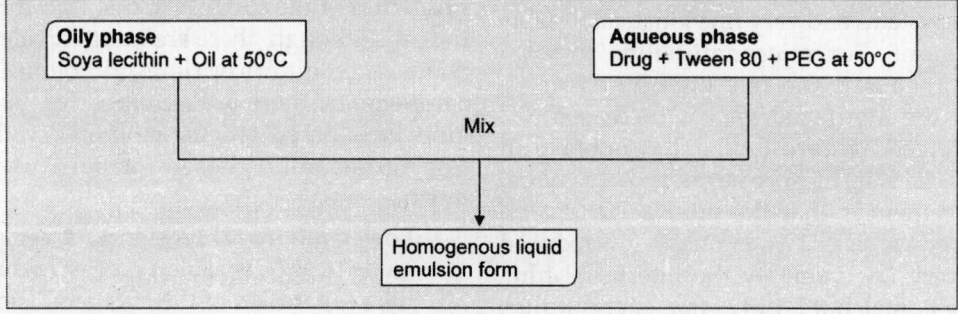

Fig. 8.4: Schematic representation of dual-targeting liposomes for the delivery of anticancer drug

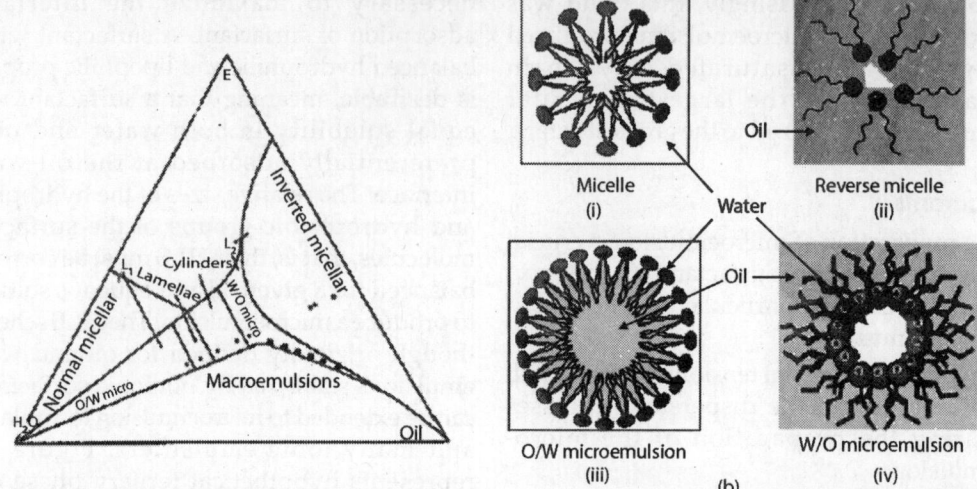

Fig. 8.5: (a) A hypothetical ternary phase diagram representing three components of the system [water, emulsifier (E) and oil] as three axios of an eqilateral triangle. Different compositions of the formulation result in the formation of different phase structures—normal micellar solution, inverted micellar solution, macroemulsion or emulsions, O/W microemulsions, W/O microemulsions and various transition phases represented by cylinders and lamellae structures. The conventionally designated L_1 phase consists of micelles and O/W microemulsions, while the L_2 phase consists of inverted micelles and W/O micromelusions. (b) Schematic representation of the dispersed phase structure of (i) micelles, (ii) reverse micelles, (iii) O/W microemulsions, and (iv) W/O microemulsions.

- A close balance between hydrophilic and lipophilic properties although slightly displaced toward the lipophilic side.
- A strong tendency to form liquid crystals notably of lamellar structure.

Microemulsion Formation

Many approaches have been used to explore the mechanisms of microemulsion formation and stability. Early theories considered interfacial aspects of microemulsions and did not distinguish between thermodynamically stable systems and very fine kinetically stable emulsions. For microemulsions to form spontaneously, the free energy involved, when the interfacial area is increased, δG (δG ¼ $g\delta A$, where δA is the increase in interfacial area) must be negative. An essential requirement is that the interfacial tension between the oil and water phases g, is reduced to a very low value by the interfacial film, giving a small but positive free-energy value. The dispersion of the droplets in the continuous phase increases the entropy of the

system. Microemulsions form because the negative free energy changes due to the entropy of the dispersion of droplets in the continuous phase overcomes the positive product of the small interfacial tension and the large interfacial area A.

The curvature of the oil-water interface in microemulsions varies from highly curved towards oil (O/W) or water (W/O) to zero mean curvature in bicontinuous structures. The type of microemulsion depends on the properties of the surfactant, cosurfactant and the oil. Although, there are no strict rules for choosing the appropriate microemulsion components, there are a number of general guidelines based on empirical observations. The surfactant(s) chosen for particular oil must:

1. Lower interfacial tension to a very low value to aid dispersion processes during the preparation of the microemulsion.
2. It should be of the appropriate hydrophile-lipophile character to provide the

correct curvature at the interfacial region for the desired microemulsion type, O/W, W/O or bicontinuous.

3. Provide a flexible film that can readily deform a round small droplets.

The analysis of film curvature for surfactant associations leading to microemulsion formation has been rationalized by Mitchell and Ninham. They used a packing ratio P defined as V/al, where V partial molar volume of the surfactant, a cross-sectional area, (i.e. size) of the surfactant head group, and l maximum length of the surfactant chain. The packing ratio provides a direct measure of HLB and is influenced by the same factors (Fig. 8.6). Oil-in-water microemulsions are favored, if the effective polar part of the surfactant is more bulky than the hydrophobic part, that is, P varies from 0 to 1, and the interface curves spontaneously towards water (positive curvature). Water-in-oil microemulsions form, when the interface curves in the opposite direction, that is, P is greater than 1 (negative curvature). At zero curvature, when the HLB is balanced and P is zero, either bicontinuous or lamellar structures may be formed according to the rigidity of the film. The critical packing parameter P is based purely on geometric considerations. Hydration of the

surfactant head group and penetration of the oil and the cosurfactant into the surfactant film also affect the packing and curvature, which also illustrates how formulation variables may be manipulated to produce a microemulsion of the desired type.

Most single-chain surfactants do not lower the oil-water interfacial tension sufficiently to form microemulsions nor they process correct molecular structures. Furthermore, short- to medium-chain length, alcohols are necessary as cosurfactants. The cosurfactant also ensures that the interfacial film is flexible enough to deform readily around each droplet as their intercalation between the primary surfactant molecules decreases both the polar head group interactions and the hydrocarbon chain interactions. Medium-chain alcohols, such as pentanol and hexanol have been used by many investigators, as they are particularly effective cosurfactants.

They are not, however, suitable for pharmaceuticals due to their high irritant potential. Double-chain surfactants, such as anionic aerosol-OT (bis-2-ethylhexyl sulfosuccinate) or cationic DDAB (didodecyl dimethylammonium bromide), which have relatively small head groups and bulky hydrophobic portions are of the required HLB to form

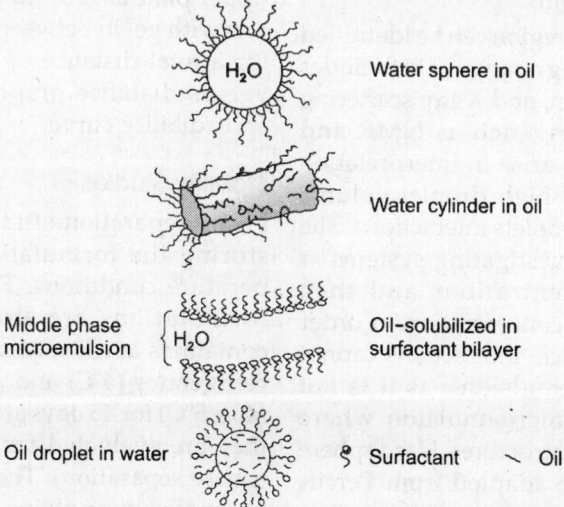

Fig. 8.6: Mechanism of phase inversion of a water-in-oil microemulsion

W/O microemulsions spontaneously without a co-surfactant. Unfortunately, these widely investigated surfactants are too toxic for general pharmaceutical or biotechnological applications.

The successful and beneficial applications of double-chain phospholipids, such as the phosphatidylcholines or lecithin have obvious possibility. Although, lecithin is too lipophilic to form microemulsions, pharmaceutically acceptable microemulsions have been prepared from double-chain phospholipids by using acceptable cosurfactants, such as ethanol, propanol, or n-butanol with isopropyl myristate. Self-emulsifying drug delivery systems are composed of triglyceride oils and surfactant mixtures that undergo spontaneous emulsification when mixed with water.

PREPARATION OF MICROEMULSIONS

As microemulsions are thermodynamically stable, they can be prepared simply by blending oil, water, surfactant, and cosurfactant with mild agitation. Once the appropriate microemulsion components have been selected, quaternary phase diagrams or ternary pseudophase diagrams may be constructed to define the extent and nature of the microemulsion regions and the surrounding two- and three-phase domains.

The microemulsion region can be identified and characterized using a range of techniques based on light, neutron, and X-ray scattering and other techniques, such as NMR and microscopy. Problems arise in interpretation of data in systems of high droplet volume fraction due to inter-droplets interactions. The normal practice of investigating systems at relatively low concentrations and then extrapolating to zero concentration in order to eliminate interparticle interactions cannot be applied to microemulsions, as it is not possible in case of microemulsion where dilution may affect the structures. Hard sphere models, such as those adapted from Percus and Yevick, have been successfully used to analyze scattering data from concentrated W/O microemulsions.

CHARACTERIZATION OF LIPID MICROEMULSION

Size, shape, and size distribution measurements: Morphology and structure of oil globules are determined with the help of transmission electron microscopy (TEM) by using negative staining with phosphotungstic acid. Size of the droplets is determined for the formulations with the master-sizer using laser light scattering technique.

Rheology of the Microemulsion

The prepared microemulsion system is studied for its rheological behavior using Brookfield viscometer. Viscosity is determined at various shear rates by subjecting the system at different torque values. The temperature is maintained constant $25 \pm 2°C$ throughout experiment. The spreadibility of formulation is determined with the parallel-plate method. The spreadibility test assembly is typically consisted of two glass plates (lower stationary and upper movable) designed to slide over each other. Approximately, 0.5 g formulations over a defined area of the lower plate is placed and covered with an upper movable plate. The upper plate is allowed to slide over the lower one with gel in between at a rate of 1 mm/sec for a total distance of 50 mm and the force versus distance graph is constructed as a spreadibility curve.

Stability Studies

Phase separation studies are conducted by storing the formulation at different temperature conditions. Three batches of same formulations are stored in sealed glass containers at room temperature $(25 \pm 5°C)$, in refrigerator $(4°C)$ and at higher temperature $(40 \pm 5°C)$ for 45 days at specific time intervals, they are evaluated for percent oil separated (phase separation). The formulation can also be studied by applying shear rate by repeated centrifugation of the formulation at 10,000 rpm and calculating the oil phase remaining after centrifugation treatment.

In Vitro Release Study/In Vitro Permeation Studies

The *in vitro* characterization of topical formulations is carried out using Franz's diffusion cell and is considered to be the most reliable method for prediction of drug transport across the skin following topical application of formulations. Drug release rate studies conducted are carried out using dialysis membrane and permeation studies are concluded measuring drug diffusion across male mouse skin.

Pharmaceutical and Biological Applications of Microemulsions

Microemulsions provide ultra-low interfacial tensions and large interfacial areas as well as the ability to concentrate and localize significant amounts of both oil- and water-soluble materials within the same isotropic medium. Over the years, attention has been focused on their potential use as novel reaction media for a wide range of chemical, biochemical, and photochemical reactions, and as carriers for chemicals and small particles. Inverse microemulsions of the W/O type are the subject of particular interest because of the rapidly emerging range of biotechnological applications based on their ability to solubilize enzymes in the aqueous domains without denaturation or loss of activity. The ability of such solubilized hydrophilic enzymes to transform hydrophobic substrates dissolved in the organic phase could lead eventually to the synthesis of new drugs. As with ordinary emulsions, microemulsions also show improved gastrointestinal absorption. They also have a number of other advantages over macroemulsions for drug delivery. Microemulsions are formed spontaneously without requiring of high shear equipment or significant heat input (heat and gentle mixing are required, only if it is necessary to melt any of the ingredients) and their microstructures are independent of the order of addition of the excipients. Optical transparency and low viscosity of microemulsions ensure that they are cosmetically elegant and easy to handle and pack, and their indefinite stabilities ensure a long shelflife. Microemulsions have thus attracted much interest for their drug delivery potential. Both o/w and W/O emulsions have been shown to enhance the oral bioavailability of drugs including, various peptides. A peroral concentrate of cyclosporine is now available commercially (Sandimmune Neoral Novartis), which forms a microemulsion in the aqueous fluids of the gastrointestinal tract. In this preparation, the rate of absorption of cyclosporin is more rapid and less variable than it is with the conventional oily dispersion.

Microemulsions have also been used for topical delivery, where they increase drug absorption. For example, cetyl alcohol, which is commonly used as an emulsifier in lotions and creams, is absorbed faster and deeper into the skin, when formulated as a component of a microemulsion. Although, efficient skin penetration may be desirable for a therapeutic agent, relatively high concentrations of surfactant (10–25%) and cosurfactant or cosolvent (5–10%) in such formulations could enhance skin absorption of potential irritants or carcinogens. In fact, the main limitations in realizing the full potential of microemulsions as drug delivery systems, are the narrow range of surfactants, cosurfactants, solvents, and other pharmaceutically acceptable materials. During the last two decades, microemulsions have been extensively researched because of their possible potential in many applications.

Oral Delivery

The development of the effective oral delivery systems has always been the goal because drug efficacy can be severely limited by instability or poor solubility in the gastrointestinal fluid. Biopharmaceutical classification system (BCS) is a useful guidance by US

FDA and it takes into account consideration of three major factors, dissolution, solubility, and intestinal permeability, which affect oral drug absorption. According to the BCS, drug substances are classified as follows:

Class I: High permeability, high solubility

Class II: High permeability, low solubility

Class III: Low permeability, high solubility

Class IV: Low permeability, low solubility

Knowledge of BCS helps the formulation scientists to develop a dosage form, based on mechanistic, rather than empirical approaches. Drug substances are considered highly soluble when the largest dose of a compound is soluble in <250 mL of water over a range of pH from 1.0 to 7.5 and highly permeable, when they show >90% absorption of the administered dose. In contrast, compounds with solubility below 0.1mg/ml provide significant dissolution related problems, and often, even compounds with solubility below 10 mg/ml present difficulties related to solubilization during formulation. A major technological hurdle for routine clinical use of many drugs is their very poor solubility in water. Microemulsions have the potential to enhance the solubility of the poorly soluble drugs and overcome the dissolution related bioavailability problems. This is particularly important for the BCS class II or class IV drugs. The successful formulation of such drugs is highly dependent on the performance of the formulated product. Microemulsions act as supersolvent for these drugs and can be optimized to ensure consistent bioavailability. In addition, they can be used for the delivery of hydrophilic drugs including macro-molecules, such as proteins and peptides. This is due to the existence of polar, nonpolar, and interfacial domains which allow encapsulation of drugs with varying solubility. More-over, these systems have been reported to protect the incorporated drugs against oxidation, enzymatic degradation and enhance the membrane permeability. Presently, Sandimmune Neoral® (Cyclosporine A),

Fortovase® (Saquinavir), Norvir® (Ritonavir), etc. are the commercially available SMEDDS formulations. A detailed illustration of their role in oral drug delivery is discussed in this section.

Bioavailability Enhancement of Poorly Water Soluble Drugs

Paclitaxel, an anticancer drug, has poor aqueous solubility and therefore, formulation of paclitaxel has proven to be difficult. Gao et al. disclosed self emulsifying compositions that generated a supersaturated paclitaxel microemulsion upon contact with water *in vivo* and permitted its rapid and efficient absorption resulting in an improved oral bioavailability. The composition comprised of a solvent, a surfactant, a substituted cellulosic polymer (e.g. hydroxypropyl methyl cellulose, hydroxypropyl cellulose, hydroxyethyl cellulose, methyl cellulose, etc.), and opti-onally a P-glycoprotein inhibitor. Paclitaxel and surfactant, were present in a ratio from about 1:3 to 1:20 by weight; and the substituted cellulosic polymer and paclitaxel, were present in a ratio from about 50:1 to about 0.1:1 by weight.

The oral administration of a commercial product, Taxol® (Bristol Myers Squibb) showed approximately 10-fold lower Cmax than that obtained with their composition in rats. Farah et al. in US Patent 6054136 provided a SMEDDS capable of forming a micro-emulsion in situ with the physiological fluid of the stomach and intestine for the enhance-ment of drug bioavailability. The SMEDDS is consisted of an active constituent, a lipophilic phase, a surfactant and a cosurfactant. The lipophilic phase consisted of a mixture of C8–C18 polyglycolized glycerides having a HLB less than 16. Surfactant was chosen from the group comprising saturated C8–C10 polyglycolized glycerides and oleic esters of polyglycerol having HLB of less than 16 (e.g. Labrasol®, Labrafac CM 10®) and a cosurfac-tant chosen from the group comprising of lauric esters of propylene glycol (Lauroglycol®), oleic esters of polyglycerol and ethyl diglycol (Transcutol®). The surfactant/cosurfactant ratio taken was between 0.5 and 6. The composition being free from aqueous phase would facilitate packaging in hard gelatin capsules. The US Patent 6312704 granted to the same inventors was the extension of their earlier patent. In that, there was an additional claim in which it was said that lipophilic phase was obtained by esterification of polyethylene glycol and glycerol with fatty acids, or by mixing of glycerol esters and condensates of ethylene oxide with fatty acids. The surfactant was selected from the group consisting of oleic esters of polyglycerol or a product obtained by esterification of glycerol and polyethylene glycol with caprylic acid and capric acid, or by mixing of glycerol esters and condensates of ethylene oxide with caprylic acid and capric acid. The use of rapamycin (macrolide antibiotic) and its structurally similar analogs, is limited by their very low solubility, low and variable bioavailability and their high toxicity. They have potent immunosuppressive activity and also antitumor and antifungal activity. Fricker et al. developed a microemulsion preconcentrate carrier medium for their effective oral delivery. The carrier medium was comprised of a reaction product of a castor oil and ethylene oxide; a transesterification product of a vegetable oil and glycerol comprising predominantly linoleic acid or oleic acid, mono-, di-, and triglycerides or a polyoxyalkylated vegetable oil; 1,2-propylene glycol; and ethanol. When administered orally high and consistent absorption was obtained. Therefore, the macrolide might be administered in lower doses, which might alleviate toxicity problems. Earlier they had described a microemulsion preconcentrate for drug delivery comprising hydrophilic component (Transcutol®, Glycofurol, 1,2-propylene glycol, or their mixtures), a lipophilic component selected from the group consisting of fatty acid triglycerides (Miglyol®, Captex®, Capmul®, etc.), mixed mono-, di-, and tri glycerides and transesterified ethoxylated vegetable oils (e.g.

Maisine®), and a surfactant which was selected from the group consisting of polyethyleneglycol, natural or hydrogenated castor oils (Cremophor EL®, Cremophor RH40®), polyethylene-sorbitan fatty acid esters (Tweens), polyoxyethylene fatty acid esters (Myrj), polyoxyethylene polyoxypropylene copolymers, and block copolymers (pluronic, polaxamers). The composition on dilution with water gave a microemulsion having an average globule size of <150 nm.

Liang et al. disclosed self-emulsifying formulations of fenofibrate or fenofibrate derivatives having an improved oral bioavailability and/or reduced food effect, when compared to by commercially available formulations such as Lipanthyl® (Groupe Fournier) or TriCor®. (Abbott Laboratories). The particle size of the active agent was not critical to the bioavailability of the product. Fenofibrate or fenofibrate derivative was dissolved in a solubilizer that allowed the complete dissolution of the fenofibrate or a fenofibrate derivative and prevented or minimized the crystallization of fibrate in the formulation. With the complete dissolution of the fibrate, the fibrate solution resulted in an increased absorption of the fibrate. Some of the earlier strategies for increasing the bioavailabilty included the use of micronized fenofibrate, and diethylene glycol monoethyl ether as solubilizer, etc.

Bioavailability for orally administered conventional crystalline or amorphous forms of cholesterol ester transfer protein (CETP) inhibitors is quite low, often having absolute bioavailabilities of less than 1%. Gumkowski et al. provided self-emulsifying or self-microemulsifying compositions, the improved solubility and bioavailability of CETP inhibitors. The formulation had a CETP inhibitor, a cosolvent, a surfactant having an HLB of 1 to 8, a surfactant having an HLB of over 8 to 20, and optionally a digestible oil.

Lambert et al. provided a composition, which could be an emulsion or a microemulsion having oil and a water phase for improving the solubility of poorly soluble drugs. Chemotherapeutic agent could be a taxoid, a taxane, or a taxine, preferably paclitaxel. Alpha-tocopherol or a tocopherol polyethylene glycol succinate was also incorporated in the oil phase. The resulting formulation was inexpensive, sterilizable by either heat or filtration, stable at least a year and accommodated a wide variety of water insoluble and poorly soluble drugs; also ethanol-free. Nonaqueous solvents and solubilizers, such as alcohol used in pharmaceutical formulations may extract toxic substances, for example, plasticizers, from their containers. This may cause adverse reactions, such as respiratory distress. This problem could be circumvented by their invention. The US Patent 6660286, described a similar composition which in addition claimed a composition consisting of paclitaxel, one or more tocopherols or their derivatives, a tocopherol polyethylene glycol derivative, polyethylene glycol, a polyoxypropylenepolyoxyethylene glycol, nonionic block polymer, and an aqueous phase.

Benameur et al. found that the incorporation of an active agent, particularly statins, into a self-microemulsifying system made it possible to reduce the first intestinal passage effect, and thus improved the systemic bioavailability of the active molecule. Earlier SMEDDS had been reported to improve the solubility of the water insoluble active principles, but there was no information given on the action of SMEDDS on intestinal metabolism. The inventors observed that the incorporation of an active principle (statins) with a strong first intestinal passage effect into a self-microemulsifying system, made it possible to reduce the first intestinal passage effect, and thus improved the systemic bioavailability of the active molecule.

The self microemulsfying carrier included a lipophilic phase, which was a mixture of glycerol mono-, di- and triesters and of PEG mono- and diesters with at least one fatty acid chosen from the group comprising C8–C18 fatty acids (Labrafil M1944CS®), a surfactant phase which is a mixture of glycerol mono-, di-, and triesters and of PEG mono- and diesters with caprylic acid (C8) and capric acid (C10) (Capryol 90®), a cosurfactant phase which was an ester of a polyvalent alcohol with at least one fatty acid chosen from the group comprising of caprylic esters of propylene glycol, lauric esters of propylene glycol and oleic esters of polyglycerol. The ratio of surfactant/cosurfactant was varied between 0.2 and 6.

The object of the invention of von Corswant was to provide a vehicle which could increase the solubility of compounds having a low solubility in water and at the same time, it should be microemulsion comprised of aqueous polar phase containing a component for adjusting the polarity of the polar aqueous phase, a surfactant film modifier generally monohydric alcohol with 2–3 carbon atoms (e.g. ethanol), a nonpolar phase, i.e. oil, and a mixture of a hydrophilic surfactant and a hydrophobic surfactant selected from the group consisting of lecithin, sphingolipids and galactolipids. The inventors found that by using at least two types of modifiers for adjusting the polarity, it was possible to minimize the amount of the surfactant and to reduce, also the toxicity. Chen et al. described a microemulsion of pyranone protease inhibitor compounds free of alcohol and propylene glycol comprising a pyranone protease inhibitor, surfactant, and a polyethylene glycol a solvent having a mean molecular weight greater than 300 but lower than 600, and a lipophilic component comprising of medium chain mono- and di-glycerides, and optionally a basic amine. The formulations of this invention provided improved solubilization, stability and/or bioavailability of the pyranone drug and permitted less arduous manufacturing processes. Gao et al. provided pharmaceutical compositions of a self-emulsifying formulation, which permitted a high loading of lipophilic compounds and also resulted in good oral bioavailability. The novel composition is comprised of a lipophilic drug, a mixture of diglyceride and monoglyceride in a ratio from about 9:1 to about 6:4 by weight, wherein the diglyceride and monoglyceride are mono- or di-unsaturated fatty acid esters of glycerol having 16–22 carbon chain length, solvent, and surfactant. The composition might be in the form of liquid to be filled in soft elastic capsules or hard gelatin capsules for oral application and might also be in the form of a liquid solution for oral, parenteral, rectal or topical application. They also provided a formulation for pyranone compounds, which was based on the use of a particular amount (0.1% to about 10% by weight) of the basic amine along with solvents, surfactants, and oil.

The invention of Bauer et al. included O/W microemulsion containing one polyglycerol ester as the emulsifier and lipophilic substance as the internal phase. The emulsifier contained a triglycerol monofatty acid ester (e.g. triglycerol monolaurate, triglycerol monocaprylate) and a lipophilic substance was selected from the group consisting of carotenoids, vitamins A, D, E and K and their derivatives and polyunsaturated fatty acids. The emulsifiers used were nontoxic, which could be used in foodstuffs in addition to the pharmaceutical field. Mishra et al. described self-emulsifying microemulsion or emulsion preconcentrate formulations containing omega-3 fatty acid oil, and a hydrophobic drug. The drug was soluble in the omega-3 fatty acid oil, and the preconcentrates were free or contained only minor amounts of a hydrophilic solvent system. US Patent 4678808 described the use of these oils to treat disorders associated with arachidonic acid metabolites, including autoimmune syndromes, acute and chronic inflammatory diseases, atherosclerosis, etc. The omega-3 fatty acid oil and drug can exert an additive or synergistic therapeutic effect or the omega-3 fatty acid oil to counteract the negative side effects of the therapeutic agent. For example, cyclosporines are soluble in omega-3 fatty acid oil and capable of exerting an additive or synergistic therapeutic effect in various autoimmune and inflammatory diseases. In addition, the omega-3 fatty acid oil mitigated the adverse side effects, such as nephrotoxicity, of cyclosporines such as cyclosporine A by reduction of its dose. The composition could be administered in soft or hard gelatin capsule. Crison et al. demonstrated a self-microemulsifying formulation for increasing the bioavailability of a drug, which included oil/lipid material, a surfactant, and a hydrophilic cosurfactant. HLB of hydrophilic cosurfactant was more than 8. The self-microemulsifying formulation could also include an aqueous solvent such as triacetin. They found that a more hydrophilic cosurfactant not only increased the dissolution of poorly water-soluble drugs, but it also increased their *in vivo* bioavailability.

Orally administered acyclovir (in tablet, capsule or suspension form) is slowly and erratically absorbed with 15–30% bioavailability. For improved patient compliance, an acyclovir preparation is required, which would permit lower dosing and less frequent administration. In one embodiment of their invention Burnside et al. provided a pharmaceutical preparation comprising of a W/O emulsion, preferably a microemulsion, containing an oil phase (such as a long chain carboxylic acid or ester or alcohol thereof), a surfactant (such as poloxamer) and an aqueous phase containing the drug acyclovir. It was found that microemulsions were ideal for oral acyclovir delivery, since they contain homogeneous and uniform droplets size of approximately 20–40 nm and had the ability to dissolve relatively large amounts of polar solutes in an overall oily environment. The outer oily phase of the microemulsion was able to incorporate into the intestinal cell matrix, thus creating channels (either paracellularly or transcellularly) through which the acyclovir could pass. Thus, poor absorption in the intestine could be circumvented. Further, the work of Rudnic et al. described a pharmaceutical preparation comprising a stable, surface-active emulsion or dispersion of a pharmaceutical agent incorporated into an emulsion having a hydrophobic discontinuous phase of a long chain carboxylic acid (e.g. lauric acid, capric acid, myristic acid, behenic acid, etc.) or ester (glyceryl monostearate, glyceryl monopalmitate, etc.) or alcohol thereof dispersed in an aqueous phase or having a hydrophilic discontinuous phase dispersed in a hydrophobic phase of a long chain carboxylic acid or alcohol. The materials when combined in accordance with the invention to form a W/O microemulsion demonstrated enhanced absorption.

Melatonin is a hormone synthesized in the epiphysis, in the retina and, presumably in the chromaffinic cells of the intestinal tract. It has immunostimulant and immunomodulatory effects. An attempt had been made by Graziella et al. to improve the oral bioavailability of melatonin. They described a microemulsion containing melatonin, L-alpha-phosphatidylcholine (emulsifier) and a solvent mixture consisting of ethanol, propylene glycol and water in which the weight ratio of L-alpha-phosphatidylcholine to melatonin was about 1:1. Eugster et al. disclosed in their invention a spontaneously dispersible concentrate which formed as an ultramicroemulsion when diluted with water or a glucose solution. The concentrate contained sterolester and/or sterolphosphor compounds, surfactant, vitamin or provitamin, free fatty acid, and a carrier or diluent. They found that the newly synthetized sterolesters and sterolphosphatides had a pronounced antitumor activity, particularly if these compounds were incorporated into spontaneously dispersible concentrates.

Ecanow proposed the drug-delivery systems, which included one or more monomeric or polymerized surface active agents (e.g. polymerized lecithin), which allowed for rapid dissolution and smooth liberation of the incorporated drug. Stable microemulsions could be produced by entrapment or encapsulation of the microemulsions in a coacervate phase matrix and/or film.

Controlled and Sustained Release of Drugs

US Patent 7147867 discloses a sustained-release dosage form for the delivery of a progestogenic steroid comprising of a capsule, a self-emulsifying drug formulation contained within a first portion of the capsule, an expandable layer contained within a second portion of the capsule. The expandable layer was so positioned that the self-emulsifying drug formulation could be expelled from the capsule upon expansion of the expandable layer and a semipermeable membrane is formed over at least a portion of an outer surface of the capsule (Fig. 8.3). The semipermeable membrane comprised of a thermoplastic polymer having a softening point of 40–180°C. The aqueous fluid dissolves the gelatin capsule embibing fluid that causes the push displacement layer to expand and push the emulsified formulation through an orifice at a controlled rate. The dosage form comprising of the liquid formulation provided various advantages, such as improved solubility, improved bioavailability, sustained release and inhibition of crystal growth during storage thereby providing improved stability. Gattefosse were granted a patent for a composition with sustained release of active agent which was capable of forming a microemulsion with an external hydrophilic phase, for example, physiological fluid or water. The composition was comprised of an inert polymeric matrix, which is not ionised at physiological pH, dispersed in the microemulsion forming system. After ingestion, polymeric matrix contacts the physiological fluid and forms a gelled polymeric matrix. The gelled barrier controls the penetration of water, making the gradual release of the microemulsified active principle by diffusion, in a continuous and prolonged manner. Fig. 8.7 shows the scheme of the functioning of polymer matrix dispersed in a SMEDDS

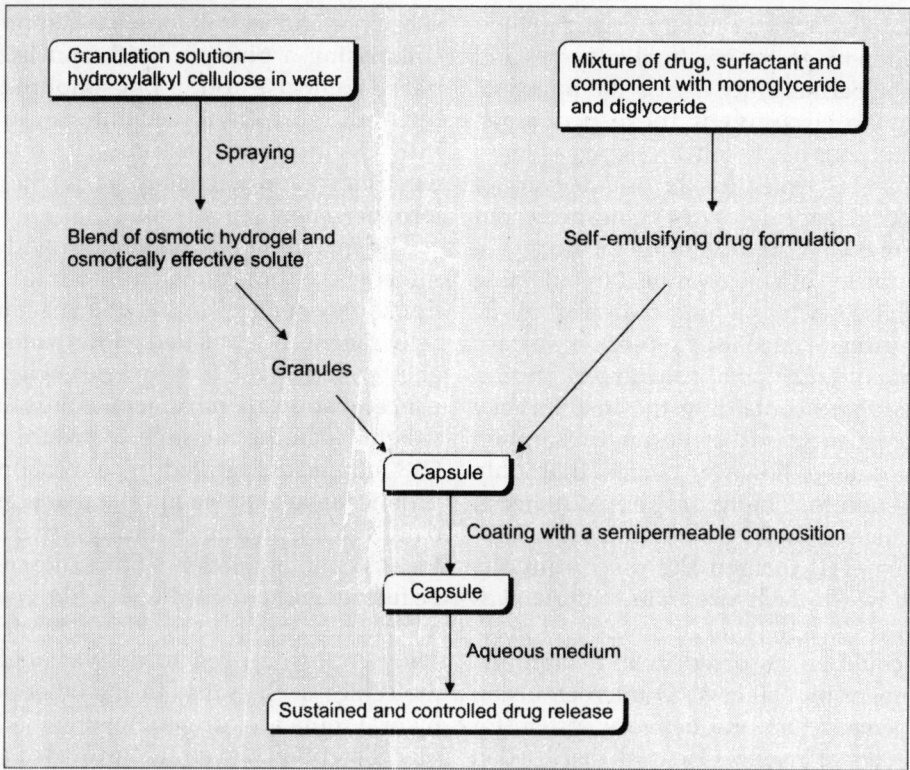

Fig. 8.7: Schematic of formulation process of sustained and controlled drug release product

formulation, the composition obtained being in the form of gel capsule. ALZA Corporation had been assigned a patent for a sustained release self-emulsifying formulation to enhance the solubility, the dissolution, and the bioavailability of the drug. The formulation process involved the following steps: (a) blending of an osmotic hydrogel and an osmotically effective solute, (b) blending a hydroxy alkylcellulose and water to provide a granulation solution, (c) spraying the granulation solution of step (b) onto the composition provided in step (a) to provide granules, (d) forming a blended, liquid mixture consisting essentially of a drug, a surfactant, and a member selected from the group consisting of a mono- and di-glyceride to provide a liquid self-emulsifying drug formulation, (e) adding the drug formulation formed in step (d) to a capsule, (f) adding the sprayed composition of step (c) to the capsule,

(g) coating the capsule with a semipermeable composition to provide a membrane permeable to an aqueous fluid and providing an exit in the membrane for delivering the drug formulation at a sustained-release and controlled rate over an extended period of time.

Protein and Peptide Drug Delivery

Numerous peptide and proteins have been identified for use as novel therapeutic agents. With the understanding of their structure and mechanism, recent research has shifted to biotechnological product. Changing scenario and increased market is imposing a need to address significant protein delivery related issues already at late discovery and early development stages. However, in spite of tremendous advances in peptide and protein development, their delivery is limited to systemic route. This is due to their low oral bioavailability, which can be ascribed to their inactivation by gastrointestinal enzymes and their poor permeability across the intestinal mucosa. To circumvent these problems, microemulsions have been developed as smart systems and patented for the oral delivery of protein and peptide drugs. One preferred embodiment of the invention of Burnside et al. comprised of a microemulsion containing an oil phase (such as a long chain carboxylic acid or ester or alcohol thereof), a surface active agent (such as a poloxamer) and an aqueous phase containing the insulin. They attempted to increase the intestinal absorption of the hormone, however could attain only limited success. The hydrophobic material formed the continuous phase and the hydrophilic material formed the discontinuous phase in which the hydrophilic material was emulsified (W/O). A large amount of polar solutes could be dissolved in an overall oily environment by using W/O microemulsion thereby creating an oral delivery system for oral delivery of insulin. Cho et al. disclosed in US Patent 5656289 that oral proteinaceous compositions comprising W/O microemulsions could form chylomicra or provide chylomicra to sites of absorption in the gastrointestinal tract. It is believed that when a biologically active material is administered in association with chylomicra or the constituents of chylomicra, it is targeted to the villae and microvillae of the intestinal wall, from where it is secreted into the lacteals and intestinal lymph and then drained into the thoracic duct and, ultimately, the circulating bloodstream. Therefore, proteinaceous active agents administrable only parenterally can possibly be given by the more preferred oral or rectal route. Formulations of the invention were suitable for the oral administration of insulin in the treatment of diabetes W/O formulation for proteinaceous compounds comprised of a hydrophilic phase dispersed in a lipophilic phase to form an emulsion/microemulsion wherein hydrophilic phase-comprises of water, a biologically active substance and lecithin or a lecithin precursor comprising a phospholipid, and lipophilic phase comprises oil, a phospholipid and a lipophilic surfactant. Lecithin can integrate into chylomicra, particularly into their membranes and ultimately carries the protein into the general circulation.

The invention of Cho et al. provided promicelle compositions (microemulsion or liposome) comprising a pharmaceutically active agent encapsulated within a membrane of esterified C12–C18 fatty acids, wherein the concentration of fatty acid is less than 15 weight %. In the intestine, exposure to C12–C18 fatty acids resulted in conversion of the promicelle to a stable micelle that effectively delivered the pharmaceutically active agent to the systemic circulation. The membrane could be further encapsulated with a film coating or an enteric coating to provide a minicapsule. They could be used to deliver acid labile molecules, such as insulin and other peptides by oral route and drugs showing inadequate oral absorption. Owen et al. provided a highly stable W/O microemulsion which readily converted in an O/W emulsion by the addition of aqueous fluid. Proteins and peptides could be stored for long periods of time at room temperature and above by using the W/O microemulsion. When required for use aqueous fluid is added, which converts the microemulsion to an O/W emulsion and releases the protein. US Patent 5688761 described the extension of the above mentioned work in which the same assignee (LDS Technologies Inc.) had included high purity short chain monoglyceride surfactant as the preferred low HLB surfactant after finding that the use of C9–13 monoglycerides as the low HLB surfactant enhanced the uptake of the active material upon administration. Desai described a microemulsion formulation for oral administration, in which a liquid polyol solvent (propylene glycol or polyethylene glycol) and lipid cosolvent containing a proteinaceous medicament, e.g. insulin formed a microemulsion in the gastrointestinal tract at sites of absorption, i.e. villi of the intestinal tract. A vital ingredient in the formulation was the protease inhibitor which inhibited or prevented the degradation of the proteinaceous material. Poli et al. presented compositions in the form of microemulsions or liposomic dispersions for the transmucosal administration of therapeutic proteins or peptidic substances. They contained in addition a thermosetting agent (Pluronic F127®), which differentiated them from the known liposomic or microemulsified compositions. The composition possessed a low viscosity at room temperature which helped in the distribution of finely absorbed divided product on a larger surface. The viscosity, however increased on reaching the mucous as a result of structural change that takes place as a function of the body temperature.

Ekwuribe et al. prepared hydrophilic and lipophilic balanced microemulsion formulations of free-form and/or conjugation-stabilized therapeutic agents such as insulin. Microemulsion described was W/O type and with a HLB value between 3 and 7. In one particular aspect, the composition comprised of insulin covalently coupled to a polymer, a linear polyalkylene glycol moiety and a lipophilic moiety, wherein insulin, the linear polyalkylene glycol moiety and the lipophilic moiety are conformationally arranged in relation to one another such that the insulin in the composition had an enhanced *in vivo* resistance to enzymatic degradation, compared to insulin plain. HLB value less than 7 provided a stable formulation for incorporating free insulin and/or insulin conjugates suitable for oral administration.

Parenteral Delivery

The formulation of lipophilic and hydrophobic drugs into parenteral dosage forms has proven to be difficult. O/W microemulsions are beneficial in the parenteral delivery of sparingly soluble drugs, where the administration of suspension is not desirable. They provide a means of obtaining relatively high blood concentration of these drugs, which usually require frequent administration. Other advantages are that they exhibit a higher physical stability in plasma than liposomes or other vesicles and the internal oil phase is more resistant against drug leaching. Several sparingly soluble drugs have been formulated into O/W microemulsion for parenteral delivery. Microemulsions can also be used as intravenous delivery systems for the fat soluble vitamins and lipids in parenteral nutrition. Dennis et al. patented an intravenous microemulsion delivery system for water insoluble or sparingly water soluble drugs that contained an oil phase comprising of the drug, a long polymer chain surfactant (e.g. lecithin, gelatin casein, tweens, macrogol ethers, etc.) and a short fatty acid surfactant (e.g. stearic acid, glyceryl monostearate, sorbitan esters, etc.) and an aqueous phase. The droplet size ranged from 10–100 nm. They found the composition to be useful for propofol, a short-acting intravenous anesthetic. Microemulsion would emulsify or partition propofol into the nonaqueous phase and preclude (or markedly reduce) stinging and allow painless injection.

Dennis et al. in their invention discussed an intravenous microemulsion delivery system comprising of a long chain polymeric surfactant component and a short fatty acid surfactant component, and an aqueous phase, wherein the amounts of the long chain polymer and short chain fatty acid surfactant components were incorporated to provide for spontaneous formation of thermodynamically stable microemulsion droplets of the oil phase having a particle size from 10–100 nm. The interfacial tension of the drug with the emulsifier combination was less than 0.1 dynes per cm. Microemulsions are generally not dilutable with aqueous fluids, such as certain fluids and buffer solutions, and form emulsions upon addition of such fluids. Various microemulsions are also sensitive to temperature and are not stable outside of room temperature conditions. US Patent

6245349 provided drug delivery compositions in both concentrated and diluted forms for use as vehicles in the administration of various active agents. The concentrated drug delivery compositions were formulated with a phospholipid component, a component selected from propylene glycol or certain polyethylene glycol compounds, a high HLB surfactant, and the drug, with water and/or an optional oil component. The concentrated drug delivery compositions could be diluted with an aqueous fluid to form an O/W microemulsion. These O/W microemulsions were characterized by their small globule size and their wide range of temperature stability, typically from about –20–50°C. They could be administered by intravenous, intra-arterial, intrathecal, intraperitoneal, intraocular, intra-articular, intramuscular or subcutaneous injection.

According to the invention of the Wretlind et al., parenteral administration of water-insoluble active agents was facilitated, when the agents were administered in the lipoid phase of a carrier microemulsion. The microemulsion comprised of a finely dispersed lipoid in an aqueous phase with a mean particle size below 1 micron. Higher concentration of the agent (diagnostic or therapeutic) could be achieved and hence a lower dose whereby a rapid onset of the pharmacological effect was accompanied by a reduced incidence of toxicity to body tissues. As the agents were present in a dissolved state in the hydrophobic phase, there was no need of affecting the pH or the osmotic pressure of the aqueous phase. Because of this, the method of administration according to the invention would cause a lower incidence of injuries to the body tissues. US Patent 7157099 described stable, biologically compatible W/O microemulsions, for the sustained release following parenteral administration of hydrophilic active ingredients. Table 8.2 enlists the patents. Microemulsions could be formulated particularly for peptide active ingredients (LHRH analogs such as leuprolide acetate, goserelin, triptorelin, somatostatin or its analogs such as

octreotide and lanreotide acetate, etc.) or biologically active oligo- or polysaccharides (unfractioned heparin or low-molecular-weight heparins), which provides protection against immediate attack by the hydrolytic enzymes as well as its release following sustained release kinetics to avoid repeated administrations. The microemulsions consisted up to 20% of an internal hydrophilic aqueous phase containing the active ingredient, 30 to 98% of a hydrophobic external phase and up to 50% of a surfactant alone or in admixture with a cosurfactant. Another technology already used for sustained release of peptides involved the use of bioerodible polymers like polymers based on glycolic acid and lactic acid.

Drawbacks of using polymers include their higher cost and the issues relating to environmental impact and safety of the pharmaceutical formulation as organic, in particular chlorinated, solvents are used in their preparation. Also, these microemulsions did not cause persistent granulomas, which were reabsorbed during the time in which the medicament was effective and did not induce local ulcerogenicity. Vigne et al. disclosed microemulsions suitable for parenteral administration of fat soluble vitamins (vitamins E, A, D, and K) and hydrophobic drugs. The microemulsions were comprised of a naturally occurring amphipathic substances and a hydrophobic lipid along with the active ingredient and were 30–100 nm sized pseudomicelles. According to them, the composition had a unique property of delivering fat soluble substances to the plasma in a form and distribution which mimicked the natural uptake in normal subjects.

Topical Delivery

Microemulsions are now being investigated for topical delivery which is evident from the publications. They have been reported to enhance the transdermal permeation of drugs compared to conventional formulations such as solutions, gels or creams. They are able to incorporate both hydrophilic (5-fluorouracil,

Table 8.2: List of some of the patents related to microemulsion

US5045337	1991	The Procter and Gamble Company, Ohio	Food microemulsion
US5160759	1992	Kao Corporation, Japan	Edible oil-in-water emulsion
US5376397	1994	Kraft General Foods Inc., Northfield, IL	Microemulsions of oil and water
US5514670	1996	Pharmos Corporation, New York, NY	Submicron emulsions for delivery of peptides
US5891490	1999	Nestec S.A. Switzerland	Edible microemulsion and method of preparing a food product treated with the microemulsion
US6165962	2000	E. I. du Pont de Nemours and Comapny, The University of Delaware.	Aqueous microemulsions
US6303662	2001	Taisho Pharmaceutical Co. Ltd., Japan	Microemulsion
US6426078	2002	Roche Vitamins Inc., US	Oil in water microemulsion
US6790435	2004	Unilever Home & Personal Care USA division of Conopco Inc.	Antiperspirant compositions comprising microemulsions
US 0165739 A1	2006	Mary Kay Inc. US	Alcohol-free microemulsion composition
US 7064114	2006	Parker Hughes Institute, US	Gel-microemulsion formulations
US 0199589 A1	2008	Cargill, Incorporated, US	Lipid microemulsions
US 0155353 A1	2009	Wyeth, N J, US	Microemulsions for pharmaceutical compositions
US 0029622 A1	2010	Neuroscienze pharmaness S.C.A.R.L., US	Microemulsions
US 0034880 A1	2010	Nanoderma Ltd. IL	Pharmaceutical compositions based on a microemulsion
US 0112115 A1	2011	Inventor-Albertina Maria Eduarda Arien et al., US	Polymeric microemulsions

apomorphine hydrochloride, diphenhydramine hydrochloride, tetracaine hydrochloride, methotrexate) and lipophilic drugs (estradiol, finasteride, ketoprofen, meloxicam, felodipine, triptolide) and enhance their permeation. Since the microemulsion is a multicomponent system and its formation requires high surfactant concentration, the skin irritation aspect must be considered especially when they are intended to be applied topically for a longer period. Several plausible mechanisms have been proposed to explain the advantages of microemulsion for the transdermal delivery of a drug:

1. A large amount of drug can be incorporated in the formulation due to the high solubilizing capacity that might increase thermodynamic activity towards the skin.

2. The permeation rate of the drug from microemulsion may be increased, since the affinity of a drug to the internal phase in microemulsion can be easily modified to favor partitioning into stratum corneum, using different internal phase, changing its portion in microemulsion.

3. The surfactant and cosurfactant in the microemulsions may reduce the diffusional barrier of the stratum corneum by acting as penetration enhancers.

4. The percutaneous absorption of drug also increases due to hydration effect of the stratum corneum, if the water content in microemulsion is high enough.

Due to the small droplet size and large amount of inner phase in microemulsions, the density of droplets and their surface area are assumed to be high. Therefore, droplets settle down to close contact with the skin providing high concentration gradient and improved drug permeation. Moreover, low surface tension ensures intimate contact to the skin. Also, the dispersed phase can act as a reservoir making it possible to maintain an almost constant concentration gradient over the skin for a long time. The liquid, transparent, multicomponents based systems according to the invention of Muller et al., containing the active agents in a solution of an oily and optionally an aqueous phase in the presence of surfactants and cosurfactants. Under certain conditions, the cosurfactants can serve as oil components or vice-versa. The efficacy of the active agents applied in the form of the multicomponent systems according to the invention was much better than active agents applied in the form of known multicomponent systems. The multicomponent systems could be used in pharmaceutical products for cutaneous, peroral, vaginal and parenteral administration of pharmaceutical active agents. The invention of Protopapa et al. referred to depilatory preparations containing proteolytic enzymes solubilized in microemulsions, formed with lecithin, aliphatic hydrocarbon, alipathic alcohol and buffer solution (pH 7–9) to be applied for permanent enzymic depilation. The invention introduced the use of microemulsions as a medium for facilitated penetration of the enzymic activity in the epithelial cells of the skin. In addition, their invention referred to a depilation method that applied the preparations of microemulsion containing the enzyme alpha-chymotrypsin, or the enzyme trypsin, for the depilation of any type of skin (fatty-resistant or dry-sensitive). The application of these preparations provided more permanent depilation than the one from other depilatory methods.

Ophthalmic Delivery

In conventional ophthalmic dosage forms, water soluble drugs are delivered in aqueous solution, while water insoluble drugs are formulated as suspensions or ointments. Low corneal bioavailability and lack of efficiency in the posterior segment of ocular tissue are some of the serious drawbacks of these systems. Recent research efforts have therefore focused on the development of new and more effective delivery systems. Microemulsions have emerged as a promising dosage form for ocular use. Bowman et al. disclosed sustained release emulsions (macroemulsions and microemulsions), in which particles of the dispersed phase were dispersed and stably maintained in physical separation by lightly crosslinked, water swellable polymers (carboxyvinyl polymers, polyvinyl pyrolidone, etc.) present in an aqueous polymeric system formulated for administration to the eye in drop or ribbon form.

Chloramphenicol, an antibiotic used in the treatment of trachoma and keratitis, in the common eyedrops hydrolyzes easily. Lv et al. investigated chloramphenicol microemulsion composed of Span 20, Tween 20, isopropylmyristate and water as potential drug delivery systems for eyedrops.

Chloramphenicol was entrapped in the O/W microemulsion free of alcohol. The authors revealed that the content of glycol (main hydrolysis product) in the microemulsion formulation was much lower than that in the commercial eyedrops at the end of the accelerated experiments. Thus, a remarkable increase in the chloramphenicol stability was observed in the microemulsion formulations. Fialho et al. prepared microemulsion based dexamethasone eye drops which showed better tolerability and higher bioavailability. The formulation showed greater penetration in the eye, which allowed the possibility of decreasing the number of applications per day. This might be useful in achieving improved patient compliance.

Nasal Delivery

Microemulsions are now being studied as a delivery system to enhance uptake across nasal mucosa. Addition of a mucoadhesive polymer helps in prolonging the residence time on the mucosa. Nasal route for administration of diazepam might be a useful approach for rapid onset of action during the emergency treatment of status epilepticus. For this, microemulsion was formulated comprising of ethyl laurate (15%), Tween 80: propylene glycol: ethanol at 1:1:1 weight ratio (70%) and water (15%). The nasal absorption of diazepam was found to be fairly rapid at 2 mg kg^{-1} dose with maximum drug plasma concentration that reached within 2–3 minutes.

Periodontal Delivery

Periodontal disease is a collective term for a number of progressive oral pathological afflictions including inflammation and degeneration of the gums, periodontal ligaments, cementum and its supporting bone. It is a major cause of tooth loss. The invention of Brodin et al. included a novel pharmaceutical composition comprising local anesthetic in oil form, surfactant, water and optionally a taste masking agent. The composition was in the form of an emulsion or microemulsion and had thermoreversible gelling properties, i.e. it was less viscous at room temperature than after introduction onto a mucous membrane of a patient. The surfactant in the formulation imparted the thermoreversible gelling properties. Preferred surfactants were Poloxamer 188®, Poloxamer 407®, and Arlatone 289®. The composition could be used as a local anesthetic for pain relief within the oral cavity in conjunction with periodontal scaling and root planning and overcame the problem with the existing topical products (jelly, ointment or spray), such as lack of efficacy due to inadequate depth of penetration, too short duration and difficulties in administration due to spread, taste etc.

Drug Targeting

Drug targeting has evolved as the most desirable but elusive goal in drug delivery. By altering the pharmacokinetics and biodistribution of drugs and restricting their action to the targeted tissue increased drug efficacy with concomitant reduction of their toxic effects can be achieved.

Drug targeting to diseased cells can be achieved by exploiting the presence of various receptors, antigens/proteins on the cell membrane, which may be uniquely expressed or over-expressed in these cells as compared to the normal cells. Specific antibodies to the surface proteins and ligands for the receptors can be used to target specific cells. The submicron size of these systems confers excellent opportunities to overcome the physiological barriers and enables efficient cellular uptake followed by intracellular internalization.

Cellular Targeting

Nucleic acids are promising therapeutics. The invention of Monahan et al. included insertion of nucleic acid into a reverse micelle for cell delivery. They referred W/O microemulsions to as reverse micelles. The reverse micelle had the property to compact the nucleic acid for easier delivery. To further enhance the delivery, other molecules such as a surfactant having a disulfide bond or a polyion might be added to the nucleic acid-micelle complex. Another advantage of the invention was the use of reverse micelles for gene delivery to the cells. The micelle containing the compacted polynucleotide could be utilized as a reaction vesicle in which additional compounds such as polycation could be added to the DNA. Additionally, the polynucleotide/reverse micelle system was used as a vesicle for template polymerization of the DNA or caging of the DNA in which the polycation was crosslinked. Another advantage was that the micelle might be cleaved under physiological conditions involved along the transfection (process of delivering a polynucleotide to a cell) pathway. Better recovery and purification of the biomolecules, which was difficult earlier could be achieved by utilizing cleavable reverse micelles. The invention of Wheeler et al. was related to cell delivery of hydrophobic compounds in microemulsion carriers. Microemulsion was comprised of a mixture of oil, a hydrophobic compound, and a polyethylene glycol-linked lipid. The purpose of polyethylene glycol-linked lipid was to enhance the stability of the microemulsion compositions. The hydrophobic compound remains in an oil environment, which is surrounded by a monolayer of a polar lipid. The polar head of the lipid face outward to provide compatibility with the external aqueous environment, while the nonpolar tail face the internal oil environment. A targeting moiety such as biotin, avidin, streptavidin or antibodies might be covalently or noncovalently attached to the lipid monolayer. The composition could also be used for diagnostic and therapeutic purposes.

Tumor Targeting

Maranhao suggested the utility of microemulsions as vehicles for the delivery of chemotherapeutic or diagnostic agents to neoplastic cells, while avoiding normal cells. They claimed a method for treating neoplasms, wherein neoplasms cells have an increased number of LDL (low-density lipoprotein) receptors compared to normal cells. The microemulsion was comprised of a nucleus of cholesterol esters, wherein more than 20% triglycerides surrounded by a core of phospholipids and free cholesterol containing a chemotherapeutic drug. Microemulsions were similar in chemical composition to the lipid portion of low-density lipoprotein (LDL), however, did not contain the protein portion. These artificial microemulsion particles incorporated plasma apolipoprotein E (apoE) onto their surface, when were injected in the bloodstream or incubated with plasma. The apolipoprotein E served as a linking element between the particles of the microemulsion and the LDL receptors. The microemulsions could then be incorporated into cells via receptors for LDL and delivered the incorporated molecules. Thus, higher concentration of anticancer drugs could be achieved in the neoplastic cells that have an increased expression of the receptors. In this way, toxic effects of these drugs on the normal tissues and organs could be avoided. In human subjects, they observed no change in the plasma kinetics of the radioactively labeled microemulsion containing carmustine or cytosine-arabinoside thereby confirming that the incorporation of these drugs did not supress the capacity of the microemulsion to incorporate apoE in the plasma and bind to the receptors. Shiokawa and coworkers reported a novel microemulsion formulation for tumor targeted drug carrier of lipophilic antitumor antibiotic aclacinomycin A (ACM). Their findings suggested that a folate-linked microemulsion may be used for tumor targeted ACM delivery. The study showed that folate modification with a sufficiently long PEG chain on emulsions is an effective way of targeting emulsion to tumor cells.

Brain Targeting

Intranasal administration confers a simple, practical, cost effective, convenient and noninvasive route of administration for rapid drug delivery to the brain. It allows a direct transport of drugs to the brain circumventing the brain barriers. Vyas et al. prepared mucoadhesive microemulsion for an antiepileptic drug clonazepam. The aim was to provide rapid delivery to the rat brain. Brain/blood ratio at all sampling points up to 8 hours followpatents related to the microemulsion.

SUGGESTED READINGS

1. Benita S, In: microencapsulation and industrial applications, Marcel Dekker, New York, 411, 1997.
2. Gasco MR, Gallarate M. and Pattarino F (1991), *Int. J. Pharm.*, 69, 193.
3. Kunieda H and Ishikawa N (1985), *J. Colloid Interface Sci.*, 107, 122.

4. Lawrence M J, Rees GD (2000), *Adv Drug Deliv Rev.*, 45:89, 121.

5. Leung R, Hou, MJ, Manohar C, Shah DO, Chun PW, Shah DO, *Ed.; American Chemical Society: Washington* DC, 325, 1981.

6. Lovell MW, Johnson, HW, Hui HW, Cannon JB, Gupta PK and Hsu CC (1994), *Int. J. Pharm,.* 109, 45.

7. Ross S and Morrison ID (1988), *Colloidal System and Interfaces*, Wiley, New York, 176.

8. Tarr B and Yalkosky SH (1989), *Pharm. Res.*, 6, 40.

9. AP Full, JE Puig, LU Gron, EW Kaler, JR Minter, TH Mourey, *J. Texter Macromolecules*, 25 (20) (1992), pp. 5157–64.

10. LM Gan, N Lian, CH Chew, GZ Li Langmuir, 10 (7) (1994), pp. 2197–2201.

11. GW He, QM Pan, GL Rempel Macromol. Rapid Commun., 24 (9) (2003), pp. 585–8.

12. T Yano, A Nakagawa, M Tsuji, *K Noda Life Sci.*, 39 (1986), pp. 1043–50.

13. C Valenta, K Schultz, *J. Control. Rel.*, 95 (2004), pp. 257–265

14. TF Vandamme Prog. *Retinal Eye Res.*, 21 (2002), pp. 15–34.

15. XL Xu, ZC Zhang, HK Wu, XW. Ge, MW. Zhang Polymer, 39 (21) (1998), pp. 5245–8.

16. XL Xu, XW Ge, YD Yin, ZC Zhang, J Zou, AZ Niu *J. Polym. Sci. Polym. Chem. Ed.*, 36 (14) (1998), pp. 2631–5.

17. XL Xu, ZC Zhang, X Wu, XW Ge, J Zuo, AZ Niu Chem. *J. Chin. Univ.*, 19(7) (1998), pp. 1166–70.

18. XL Xu, ZC Zhang, X Wu, XW Ge, J Zuo, AZ Niu, *J. Chem Chin Univ*, 19 (1998), pp. 1166–70.

19. S Roy, S Devi Polymer, 38 (1997), pp. 3325–31.

20. XJ Xu, CH Chew, KS Siow, MK Wong LM Gan Langmuir, 15 (1999), pp. 8067–71.

21. A Aguiar, S Gonzalez-Villegas, M Rabelero E. Mendizábal JE Puig JM, *Dominguez et al. Macromolecules*, 32 (1999), pp. 6767–71.

22. N Sosa, RD Peralta RG López LF Ramos I Katime, C *Cesteros et al. Polymer*, 42 (2001), pp. 6923–8.

23. M Barrere, SCd Silva R, Balic F. Ganachaud Langmuir, 18 (2002), pp. 941–4.

24. Y Dan YH Yang SY, *Chen Chem Res Chin Univ,* 17 (2001), pp. 325–30.

25. Y Dan, YH Yang, SY, *Chen J Appl Polym Sci,* 85 (2002), pp. 2839–44.

26. XJ Xu, KS Siow, MK Wong, LM. *Gan Colloid Polym Sci,* 279 (2001), pp. 879–86.

27. XJ Xu, PY Chow, CH Quek, HH Hng, LM Gan, *J. Nanosci Nanotechnol,* 3 (2003), pp. 235–40.

28. AG Ramirez, RG López, K, *Tauer Macromolecules,* 27 (2004), pp. 2738–47.

29. KD Hermanson, EW Kaler Macromolecules, 36 (2003), pp. 1836–42.

30. D Morgan, KM Lusvardi, EW Kaler Macro-molecules, 30 (1997), pp. 1897–905.

9

Implants and Inserts

INTRODUCTION

Implantable drug delivery devices do not suffer the limitations associated with oral, intravenous or topical drug administration. Additionally, subcutaneously implantable drug delivery devices offer a unique advantage of a retrievable or withdrawal opportunity. This feature enables a readily reversible termination of drug administration, whenever required. Some desirable properties of effective subcutaneous controlled release drug delivery systems are:

- It should improve patient compliance by reducing the frequency of drug administration over the entire period of treatment.
- It should be free from any major surgical procedure and ideally should be readily administered.
- It should release the drug in a rate-controlled manner, leading to enhanced effectiveness and reduction in side effects.
- It should be retrievable by medical personnel to terminate medication, in case so needed.
- It should be easy to sterilize.
- It should be easy to manufacture and relatively inexpensive.
- It should be stable and safe, and should have good mechanical strength.

CLASSIFICATION

Transdermal implantable systems
- Subdermal implantable systems
- Implantable polymeric matrix

Subdermal implants are of various types, namely pellets, rods, and fibers of biodegradable and nonbiodegradable polymers. They provide a means to avoid the first pass metabolism and to deliver sustained release of drugs in relatively smaller and safer quantities. A subdermal delivery system can provide constant and efficacious blood levels of drugs over a desired period with little likelihood of either drug insufficiency or accumulation due to imbalance between drug availability (absorption) and depletion (elimination). Such a system would be easily administered, disallowing patient intervention with increased patient compliance. It would be effective for an extended period of time or treatment. Biologically compatible polymers are used in the fabrication of subdermal implants for delivering drugs at an optimum rate and concentration.
- Implantable devices
- Implantable infusion pumps
- Vapor pressure powered devices
- Peristaltic pumps
- Solenoid pumps

- Electronic pumps
- Implantable mini-osmotic pump (Alzet®)
- Ocular implantable system
- Vaginal implants
- Intra-arterial catheter infusion drug delivery systems
- Needle injection catheter
- Microcatheter
- Helical catheter
- Porous balloon catheters
- Implantable drug delivery pump

CLASSIFICATION-BASED ON MECHANISMS OF DRUG RELEASE FROM IMPLANTS

Diffusion Controlled

Reservoir

This type of system consists of a core of drug surrounded by a polymer, where diffusion of the drug across the polymer layer is the rate-limiting step to drug dissolution or release. Zero-order release kinetics can easily obtained from reservoir type systems, which could be modified to meet the drug requirement in terms of rate of availability. These systems are generally nonbiodegradable, therefore must be surgically removed on completion of treatment or when they are exhausted of their drug content. They are however relatively expensive and may leak the contents, in a uncontrolled manner, hence could lead to severe toxic manifestations.

Matrix

These systems rarely provide zero-order release rate, which can be achieved by compensating for the increased diffusional distance with an increasing area and pathway of the drug diffusion. Applications of these systems include cases of drugs, which are distributed uniformly in the matrix or chemically bound to a polymer backbone chain. It has been reported that if the kinetics of the biodegradation of polymer is known, a zero-order release can be generated by manipulation of geometry of the device, where the surface area remains unchanged with time. The most frequently used biodegradable polymer is polylactic acid or lactic-glycolic acid copolymers.

Chemically Controlled

These systems are analogous to diffusion-controlled implantable delivery systems except the drug is distributed uniformly throughout the bioerodible polymer; the erosion of the polymer decreases the geometry/dimension with time, thus allows for the drug release at the constant rate. Degradation products of the polymer should not be toxic. A zero-order kinetics can be achieved, if the surface area remains unchanged with time.

Three dissolution mechanisms discussed by Heller [1980] are:

- Water-soluble polymers are made or modified to be water insoluble, however water-loving and swellable through biodegradable chemical cross linking
- Water-insoluble polymers are solubilized by hydrolysis, ionization or protonation of the side groups, and
- Water-insoluble polymers are solubilized by backbone chain cleavage to small water, soluble molecules.

Swelling Controlled

In case of swelling-controlled systems, the release rate is equal to the product of surface area and a rate constant that corresponds to rate of advancement of the boundary separating the outer shell from central core (Fig. 9.1). The release rate is constant provided

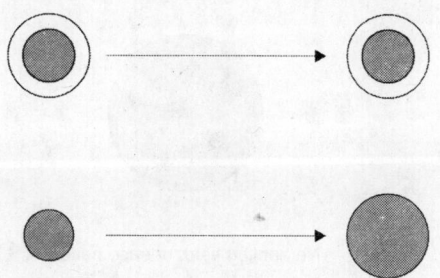

Fig. 9.1: Swelling-controlled delivery system

the absorption rate of the environmental fluid is constant. In this system the rate-limiting step largely depends on ingression of an external agent and not on the diffusive or physico-chemical properties of the incorporated drug.

Osmotically Controlled

This type of system utilizes osmotic pressure as a driving force for delivery of drugs/bioactive. The systems are typically matrix type (Fig. 9.2), where the core is surrounded by a semipermeable film. Zero order drug release is difficult to achieve, however, system could be fabricated to be a pump containing a laser-drilled hole at the outlet deliver. The

drug release under osmotic pressure follows a zero-order kinetics. A typical example is Alzet® osmotic minipump (Alza).

Magnetically Controlled

This type of system (Fig. 9.3) is consisted of the drug and small magnetic beads uniformly dispersed throughout a polymer matrix. In contact to aqueous media, the drug is released in a diffusion-controlled manner and the rate can be increased on application of an oscillating external magnetic field. A typical application of this type of system is demanded or needed for drug delivery designed to correspond with the changes in steroid

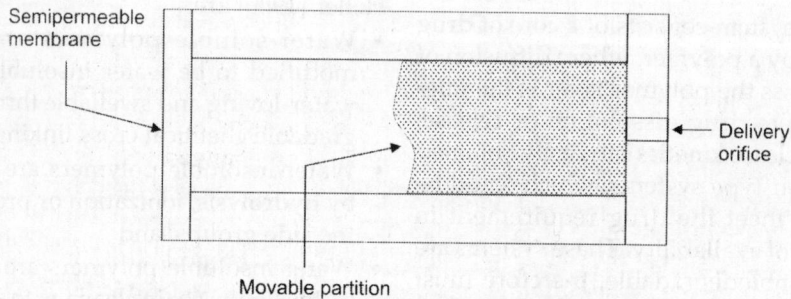

Semipermeable membrane

Delivery orifice

Movable partition

Fig. 9.2: Schematic representation of osmotic pump

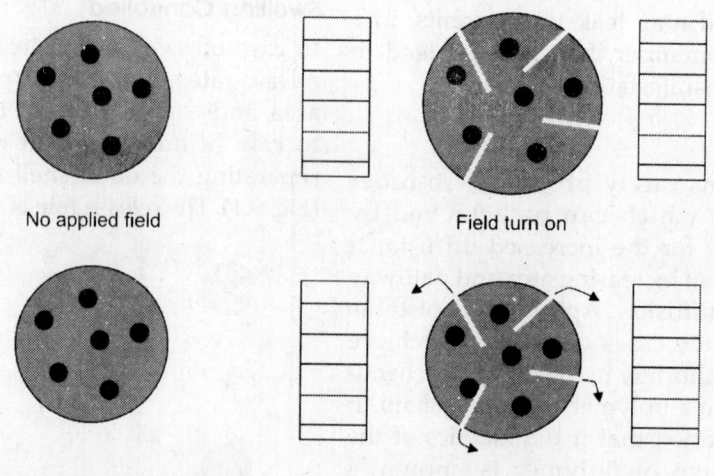

No applied field

Field turn on

No applied field, release halted

Drug release occurs

Fig. 9.3: Drug release from magnetically-controlled delivery system

secretion particularly during the menstrual cycle.

Controlled Drug Delivery

The therapeutic benefits of implantable-controlled release drug administration can be assessed by comparing the biological activity and duration of application of subcutaneous-controlled release drug delivery system with those produced by subcutaneous injection. Table 9.1 illustrates implantable drug delivery devices with their use.

IMPLANTABLE INFUSION PUMP

The rapidly expanding field of genetically engineered drugs synthesized or produced by recombinant DNA techniques places an urgent need for an effective system for therapeutic delivery of drugs to the specific site of action. These new drugs present a challenge to the developing delivery systems because of their potency, high molecular weight, and sensitivity to environmental agents poor oral activity. Despite many obstacles, investigators are developing many potential solutions to the delivery problems posed by theses new drugs.

With the advent of implantable infusion pumps, drug delivery rate can be controlled and provided to almost every or only location within the body. Currently, in clinical uses, there are three basic types of implantable infusion pumps. They are the vapor-pressure powered pump, which are relatively simple mechanical devices, which utilize peristaltic and solenoid pumping mechanisms.

Vapor Pressure Powered Devices

A vapor pressure powered pump was invented in August 1969. This device consists of two chambers and is disk shaped with an inexhaustible volatile liquid power source.

Table 9.1: Implantable drug delivery devices with their use

Delivery system	Drug	Purpose
Reservoir type	Progestin + Estradiol	Contraception
Implantable system	Megestrol	Contraception
	Norgestrel	Contraception
	Norethynodrel	Contraception
	Ibuprofen	Polyarthritis
	Norprofen	Polyarthritis
	Phenylbutazone	Polyarthritis
	Indomethacin	Polyarthritis
	Cyclophosphamide	Cancer
	5-flurodeoxyuridine	Cancer
	Merchloroethamine	Cancer
	Triethylenemelamine	Cancer
Polymeric pellet	Deoxycoryticosterone	Antihypertension studies
	Morphine	Narcotic addiction studies
	Insuline	Diabetes
Implantable infusion pump	Heparin, insulin antineoplastic drugs. intraspinal morphine	Anticoagulation treatment, diabetes, Solid tumor
Ocusert®	Pilocarpine	Glaucoma
Ocualr implantable silicone device	1,3-bis-(-2-chloroethyl)-1-nitroso urea (BCNU)	Tumor studies

The basic principle of operation is based on a physicochemical concept that at a given temperature, a liquid in equilibrium with its vapor phase exerts a constant pressure that is independent of enclosing volume. The selected volatile charging fluid thus provides an appropriate vapor pressure at physiological temperature. This fluid is sealed in a chamber then drug to be infused is filled in second chamber. The two chambers are separated by a flexible metal vestibule, which eventually leads to delivery of infusate through a bacterial filter, a capillary flow restrictor, and an infusion cannula into the desired body site. When the reservoir of the pump is refilled, the expansion of vestibule compartment or bellows compresses and subsequently condenses the charging fluid vapor. A typical example of this type of pump is Infusaid pump of model 100 series. Another novel implantable pump has been devised containing fluorocarbon propellent that generates the vapor pressure. Pump is divided into two chambers by using a titanium bellows. The bottom chamber contains fluorocarbon propellent that liquefies, when the chamber is compressed by forcing drug solution into the upper chamber. The generated constant pressure pumps the drug solution from the upper chamber through a catheter. Refilling of the infusate chamber is done with new drug solution every three months with the help of a hypodermic syringe. This pump is implanted in several patients who need long term heparin based anticoagulant or insulin treatment (Fig. 9.4).

Peristaltic Pumps

Peristaltic pumps consisted of a flexible tube placed in a U-shaped chamber with rollers that press against the tube with sufficient force to occlude its lumen. A motor rotates the rollers that are mounted on a rotor. With the movements of rollers, the lumen of tube compresses, which causes flow of fluid towards the exit. The rollers and housing are arranged, so as to prevent the backflow of the infusate, this is

achieved, when second roller begins to squeeze the tube before the first disengages. This type of system is exemplified by Seimens pumps, Medtronic pump and Sandia pump.

Solenoid Pump

The programmable implantable pump has been developed at the Johns Hopkins University Applied Physics Laboratory (APL). This programmable implantable medication system (PIMS) includes an implantable infusion device, an external physician's console and hand held unit with which patients can initiate preprogrammed doses of drugs to be delivered as required. The implantable device referred to as the implantable programmable pump (IPIP) uses a

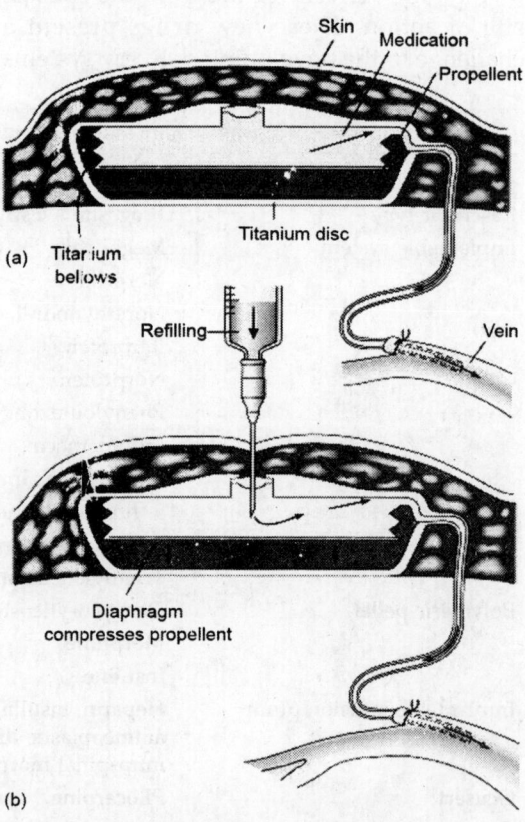

Fig. 9.4: An implantable propellent driven pump system during operation (a) and during refilling (b)

solenoid driven reciprocating chamber wherein a check valve operates to move the infusate from the reservoir out through a delivery catheter. PIMS includes a command system, a telemetry system, a miniature, long-life power supply, and very large-scale integrated circuit chips.

Command System

Implantable electronic devices use command systems that operate from a radio signal originating in a physician console that it is exterior to the patients, examples of control command in a modern pacemakers that is used to change the stimulation pulse rate, pulse voltage, or pulse width; to enable or disable an electrical signal from the atrium and to adjust the sensitivity for an electrical signal from the ventricle. The PIMS commands system is used to change basal delivery rate, to turn the device on and off, and also to set limits on use of medication. A command system enables the implant to adapt according to the need of patient.

Telemetry System

This system involves the transmission of data from a remote location. Typical implant telemetered data might be the confirmation of the parameters that have been incorporated and commanded into it, the battery voltage and the rate of delivery of infusing medication.

Power System

Power system for implants must be small in size and long lasting. They use rechargeable nickel-cadmium cells to store energy and operate the system between recharges. With time and age, the power demand of implantable medical electronic devices reduced to an extent that a single, AA size, lithium primary cell can efficiently operate the device for more than 5 years.

Microminiaturization

Extensive research is continued in order to reduce the size and weight, while at the same time, attempts are directed to increase the operating efficiency. The first pacemaker with two transistors, measuring 3-inch in diameter and 1 inch width and weight approximately 250 g was developed. Nowadays multi programmable pacemakers which contain 100,000 transistors and one-fifth the weight of the first pacemaker, making it compact and convenient to implant even in newborn babies have been developed.

Functioning of Programmable Implantable Medication System (PIMS)

Computer-controlled implantable medication system are not so common. The patient is provided with a handset called patient's programming unit, by which he/she can start self-medication from the IPIP within the constraints of programme into IPIP already fed by the physician. The most important part of the medication programming system is a computer terminal employed for programming the IPIP. The medication injection unit is used for refilling the IPIP. Telephone communication system provides the major portion of PIMS, by means of which the patient at a location remote from the medication programming system can have the IPIP reprogrammed with a new prescription protocol.

Electronic Pumps

A small pumping device has been developed that is driven by the electrolysis of a solution of hydrazine sulfate to produce nitrogen and hydrogen. These gases produced at the electrodes and push a piston, which in turn pumps the drug solution. The current flowing through the electrolyte determines the volume of gas produced, hence altering this current can change the pumping rate. An automatic cut off is included in this device that shows the electrodes at the end of a run, so as to prevent further generation of gas beyond the piston.

IMPLANTABLE MINI-OSMOTIC PUMP (ALZET)

Alzet mini-osmotic pump is a well developed and marketed system employs osmotic pressure as a release mechanism. Simply, it is containing drug reservoir enclosed in by a semipermeable membrane that is associated with a flow moderator. The drug in solution form is filled in the drug reservoir and inserted into the body. The drug reservoir is cylindrical in shape surrounded by osmotic agent (osmogens), which is covered by a semipermeable membrane (Fig 9.5).

When the system contacts an aqueous environment, water permeates through semipermeable membrane and dissolves osmotic agent to produce osmotic pressure. The generated pressure compresses the drug reservoir to expel the drug solution through flow moderator. A variety of flow rate levels and volumes is available with different treatment periods.

OPHTHALMIC INSERTS

Ophthalmic diseases require frequently localized administration of drugs to the tissues around the ocular cavity. The most prescribed dosage form is the eye drop solution, however it suffers from inherent drawbacks like a major part of the medication is immediately diluted in the tear and rapidly drained or cleared away from the ocular cavity by constant tear flow, hence frequent instillation of eyedrops is required in order to maintain a, required constant level of medication. Unfortunately, this results in a massive and unpredictable medication. This makes it necessary to look for a continuous and controlled administration of drugs to eye. With the advent of ophthalmic inserts, it is now possible to administer drugs in a truly continuous and controlled manner.

Drug Delivery Kinetics from Ophthalmic Inserts

The ophthalmic inserts have been classified on the basis of their physicochemical behavior, i.e. soluble (s) or insoluble (I). Insoluble inserts can be modified to deliver drugs at a controlled and predetermined rate, however they need to be removed from eye when exhausted. Soluble inserts are also generally defined as erodible systems (E), which undergo gradual solubilization in the process of drug release and thereby need not to be removed. The terms 'soluble' and 'erodible' are not interchangeable, true dissolution occurs mainly due to swelling, whereas erosion involves chemical, enzymatic, or hydrolytic degradation of polymer(s).

Swelling-controlled release devices consist of homogeneously dispersed active agent in a

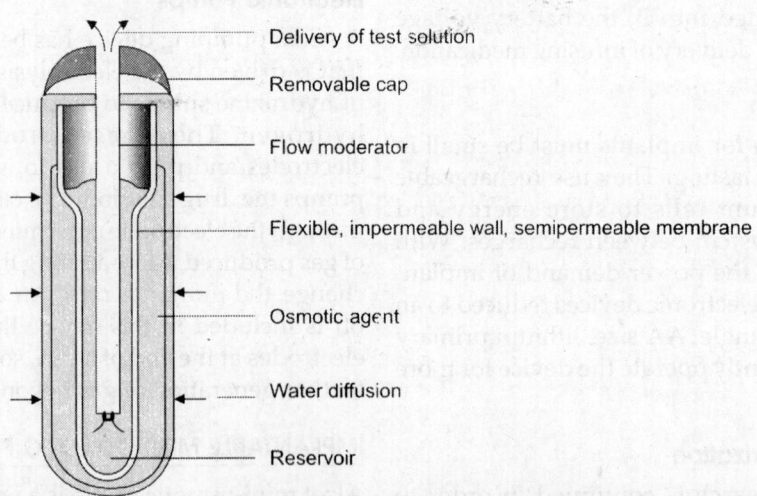

Delivery of test solution

Removable cap

Flow moderator

Flexible, impermeable wall, semipermeable membrane

Osmotic agent

Water diffusion

Reservoir

Fig. 9.5: Alzet miniosmotic pump

glassy polymer. When the devices are placed in the eye, tear fluid begins to penetrate the matrix causing swelling and subsequently polymer chain relaxation, which allows drug diffusion to occur. The dissolution of matrix depends on polymer structure; linear polymers dissolve faster followed by cross-linked or partially crystalline polymers. Release from these devices in general follows Fickian Square root of time kinetics, however in some cases zero order kinetics have been observed. The erodible or E-type devices exhibit controlled release of drug due to chemical or enzymatic hydrolytic reaction that brings about polymer solubilization, or degradation to smaller water-soluble molecules. These systems may display zero-order release kinetics provided the devices maintain a constant surface geometry and the drug is poorly water-soluble.

Antiglaucoma drugs appear to be the most promising class of therapeutic agents that require long-term application for optimal action on receptors and similarly, antimicrobial drugs recommended for short-term use, however require high-drug concentration in treated tissues.

In fact, ophthalmic inserts offer many advantages including increased ocular residence, possibility of releasing drugs at a slow, and constant rate, accurate dosing, exclusion of preservatives and increased shelflife compared to aqueous solutions. Moreover, the use of these devices reduces systemic absorption, which otherwise often occurs freely in case of eyedrops. The ocular systems ensure better patient compliance due to reduced frequency of administration and lower incidences of side effects. It is also possible to target internal ocular tissues through conjunctival sclera routes. These devices can also be employed for incorporating various novel chemical approaches, such as prodrugs, permeation enhancers, mucoadhesives and microparticulates. Ophthalmic inserts suffer from some disadvantages mostly due to their 'solidity', they

are felt as an extraneous body in the eye by patients, and this may contribute to a formidable physical barrier for user compliance and acceptance. Discomfort, movement around the eye, occasional inadvertent loss during sleeps or while rubbing eyes, interference with vision and difficulty in placement are some of the drawbacks associated with ocular inserts.

There are two ocular inserts presently available commercially, soluble ophthalmic drug insert (SODI) and Ocusert®, others like collagen shields, Ocufit, NODS and minidisc are in advanced stages of development.

Soluble Ophthalmic Drug Inserts (SODI)

The SODIs are the modern revival of the gelatin 'lamellae'. The system was developed by collaborative efforts of eminent Russian chemists and ophthalmologists, which eventually led to the development of a new soluble copolymer of acrylamide, N-vinyl pyrrolidone and ethyl acrylate (0.25:0.25:0.5) in 1976, popularly known are ABE.

Large scale preclinical and clinical trials have been conducted on ABE copolymer. The SODIs were then prepared on the industrial scale using this ABE copolymer. The SODIs were then prepared using this ABE copolymer. SODIs prepared were in the form of sterile thin films, oval in shape (9.4 × 4.5 mm, thickness 0.35 mm), weighing 15–16 mg. Insertion of SODI into the upper conjunctival sac, leads to softening in 10–15s and conforming to the shape of the eyeball, followed by formation of a polymer clot within next 10–15 min, which gradually dissolves in next 1 hour with concomitant release of incorporated drug. It was observed that sensation of an extraneous body in the eye vanishes in 2–15 min.

A prolonged release of the drug, has been observed from SODIs. Nevertheless, the ocular tissues serve as drug reservoirs thereby a single SODI application could effectively replace 4–12 times drop instillation or 3–6 applications of ointment This enables SODI to become a valid once-a-day therapy even which may be implicated for long-term treatment of glaucoma.

Ocusert®

In Ocusert® system zero order release is achieved by diffusion of drugs from a reservoir through a rate-controlling membrane over a specific time till the drug reservoir is depleted of drug. The rate-controlling membrane is typically composed of ethylene vinyl acetate, a copolymer that is biocompatible with eye tissues. Ocuserts are available as Pilo-20, Pilo-40. The former delivers the drug at a rate of 20 µg/h for 7 days, whereas the later at a rate of 40 µg/h. OcusertÒ consists of a reservoir containing pilocarpine and alginate sandwitched between two thin ethylene vinyl acetate (EVA) membranes. The insert is encircled by a retaining ring of the same material, impregnated with titanium dioxide. The membranes of both the systems are the same, but to obtain a higher release rate, the reservoir in the case of 40 µg/h system contains about 90 mg of di-(2-ethyl hexyl) phthalate used as a flux enhancer. Patients suffering from glaucoma can place the system loaded with pilocarpine in the cul-de-sac once a weak. They are well retained and tolerated allowing for continuous use without much difficulty. Intraocular pressure is controlled appropriately with minimal side effects. The pilocarpine Ocusert® system thus enables the glaucoma patients to be treated effectively with one-fourth to one-eighth the dose required in the case of eyedrops.

A major advantage is that two disturbing side effects of pilocarpine, i.e miosis and myopia, are reduced to minimum levels, while intraocular pressure (IOP) in glaucoma patients is fully maintained, at the desirable level.

Collagen Shields

Collagen represents a unique class of structural protein and found in bones, tendons, ligaments, and skin. It comprises more than 25% of the total body protein in mammals. Collagen corneal bandages were firstly introduced by Fyidorov et al., (1985) in the shape of a contact lens as an alternative to contact lenses to protect postsurgery corneal epithelium. The corneal shields, currently available for clinical use do not contain drugs and are fabricated to function as disposable, therapeutic corneal bandages.

Collagen inserts have been suggested as tear substitutes and as drug delivery systems for gentamycin. For drug delivery, the sterile packed and dehydrated shields are rehydrated in the aqueous solution of the drug, which lead to absorption of drug by the protein matrix. The drug is delivered once the shield is placed in the eye. Hydrophobic drugs are better candidates to be incorporated into the shields at the time of manufacture. Some novel approaches like incorporation of drug-loaded poly (butyl-cyanoacrylate) nanoparticle and liposomal formulations in collagen shields have also been reported. Delivery of antibiotics, antimicrobials, antifungals, steroids, fibrinolytics, immunosuppressants and antivirals have been attempted using collagen shields. Use of collagen shields produces higher drug concentrations in the cornea and aqueous humor compared to eyedrops and soft contact lenses.

Collagen shields, however suffer from certain drawbacks like the cornea is to be anesthetized and needs the use of forceps by physician to insert the hydrated or unhydrated shields. Collagen shields often produce some discomfort and interference with vision. Due to these constraints collagen shields are mostly limited for their use as a bandage lense and their use as drug delivery systems is still in developing stage. Collasome, a new system consisting of small pieces (1 mm, 2 mm, 0.1 mm) of collagen suspended in a 1% methylcellulose vehicle has been reported to provide high and sustained levels of drugs and lubricants to the cornea as in case of collagen shields, while collagen shield related disadvantages as discussed, are largely resolved and addressed.

Ocufit

The Ocufit SR is a rod-shaped sustained release device made up of silicone elastomer and is designed to fit within the shape and size of the human conjunctival formix. Usually, its size does not exceed 1.9 mm in diameter and 25–30 mm in length. Lacrisert (Merck and Co. Inc.), a cellulosic device is a typical example of rod-shaped insert used to test dry-eye patients (Lambert et al., 1978). Long retention and sustained drug releases are the two important features of the insoluble Ocufit. Placement of timolol loaded cylindrical prolonged-release device in the upper conjunctival sac of rabbits showed an increased corneal and ocular absorption of drug, as compared with application in the inferior conjunctival sac.

Minidisc Ocular Therapeutic System (MOTS)

MOTS is a miniaturized contact lens (diameter 4–5 mm), with a convex and a concave face. This small size and shape allows an easy placement of the device under the upper or lower lid without compromising vision, comfort or oxygen permeability. Minidisc has been reported to require less time and less manual dexterity for insertion compared to Lacrisert. MOTS have been formulated in different versions like nonerodible hydrophilic, non-erodible hydrophobic, and erodible systems.

Hydrophilic MOTS based on polyhydroxy-methyl methacrylate released sulfisoxazole for 118 hours, while hydrophobic system released gentamycin sulfate for more than 320 hours. These devices have been well tolerated, when placed either in the upper or lower conjunctival sac. The erodible MOTS made up of hydroxyl propyl cellulose compares well with the Lacrisert for ease of insertion in eye and comfort.

New Ophthalmic Delivery System (NODS)

A new ophthalmic delivery system NODS delivers precise amount of water soluble drugs into the eye. The device consists of medicated flag (4 mm × 6 mm, thickness 20 µm, weight 0.5 g), which is attached to a paper-covered handle by means of a short (0.7 mm) and thin (3–4 µm) membrane. All components are made of water soluble polyvinyl alcohol (PVA) and the devices are individually packed, sterilized by gamma radiation. The flag is touched onto the surface of the lower conjunctival sac for use followed by dissolution of membrane, which leads to release of flag which swells and dissolves in the lacrimal fluid, delivering the drug. The drawback associated with the system is that it is difficult to achieve slow and predetermined release. NODS have been reported to produce 8-fold higher in bioavailability of pilocarpine as compared to standard eyedrop formulations. In human volunteers improvement in bioavailability of tropicamide and chloramphenicol in NODS as compared to solutions, were also demonstrated. NODS are well tolerated, easy to use, and convenient.

EVALUATION OF IMPLANTABLE POLYMERIC MATERIALS

Newer drug delivery devices and materials are continually being developed for various biomedical applications. Initially, the basis of selection of materials had been for biological applications, their physical properties, biological activity, and biological acceptance (biocompatibility) of the material were not taken into account. Plastic containers were used frequently with a convention that these are quite inert against harsh acid and base treatments. However, studies indicated that plastics adversely affect the biological milieu. The adverse effects include thrombogenicity, cellular necrosis, carcinogenicity, etc. Numerous clinical reports and continuous studies indicating adverse reactions from plastic materials, have created concern as to whether or not the patient does feel better from use of the device than without use of the device. However, nowadays emphasis is being placed on the fact that patient should receive maximum benefit from use of the device, while being exposed to minimum risks or disadvantages.

Acute Toxicity Evaluations

Acute biological incompatibilities mostly arise due to presence of biologically active leachable substances in the medical material. The most common short-term response of the tissues to an implanted material is its encapsulation by fibrous tissue within few weeks.

A leachable is a substance or component in the biomedical material or device, which may migrate (diffuse) from the material/device to the surrounding medium. The medium may be tissue fluids surrounding the implanted device, blood stored in a blood bag, therapeutic preparations with their solvent given by solution administration set etc. Leachables may be divided into two main categories, intentional or unintentional. Intentional additives include those substances which are incorporated into the formulation to provide some specific characteristics to the device like, plasticizers, radiopaque materials, UV absorbers, fillers, colorants, stabilizers, antioxidants etc. Unintentional leachables are introduced into the material in a number of ways during its manufacturing, fabrication, sterilization, etc. Some examples of unintentional incorporation of leachables include contaminated starting materials used for polymer synthesis, unreacted monomers, contaminants from processing equipment, adhesive or sealants etc.

Tests for Biological Compatibility

Acute tests mostly evaluate a material for biocompatibility with respect to the presence of biologically active leachables. The biological activity, which is observed in most of these tests, represents the combination of the concentration of the substance that reaches the target cells and the intrinsic activity of the substance upon these cells.

Acute safety evaluation of biomedical devices can be made by using or applying a number of biological tests. Biomedical devices made up of two or more polymers or multiple parts may be evaluated as an intact unit by some tests using extracts of the device. Acute safety tests can either be conducted directly upon the material, perse or performed on the extracts (elutes) of the material or device.

Rabbit Muscle Implant

This is a simple test conducted for short term compatibility of a biomedical material with living tissues. The test, when supported by careful histopathological examination of adjacent tissue, provides considerable information regarding biocompatibility of the material/device.

Healthy New Zealand albino rabbits of either sex are lightly anesthetized by slowly injecting 25 mg/kg of pentobarbital sodium intravenously via ear marginal vein. One negative control, one positive control and two test samples are inserted through the skin (at 90° to the surface) and into the paravertebral muscles to a sufficient depth. 7 days after implantation, the rabbit is sacrificed by an overdose of pentobarbital sodium intravenously and implant site along with adjacent tissues are examined and appropriately scored for the severity of response. This test primarily detects histopathological abnormalities of the muscle tissue adjacent to the implanted sample and adds to the sensitivity of the test.

Agar Overlay Cell Culture

This is a relatively inexpensive and rapid test used to detect the presence of leachable cytotoxic substances in a material/device. This test can be conducted to assess the cytotoxicity of almost any compound, which is capable of diffusing through the agar layer. In this test, a 24-hour confluent monolayer of mouse fibroblast cells (L cells) is grown on Eagle's medium in petri dishes. The nutrient medium is replaced with agar composed of equal part of double strength Eagle's medium and 3% agar, cells are pink stained with a neutral red stain, and four samples, one negative control, one positive control and two test samples are placed on the agar. The petri dishes are incubated at 37°C for 24 hours in an atmosphere of 5% CO_2 and 95% air. After 24 hours each site is examined for cytotoxic activity. A clear zone with loss of pink color produced by cytotoxic reaction around the 'toxic' sample which 'nontoxic' sample gives a pinkish, translucent appearance around.

A semiquantitative scoring system was developed for primary acute toxicity screening in which size of the clear zone (zone index) and degree of lysis within the zone (lysis index) were observed and combined to get response index.

This basic test has shown good correlation with the rabbit muscle implant test, moreover the test is somewhat more sensitive compared to muscle implant test. In addition to these tests, many other tests are performed on the extracts of materials like cell culture test, intradermal irritation, systemic toxicity, isolated perfuse heart and sensitivity testing. However, whether the biological activity shown at the levels present would be toxic, beneficial or without any therapeutic effect to the patient is not answered directly by these tests. Nevertheless, positive test indicates the presence of toxicologically active substance.

Evaluations of Chronic Toxicity

Biomaterials or devices may release leachables, which elicit a mild, temporary effect or may produce irreversible damage to the organs or tissues and their prolonged release may lead to progressive organic damage. This suggests that some acute subtle effects may become quite apparent in chronic studies. Polymeric material in contact with living tissues and biological fluids for long term may result in bidegradation. Long-term implantation of solid materials also raises other potential problems of carcinogenesis. Some investigators have suggested that biodegradation of a polymer produces free radical species which may be carcinogens, however no data available indicating that the degradation products produce significant adverse effects in man and animals, except for those resulting from mechanical failure of the device and subsequent dose dumping.

Some studies conducted in 1940s reported that local sarcomas were developed when bakelite disks were implanted subcutaneously in rats. Tumors of this etiology were called material induced cancers, solid-state cancers, foreign body cancers, and smooth-surface cancers. The risk of solid tumor formation can be reduced by selection of appropriate materials and/or devices. The true risk of material induced tumors is still unknown in case of human beings. Estimates made from published reports and from surveys of certain groups of patients suggest that the incidences of material associated tumors are quite small in human beings. Until, more accurate data are available on long term use of implants in human, it would be worthwhile to limit such implants to the situation of decided therapeutic benefit.

THERAPEUTIC APPLICATIONS OF IMPLANTS AND INSERTS

Ocusert®

A truly continuous, controlled and zero order release kinetic was achieved using Ocusert®. First marketed by Alza Corporation California, the pilocarpine Ocuserts improved the noncompliance, low intraocular drug bioavailability and potential systemic side effects of pilocarpine. The system consists of a pilocarpine-alginate core (drug) sandwiched between two transparent, rate-controlling ethylene-vinyl acetate copolymer based thin membranes. When this is placed under the upper or lower eyelid, the pilocarpine molecules after getting dissolved in the lacrimal fluid are released through the rate-controlling membranes at a preprogrammed defined rate.

A mixture of pilocarpine and alginic acid in the drug reservoir releases the drug for almost one week. A thin membrane of ethylene-vinyl acetate (EVA) copolymer encloses the reservoir from above and below. A retaining ring of the same material impregnated with titanium dioxide encloses the drug reservoir circumferentially (Fig. 9.6). The

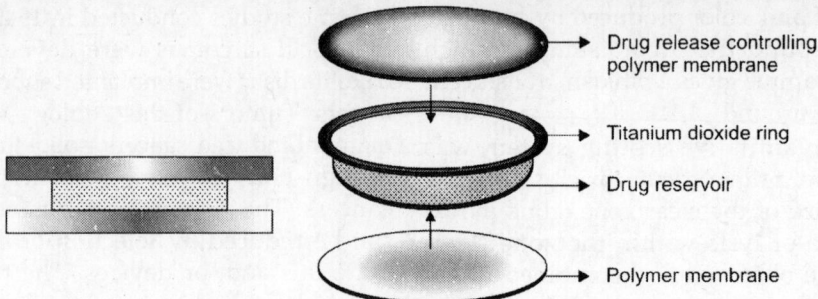

Drug release controlling polymer membrane

Titanium dioxide ring

Drug reservoir

Polymer membrane

Fig. 9.6: Schematic representation of Ocusert®

typical dimensions of the elliptical devise are—major axis, 13.4 mm, minmor axis, 5.7 mm, thickness, 0.3 mm. Two types of Ocusert® are available, Ocusert® Pilo-20 and Ocusert® Pilo-40. The Ocusert® Pilo-20 can release pilocarpine at a rate of 20 g/hr for 7 days (total amount of drug released, 3.4 mg) and Ocusert® Pilo-40 at a rate of 40 g/hr for 7 days (total amount of drug released, 6.7 mg). Ocusert® Pilo-20 contains 5.0 mg drug and Ocusert® Pilo-40, 11.0 mg of drug to maintain a constant release rate from the drug reservoir. Ocusert® Pilo-40 contains about 90 g of di-(2-ethylhexyl) phthalate as flux enhancer to maintain the higher release rate (40 g/hr).

Osmotic Pumps

Osmotic pumps are controlled drug delivery devices based on the principle of osmosis. Wide spectrums of osmotic devices are available, out of them osmotic pumps are unique, dynamic and widely employed in clinical practice. Osmosis is a universal bio-phenomenon, which is exploited for development of delivery systems with every desirable property of an ideal controlled drug delivery system. Osmotic pumps offer many advantages like they are easy to formulate and simple in operation, improved patient compliance with reduced dosing frequency, more consistent and prolonged therapeutic effect is obtained with uniform blood concentration. Further more, they are inexpensive and their industrial adaptability vis-a-vis production scale up is easy.

An elementary osmotic pump developed by Alza is OROS, for controlled release oral drug delivery formulations. The elementary osmotic pumps essentially contain an active agent having suitable osmotic pressure, compressed into a tablet, coated with a semi-permeable membrane usually of cellulose acetate. A small orifice is drilled through the coating by using LASER or a high-speed mechanical drill (Fig. 9.7). In fact, this system represents a coated tablet with an aperture. When exposed to an aqueous environment, the osmotic pressure of the soluble drug within the tablet draws water through the semipermeable coating, resulting in the formation of a saturated aqueous drug solution within the device. The membrane is non-extensible. Therefore, an increase in volume due to imbibitions of water raises inner hydrostatic pressure, eventually leading to flow of saturated solution of active agent out of the device through small orifice. Solubility of drug in water plays a critical role in the functioning of an osmotic pump. Ideally the solubility of drug delivered by these pumps should be at least 10 to 15% w/v.

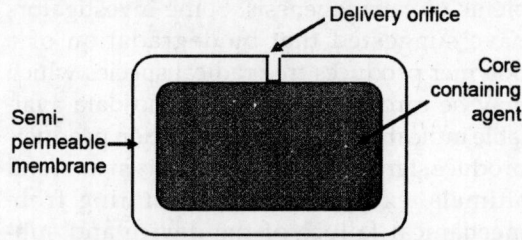

Delivery orifice

Core containing agent

Semi-permeable membrane

Fig. 9.7: An elementary osmotic pump

The choice of a rate-controlling membrane is an important determinant in the formulation development of oral osmotic systems. Since the membrane in osmotic systems is semi-permeable in nature, any polymer that is permeable to water but impermeable to solute can be selected. Some of the polymers that can be used include cellulose esters such as cellulose acetate, cellulose diacetate, cellulose triacetate, cellulose propionate, cellulose acetate butyrate, etc. cellulose ethers like ethyl cellulose and eudragits. Cellulose acetate is a commonly employed semipermeable polymer used in the preparation of osmotic pumps. It is available with different acetyl content grades. In general, the acetyl contents 32% and 38% are widely used. Cellulose acetate is having degree of substitution (DS), i.e. the average number of hydroxyl groups on the anhydro-glucose unit of the polymer replaced by substituting group. If it is up to 1, the acetyl content up to 21%. Cellulose diacetate is having a DS of 1–2 and an acetyl content of 21–35%. Cellulose triacetate has a DS of 2–3 and an acetyl content of 35–44.8%.

Apart from cellulose derivatives, some other polymers, such as agar acetate, amylose triacetate, betaglucan acetate, poly-(vinyl methyl)-ether copolymers, poly (orthoesters), polyacetals and selectively permeable poly-(glycolic acid) and poly-(lactic acid) derivatives can be used as semipermeable film forming materials. The permeability is the important criteria for the selection of semi-permeable polymers.

Second type of osmotic device is a small osmotic pump sold under the trade name Alzet® (Alza Corporation) that is implanted in the tissue of animals, where it delivers a chosen therapeutic agent at predetermined rate. The active agent is placed in an impermeable flexible walled reservoir that is surrounded and sealed within a rigid cellulose acetate membrane. When device comes in contact with an aqueous environment, water is osmotically driven across the cellulose acetate membrane and the resultant pressure on the reservoir wall forces the agent out of the orifice (Fig. 9.8).

Intrauterine Devices (IUDs)

Intrauterine devices belong to novel therapeutics commonly used for the delivery of contraceptive steroidal hormones. Medicated IUDs are those that serve as carriers or vehicles for pharmacologically effective antifertility agents, such as the copper-bearing IUD and the progesterone-releasing IUD. The advantages of these delivery systems include prolonged drug release, minimum side effects and increased bioavailability. Copper and other metals such as zinc, cadmium, lead etc., have been reported to enhance the contraceptive effectiveness of an IUD. Zipper and his

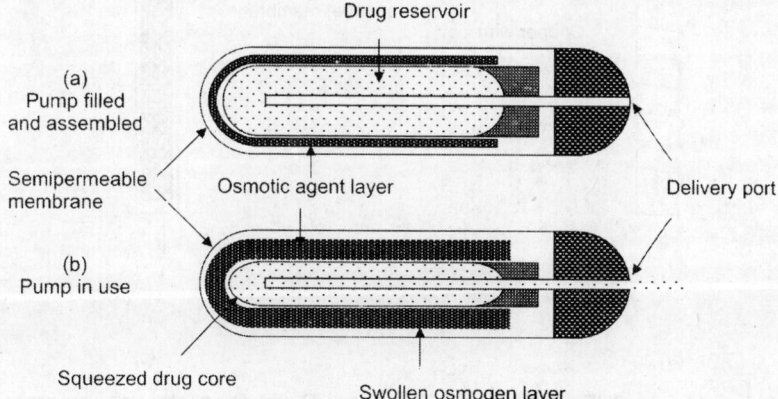

Fig. 9.8: Alza mini-osmotic pump (Alzet®)

associates in 1969, were first to conduct clinical studies on a T-shaped polyethylene plastic device with 30 mm^2 of copper wire (CU T-30) (Fig. 9.9a). The pregnancy rate was declined as low as up to 5% as compared to the 18% level as achieved with nonmedicated T-shaped device. It has been reported that the copper-bearing IUD is more efficacious when the copper wire is located on the transverse arms of the device, which remain in contact with the fundus after insertion. This facts led to the development of new generation of copper bearing-T-shaped IUDs, CU-T 380A having two sleeves of copper located on the transverse arms resembling the letter 'T'. The additional surface area of 30 mm^2 and relatively small surface area of copper (2 × 30 mm^2) comes in close contact with the upper portion of the endometrial cavity resulting into significantly enhanced antifertility efficacy of copper-bearing IUD.

In progesterone-releasing device (Progestasert® IUD), the drug reservoir exists as a dispersion of progesterone crystals in silicone (medical grade) fluid encapsulated in the vertical limb of a T-shaped device walled by a nonporous membrane of ethylene-vinyl acetate copolymer (Fig. 9.9 b).

Contraceptive Implants

Contraceptive implants work in a similar way to contraceptive pills. They contain one of the hormones of contraceptive pills. This hormone prevents pregnancy. But instead of being in a pill, this hormone is contained in a small, thin flexible rod. It is 4 cm long and made of plastic. It is inserted just under the skin on the inside of a woman's arm.

The implant steadily releases a small amount of hormone. This prevents pregnancy for 3 years. The implant must be removed at the end of 3 years. However, it can be taken out at any time by a doctor familiar with the removal technique.

The implant prevents pregnancy by either of two mechanisms: (1) stopping a woman's ovaries from making an egg each month, (2) thickening the mucus that women have in their cervix (entrance to the womb). This makes it hard for sperm to get through and fertilise an egg. The contraceptive implant is more than 99% effective in preventing pregnancy.

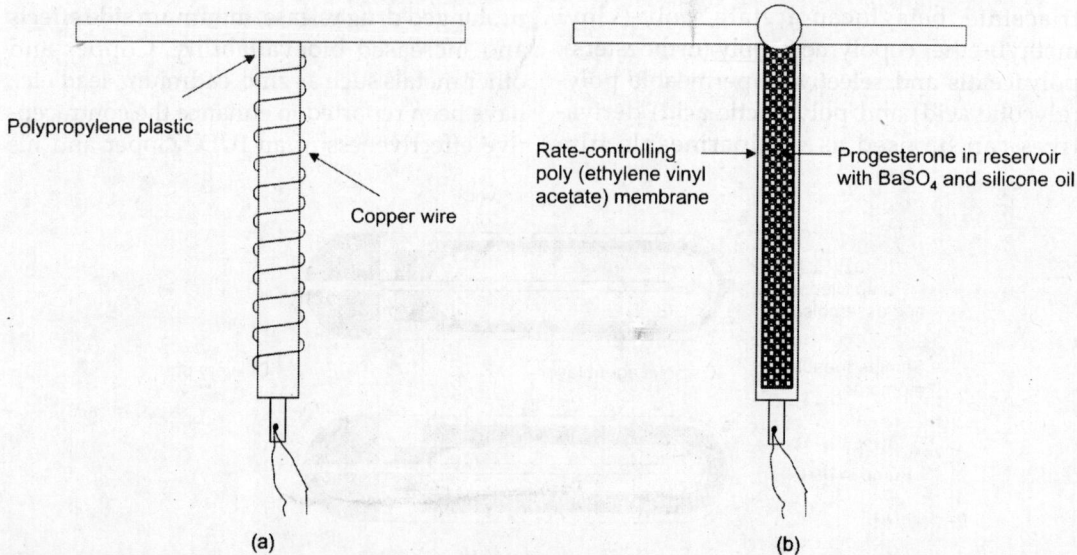

Polypropylene plastic

Copper wire

Rate-controlling poly (ethylene vinyl acetate) membrane

Progesterone in reservoir with BaSO$_4$ and silicone oil

(a)

(b)

Fig. 9.9: Intrauterine devices (IUDs)—(a) copper-bearing IUD, (b) Progestasert®, progesterone-releasing IUD

Advantages

- Effective contraception for 3 years. It comes in the form of a small stick of the size of a matchstick, which, once inserted under the skin diffuses progestin.
- Excellent efficiency: 99%.
- Tolerance is good and the side effects are not systematic. They usually disappear over a few months after administration or implantation.
- One has not to remember to use contraception every day.
- Doesn't interfere with sexual intercourse.
- Does not contain estrogen, indeed, the implant contains a progestin—only reservoir, like a conventional pill, blocks ovulation and changes the cervical mucus to oppose the progress of sperm.
- The effect is immediate, within 24 hours after installation.
- As with other contraceptive methods, the retrieval of fertility is rapid after removal of the implant. Hormone levels return to their normal values in less than a week.
- Low cost.

Disadvantages

- Women using implants encountered changes in their periods.
- Most women have less bleeding than before the implant, but some have more frequent or longer periods.
- Some women have side effects that may include headache and acne.
- Doesn't protect against sexually transmitted infections, HIV/AIDS or hepatitis B.

Subcutaneous Implants

Nondegradable subcutaneous implants are essentially diffusion-controlled drug delivery systems, including Norplant. Unlike, biodegradable implants with long-term toxicological concern for metabolism of the polymer, nondegradable implants cannot avoid removal of the system after use. Norplant, a female contraceptive implant, contains a set of six flexible closed capsules of levonorgestrel and uses silastic as the rate-controlling membrane. The capsules are inserted by a physician beneath the skin and removed at the end of 5-year therapy period. Clinical studies have shown plasma concentrations of 0.30 ng/ml over 5 years, but are highly variable as a function of individual metabolism and body weight. The typical failure rate with this implant in the first year is only 0.2% compared with 3% in case of oral contraceptives. Another synthetic female contraceptive subcutaneous implant is under development (Akzo Nobel). It would release 40 mg/day etonogestrel. A subcutaneous silicone implant of norgestomet has been evaluated in synchronizing estrus and diagnosing pregnancy in ewes, permitting the diagnosis of pregnancy status with 100% accuracy with no adverse effects on established pregnancy.

The element of targeting or site-specific delivery is often linked with novel-controlled released systems. For example, as fused with a lipoid carrier or encapsulated in microcapsules or in silastic capsules, breast implants of antiestrogens and prostatic implants of androgen-suppressive drugs render a constant slow release of drugs to the target tumor tissue for extended periods and minimize systemic toxicity. There are various approaches that could be used to regulate the growth factor released from polymer scaffolds in tissue engineering as well as in cell transplantation. Diffusion-controlled DNA delivery from implantable EVAc matrices is useful for DNA vaccination and gene therapy. However, these fields are in their initial developing stage and need specific problems identified for them to be developed.

INTRA-ARTERIAL CATHETER INFUSION DRUG DELIVERY SYSTEM

To deliver the drug to the target sites, such as cancer tissue blood vessels, infusion pumps have been developed. The intra-arterial infusion pumps deliver the drug with a specific flow rate by means of a catheter. A catheter based system should be devoid of any possibility of thrombosis. It should infuse the therapeutic agent into the specific sites with maximum response and minimum toxicity.

Type of Catheters

Needle Injection Catheter

This V shape is made with 6 circumferential needles, which were used to infuse the drug into vascular walls and adventitia. All 6 outer needles (250 mm) positioned symmetrically. Flexible polyethylene was used to make this device with a center lumen for a guide wire. The needles are advanced by a mechanism provided at the external level of the catheter, when it is placed on the vascular lumen. Thus, the needles were extended proximally, so that they encompass a diameter of 5.5 mm. The needles are shaped with a cover at the end, hence they can penetrate laterally into the media or perivascular area. Drug delivery into the adventitia creates a depot, which may provide a prolonged therapeutic action.

Microcatheter

This is a small sized catheter made up of shafts of different thickness with a flexible supply distal extremity. The external diameter is 0.5–0.85 mm. To increase the opacity under fluoroscopy, a gold or platinum ring is inserted in the tip. They employ sterilizable micro guide wire for torque advancement by which the sixth division branches of arteries can be accessed and reached. They have narrow distal aperture, hence only liquids or particles of diameter less than 300 μm can be infused. Flow of nonspherical particles is, however difficult to control.

Helical Catheter

They are devised for local delivery of endo-vascular drugs by placing near to the vessel wall proximal to the diseased area, such as thrombosis or vascular lesion. Markou et al.

(1998) made these devices by using poly-ethylene tubing of an outer diameter of 0.356 mm and internal diameter of 0.203 mm. The catheter end shaped helix, used to make contact with vessel wall. The coils of catheter are laser drilled to form many small holes for drug infusion to be affected. Due to small holes, drug infusion lies in solely moving layers of blood near the wall.

Porous Balloon Catheters

To infuse drug with high pressure, the balloon catheters have been developed with pores. Gonchior and Clemens (1995) made a catheter designed with 35 perforations, which are arranged radially around the circumferance and along the length of the balloon catheter.

They can withstand the hydraulic pressure from 6–10 atm, which is needed to inflate the balloon and to develop outward flow of drug solution through the pores. Another design involved a porous balloon that functions or operates through mechanical expansion before the infusion of drugs. The balloon contains 50 holes with a diameter of 75 mm and covers a graded cure cage. The operator enlarges the mechanical cage and expands the balloon against the vascular wall by using a rotation knob without infusing the drug. Direct infusion of the drug is achieved (with infusion pressure of 6 atm), following the mechanical inflation (Figs 9.10 and 9.11).

Implantable Drug Delivery Pump

These pumps have been used for the hepatic arterial chemotherapy. This pump employs a small flexible silastic catheter of 0.92 inch in

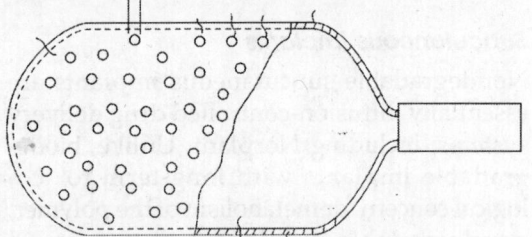

Fig. 9.10: Porous balloon catheter

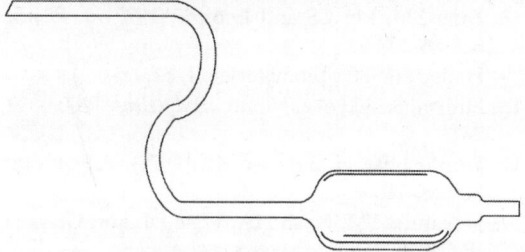

Fig. 9.11: Balloon catheter having metal balloon

diameter and is implanted to infuse the entire liver arterial vasculature. One end of the catheter is connected to a subcutaneous Infusaid pump (Buchwald and Grage, 1980). Pump consisted of a side port with an auxiliary system. It is disc shaped and separated into two chambers, where inner chamber contains the drug solution and outer charging chamber contains a chlorocarbon liquid in equilibrium to produce a vapor pressure. The exerted vapor pressure on bellows forces the drug solution via a flow regulator. Pump volume and flow rate is 50 ml, 3–6 ml per day respectively.

Pump can be refilled every 8–16 days through a side port with the help of a percutaneous injection.

Problems in the use of catheters are as follows:

- Patient inconvenience
- Incidence of bleeding, catheter thrombosis or infection
- Other problems such as clotting ,leaking, dislodgment, septicemia or hemorrhage and fever
- Need of more number of personals for maintenance

PRESENT STATUS AND FUTURE PROSPECTS

The implantable system represents versatile devices especially well suited for long-term delivery of drugs. Table 9.2 enlists the patents. Steroidal contraceptive agents are delivered as subdermal implants for drug delivery at an optimum rate and concentration. Implantable systems effectively prevent pregnancy by delivering the agent at predetermined rate and by simulating the condition and hormonal status during menstrual cycle. Implantable infusion pumps are especially well suited for long-term delivery of drug in application in which drug activity is enhanced by delivery of drug(s) directly into intravenous, intra-arterial, intrathecal, subdural,

Patent no.	Year	Original assignee/inventor	Title
Table 9.2: List of some of the patents related to various implants and inserts			
US7232423	Jun 19, 2007	M2 Medical A/S	Infusion pump system, an infusion pump unit and an infusion pump
US7374556	May 20, 2008	Tandem Diabetes Care	Infusion pump and method for use
US7699834	Apr 20, 2010	Searete LLC	Method and system for control of osmotic pump device
US7933780	Apr 26, 2011	Telaric, LLC	Method and apparatus for controlling an infusion pump or the like
US8137083	Mar 20, 2012	Baxter International Inc.	Infusion pump actuators, system and Baxter Healthcare S.A. method for controlling medical fluid flow rate
US8206736	Jun 26, 2012	Allergan Inc.	Hypotensive lipid-containing biodegradable intraocular implants and related methods
US8147865	Apr 3, 2012	Allergan Inc.	Steroid-containing sustained release intraocular implants and related methods
US8119154	Feb 21, 2012	Allergan Inc.	Sustained release intraocular implants and related methods

intraventricular, intraperitonial or other body location with minimal risk of infection—an interference with the patient's life. This system provides a means of accurately delivering therapeutic agents across the blood brain barrier, vis-a-vis the successful treatment of disease. PIMS allow a precise medication rate and enhanced patient's compliance.

Next generation of PIMS is the sensor actuated medication system (SAMS) a macro-computer controls close loop system by which a physiological parameter like increase in blood glucose or blood pressure is sensed and drug(s) are installed into the IPIP.

Many diseases like glaucoma or any infection associated with ophthalmic cavity need localized treatment with pilocarpine and other antibiotics. The problem associated with conventional ocular doses forms have been obviated by Ocusert® system. With emerging improvement in design, construction and advancement in bioerodible polymer technology, significant changes in the use of devices for ocular drug delivery are expected to come into effect. Implantable drug delivery devices are versatile in nature and have wide spectrum of applications with large potential in immediate future.

SUGGESTED READINGS

1. Ariel IM (1965), *Cancer* 18, 1489.
2. Baker RW and Lonsdale HK (1974), In: Controlled release of biologically active agents, A tanquary and RE Lacey (Eds), Pleum, New York, 15.
3. Bawa R (1993), In: Ophthalmic Drug delivery Systems, AK Mitra (Ed.), Marcel Dekker, New York, 223.
4. Clark BF (1973), *J. Endocrinol.* 58, 555.
5. Cyril Desevaux, Vincent Lenaerts, Christiane Girard, Pascal Dubreuil Journal of Controlled Release (2002), 82, 95.
6. Dash AK and Cudworth II GC (1998), *J Pharmacol Toxicol Methods* 40, 1.
7. Duncan GW (1970), US Patent 3, 545, 439.
8. Fang SM, Lin CS and Lyon V (1977), *J. Pharm. Sci.* 66, 1744.
9. Heller J (1980), Biomaterials 1, 51.
10. Hitoshi Sasaki et al *J. Controlled Release* (2003), 92, 241.
11. Hopfenberg H and Hsu KC (1978), *Polym. Eng. Sci.* 18, 1186.
12. Jackanicz TM, Nash HA, Wise DL and Gregory JB (1973), *Contraception* 8, 227.
13. Kelly J, Molyneux PD, Smith SA and Smith SE (1989), *Br. J. Ophthalmol* 7, 360.
14. Loewit K (1971), *Contraception* 3, 219.
15. Maichuk YF (1976), In: Ocular Therapy, IH Leopold (Ed)., Wiley, New York, 1.
16. Markou CP, Brown JE, Puresley MD and Hanson SP (1998), *J. Control. Rel.* 53, 281.
17. G Legendre Fertil Steril 94 (2010), pp. 2732–2735.
18. F Pachy J Gynecol Obstet Biol Reprod (Paris), 38 (2009), pp. 321–7.
19. Galen J Minim Invasive Gynecol, 18 (2011), pp. 338–42.
20. RB Rosenfield Fertil Steril, 83 (2005), pp. 1547–1550
21. PA Campochiaro, G Hafiz, SM Shah. Ophthalmology, 117 (2010), pp. 1393–9.
22. PA Pearson, TL Comstock, M Ophthalmology, 118 (2011), pp. 1580–87.
23. VHL Lee, *J. Ocul. Pharmacol.*, 6 (1990), pp. 157–64.
24. R Bawa AK Mitra (Ed.), Ophthalmic Drug Delivery Systems, Marcel Dekker, New York (1993), pp. 223–59.
25. Sershen S and West J (2002), *Adv. Drug Deliv. Rev.* 54, 1225.
26. Tatum HJ (1970), US Patent 3, 533, 406.
27. Zaffaroni A (1974), US Patent 3, 854, 480.
28. SM Kurtz, CM Rimnac, WJ Hozack et al. J Bone Joint Surg Am, 87A (2005), pp. 815.
29. JF Kerin Hum Reprod, 18 (2003), pp. 1223–1230.
30. YW Chien Novel Drug Delivery Systems, Marcel Dekker, New York (1982), pp. 13–50 Ch. 2.
31. L Salminen MF Saettone, G Bucci, P Speiser (Eds.), Ophthalmic Drug Delivery: Biopharmaceutical, Technological and Clinical Aspects, Fidia Research Series (2nd ed.), Vol. 11, Liviana Press, Padua (1987), pp. 161–70.
32. YF Maichuk. Invest. Ophthalmol., 14 (1975), pp. 87–90.
33. YF Maichuk Lancet I (1975), pp. 173.

10
■ Micellar Systems

INTRODUCTION

Colloidal carriers are frequently used to transport and deliver drugs through the body for the reason of protecting the drug against degradation and/or excretion, to prevent adverse side effects of toxic drugs, or to accomplish targeted drug delivery. Examples of such carriers are micro/nanospheres, polymer-drug conjugates, liposomes, and micelles. After micelles were first proposed as drug carriers by Ringsdorf in 1984, they have been emerged as a convenient carrier system.

A notable feature of surfactant is their ability to self-associate to form micelles. Since micelles consist of surfactant molecules packing in a space-filling manner, numerous parameters of the surfactant solution change at the critical micellization concentration (CMC). The main driving force for micelle formation in aqueous solution is the effective interaction (cohesive binding) between the hydrophobic parts of the surfactant molecules, whereas interaction opposing micellization may include electrostatic repulsive interaction between charged head groups of ionic surfactants, repulsive osmotic interactions between chainlike polar head groups, such as oligoethylene oxide chains, or steric interaction between bulky head groups. In aqueous solution, surfactants aggregate in different

forms, such as spherical micelles, wormlike micelle, bilayer fragments, vesicles, or inverted structures. The way surfactant molecules aggregate is mainly determined by the attraction between the hydrophobic tails and electrostatic repulsions of the hydrophilic head groups, which are present in the surfactant molecules.

The type of aggregated surfactant can be determined by the packing parameter P as in the following equation:

$$P = \frac{V}{a_o l}$$

in which V is the volume of the hydrocarbon part of the surfactant, l is the chain length of alkyl tail, and a_o is the mean cross-sectional head group surface area. A value of P smaller than $1/3$ is indicative of the formation of micelles; P between $1/3$ and $1/2$ indicates the formation of wormlike micelles, whereas surfactants with P between $1/2$ and 1 form vesicles. Inverted structures are formed when P is larger than 1 (see Table 10.1). Recently, micelles have attracted the attention of researchers as drug delivery systems, because of their nanoscopic size, ability to solubilize hydrophobic drugs and site-specific delivery by passive and active targeting. Amphiphilic block copolymers with biodegradable and/or biocompatible chains have been used to

Table 10.1: The different types of surfactant aggregation with relation to their shapes

Effective molecule	Shape of the surfactant	Parameter	Packing aggregation	Types of schematic structure
	Cone	<1/3	Spherical micelles	
	Truncated cone	1/3–1/2	Wormlike micelles	
	Cylinder	1/2–1	Bilayers, vesicles	
	Inverted (truncated) cone	> 1	Inverted micelles	

incorporate hydrophobic drugs and target them to their sites of action upon parenteral administration. Block copolymers, which have both hydrophilic and hydrophobic polymer chains in a molecule form micelles, in water, with hydrophilic chains outside and hydrophobic chains inside. The micelles are excellent drug carriers, because they can hold drugs firmly in their inner cores and control the drug release by changing the molecular structure of the inner cores. Protein antigens are mixed with detergent and the detergent slowly removed by dialysis. The antigenic proteins orient with the hydrophilic residues facing outside and the hydrophobic residues inward. Since polyethyleneglycol (PEG) is used for the hydrophilic chains, the immune system does not recognize the micelles as foreign materials. The micelles also have an enhanced permeability and retention effect, useful for tumor targeting. Micelles are also used as nonviral carrier system for gene delivery. Polyethylene glycol-poly-aspartic acid as anion block copolymer mixed with polyethylene glycol-poly L-lysine (PEG-PLL) as cation block copolymer generates PIC with a diameter of nanometers with a sharp size distribution. Micelles (80 nm in diameter) were formed with plasmid DNA and PEG-PLL. Higher expression of luciferase in cultured cells was obtained with the micelles, compared with conventional. Although, pH-sensitive micelles may be advantageous for oral drug delivery as they can prevent burst drug release and precipitation upon dilution in the upper part of gastrointestinal tract. Upon oral administration, these drug-loaded self-assemblies will remain in the aggregated form at low pH of stomach reducing the drug release. This may benefit the oral bioavailability of incorporated drug by enhancing its transport across the gut wall into the systemic circulation. Moreover, such micelles are advantageous over conventional nanoparticles because of the possibility of forming drug-loaded self-assemblies with an amphiphilic diblock copolymer as sole excipient. Thus, it is of interest to explore the potential of pH-sensitive micelles for improving oral bioavailability of poorly water-soluble drugs.

FORMATION OF MICELLES

At very low concentration (e.g. 10–4 M) many surfactants are soluble in water, forming solutions; if they are ionic, like fatty acid soaps or alkyl sulfate detergents, they will be dissociated as weak or strong electrolytes. As the concentration increases, the adsorption at the air in solution interface becomes stronger. Saturation is reached when the molecules are packed close together, with strong lateral interactions occurring between the hydrophobic chains, which tend to stick up cohesively [*see* Figs 10.1 (a) and (b)]. When the concentration of surfactant solute in the bulk of solution exceeds a limiting value, the formation of micelles begins, globular or spherical structures, which are, organized aggregates of a large number of molecules.

In the micelle, the hydrocarbon tails of the surfactant molecules align to orient toward the center of the sphere and the polar heads towards the water at its surface. The minimum concentration at which micelles formation begins in the solution is referred as critical micellization concentration or CMC. Micelle size is expressed as the micellar molecular weight or, more generally, as the aggregation number, i.e. the number of monomers making up the micelles. Generally, this number is between 20 and 100 for single-chain anionic and cationic surfactants. Large aggregation numbers (>1000) have been reported for non-ionic micelles, especially near the cloud point. In these structures the hydrophobic portions of the surfactant molecule associate to form regions from which the solvent (water) is effectively excluded. The hydrophilic head groups remain on the outer surface to favor and maximize their interaction with water and, in the case of ionic amphiphiles, with the oppositely charged ions (counterions). A significant fraction of the counterions remains strongly bound to the head groups, so that the lateral repulsive force between those groups is greatly reduced. The precise structure of the micelle depends upon the temperature and concentration, but also on the molecular structure, i.e. the size of head group, the length and number of hydrocarbon chains, the presence of branches, double bounds or aromatic rings etc., are some of the factors that determine the shape of a micelle. Increasing the concentration of the surfactant leads to the formation of wormlike micelles and, subsequently, liquid crystals.

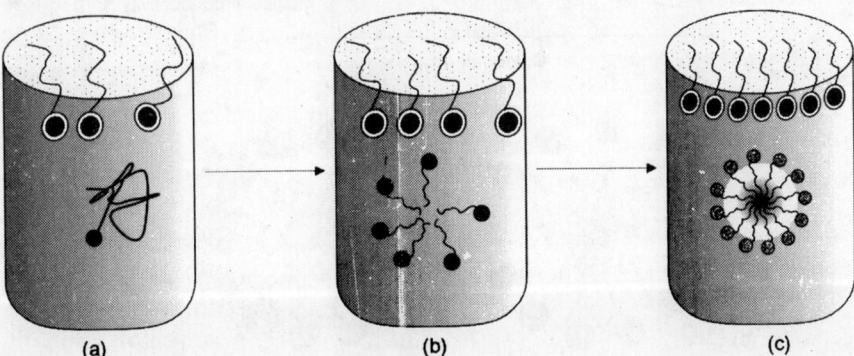

(a)　　　　　　(b)　　　　　　(c)

Fig. 10.1: Formation of micelles—(a) amphiphilic molecules at low concentration, (b) amphiphile at higher concentration ≤ critical miceller concentration (CMC), (c) aggregated amphiphiles at above CMC

CRITICAL MICELLAR CONCENTRATION (CMC)

The CMC is the concentration at which micelles first appear in the solution. Below this critical value, additional surfactant molecules added to the solution remain in monomeric form, and above this, essentially all additional surfactant form micelles. This transition from premicellar to micellar solution at the CMC occurs over a narrow concentration range. Surfactant solutions exhibit a striking characteristic, when quantitative data of their physical properties are plotted against concentration. Each curve shows a break, an inflection, occurring within a narrow concentration range. Among the properties that have been employed to determine the CMC are surface tension, optical turbidity, electric conductivity, osmotic coefficient, density, sound velocity, diffusion, viscosity, solubilization, and NMR chemical shifts. Usually, a selected property is plotted against amphiphile concentration; the functions are

selected so that the graph resembles as close as possible to a pair of straight lines, whose intersection can be taken as the CMC. The cmc can be used quantitatively as well as qualitatively to determine the average molecular weight and the net charge (if the amphipathic species are ionic) of the micelle.

Factors that affect the CMC are the nature of the hydrophilic group and of the counterion, the presence of organic molecules, and the effect of temperature and pressure (Fig. 10.2).

A low CMC indicates that it is thermodynamically favorable for the hydrophobic domain of the surfactant molecule to leave the aqueous solution, which will result in both an excess concentration at the interface and the formation of micelles. This ability to adsorb at an interface and reduce interfacial tension is of great importance for many processes of technological interest, such as emulsification, foaming, wetting, solubilization, detergency, particle suspensions, and surface coatings.

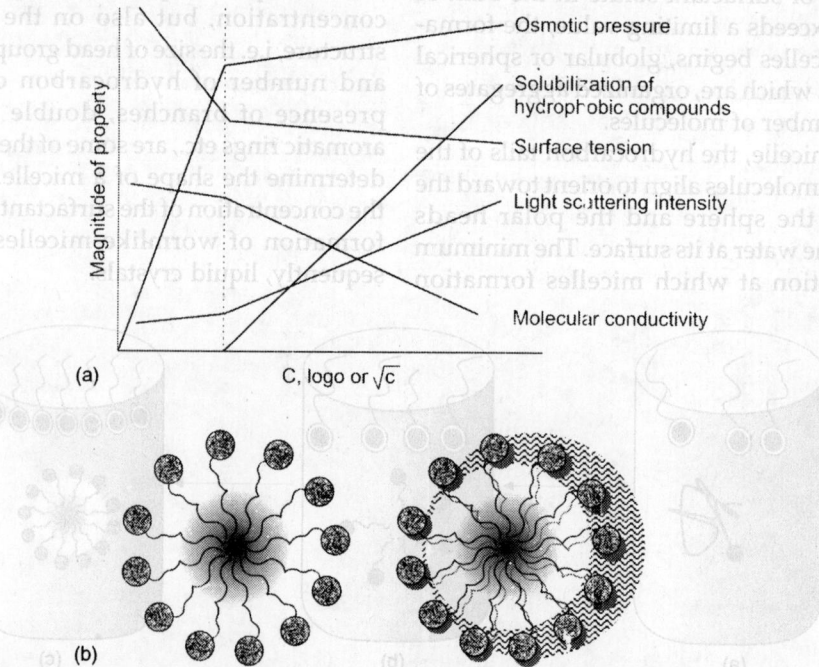

Fig. 10.2: (a) Schematic illustration of how a range of experimentally accessible parameters changes with the surfactant concentration and how this can be used to detect the CMC, (b) schematic illustration of spherical micelles

Characterization of Polymeric Micelles (CMC)

In aqueous media, amphiphilic polymers can exist in the form of micelles, when the concentration is higher than CMC, and when diluted below this concentration, the micelles may collapse. Hence, CMC is the key parameter for the formation and the static stability of polymeric micelles. Some of the methods used for determination of CMC in aqueous dispersions of micelles include surface tension measurements, chromatography, light scattering, small angle neutron scattering, small angle X-ray scattering, differential scanning calorimetry, viscometry, and utilization of fluorescent probes. For easy practical determination, CMC is obtained from plots of the surface tension as a function of the logarithm of the concentration. The CMC is said to be attained when surface tension stops decreasing and reaches a plateau value. Most of the researchers have relied upon use of pyrene as a fluorescent probe for estimating CMC.

Size and Shape Determination

After the preparation of the micelles useful information regarding the polydispersity index of the prepared structures is obtained by examining the micellar solution with quasi-elastic light scattering technique. Monodispersed micelles produce blue color from light scattering which indicates good micellar preparation, as contrasted with the white color shown by aggregates.

Size of polymeric micelles usually falls in the colloidal range. Scanning electron microscopy (SEM) and transmission electron microscopy (TEM) techniques have been widely used for past many years for the direct visualization, size and shape determination of block copolymer, i.e. micelles. More recently developed cryo-TEM technique has increasingly started gaining importance for characterization of block copolymer, i.e. micelles in aqueous medium. SEM or atomic force microscopy (AFM) reveals information

regarding size distribution, when chemically attached micelles to surfaces are presented.

Direct visualization of block copolymer micelles either in the dried state or directly 'in situ' within a liquid cell can be directly seen or captured by AFM. Hydrodynamic diameters and polydispersity indices of micelles are obtained using photon correlation spectroscopy. Recently, size characterization of drug-loaded polymeric micelles was done using asymmetrical flow field-flow fractionation and the structure of assemblies was determined by small angle neutron scattering.

In Vitro Drug Release Behavior

In vitro drug release behavior from micelles is easily studied by placing the micellar solution in a dialysis tube. The dialysis bag is immersed into a flask containing release medium, kept at a constant temperature. At predetermined time intervals, aliquots of the release medium are withdrawn and replaced by fresh medium. The drug released in the medium can be measured by spectroscopic or other suitable method.

STABILITY OF POLYMER MICELLE

The aqueous stability is a issue needs to be resolved before development of effective polymer micelles. Because a polymer micelle is a physically assembled structure in water, thermodynamic equilibrium and kinetic stability should be considered for practical application. Especially, the stability under biological condition is very important to accomplish successful delivery of therapeutic drugs.

Stability of Polymer Micelle in Water and Buffers

Micelle Stability in Water

The obstacle in the development of effective micellar drug carriers is the poor stability of micelles in an aqueous environment. Even though multiple interactions may coexist to improve the drug loading capacity, the polymer micelle still remains a physically assembled structure. In aqueous medium, the micelle stability is influenced by many factors, such as polymer concentration, molecular mass of the core-forming block, and drug incorporation. It is well known that the micelle stability depends on the polymer concentration. A polymer micelle has a critical micelle concentration (CMC) that is the lowest concentration limit for polymers to produce a micelle structure. When diluted below CMC, polymer micelles are gradually disintegrated into unimers. The value of CMC is determined primarily by the molecular mass (size) and the hydrophobicity of the core-forming block of copolymers. For example, poloxamer block copolymers decrease their CMC values by increasing the molecular mass of hydrophobic poly (propylene oxide) block. Also, Attwood et al. found that different species of core-forming block led to different CMC values as a function of the degree of polymerization. They showed that the CMC of block copolymer consisting of e-caprolactone exceeds that of lactic acid, with that of polypropylene oxide being the least, in accordance with the hydrophobicity of the repeating units.

Polymeric micelle is a dynamic structure. In addition to the thermodynamic aspect, the kinetic stability stems from the unimer exchange between micelles. The Aniansson-Wall equation describes the exchange rate between unimers and micelles. The exchange rate could be experimentally determined by nonradiative energy transfer (NET), which is now known as the Forster resonance energy transfer (FRET). The FRET is a physical property of energy transfer from a donor dye to an acceptor dye. If both dyes exist within a range of Forster distance, nonradiative fluorescence from the excited donor dye can be effectively used as the excitation energy of the acceptor dye, resulting in emission of acceptor fluorescence. The unimer exchange is determined not only by the explusion/insertion of unimers, but also by the fusion/split of micelles. Halioglu

and coworkers identified that, where the explusion/insertion of unimers occurs at a lower concentration of polymer, however the fusion/split of micelles is the major mechanism of unimer exchange at higher concentration.

It should be noted that those studies on the kinetic stability, were conducted without loading hydrophobic drugs. It is believed that incorporation of drugs makes polymeric micelles more stable. As the CMC is proportional to the standard free energy and also the free energy is important to the miscibility between polymers and drugs, (i.e. LSER equation), polymer micelles loading lipophilic drugs can be stabilized much more effectively than blank micelles. Therefore, it is necessary to identify the unimer exchange rate in the presence of hydrophobic drug for clear understanding of the kinetic stability.

Micelle Stability in Biological Environments

After systemic injections, polymer micelles become much diluted by blood. Furthermore, the polymer micelles are confronted with numerous blood components, such as proteins and cells. A conventional polymeric micelle of PEG-b-PCL is unstable in serum-containing culture media with or without cells, but stable in phosphate-buffered saline. The polymer micelles that conjugated with a fluorophore at the end of the PCL segment are slowly disintegrated on incubation in the cell culture media, and the disintegration could be quantified by measuring released dye content due to hydrolytic degradation.

Recently, conventional polymer micelles made up of PEG-b-PDLLA were found to be unstable in blood. The FRET technique was used to monitor the stability of polymer micelles in real time after intravenous administration. The micelles were loaded with a pair of FRET dyes. The FRET ratio detected in the blood vessels of the mice ears was reduced to half of the initial value at 15 min postintravenous injection, indicating that the dyes were released from the core of the micelles. It was further revealed that the main components responsible for the release of lipophilic dyes from micelles into the blood are α and β globulins rather than γ-globulin or serum albumin.

In polymeric micelles, PEG is commonly used to construct the hydrophilic shell. Although, PEG is known to be biocompatible, many researchers have reported inter actions between PEG and proteins. According to Xia et al. PEG interacts with pepsin in buffer solutions, which was observed by the quasielastic and electrophoretic light scattering methods. The interaction was mediated by hydrogen bonding between carboxyl groups of the protein and oxygen atoms in the PEG backbone. Interactions between PEG with other proteins such as α-chymotrypsin and hen-egg-white lysozyme were also reported. Indeed, it is not surprising that PEGs interact with serum proteins because PEG was detected along soluble immune complexes formed due to inflammatory diseases, such as systemic lupus erythematosus (SLE) and rheumatoid arthritis (RA). The immune complexes are precipitated in the presence of PEG and the agglomeration is mediated by fibronectin. Serum albumin has also shown direct interaction with PEG. The hydrogen bonding between PEG and albumin was revealed by Fourier transform infrared (FTIR) spectroscopy, and the van der Waals' interactions between PEG and albumin were detected using binding force measurements. Furthermore, crystal structure analysis of PEG-protein complexes showed that multiple coordinations between PEG backbone and positively charged amino acids, that is, Lys, Arg, His, serve as another interaction force. The formation of complex between PEG and proteins possibly induces micelle aggregation as well as unimer extraction, which may significantly affect the micelle stability *in vivo*. There exist some evidences that proteins possibly penetrate the hydrophilic shell of the micelles. For example, it was observed that a micelle consisting of PEG-b-PCL block copolymer was slowly degraded in the presence of lipase K. To hydrolyze ester bonds of PCL, the lipase should directly come in contact with PCL molecules. Therefore, the micelle degradation by lipase K, implies that serum proteins seem to overcome the hydrophilic corona and reach the micelle core. Enzymatic degradation of a polymer micelle composed of PEG-b-poly (3-hydroxybutyrate) -b-PEG (PEG-b-PHB-b-PEG) depends on enzyme (PHB depolymerase) concentration, polymer concentration, and PHB block length. In addition to the enzyme penetration, micelles can be degraded by enzymatic hydrolysis of unimers dissociated from micelles.The possible mechanisms accounting for the instability of micelle include induction by serum proteins, protein adsorption, protein penetration, and drug extraction. Although the effect of drug extraction on micelle stability has not been investigated yet, the loss of drug from a micelle may inevitably provoke micelle disassembly because drug-containing polymer micelles are more stable than blank micelles.

Thermodynamic Stability

Micelle is a structure in thermodynamic equilibrium, and in general, a closed association model is employed to explain micelle formation. The strict closed association model is based on an all-or-none process, in which block copolymers (unimers) generate homogeneous micelles in size. As a result, an aqueous medium contains only unimers and monodisperse micelles. In pure water, the standard free energy change of micellization is

$$G = RT \ln(CMC)$$

where, CMC is the critical micelle concentration. The CMC has significance in micelle stability. It may be reasonable, therefore, that micelles at equilibrium state will be destabilized (i.e. dissociated into unimers), when diluted. In general, higher MW of hydrophobic block provides the lower CMC value, which means more 'stable.'

Attwood et al. scored hydrophobicity of core-forming polymer blocks based on the analysis of CMC change as a function of the degree of polymerization (DP). For example, the hydrophobic ratio of propylene oxide: lactic acid: e-caprolactone is 1:4:12. Logarithm curve of CMC versus DP of a polyester (=block length) shows two transition points. As the DP increases, it is hypothesized that a long and linear chain of hydrophobic blocks spontaneously collapses, leading block copolymers to form unimeric or oligomeric micelles. The reports support the 'bunchy micelle' model, in which the micellization occurs by aggregation of unimers with collapsed hydrophobic segments. Since the stable geometry of the collapsed segments is a sphere, the micelle core may have many pores that are filled with solvents or drugs. However, it has been considered that the micelle core is a molten globule. Usually, micelles are prepared from polymer solution of high concentration followed by removal of the solvent. Even though the preparation method is a thermodynamically quenching process, long polymer chains, especially hydrophobic polymer chains, are liable to be entangled together. If the time scale is infinite, then all hydrophobic polymer chains can be converted to globular structures. As a result, micellization may be explained by combining the molten liquid core model and the bunchy micelle model together (Fig. 10.3).

CMC depends on the hydrophobicity of the core-forming block. However, it is also influenced by the crystallinity of hydrophobic blocks. For instance, the PDLLA, a kind of polyester, is an amorphous polymer, which has its glass transition temperature (T_g) around 55°C. Likewise, poly-(lactide-co-glycolide) (PLGA) is an amorphous polymer $(T_g \sim 50-60°C)$. However, poly-(L-lactide) (PLLA) has high crystallinity with melting temperature (T_m) and T_g around 130°C and 60°C, respectively. Poly-(ε-caprolactone) (PCL) is a semicrystalline polymer. T_m and T_g of PCL are ~55–65°C and ~60°C, respectively. Isomers of D-and L-lactic acid in PDLLA

influence the molecular configuration, which makes packing structure more spacy, i.e. more mobility of each PDLLA molecule. Glycolic acid, results on loss of a methyl group from lactic acid, is more hydrophilic, and also provides more space for the packing structure of PLGA. Therefore, D-lactic acid and glycolic acid play the role of crystal structure breakers. Void volume at the micelle core is possessed by water molecules during micelle formulation. Therefore, micelle dissociation (relaxation) process can be more facilitated in short-term application to a diluted environment.

Block length ratio of diblock copolymers also controls CMC. The hydrophilic-lipophilic balance (HLB) is another expression of the block length ratio. For surfactant molecules containing PEG block, the HLB is equivalent to the mass percentage of oxyethylene content (E) divided by 5 (HLB = E/5). Block copolymer with higher HLB value (more hydrophilic) generally decreases the CMC and increases the micelle size due to loose packing density. Diblock copolymer with HLB <10 has a conical shape in water, which produces micellar structure by assembly. Polymers with HLB >10, can generate different shapes of supramolecular structure. If the hydrophobic block is long enough to be of cylinder shape in water, copolymer generates polymersome, which is very similar to the conformation of phospholipids.

Kinetic Stability

Micelle association and dissolution are kinetic processes. Aniansson and Wall (A-W) interpreted the dynamic mechanism of micelle relaxation. The A-W equations show that the exchange of unimers between micelles is a fast process and the decomposition of micelles into unimers is a slow process. The relationship between the number of unimers in a micelle and the concentration of micelles shows three continuous regions, i.e. the initial association (unimer-abundant) region, the intermediate region with unimer aggregates, and the

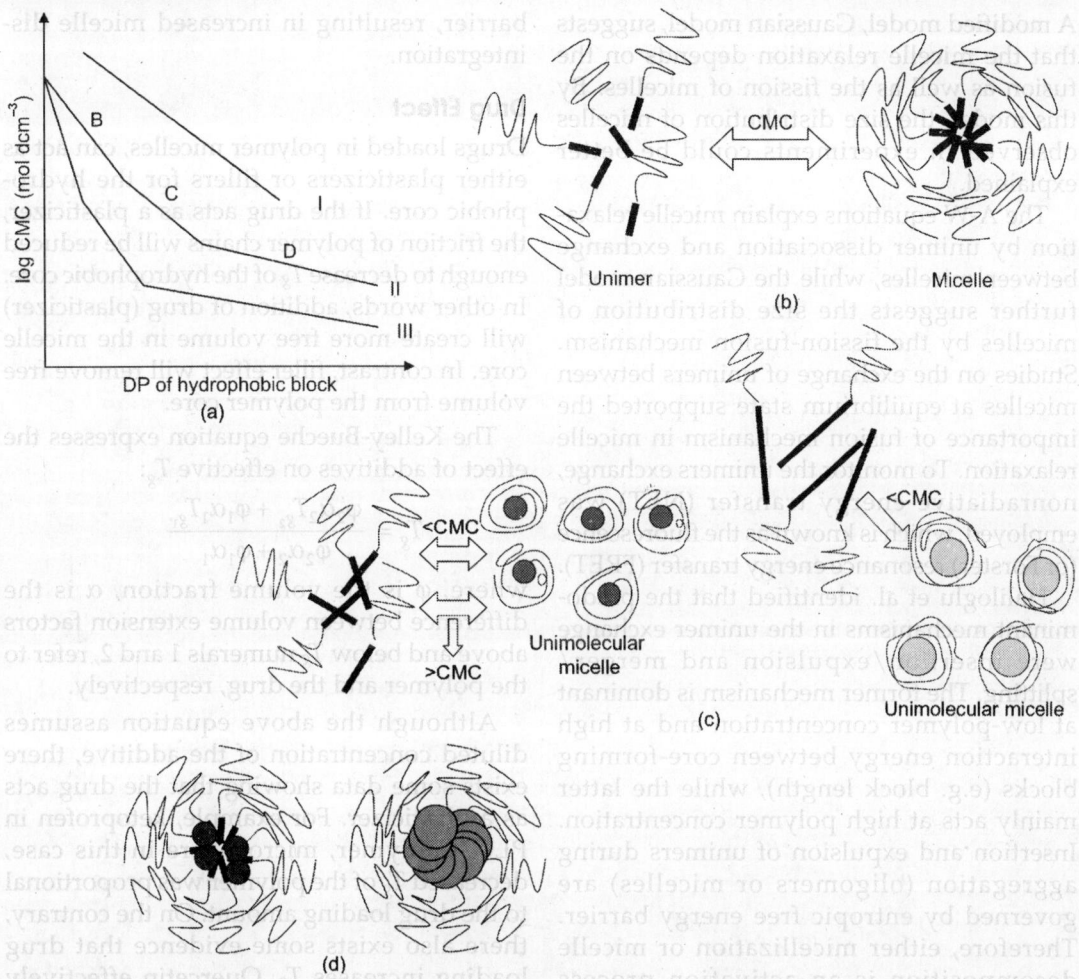

Fig. 10.3: A hypothesis to explain unimolecular and multimolecular micelles. (a) Relationship between log CMC and the degree of polymerization (DP) of the hydrophobic block. The log CMC decreases as the hydrophobicity of the core-forming block increases [e.g. (i) polypropylene, (ii) poly-(d, I-lactide), (iii) poly-(e-caprolactone)]. (b) If the block length is short, there exists only unimer-micelle equilibrium, (c) as DP of the hydrophobic block increases, unimers collapse to unimolecular micelles. Over the CMC, multimolecular micelles are generated, (d) Hydrophobic block with high DP is spontaneously collapsed, and most of the unimers exist as unimolecular micelles. At higher polymer concentration, the unimolecular micelles aggregate further to form multimolecular micelles.

micelle-abundant region. Because the aggregation process is very fast, micelle-containing solution will show a sharp bimodal distribution of the micelle size (either unimer- or micelle-dominant distribution) and, dissociation of unimers from micelles is governed by the internal free energy of micelles that is proportional to the length of hydrophobic blocks. However, experimental data have shown that this model (A-W model) of micelle relaxation is not always a well-fit. This was because drastically simplified assumptions were made to explain the micelle relaxation process. The A-W model did not consider the micelle-micelle interaction, but only the fission process was taken in account.

A modified model, Gaussian model, suggests that the micelle relaxation depends on the fusion as well as the fission of micelles. By this model, the size distribution of micelles observed in experiments could be better explained.

The A-W equations explain micelle relaxation by unimer dissociation and exchange between micelles, while the Gaussian model further suggests the size distribution of micelles by the fission-fusion mechanism. Studies on the exchange of unimers between micelles at equilibrium state supported the importance of fusion mechanism in micelle relaxation. To monitor the unimers exchange, nonradiative energy transfer (NET) was employed, which is known as the fluorescence (or Forster) resonance energy transfer (FRET).

Haliloglu et al. identified that the predominant mechanisms in the unimer exchange were insertion/expulsion and merger/splitting. The former mechanism is dominant at low-polymer concentration and at high interaction energy between core-forming blocks (e.g. block length), while the latter mainly acts at high polymer concentration. Insertion and expulsion of unimers during aggregation (oligomers or micelles) are governed by entropic free energy barrier. Therefore, either micellization or micelle decomposition is an activation process involving collective energy barriers, which can be explained by the internal free energy of micelle. The internal free energy of micelle suppresses association of too many unimers in a micelle (internal free energy of association, F_a) and dissociation of unimers from a micelle (internal free energy of dissociation, F_d). Due to F_a, a thermodynamic equilibrium of the micellization requires a very long time, which is not achievable in practical situations. As a result, micelles are loosely aggregated under experimental conditions. The F_d tends to prevent micelle disintegration. However, a 'jump' condition, such as either dilution or increased temperature, provides enough energy for micelles to overcome the energy barrier, resulting in increased micelle disintegration.

Drug Effect

Drugs loaded in polymer micelles, can act as either plasticizers or fillers for the hydrophobic core. If the drug acts as a plasticizer, the friction of polymer chains will be reduced enough to decrease T_g of the hydrophobic core. In other words, addition of drug (plasticizer) will create more free volume in the micelle core. In contrast, filler effect will remove free volume from the polymer core.

The Kelley-Bueche equation expresses the effect of additives on effective T_g:

$$T_g = \frac{\varphi_2\alpha_2 T_{g_2} + \varphi_1\alpha_1 T_{g_1}}{\varphi_2\alpha_2 + \varphi_1\alpha_1}$$

where, φ is the volume fraction, α is the difference between volume extension factors above and below T_g numerals 1 and 2, refer to the polymer and the drug, respectively.

Although the above equation assumes diluted concentration of the additive, there exists some data showing that the drug acts as a plasticizer. For example, ketoprofen in PLGA polymer, microsphere in this case, decreased T_g of the polymer was proportional to the drug loading amount. On the contrary, there also exists some evidence that drug loading increases T_g. Quercetin effectively increased T_g of PCL block in PEG-b-PCL micelles, which was proportionally depended on the drug-loading amount. It was suggested that the increased T_g would be due to the hydrogen bonds between drug and carbonyl groups of PCL. Also, a poly-(N-isopropylacrylamide-co-N,N-dimethylacrylamide)-b-PLGA (P(NIPAAm-co-DMAAm)-b-PLGA) micelle increased T_g of PLGA block by addition of paclitaxel. As discussed previously, T_g of core-forming polymers should be important for micelle stability (Fig. 10.4). It has been believed that hydrophobic drugs may enhance the micelle stability primarily due to the hydrophobic effect, but there is not enough evidence to support this. It is more reasonable that the

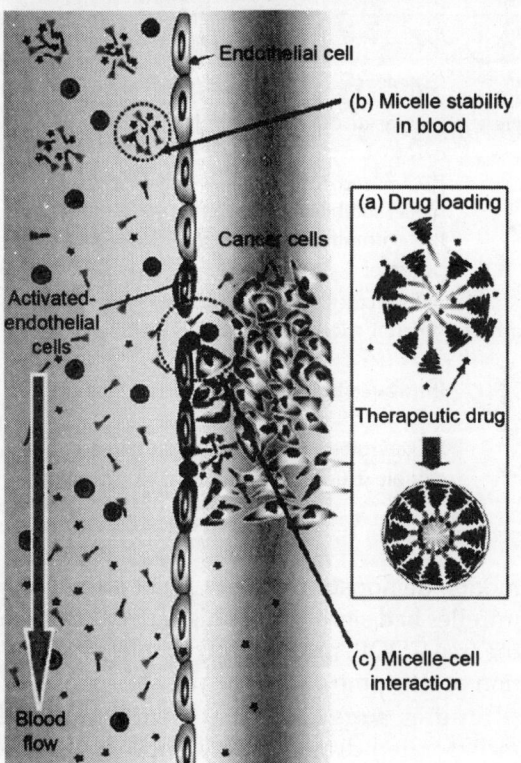

(b) Micelle stability in blood

(a) Drug loading

Therapeutic drug

(c) Micelle-cell interaction

Endothelial cell

Cancer cells

Activated-endothelial cells

Blood flow

Fig. 10.4: Three major problems in developing an effective micellar drug delivery system. (a) A low drug loading content and efficiency, (b) poor stability in bloodstream, (c) cell membrane as barrier in the intracellular drug delivery

role of drugs is determined by the miscibility with hydrophobic polymer block. Actually, one unsolved problem of drug-loaded polymer micelles is the aqueous stability. Frequently, drug precipitation is observed, when the micelles are stored in an aqueous medium, though the micelle structure is not disrupted. It is explained by phase separation out of poor miscibility between the drug and the polymer.

APPLICATION OF MICELLES IN PHARMACEUTICAL SCIENCE

Solubilization

The micellar core is a compatible microenvironment and a hub for incorporating water-insoluble guest molecules. The hydrophobic molecules can be covalently coupled to the block copolymers or physically incorporated into the hydrophobic core of micelles. The solubilization process leads to enhancement of their water solubility and thereby bioavailability. It is often observed that the gastrointestinal (GI) uptake of particles is affected significantly by particle size A 15 to 250-fold higher uptake efficiency of particles approximately 100 nm in diameter by the GI tract was noted than that of the micrometer-sized particles. Thus, polymeric micelles (nanosized) enhance the uptake and the bioavailability. The extent of solubilization depends upon the micellization process, the compatibility between the drug and the core-forming block, chain length of the hydrophobic block, concentration of polymer, and temperature. Above CMC, there is a sharp increase in the solubility of drug as it gets more space to occupy in the aggregates of the hydrophobic part of the micelle. The occupancy of the core region by drug leads to an increased R_c of the micelle. It is worth mentioning that the core region has limited capacity for accommodation, for instance, pluronic P85 has a core region, which is 13% of the whole micelle weight. The influence on solubilization capacity of hydrophobic block length, has been examined for griseofulvin in polyoxyethylene and polyoxybutylene copolymer micelles with varying number of hydrophobic block lengths and hydrophilic block lengths sufficient for formation of spherical micelles. It was found that the solubilization capacity was dependent on the hydrophobic block length up to a certain extent (15 units of hydrophobic block), after which the solubilization capacity became independent of the same. Dong and coworkers also studied the effect of hydrophobic block length on solubilization of toluene in diblock and triblock polyurethane surfactants. It was concluded that solubilization capacity of polyurethane surfactants increased with an increase in the hydrophobic segment for the same block chain structure. Some noteworthy contributions for solubilization of drugs are recorded in Table 10.2.

Table 10.2: Examples of improvement in solubility of drugs using polymeric miceller system

Drug	Amphiphilic polymer	Comment
Camptothecin	Pluronic P105, d-α-tocopheryl polyethylene glycol 1000 succinate	Increased miceller stability; increased cytotoxicity
Docetaxel	Poly-(ethylene oxide)-block-poly-(styrene oxide) (PEO-b-PSO) and PEO-b-poly (butylenes oxide) (PEO-b-PBO)	PSO-based copolymer were associated with higher solubilizing capacities than PBO due to the aromatic structure of the core-forming polymer
Griseofulvin	EmB copolymer (E = oxyethylene, B = oxybutylene, subscripts denote number-average block lengths in repeat units)	Solubilization independent of B block length when it exceeds about 15 B units
Paclitaxel	N-octyl-O-sulfate chitosan	Improved bioavailability and reduced toxicity
Paclitaxel	Mixed micelles of polyethylene glycol-phosphatidyl ethanolamine (PEG-PE) and vitamin E	Mixed micelles efficiently solubilized poorly soluble drug as compared to PEG-PE micelles

Drug Delivery Applications

The studies on the application of polymeric micelles in drug delivery have been mostly focused on the following areas that are considered below—(1) delivery of anticancer agents to treat tumors; (2) drug delivery to the brain to treat neurodegenerative diseases; (3) delivery of antifungal agents; (4) delivery of imaging agents for diagnostic applications; and (5) delivery of polynucleotide therapeutics.

Chemotherapy of Cancer

To enhance chemotherapy of tumors using polymer micelles, four major approaches have been employed—(1) passive targeting of polymer micelles to tumors through EPR effect; (2) targeting of polymer micelles to specific antigens overexpressed at the surface of tumor cells; (3) enhanced drug release at the tumor sites having low pH; and (4) sensitization of drug resistant tumors by block copolymers.

In a series of studies polymer micelles have been used for passive targeting of various anticancer agents and chemotherapy of tumors. One notable recent example reported involves polymer micelles of PEO-b-poly (L-aspartic acid) incorporating CDDP. Evaluation of anticancer activity using murine colon adenocarcinoma C26 as an *in vivo* tumor model, demonstrated that CDDP in polymer micelles had significantly higher activity than the free CDDP, resulting in complete eradication of the tumor.

Studies suggested that various micelle incorporated drugs display improved therapeutic index in solid tumors, which correlates with enhanced passive targeting of the drug to the tumor sites, as well as decreased side effects, compared with conventional formulations of these drugs.

A cyclic pentapeptide, cRGD was used as a targeting ligand that is capable of selective and high affinity binding to the avb3, integrin. Micelles of PEOb-poly-(e-caprolactone) loaded with doxorubicin were covalently bound with cRGD.

Micelles conjugated with antibodies or antibody fragments capable to recognize tumor antigens were shown to improve therapeutic efficacy *in vivo* over nonmodified micelles. This approach can result in high selectivity of binding, internalization, and effective retention of the micelles in the tumor cells. In addition, recent advances in antibody engineering allow for the production of humanized antibody fragments, reducing problems with immune response against mouse antibodies. The micelles were used for incorporating various poorly soluble anti-cancer drugs including tamoxifen, paclitaxel and dequalinium. It was shown that pacli-taxel-loaded 2C5-immunomicelles could specifically recognize a variety of tumor types. The binding of these immunomicelles was observed for all cancer cell lines tested, i.e. murine Lewis lung carcinoma, T-lymphoma EL4, and human breast adenocarcinomas, BT-20 and MCF7. Moreover, paclitaxel-loaded 2C5 immunomicelles demonstrated highest anticancer activity in Lewis lung carcinoma tumor model in mice, compared with plain paclitaxel-loaded micelles and the free drug. The increased antitumor effect of immunomicelles *in vivo* correlated with the enhanced accumulation of the drug delivered with the immunomicelles inside the tumor (Fig. 10.5).

Tumors often display low pH of interstitial fluid, which is mainly attributed to higher rates of aerobic and anaerobic glycolysis in cancer cells than in normal cells. This phenomenon has been employed in the design of various pH-sensitive polymer micelle systems for the delivery of anticancer drugs to the tumors.

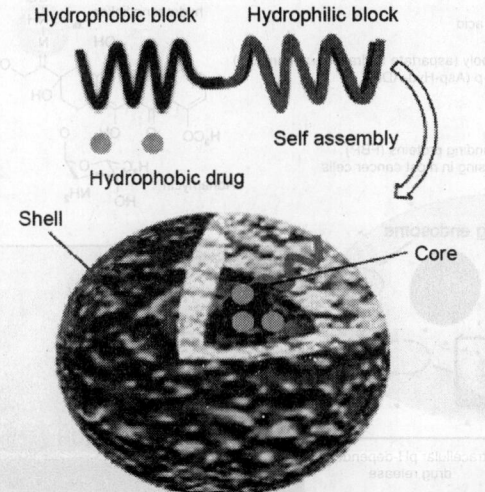

Fig. 10.5: Schematic representation of the self-assembly of amphiphilic block copolymers to poly-meric micelles

One approach was based on the chemical conjugation of anticancer drugs to the block copolymers through pH-sensitive cleavable links that are stable at neutral pH, but are cleavable in the mildly acidic pH. For example, several groups used hydrasone-based linking groups, to covalently attach doxorubicin to PEO-b-poly-(DL-lactic-co-glycolic acid) block copolymer, PEO-b-block-poly-(allyl glycidyl ether) or PEO-b-poly-(aspartate hydrazone) block copolymer. It was suggested that doxorubicin will remain in the micelles in the blood stream, and will be released at tumor sites at lower pH. An alternative mechanism for pH-induced triggering of drug release at the tumor sites consists of using pH-sensitive polyacids or polybases as building blocks of polymer micelles. For example, mixed micelles of PEO-b-poly-(L-histidine) and PEO-b-poly-(L-lactic acid) block copolymers incorporate pH sensitive poly-base, poly-(L-histidine) in the hydrophobic core. The core can also solubi-lize hydrophobic drugs such as doxorubicin. The protonation of the polybase at acidic conditions resulted in the destabilization of the core and triggered release of the drug. This system was also targeted to the tumors through the folate molecules as described earlier and has shown significant *in vivo* antitumor activity and less side effects as compared with the free drug. Notably, it was also effective in *in vitro* and *in vivo* against multidrug resistant (MDR) human breast carcinoma MCF7/ADR that overexpresses P-glycoprotein (Pgp). Pgp is a drug efflux transport protein that serves to eliminate drugs from the cancer cells and significantly decreases the anticancer activity of the drugs. The micelle incorporated drug was released inside the cells, and thus avoided the contact with Pgp localized at the cell plasma mem-brane, which perhaps contributed to the increased activity of pH sensitive doxorubicin micelles in the MDR cells. A different approach using pluronic block copolymer micelles to overcome MDR in tumors has been developed. It was demonstrated that pluronic block copolymers can sensitize MDR cells, resulting in an increased cytotoxic activity of doxorubicin, paclitaxel, and other drugs by 2, 3 orders of magnitude. Remarkably, pluronic can enhance drug effects in MDR cells through multiple effects including (1) inhibiting drug efflux transporters, such as Pgp and multidrug resistance proteins (MRPs), (2) abolishing drug sequestration within cytoplasmic vesicles, (3) inhibiting the glutathione/glutathione S-transferase detoxification system, and (4) enhancing proapoptotic signaling in MDR cells. Similar effects of pluronics have also been reported using *in vivo* tumor models (Fig. 10.6).

Drug Delivery to the Brain

By restricting drug transport to the brain, the blood brain barrier (BBB) represents a formidable impediment for the treatment of brain tumors and neurodegenerative diseases, such as HIV-associated dementia, stroke, Parkinson's and Alzheimer's diseases. Two strategies using polymer micelles have been evaluated to enhance the delivery of biologically active agents to the brain. The first strategy is based on the modification of polymer micelles with antibodies or ligand molecules capable of transcytosis across brain microvessel endothelial cells, comprising the BBB. The second strategy uses pluronic block copolymers to inhibit drug efflux systems, particularly, Pgp, and selectively increase the permeability of BBB to Pgp-substrates. An earlier study used micelles of pluronic block copolymers for the delivery of the CNS drugs to the brain. These micelles were surface-modified by attaching to the free PEO ends, either polyclonal antibodies against brain-specific antigen, α^2-glycoprotein, or insulin to target the receptor at the lumenal side of BBB. The modified micelles were used to solubilize fluorescent dye or neuroleptic drug, haloperidol, and these formulations were administered intravenously in mice. Both, the antibody and insulin modification of the micelles resulted in enhanced delivery of the fluorescent dye to the brain and significant increases in neuroleptic effect of haloperidol in the animals. Subsequent studies using

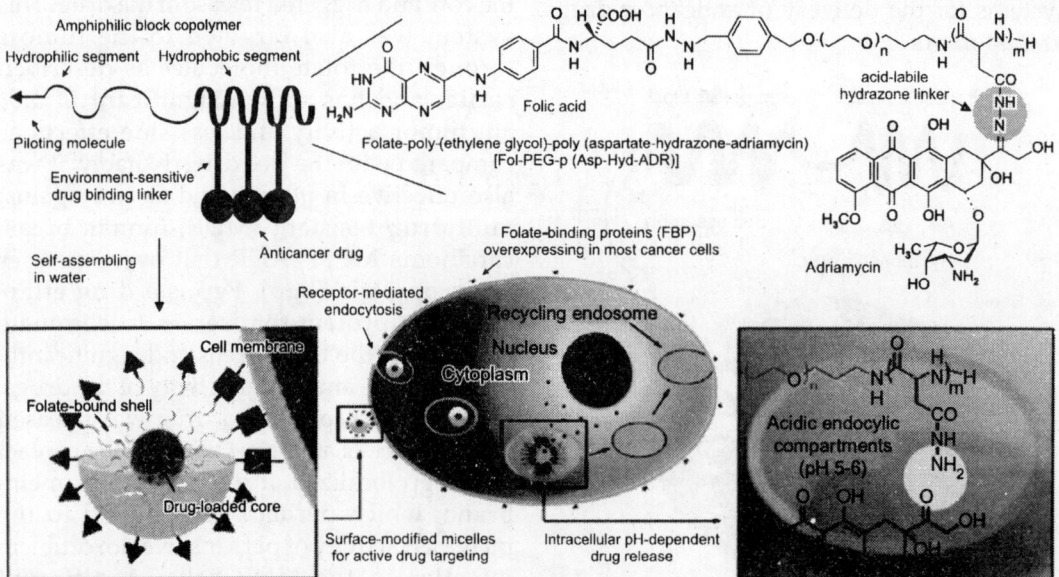

Fig. 10.6: Preparation of multifunctional folate-PEO-P-(Asp-Hyd-DOX) polymeric micelles with tumor selectivity for active drug targeting and pH-sensitivity for intracellular site-specific drug release (reproduced from Bae et al. 2005)

in vitro BBB models demonstrated that the micelles, vectorized by insulin, undergo receptor-mediated transport across brain microvessel endothelial cells. Based on one of these observations, one may expect development of novel polymer micelles that target specific receptors at the surface of the BBB to enhance transport of the incorporated drugs to the brain.

The studies have also demonstrated that selected pluronic block copolymers, such as pluronic P85, are potent inhibitors of Pgp, and they carry across and allow an increased entry of the Pgp-substrates to the brain across BBB. Pluronic did not induce or may cause toxic effect in BBB, as revealed by the lack of alteration in paracellular permeability of the barrier, and in histological studies, using specific markers for brain endothelial cells. Overall, this strategy has potential in developing novel modalities for the delivery of various drugs to the brain, including selective anticancer agents to treat metastatic brain tumors, as well as HIV protease inhibitors to eradicate HIV virus in the brain.

The modified micelles were used to solubilize fluorescent dye or neuroleptic drug, haloperidol, and these formulations were administered intravenously in mice. Both the antibody and insulin modification of the micelles resulted in enhanced delivery of the fluorescent dye to the brain and significant increases in neuroleptic effect of haloperidol in the animals. Subsequent studies using *in vitro* BBB models demonstrated that the micelles, vectorized by insulin, undergo receptor-mediated transport across brain microvessel endothelial cells. Based on one of these observations, one may expect development of novel polymer micelles that target specific receptors at the surface of the BBB to enhance transport of the incorporated drugs to the brain.

Unimolecular Micelles

Unimolecular micelles are single-molecular micelles, which possess a distinct core and shell that are covalently bound together. Comparing with conventional multimolecular micelles in terms of dynamic equilibrium in solution, unimolecular micelles are covalently reinforced core-shell nanostructured materials which exhibit excellent stability to environmental changes such as pH, temperature, ionic strength, high dilution condition and other microenvironment changes, enabling them as stable micelles for pharmaceutical applications etc. Various types of architectural materials that have been used in the prepration of unimolecular micelles, such as single macromolecular amphiphilic polymers, dendrimers, hyperbranched, dendritic, star, brush-like and cyclic polymers. The unimolecular micelle formation does not rely on self-assembly. Thus, structuring of these sophisticated materials help overcome many challenges of using micelles as delivery carriers in biomedical applications. For example, the premature disassociation of the self-assembled multimolecular micelles during circulation in the bloodstream can result into a burst release of highly toxic drugs and further may cause potential systemic toxicity and insufficient tumor-targeting ability. Another advantage is the highly branched structure in unimolecular micelles, which can provide many possibilities for further functionalization to adapt specific applications. The most investigated biomedical applications in using unimolecular micelles, as drug carriers have been for controlled release or targeted delivery. The utilization of unimolecular micelles in catalysis and as a template for preparation of inorganic particles has also been investigated (Loh et. al., 2016).

The mechanism explaining endocytosis of polymer micelles has not been fully clarified. One possibility focuses on the role of the labeled dye. In fluorescence imaging studies, one should be cautious about the change of polymer property by fluorophore labeling. As the TRITC is positively charged, TRITC labeled PEG-b-PCL also has positive charge. It is known that positively charged macromolecules can be effectively internalized by electrostatic interaction with heparin sulfate on cell surface. To revisit the endocytosis of micelles, a recent study by Chen et al. revealed that PEG-b-PDLLA micelles consisting of fluorescein isothiocyanate (FITC)-labeled PEG-b-PDLLA could not be endocytosed into cultured HeLa cells. The authors performed a dual-color imaging experiment in which the copolymer was conjugated with FITC, and another dye, DiI, was physically incorporated into the micelles. As a result, the DiI was found inside cells within 30 min, whereas the FITC remained outside the cells even after 24 hours. This indicates that DiI may be released from the micelle and enter tumor cells separately.

Chen et al. loaded a FRET pair (DiI/DiO) into the micelle. By monitoring the FRET efficiency, they demonstrated that core loaded probes are released to the cell plasma membrane during incubation, indicating that plasma membrane mediates the cellular uptake of the hydrophobic molecules loaded in polymer micelles. On the other hand, polymer micelles are shown to increase the drug accumulation inside cells without endocytosis. For example, polymer micelle made of pluronic (Poloxamer; BASF Corp., NJ, USA) P-85 or P-105 enabled effective accumulation of a hydrophobic dye inside cells by inhibiting P-glycoprotein (Pgp). The Pgp is an important protein that endows the MDR phenotype to cancer cells. A polymer micelle consisting of PEG-b-PCL also showed a similar effect on blocking the Pgp function. It is, however, noticed that the Pgp inhibition can be facilitated only at low polymer concentration, usually CMC. Hence, the MDR inhibition seems to be caused by an action of unimers rather than polymer micelles. As the Pgp pump is effectively blocked by block copolymers with relatively long hydrophobic block (HLB <20) and owing to the fact that P105 increases the membrane permeability, it is highly suspected that unimers dissociated from micelles may perturb the plasma membrane resulting in acceleration of drug penetration through cell membranes. Notably,

there is no evidence showing that polymer micelle or unimer directly binds to Pgp molecules, implying that the MDR inhibition may be due to a downstream effect for suppressing the phenotype. In summary, the micelle-cell interaction as well as the cellular uptake of polymer micelles could be mediated by means of complicated molecular and cellular events, which needed to be clarified by continuous research.

The targeting moiety onto micelle surface provides one solution to deal with the cellular uptake problem. In parallel to or in combination with the stimuli sensitivity, tagging the targeting molecule has been a major strategy to enhance the therapeutic effect of micellar drug carriers. Micelles conjugated with different targeting moieties such as biotin, folate, antibodies, growth factors, or homing peptides have been developed. These micelles are designed especially for intracellular delivery of anticancer drugs. However, most of the micelles are based on the physical assembly of block copolymers so their stability in blood is not ensured. If a polymer micelle having a highly specific homing molecule on its surface, is rapidly disintegrated in the bloodstream, the therapeutic effect cannot be maximized. Therefore, improving the micelle stability in blood should be considered in order to optimize the active targeting strategy using targeting moieties.

In Vivo Fate of Polymer Micelles

Pharmacokinetics and pharmacodynamics of drugs formulated using polymer micelles have been widely studied, and have been excellently summarized by Aliabadi and colleagues. *In vivo* fate of polymer micelles has also been investigated. The radioisotope has been a chief tool to monitor the biodistribution of polymer micelles. Without loading any therapeutic drug, polymer micelles are mostly located in liver, kidney, spleen and blood. This means that micelles seem to prolong the circulation time in blood, which has been an important rationale to develop micellar formulation of lipophilic drugs. However, it is not obvious whether the trace of isotope in blood indicates unimers or micelles. To define clearly the biodistribution of polymer micelles, other methods that can inform the structural integrity of the polymer micelles in blood should be considered. On the other hand, micelles (or unimers) are highly distributed to organs that have excretion and metabolism functions. Assuming that micelles circulate stably along the bloodstream for a certain period of time, a high toxicity of the loaded drug would be expected owing to slow drug release at those organs. Therefore, although micelles can be used as a drug carrier of high loading efficiency, one should be cautious to avoid increasing toxicity to healthy organs. To clarify the *in vivo* toxicity-biodistribution relationship of drug-containing polymer micelles, their structural integrity and fate in the body should be visualized by many means.

Often, pharmacokinetic data are translated to the biodistribution of polymer micelles. However, if *in vivo* stability of micelles is not guaranted, the biodistribution data cannot represent the real location of the polymer micelles. Recent advances in imaging technology may provide useful tools to monitor the micelle stability and biodistribution of drugs at the same time. List of patents related to micellar system are shown in Table 10.3.

CONCLUSION

In parallel with the mechanism, attempts have been made to improve drug-loading content/ efficiency, stability in blood and cellular uptake of polymer micelles. The stimuli-sensitive polymer micelle showed an alternative solution to figure out the inherent problems in case of polymer micelles. Controllability of micelle disintegration using environmental

Table.10.3: List of some of the patents related to micellar drug delivery system

Citing patent	Issue date	Original assignee	Title
US8173167	May 8, 2012	Wisconsin Alumni Research Foundation	Micelle composition of polymer and passenger drug.
US7018655	Mar 28, 2006	Labopharm Inc.	Amphiphilic diblock, triblock and star-block copolymers and their pharmaceutical compositions.
US6623729	Sep 23, 2003	Korea Advanced Institute of Science and Technology	Process for preparing sustained release micelle employing conjugate of anticancer drug and biodegradable polymer.
US7897563	Mar 1, 2011	Soane Family Trust	Use of oligomers and polymers for drug
US6623729	Sep 23, 2003	Korea Advanced Institute of Science and Technology	Process for preparing sustained release micelle employing conjugate of anticancer drug and biodegradable polymer
US7875677	Jan 25, 2011	The University of British Columbia	Micellar drug delivery systems for hydrophobic drugs
US7897563	Mar 1, 2011	Soane Family Trust	Use of oligomers and polymers for drug solubilization, stabilization, and delivery
US7875677	Jan 25, 2011	The University of British Columbia	Micellar drug delivery systems for hydrophobic drugs
US7655258	Feb 2, 2010	Industrial Technology Research Institute	Biodegradable copolymer, and polymeric micelle composition containing the same
US7311901	Dec 25, 2007	Samyang Corporation	Amphiphilic block copolymer and polymeric composition comprising the same for drug delivery

stimuli can enhance the therapeutic effect. Also, the ligand-conjugated polymer micelle could increase the probability of cellular uptake of polymer micelles, which is useful for the intracellular drug delivery. A combination of stimuli sensitivity and targeting moiety has been frequently used to maximize the specificity and selectivity of therapeutic effect at disease sites.

Crosslinked micelles have given a clue to increasing stability of physically-assembled polymer micelles in blood. Chemically or electrostatically crosslinked polymer micelles prevent micelle disintegration in the bloodstream. However, crosslinking between polymer chains may result in another problem of drug-controlled release owing to the lack of a biodegradation mechanism. To circumvent this problem, one pilot study based on disulfide-mediated crosslinking, this can be reversely disintegrated by reducing agent. Further an effort on combination of targeting moiety, stimuli sensitivity and crosslinking strategy may promise a polymer micelle as an effective drug delivery carrier. Another approach to improve the *in vivo* stability is to generate unimolecular micelles. Recently, a new strategy to prepare multiarm unimolecular micelles based on hyperbranced copolymers. These polymer micelles were constructed by polymerization of L-lactide from Boltorn H40, a dendritic polymer containing 64 primary hydroxyl groups, and then coupled with MPEG, thus forming a highly stable unimolecular micelle with high molecular mass ($\sim 10^9$ kDa). The H40-PLA-b-MPEG micelle showed an initial burst of 5-fluorouracil (5-FU), an anticancer drug, followed by a sustained release. Micelles were slowly degraded within 6 weeks. Moreover, introduction of folate by PEG tethers showed improved tumor-targeting ability of the unimolecular micelle. The micelle degradation was accelerated under acidic environment provided by solid tumors and endosomal vesicles, which might provide more efficient therapeutic effect.

Unimolecular micelle conjugating DOX by means of hydrolysable hydrazone bond presented a high sensitivity to environmental pH and significantly enhanced the cellular uptake as well as selective to toxicity of the drug micelle. Recent advances in molecular imaging have provided indepth insight into the micelle stability and its interaction with cells. As described earlier, the FRET technique, as one of the optical imaging methods, suggested the possibility of clarifying the mechanisms of micelle disintegration under physiological conditions and simultaneously elucidating the fate of micelles and drugs. Optical imaging techniques have now been expanded to visualize the *in vivo* fate of polymer micelles, which was typically examined using radioisotopes. In particular, the development of fluorescent probes with a long wavelength (e.g. near infrared light) is desirable for small animal imaging due to minimized autofluorescence from living tissues. The multifunctional polymer micelle includes not only multiple targeting strategies, (i.e. stimuli sensitivity and targeting ligand), but also imaging probes to visualize *in vivo* behavior. In addition, the use of imaging modalities makes it possible to follow up the therapeutic effect after drug treatment. Therefore, diagnosis, therapy, and prognosis of a certain disease can be accomplished using a single micellar drug delivery system. For this reason, the multifunctional polymer micelle is a good candidate to realize personalized medicine. Pharmacogenomics, high-through-put screening, biopanning and combinational chemistry have continuously discovered small molecular therapeutic drugs, ligands highly selective to a specific disease, and pathophysiological microenvironment distingui-shed from normal condition. Therefore, polymer micelles will evolve further by actively combining and using these findings.

SUGGESTED READINGS

1. Allen C, Maysinger D, Eisenberg A (1999), *Colloids Surf.* 16, 3.
2. Antonietti M, Goltner C, (1997), *Angew. Chem. Int. Ed. Engl.* 36, 910.
3. Bader H, Ringsdorf H, Schmidt B, (1984), *Angew. Makromol. Chem.* 123/124 457.
4. Cammas-Marion S, Okano T, Kataoka K, (1999), *Colloids Surf.* B 16, 207.
5. Israelachvili JN, Mitchel DJ, and Ninham BW, (1976), *J. Chem. Soc., Faraday Trans. II.* 72, 1525.
6. Kataoka K, Harada A, Nagasaki Y (2001), *Adv. Drug Deliv. Rev.* 47, 113.
7. Kataoka K, Kwon GS, Yokoyama M, Okano T, Sakurai Y (1993), *J. Controlled Release* 24, 119.
8. Kramarenko EY, Potemkin II, Khokhlov AR, Winkler RG, Reineker P, (1999). *Macromolecules* 32, 3495.
9. Kunitake T, (1992), *Angew. Chem.* 104, 692.
10. Lobanov PC TVS, Katritzky AR, Shah DO, and Karelson M (1996), *Langmuir*, 12, 1462.
11. Lynn JL and Bory BH (1999), *In: Concise Encyclopaedia of Chemical Technology*, R Kirk, Ed., Wiley, New York, p. 1949.
12. Mackeben S, Muller-Goymann CC, (2000), *Int J Pharm* 196, 207.
13. Moffitt M, Khougaz K, Eisenberg A (1996), Micellization of ionic block copolymers, *Acc. Chem. Res.* 29, 95.
14. Munk P, Prochazka K, Tuzar Z, Webber SE (1998), *Chemtech* 28, 20.
15. Nostrum CFV (2004), *Adv Drug Deliv Rev* 56, 9.
16. Preston WC, (1948) *J. Phys. Colloid Chem.* 52, 84. Drug Deliv. Rev. 53, 95.
17. Tuzar Z, Kratochvil P, (1993). *Surf. Colloid Sci.* 15, 1.
18. Yang L, Alexandridis P, (2000). *Curr. Opin. Colloid Interface Sci.* 5, 132.
19. Zana R, editor. Boca Raton, FL 33487–2742: CRC Press, Taylor and Francis Group; 2005.
20. Moroi Y Micelles: Theoretical and applied aspects. Springer international ed. New York: Springer; (2005).
21. Jones MC, Leroux JC. *Eur J Pharm Biopharm* (1999), 48: 101–11.
22. Bromberg L. *J Control Release* (2008), 128: 99–12.
23. Peng X, Zhang L, Langmuir (2007), 23: 10493–98.
24. Mahmud A, Xiong XB, Aliabadi HM, Lavasanifar A. *J Drug Target* (2007), 15: 553–84.
25. Kataoka K, Harada A, Nagasaki Y. *Adv Drug Del Rev* (2001), 47: 113–31.
26. Zhang J, Ma PX. *Angew Chem Int Ed Engl* (2009), 48: 964–8.
27. Moughton AO, O'Reilly RK. *J Am Chem Soc* (2008), 130: 8714–25.
28. Wang M, Zhang G, Chen D, Jiang M, Liu S. (2001), 34: 7172–8.
29. Webber SE. *J. Phys Chem B* (1998), 102: 2618–26.
30. Martin (ed.), Physical Pharmacy. Lippinkott, Williams and Wilkins, Philadelphia, 1993.
31. Gohy JF. *Adv Polym Sci* (2005), 190: 65–36.
32. Yalkowsky SH. Techniques of Solubilization of Drugs, 2ed. New York, NY : M Dekker; 1981.
33. Torchilin VP. *Cell Mol Life Sci* (2004), 61: 2549–59.
34. Lukyanov AN, Torchilin VP. *Adv Drug Del Rev* 2004; 56: 1273–89.
35. Zhang Y, Jiang M. *Front Chem* (2006), 4: 364–68.
36. Nishiyama N, Kataoka K. Pharmacol Therap (2006), 112: 630–48.
37. Jones and J Leroux. Eur. *J. Pharm. Biopharm.* 48: 101Y111(1999).
38. Xiaoshan Fan, Zibiao Li, Xian Jun Loh. Recent Development of Unimolecular Micelles as Functional Materials and Applications. *Polym. Chem.*, 2016, 7, 5898–919.

11

Liposomes

INTRODUCTION

Liposomes are concentric bilayered vesicles in which an aqueous core is entirely enclosed by a membranous lipid bilayer mainly composed of natural and synthetic phospholipids. The lipid molecules are usually phospholipids-amphipathic moieties with a hydrophilic head group and two hydrophilic lipidic tails. On addition of excess water, such lipidic moieties spontaneously orient to give the most thermodynamically stable conformation, in which polar head groups face outwards into the aqueous medium, and the lipidic chains turn inwards to avoid the water phase, giving rise to double layer or bilayer lamellar structures. Both water and lipid soluble drugs can be entrapped into the liposomes. Hydrophilic drugs can be entrapped in the aqueous environment and lipophilic drugs intercalate within the bilayer region. Liposomes may also contain the glycerol, glycolipids, organic acids, membrane proteins, hydrophilic polymers and other agents depending upon the type of vesicle required.

Some of the advantages of liposomes are as follows:

- Provide selective passive targeting to tumor tissues (liposomal doxorubicin).
- Increased efficacy and therapeutic index.
- Increased stability via encapsulation.

- Reduction in toxicity of the encapsulated agent.
- Site specific effect.
- Improved pharmacokinetic effects (reduced elimination, increased circulation life times)
- Flexibility to couple with site-specific ligands to achieve active targeting.

MECHANISM(S) OF LIPOSOMES FORMATION

In order to understand, why liposomes are formed, when phospholipids are hydrated, it requires a basic understanding of physico-chemical features of phospholipids.

Phospholipids are amphipathic (having affinity for both aqueous and polar moieties) molecules, as they have a hydrophobic tail and a hydrophilic or polar head. The hydrophobic tail is composed of two fatty acid chains containing 10–24 carbon atoms and 0–6 double bonds in each chain. The polar end of the molecule is mainly phosphoric acid bound to a water-soluble molecule. The hydrophilic and hydrophobic domains/segments within the molecular geometry of amphiphilic lipids orient and self-organize in ordered supramolecular structures, when confronted with solvents (Lasic, 1988).

In aqueous medium, the molecules in self-assembled structures are orientated in such a way that the polar portion of the molecule remains in contact with the polar environment and at the same time shields the nonpolar part. Among the amphiphiles used in the drug delivery, viz. soaps, detergents, polar lipids, the latter (polar lipids) are often employed to from concentric bilayered structures. However, in aqueous mixtures, these molecules are able to form various phases, some of them are stable and others remain in the metastable state (Lasic, 1993). At high concentrations of these polar lipids, liquid-crystalline phases are formed that upon dilution with an excess of water can be dispersed into relatively stable colloidal particles. The macroscopic structures most often formed include lamellar, hexagonal or cubic phases dispersed as colloidal nanoconstructs (artificial membranes) referred to as liposomes, hexasomes or cubosomes, respectively (Lasic, 1998).

Molecules of PC are not soluble (rather dispersible) in aqueous milieu in the physical chemistry sense, as in aqueous media they align themselves closely in planer bilayer sheets to minimize the unfavorable interactions between the bulk aqueous phase and long hydrocarbon fatty acyl chain. Such interactions are completely eliminated, when the sheets fold over themselves to form closed, sealed, and concentric vesicles. The large free energy change between an aqueous and hydrophobic environment explains the most favored orientation of lipids to assemble as concentric bilayer structures that excludes confrontation between aqueous and hydrophobic domains. This distinctive behavior derives the lowest free energy state and hence ensures the maximum stability to self-assembled structures (Lasic, 1993). The phosphatidylcholine and its synthetic analogues differ markedly from amphiphilic molecules of other origin (soaps, detergents, lysolecithin) in that they preferably orient to form bilayer sheets rather than miceller structures. This presumably attributed to the double fatty acid chain that imparts the molecule an overall tubular shape, more suitable for assemblage in planer sheets.

In contrast, the detergent molecules with a polar head and single acyl chain acquire a conical shape and facilitate the formation of spherical miceller structures. Depending on the hydrophobic environment and aqueous phase, homogeneous smectic phases of parallel lipid bilayers (lyotropic phases) or heterogeneous dispersion of multilamellar or single-walled liposomes can be observed. At lower water content and higher temperature, other lyotropic liquid crystalline phases exist, such as the hexagonal, the cubic and the ribbon phases (Fig. 11.1).

Phase transition of lipids from a rather closely packed, relatively ordered state (gel phase) to a more loosely packed, less ordered liquid crystal state (fluid phase), where the side chains are capable of more rotational motion that occurs at a very narrow temperature range. Thus, the amphipathic (amphiphilic) nature of phospholipids and their analogs renders them the ability to form closed concentric bilayers in the presence of water. Liposomes (lipid vesicles) are formed, when thin lipid films or lipid cakes (of amphiphilic nature) are hydrated and stacks of liquid crystalline bilayers become fluid and swell. The hydrated lipid sheets detach during agitation and self-close to form large, multilamellar vesicles (MLVs), which prevent interaction of water with the hydrocarbon core of the bilayer at the edges. Once these vesicles are formed, a change in the vesicle shape and morphology requires energy input in the form of sonic energy (sonication to get small unilamellar vesicles, SUVs) and mechanical energy (extrusion to get large unilamellar vesicles, LUVs) (Juliano and Lyton, 1980; Deamer and Uster, 1983) (Fig. 11.1). In order to explain the mechanisms or factors involved in the formation of concentric bilayers, the relationships between self- assemblages of amphiphiles, cholesterol, and energy balance are pivotal. Some of the physicochemical forces responsible for bilayer orientation are discussed in Table 11.1.

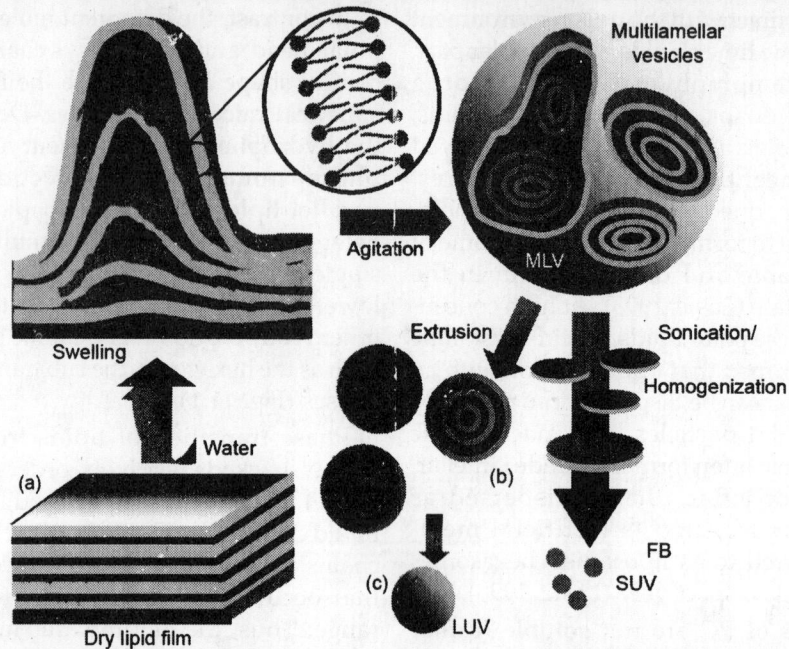

Fig. 11.1: Mechanism of liposome formation and subsequent processing to get various types of vesicles

Table 11.1: The effect of molecular geometry on the structures of amphiphilic aggregates. Cone-like molecules tend to pack into structures with high radii of curvature and inverse cone-like molecules form structures with large negative curvatures. Cylindrical molecules organize into flat lamellar bilayered structure.

Species	Shape	Organization	Phase
Soaps Detergents Lysophospholipids			Isotropic hexagonal 1
Phosphatidylcholine Phosphatidylserine Phosphatidylinositol Sphingomyelin Dicetylphosphate			Lamellar cubic
Phosphatidylethanolamine Phosphatidic acid Cholesterol Cardiolipin Lipid A			Hexagonal 2

Rigidization of Fluid Phase Vesicles with Cholesterol

Cholesterol is known to have important modulatory effect on the bilayer membrane (Papahadjopoulos et al., 1973; Kirby and Gregoriadis, 1980; New, 1989). Cholesterol acts as 'fluidity buffer', since below the phase transition, it tends to make the membrane less ordered while above the transition it tends to make the membrane more ordered, thus suppressing the tilts and shift in membrane structure specifically at the phase transition (Table 11.2).

Though, cholesterol itself does not form bilayers, but it can be incorporated into

Table 11.2: Role of cholesterol (Chol) in bilayer formation

- Acts as a fluidity buffer.
- After intercalation with phospholipid molecules alters the freedom of motion of carbon molecules in the acyl chain.
- Restricts the transformations of trans-to Gauche-conformations.

phospholipid membrane in very high concentrations up to 1:1 or even 2:1 molar ratio of cholesterol to PC. Being an amphipathic molecule, cholesterol inserts into the membrane with its hydroxyl group oriented towards the aqueous surface, and the aliphatic chain aligned parallel to the acyl chains in the centre of the bilayer. Above a certain concentration of cholesterol, the membrane area occupied by the combination of acyl chains and cholesterol is greater than (or equal to) that taken by the phosphocholine head-group.

This could be the possible mechanism for phospholipid membranes with high levels of cholesterol that does not exhibit the chain tilt. The tilt is observed in the gel phase of liposomes composed of pure PC that favors maximum lipid chain interactions. Addition of cholesterol to PC membranes at lower

concentration, has a marginal effect on the transition temperature, but with increased concentration (~50 mole % cholesterol), it eliminates evidence of a phase transition at original T_c altogether by reducing the enthalpy of phase change to zero value. In doing so, it alters the fluidity of the membrane both below and above the phase transition temperature. Below this temperature, the phospholipids are pushed apart, the packing of the head groups is weakened, and the fluidity of the ordered phase is increased. Above the transition temperature, the reduction in freedom for bending of acyl chains causes the membrane to condense and rigidize, with a reduction in area through closer packing and resultant decrease in fluidity. These changes in the fluidity are paralleled by changes in the permeability of the membrane, i.e. decreased by high cholesterol at temperatures higher than the T_c, but increased at lower temperatures. At a ratio of 1:1 of cholesterol to PC, space-filling models show consistent and efficient packing of components in two-dimensional lattice in the form of linear arrays, with rows of cholesterol molecules alternating with rows of phospholipids, such that both cholesterol-cholesterol and cholesterol-PC interactions are favorably possible (Fig. 11.2).

Thus, cholesterol interacts preferentially with the component having the lower transition temperature, i.e. with more fluid phase (and presumably in Gauche-confirmation),

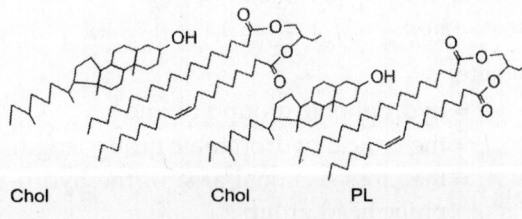

Chol   Chol   PL

Fig. 11.2: The orientation of cholesterol (Chol) in phospholipid (PL) bilayers

which is rigidized in the gel phase with a resultant restriction of the transformations of trans- to Gauche-conformations (New, 1989). It should be emphasized however, that concentration of cholesterol above 50 mole % is difficult to incorporate without disrupting the bilayer configuration and conventional linear structure as it reduces the number of specific intermolecular interactions. The addition of cholesterol to membranes composed of heterogeneous lipids abolishes the phase transitions and alters permeability and fluidity The micelle-forming amphiphiles show relatively high solubility in water (CMC corresponds to CMC about 10^{-3} mol L^{-1}); the concentration in case of membrane forming lipids is significantly low (CMC about 10^{-8} mol L^{-1}). Unfortunately, the prediction of vesicle formation characteristics is not merely a matter of HLB numbers (as in the case of soaps, detergent, etc.), it involves several other factors as suggested by Israelachvili (1991), who described the parameters of self assemblages as a critical packing parameter (CPP). Their self-organization in water is mainly the result of the hydrophobic effect, as in the case of soap and detergent, however, it also depends on the relative proportions of hydrophobicity and hydrophilicity of the lipid, as well as mesogen molecular geometry. The symmetry of lipid self-assembly and liquid crystalline-phase formation shows strong dependence on the molecular shape of the mesogen/amphiphiles. The different shapes and volumes constructing different phases are characterized as dimensionless critical packing parameter (CPP):

$$CPP = n/I_c A_c = A_{hp}/A_p$$

where,

n = hydrophobic group volume

l_c = the critical hydrophobic group length

A_p = the cross-sectional area of the hydrophilic head group

A_{hp} = the cross-sectional area of hydrophobic group.

A CPP below 0.5 (indicating a large contribution from the hydrophilic head group area) is said to give spherical micelles and above 1 (indicating a large contribution from the hydrophobic group volume) should produce inverted micelles. A CPP of between 0.5 and 1 indicates that the cross hydrophilic domains suggests for geometric configuration that is most stable surfactant sectional geometry is hydrophobic; it is likely to form vesicles. For $A_{hp} > A_p$, structures with high curvature (such as micelles) are formed. When the areas are comparable $A_{hp} A_p$, a bilayered configuration is the most stable form, while for $A_{hp} > A_p$, inverse micelles (with negative surface curvature) are formed. Furthermore, in self-assembled multi-component systems, one can define an average value for the two parameters, A_{hp} and A_p, which are typically a linear combination of individuals' areas multiplied by the mole fraction of a contributing molecule.

The molecular shape analysis and the concept of shape parameters (A_{hp}/A_p) are very useful for qualitative understanding of the topology of lipid vesicles based on different lipid compositions. However, one must be careful not to attempt accurate thermodynamic analysis of liposomal models based on these concepts, because such an analysis is generally applied to systems that are at thermodynamic equilibrium. If applied to liposomes containing lipids with a given shape parameter, such an analysis should yield a very narrow size distribution, rather a quite shallow profile as observed in real practice. Such thermodynamic models also predict the spontaneous formation of liposomes; however, a high-energy process is typically needed to produce liposomes (Lasic, 1998).

CLASSIFICATION OF LIPOSOMES

Liposomes may be produced by a wide variety of methods. Their nomenclature also depends upon the method of preparation, structural parameters or special functions assigned to them (Table 11.3). Liposomes are manufactured in majority using various procedures in which the water soluble (hydrophilic) materials are entrapped by using aqueous solution of these materials as hydrating fluid or by addition of drug/drug solution at some stage during the manufacturing of the liposomes. The lipid soluble (lipophilic) materials are solubilized in the organic solution of the lipid dried as film followed by its hydration. These methods involve the loading of the entrapped agents before or during the hydration and preparation (passive loading). However, certain types of compounds with ionizable groups, and those, which display both lipid and water solubility, can be introduced into the liposomes after the formation of intact vesicles (remote loading).

Passive Loading Techniques

Passive loading techniques include three different groups of methods working on different principles namely, mechanical dispersion, solvent dispersion, and detergent solubilization.

Mechanical Dispersion Methods of Passive Loading

All methods covered under this category begin with a lipid solution in organic solvent and end up with lipid dispersion in water. The various components are typically combined by codissolving the lipids in an organic solvent and the organic solvent is then removed by film deposition under vacuum. When the solvent is removed completely, the solid lipid mixture is hydrated using aqueous buffer. The lipids spontaneously swell and hydrate to form liposomes. At this point, methods

Type of vesicles	Size
Table 11.3: Classification of liposomes	
1. Based on the size and number of lamellae	
Multilamellar vesicles (MLVs)	500
Oligolamellar vesicles (OLVs)	100 to 1000
Unilamellar vesicles (ULVs)	20 to >1000
Multivesicular system (MVs)	>1000
Double liposomes	>1000
Depofoam	>1000
2. Based on the method of liposome preparation	
REV	Single/oligomer vesicles made by reverse phase evaporation method
SPLV	Stable plurilamellar vesicles
FATMLV	Frozen and thawed MLV
VET	Vesicle prepared by extrusion technique
DRV	Dehydration-rehydration vesicles
3. Based on composition and application	
Conventional liposomes	Natural or negatively charged phospholipid and cholesterol
Fusogenic liposomes	Reconstituted Sendai virus envelop
pH sensitive liposomes	Phospholipid such as PE or DOPE with CHEMS or OA
Stealth liposomes	PEGylated long circulatory liposomes
Immunoliposomes	Monoclonal antibody anchored liposomes

incorporate some diverge processing parameters in various ways to modify their ultimate properties. These posthydration treatments include vortexing, sonication, freeze thawing, and high-pressure extrusion.

Thin Film Hydration using Handshaking (MLVs) and Nonshaking Methods (ULVs)

In these methods, the mechanical energy required for the swelling of lipids and dispersion of casted lipid film is imparted by manual agitation (hand shaking technique) (Fig. 11.3) or by exposing the film to a stream of water-saturated nitrogen for 15 min followed by swelling in aqueous medium without shaking (nonshaken vesicles).

Proliposomes

In order to increase the surface area of dried lipid film and to facilitate instantaneous hydration, the lipid is dried over a finely divided particulate support, such as powdered sodium chloride, or sorbitol or other polysaccharides. These dried lipid coated particulates are called proliposomes. Proliposomes form dispersion of MLVs on adding water into them, where support is rapidly dissolved and lipid film hydrates to form MLVs. Size of the carriers influences the size and heterogeneity of the liposomes. This method also overcomes the stability problems of liposomes encountered during their storage as dispersion, dry or frozen form. It is ideally suited for preparations, where the material to be entrapped incorporated into lipid membrane. The method is applicable in cases, where 100% entrapment of components is not a requirement rather the stability is an important consideration.

Mechanical Treatment of MLVs

Multilamellar vesicles formed on hydration of dried lipids could be further engineered or modified for their size and other characteristics. A large number of methods are devised to reduce their size and to convert liposomes of the large size range into smaller homogenous vesicles. These include techniques such as microemulsification, extrusion, ultrasonication and use of French pressure cell. A second set of methods is designed to increase the entrapment volume of hydrated lipids, and/or reduce the lamellarity of the vesicles formed. These include procedures such as freeze-drying, freeze thawing, or induction of vesiculation by ions or pH change.

Sonicated Unilamellar Vesicles (SUVs)

At high energy level, the average size of the vesicles is further reduced. This was first

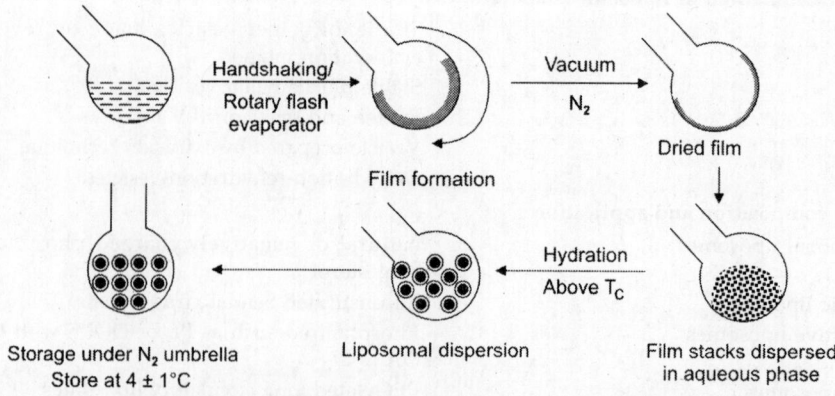

Fig. 11.3: MLVs formed either by handshaking technique using rotary flash evaporation

achieved on exposure of MLVs to ultrasonic irradiation. It still remains the method most widely used for producing small vesicles. Sonication of an MLV dispersion is accomplished by placing a test tube containing the dispersion in a bath sonicator (or placing the tip of the sonicator in the test tube in a probe sonicator) and sonicating for 5–10 min (1,00,000 g) above the T_c of the constituent lipid. The lipid dispersion should begin to clarify to yield a slightly hazy transparent solution. The haze is due to light scattering induced by residual large particles remaining in the dispersion. These particles can be removed using centrifugation to yield a clear SUVs dispersion.

French Pressure Cell Liposomes

The ultrasonic radiation not only degrades the lipids, but also macromolecules and other sensitive compounds, which are to be entrapped in liposomes. One of the first and still very useful methods developed is extrusion of preformed large liposomes using a French press under very high pressure. This technique yields rather uni- or oligolamellar liposomes of intermediate size (30–80 nm in diameter depending on the applied pressure). These liposomes are more stable as compared to sonicated liposomes. The method however, suffers some drawbacks, which include high initial cost of the press that consists of an electric hydraulic press and pressure cell (Fig. 11.4).

Vesicles Prepared by Extrusion Techniques (VETs)

In membrane extrusion method, the size of liposomes is reduced by gently passing them through membrane filter of defined pore size. This can be achieved at much lower pressure (<100 psi.) than required in case of French pressure cell. The membrane extrusion technique can be used to process LUVs as well as MLVs. In this process, the vesicles contents are exchanged with the dispersion medium during breaking and resealing of phospholipid

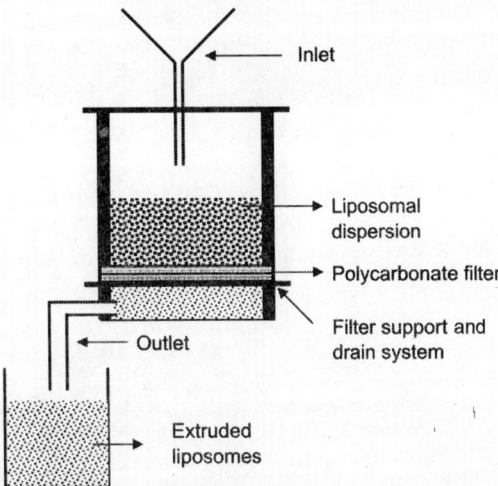

Fig. 11.4: Liposomes preparation using extrusion based on polycarbonate filters

bilayers as they pass through the polycarbonate membrane. In order to achieve high entrapment, the water-soluble compounds should be present in suspending medium during the extrusion process. The liposomes produced by this technique have been termed LUVETs. The capture volume up to 30% can be obtained using high lipid concentration (300 mM PC). The trapped volume in this process is 1–2 litre/mol of lipids.

Dried-reconstituted Vesicles (DRVs)

This method starts with freeze drying dispersion of empty SUVs followed by rehydration using aqueous fluid containing the drug to be entrapped. This leads to a dispersion of solid lipids in finely subdivided form. However, the step of freeze-drying is used to freeze and lyophilize a preformed SUVs dispersion rather than to dry the lipids from an organic solution (as in the case of other methods). This leads to an organized membrane structure as compared to random matrix structure, which on addition of water (one-tenth the volume of the original SUVs) can rehydrate, fuse and reseal to form vesicles with high capture efficiency (Fig. 11.5). The

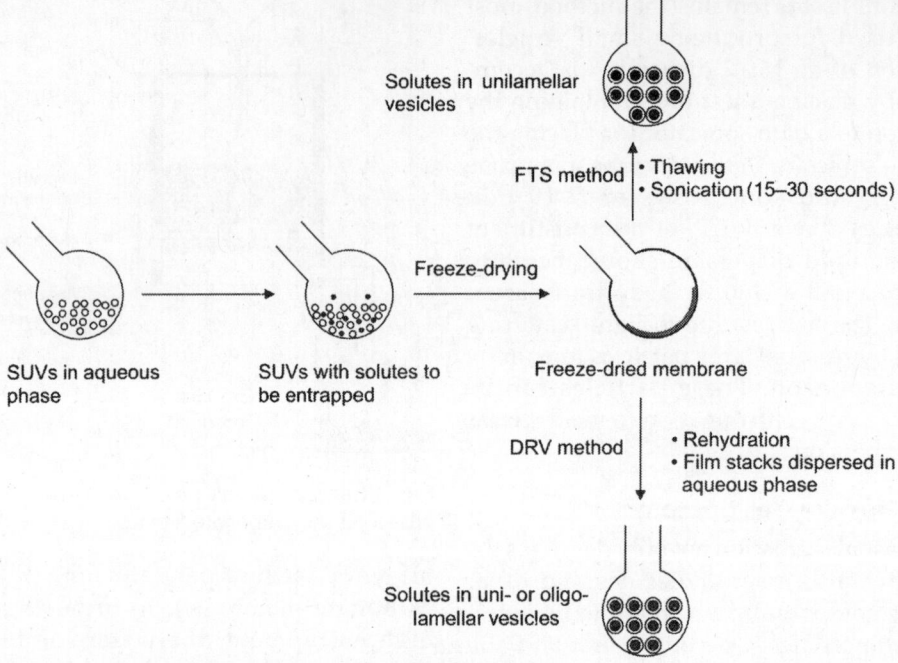

Fig. 11.5: Preparation of dried-reconstituted vesicles (DRVs). Membrane restructures enclosing a proportion of solute, which was originally present in extraliposomal medium

water-soluble materials to be entrapped are added to the dispersion of empty SUVs and they are dried together, so the material for inclusion is present in the dried precursor lipid before the final step of addition of aqueous medium. Liposomes obtained by this method are usually uni- or oligolamellar of the order of 1.0 μm or less in diameter. Entrapment yield can vary, but 40% is fairly standard compared with 2–10% for MLVs prepared by hand-shaking method.

Various advantages proposed for the DRVs technique are high entrapment of water soluble component and the use of mild conditions for the preparation and loading of bioactives. However, this method is suitable only for unilamellar vesicles, (i.e. SUVs), i.e. the liposomes to be freeze-dried should be in the form of unilamellar vesicles as the incorporation rates with multilamellar vesicles are noticeably low.

Freeze Thaw Sonication (FTS) Method

The FTS method is an extension of classical DRV method. The method is based upon freezing of unilamellar (mainly SUVs) dispersion and then thawing by standing at room temperature for 15 min (DRVs method, where the freeze-dried lipids are rehydrated with aqueous buffer) and finally subjected to a brief sonication cycle. Thus, the process ruptures and re-fuses SUVs during which the solute equilibrates between inside and outside, and also inter liposomal fusion takes place with an increase in size. The entrapment volume can be up to 30% of the total volume of the dispersion (10 μl/mg phospholipids). Similar to DRVs, the starting preparation of empty liposomes can be made by sonication and after thawing; the liposomes are subjected to brief sonication again. The second step sonication considerably reduces the permeability of the liposome membrane, perhaps by accelerating the rate at which packing defects are eliminated. In order to prepare giant vesicles of diameter between 10 μm and 50 μm, the freeze thaw technique has been modified to incorporate a dialysis step against hypo-osmolar buffer in place of second step sonication. In this case, SUVs (prior to freeze-thawing step) are first mixed with salt solution followed by freeze-thawing several times. During subsequent dialysis, the large vesicles formed by freeze-thawing swell and rupture, as a result of osmotic lyses, where upon they fuse with each other to yield a large number of giant vesicles. The inclusion of some negatively charged lipids gives yet higher trapped volume (20 μl/mg as compared with 10 μl/mg for neutral phospholipids). The FTS method has several disadvantages compared to DRVs in regard to encapsulation efficiency. Since, the presence of charge is required for the formation of ice crystals to aid in the rupture/fusion process, neutral liposomes cannot be subjected to freezing and thawing method. For similar reasons, sucrose (a cryo-protectant), divalent metal ions (which can neutralize the surface charge) and high ionic-strength salt solutions cannot be entrapped efficiently. Nevertheless, the method is simple, rapid, and mild for entrapped solutes, and results in a high proportion of large unilamellar vesicles formation, which are useful for study of membrane transport phenomenon.

Liposomes from Preformed Vesicles

Several methods of liposome preparation use preformed vesicles and are intended mostly to increase the encapsulation efficiency of the preformed vesicles by using fusion of SUVs by fusogenic agents or by change in the microenvironment of the system.

pH-induced Vesiculation

This method is used to transform MLVs to LUVs using a change in the pH of the dispersion, thus avoids the use of sonication or high-pressure application. The process is an electrostatic event and termed 'pH- induced vesiculation'. The transient change in pH brings about an increase in the surface charge density on the lipid bilayer, which induces spontaneous vesiculation.

The preformed MLVs (prepared using hand shaking followed by freeze-thawing and having a pH of 2.5–3.0) are exposed to high pH (1 M NaOH) to bring the pH 11.0. The period of exposure of liposomes to high pH should be less than 2 min. The exposure time should not be long enough to cause any detectable degradation of the phospholipids. Then the pH is reduced by addition of 0.1 M HCl until a value of pH 7.5 is achieved.

Calcium-induced Fusion

Calcium induced fusion method is principally based upon the concept of aggregation and fusion of acid phospholipid vesicles in the presence of calcium. In this method, SUVs are formed using sonication buffer (NaCl 0.385 g, histidine 31.0 mg, Tris-base 24.2 mg, EDTA 3.72 mg, water 100 mL, pH 7.4) as the hydrating fluid. The large liposomes and lipid particles are removed by centrifugation at 100,000 g. Equimolar proportion of calcium solution ($CaCl_2$) is added to phospholipids in the supernatant resulting in the formation of a white flocculent precipitate. It is incubated for 60 min at 37°C and the precipitate (pellet) is separated by spinning the contents at 3000 g for 20 min at room temperature, where the supernatant is discarded. The pellet is re-suspended in a buffered saline containing the material to be entrapped, and incubated at 37°C for 10 min. The addition of EDTA to the pellet suspension with mixing, results in the formation of a cloudy dispersion, which clears rapidly and incubated for 15 min at 37°C and further 15 min at room temperature. Finally, the Ca-EDTA complex is removed by dialysis of the dispersion overnight against a liter of phosphate saline buffer.

The method has the advantage, that it does not expose lipids or entrapped materials to deleterious chemical or physical conditions. Its principal drawback is the requirement of acidic phospholipids and the residual presence of calcium inside the liposomes, even after dialysis.

Cochleate Method

Cochleates are formed when small unilamellar vesicles made from negatively charged lipids mainly phosphatidylserine (PS) fuse into cylindrical rolls, termed as cochleate cylinders, upon addition of Ca^{++} ions. Subsequent removal of Ca^{++} by EDTA or by ion exchange or precipitation, results in the formation of large unilamellar vesicles. Concentration of Ca^{++} required to reproduce such effects vary for the nature of lipids used, for PS, it should be slightly above the half of the lipid concentration, while cardiolipin (CL) and especially for PG higher overages (conc. of Ca^+) are required.

Solvent Dispersion Methods for Passive Loading

In solvent dispersion method, lipids are first dissolved in an organic solution, which is then brought into contact with an aqueous phase containing materials to be entrapped within the liposomes. The lipids align themselves at the interface of organic and aqueous phase forming monolayer of phospholipids, which forms the half of the bilayer of the liposome. Methods employing solvent dispersion can be categorized on the basis of the miscibility of the organic solvent and aqueous solution. These include the conditions, where the organic solvent is miscible with the aqueous phase; the organic solvent is immiscible with the aqueous phase, the latter being in excess; and the cases, where the organic solvent is in excess, and immiscible with the aqueous phase.

Ethanol Injection

This method has been reported as one of the alternatives used for the preparation of SUVs without sonication. An ethanol solution of lipids is injected rapidly through a fine needle into an excess of saline or other aqueous medium. The rate of the injection is usually sufficient to achieve complete mixing, so that the ethanol is diluted almost instantaneously in water, and phospholipid molecules are dispersed evenly throughout the medium (Fig. 11.6). This procedure yields a high proportion of SUVs (~25 nm), although lipid aggregates and larger vesicles may form, if the mixing is not thorough enough. This method is extremely simple and has low risk of degradation of sensitive lipids. The major short coming of the method is the limitation of the solubility of lipids in ethanol and volume of ethanol that can be introduced into medium (7.5% v/v maximum), which in turn limits quantity of lipid dispersed, so that resulting liposomal dispersion gets diluted. Another drawback is residual ethanol from phospholipid membrane that is difficult to remove.

Ether Injection

Ether injection method is similar to the ethanol injection method, however, it contrasts markedly with ethanol injection in many respects. It involves injecting the immiscible organic solution into an aqueous phase through a narrow needle at the temperature, at which organic solvent vaporizes (Fig. 11.6). This method may also treat sensitive lipids very gently. It has little risk of causing oxidative degradation provided ether is free from peroxides. The disadvantages of the technique are the long-time taken to produce a batch of liposomes and a careful control needed for introduction of the lipid solution, requiring a mechanically operated pump. If substances are degraded at elevated temperature (60°C), then the fluorinated hydrocarbons (Freons) may be used instead of ether. The efficiency of encapsulation is relatively low, although the captured volume per mole of lipid remains high, 8–17 L/mol.

Rapid Solvent Exchange Vesicles (RSEVs)

Rapid solvent exchange method has been a recent addition to the field of methodology used in liposome preparation. In this method principally, the lipid mixture is quickly

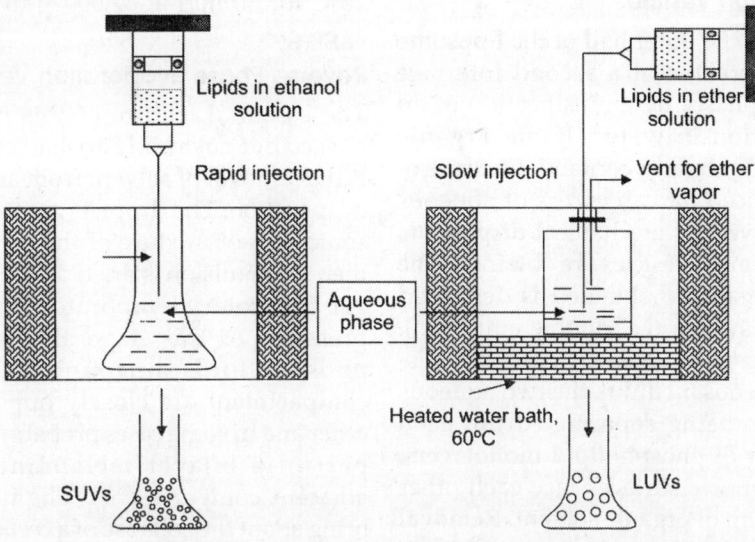

Fig. 11.6: Principle of vesicle formation by ethanol and ether injection

transferred between an essentially pure solvent environment and a pure aqueous environment. This method is specifically designed to form compositionally homogenous dispersion by sudden precipitation of a lipid mixture in an aqueous buffer. Phospholipid/cholesterol dispersion turns to be free of artifactual crystals, when prepared by rapid solvent exchange method.

The method involves passing the lipids solution (organic) through the orifice of blue-tipped syringe (injection needle) under the vacuum into a tube containing aqueous buffer. The tube is mounted on a vortexer. Bulk solvent vaporizes and removed within seconds before coming in contact with aqueous environment, while the lipid mixture rapidly precipitates in aqueous buffer. Since the method is devised specifically for the fast and efficient removal of organic solvent, it does not require a highly volatile solvent. RES liposomes require not more than a minute for preparation and manifest high entrapment volumes with a high fraction of external surface area with no evidence of artifactual demixing as observed with conventional solvent dispersion methods.

De-emulsification Methods

This method requires two steps for the preparation of liposomes, first the inner leaflet of the bilayer, then the outer half. The common feature of this method is the formation of 'water in oil' emulsion by introduction of a small quantity of aqueous medium containing material to be entrapped into a large volume of immiscible organic solution of lipid. This was followed by mechanical agitation to break-up the aqueous phase into microscopic water droplets. These droplets are stabilized by the presence of phospholipid monolayer at the interface. The size of droplets is determined by the intensity of mechanical energy used to form the emulsion and amount of lipid relative to the volume of aqueous phase, since each droplet requires a complete monolayer of phospholipid covering its surface in order to prevent the possible coalescence with other droplets. The aqueous solution surrounded by the monolayer of phospholipid forms the central core of the final liposome. There are number of methods, which could be used for preparing droplets including double emulsion, reverse phase evaporation and sonication methods.

Double Emulsion Vesicles

In this method, the outer half of the liposome membrane is created at a second interface between two phases by emulsification of an organic solution in water. If the organic solution, which already contains water droplet, is introduced into an excess of aqueous medium followed by mechanical dispersion, multi-compartment vesicles are obtained. The ordered dispersion so obtained is described as a W/O/W system (i.e. double emulsion). These vesicles with aqueous core are suspended in aqueous medium, the two aqueous compartments being separated from each other by a pair of phospholipid monolayers, whose hydrophobic surfaces face each other across a thin film of organic solvent. Removal of this solvent clearly results in an intermediate-sized unilamellar vesicle. The theoretical entrapment may reach up to 90% (Fig. 11.7).

The double emulsion is prepared by rapidly injecting the dispersion of microdroplets into hot aqueous solution of Tris-buffer with the help of 22-gauge hypodermic needle under vigorous stirring. Organic solvent is evaporated using strong jet of nitrogen, thus forming double emulsion. Organic solvent is removed completely by evaporation and finally the volume is adjusted by adding extra-distilled water and then the product is centrifuged at 20°C for 30 min at 37,000 g to remove lipid aggregates.

Reverse Phase Evaporation Vesicles

The essential feature of this method, established by Szoka and Papahadjopoulos (1978), is the removal of solvent from an emulsion by evaporation. The droplets are formed by bath sonication of mixture of the two phases, and then the emulsion is dried down to a semisolid gel in a rotary evaporator under reduced pressure. At this stage, the monolayers of phospholipids surrounding each water compartment are closely opposed by each other and in some cases probably already form part of a bilayer membrane separating adjacent compartments. The next step is to bring about the collapse of a certain proportion of the water droplets by vigorous mechanical shaking using a vortex mixer. In these circumstances, the lipid monolayer, which enclosed the collapsed vesicle, is contributed to adjacent intact vesicle to form the outer leaflet of the bilayer of a large unilamellar liposome. The aqueous content of the collapsed droplet provides the medium required for dispersion of these newly formed liposomes. After conversion of the gel into a homogenous free flowing fluid, the dispersion is dialyzed to remove the last traces of solvent. The vesicles formed are unilamellar and have

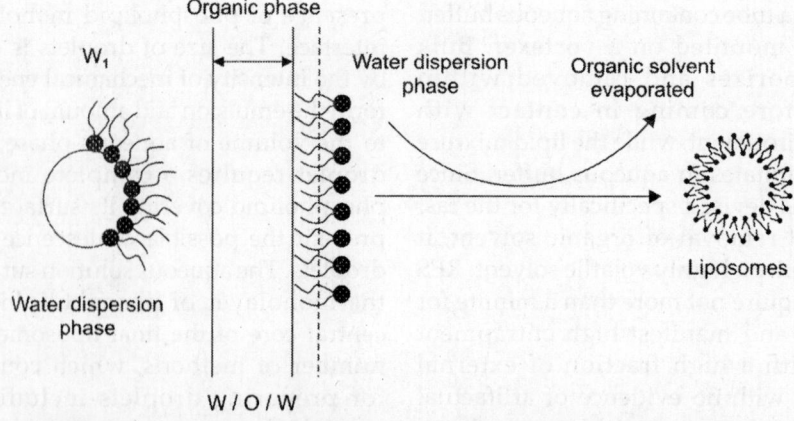

Organic phase

W_1

Water dispersion phase

Organic solvent evaporated

Liposomes

Water dispersion phase

W / O / W

Fig. 11.7: Formation of liposomes by double emulsion vesicle method

an average diameter of 0.5 micrometer. The encapsulation efficiency is found to be nearly 50% (Fig. 11.8).

Stable Plurilamellar Vesicles (SPLVs)

The method of plurilamellar vesicle formation involves preparation of water-in-organic phase dispersion with an excess of lipid followed by drying using continued bath sonication with an intermittent stream of nitrogen. The redistribution and equilibration of aqueous solvent and solute occurs in between the various bilayers in each plurilamellar vesicle. The internal structure of SPLVs is different from that of MLV-REVs, in that they lack a large aqueous core, the majority of the entrapped aqueous medium being located in the compartments in between adjacent lamellae. The percent entrapment normally ranges around 30% (compared with > 60% for MLV-REVs).

Detergent Depletion (Removal) Methods of Passive Loading

In these methods, the phospholipids are brought into intimate contact with the aqueous phase via detergents, which associate with phospholipid molecules and serve to screen the hydrophobic portions of the molecule from water. The structures formed as a result of this association are known as micelles, and can be composed of several hundreds of component molecules. Their shape and size depend on chemical nature of the detergent, the concentration and other lipids involved. The concentration of detergent in water at which micelles just start to form is known as the 'critical micelle concentration' (CMC). Below the CMC, the detergent molecules exist entirely in free solution. As detergent is dissolved in water in concentration higher than the CMC, micelles form in more and more numbers, while the concentration of detergent in the free form remains essentially the same as it is at the CMC. Micelles containing other participating components in addition to the detergent (or composed of two or more detergents) in their formation are known as 'mixed micelles'. As a general rule, membrane-solubilizing detergents have a higher affinity for phospholipid membranes than for the pure detergent micelles. Thus, as detergent is added in increasing amounts to the membrane preparation, more and more detergent gets incorporated into the bilayer, until a point is reached, where a transition from the lamellar to the spherical micellar phase configuration takes place. As the detergent concentration increases further, the

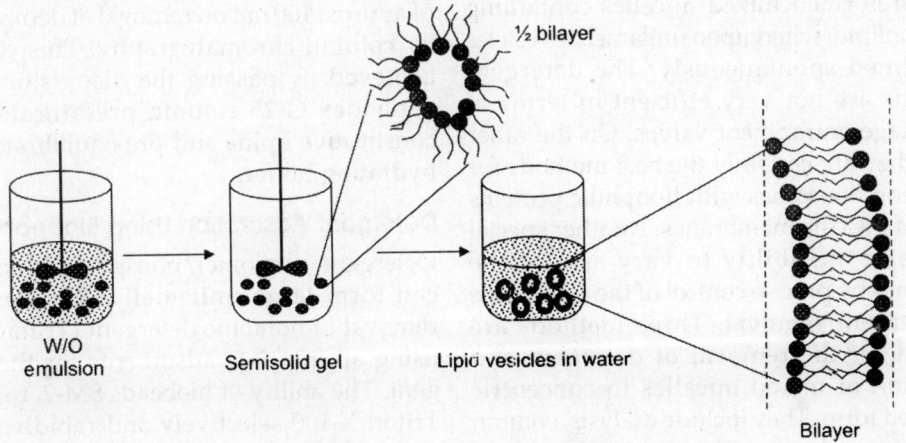

½ bilayer

W/O emulsion   Semisolid gel   Lipid vesicles in water   Bilayer

Fig. 11.8: Preparation reverse phase evaporation vesicles

micelles are reduced in size until they become saturated with detergent, whereupon the concentration of free molecules equals the CMC and simple detergent micelles are formed. It is usually found that a high concentration is advantageous for solubilizing membrane phospholipids, although one might expect the converse, since a high affinity for lipid membranes should be reflected by a low CMC. A three-stage model for the interaction of detergents with the lipid bilayers with increasing detergent/lipid ratio was proposed.

- At low (sublytic) concentrations detergent equilibrates between vesicular lipid and water phase (stage-I). At this stage, mean vesicle size increases with changing functional properties of the bilayer.
- After reaching a critical detergent concentration ('saturation' of the bilayers), membrane structure tends to be unstable and transforms gradually into micelles (stage-II). In this stage detergent saturated bilayers coexist with lipid-saturated micelles.
- At stage-III, all lipids exist in mixed micelle form.

Invariably in all methods, which employ detergent in the preparation of liposomes, the basic feature is to remove the detergent from preformed mixed micelles containing phospholipid, whereupon unilamellar vesicles are formed spontaneously. The detergent methods are not very efficient in terms of percentage entrapment values. On the other hand, they are certainly the best methods for preparing liposomes with lipophilic proteins inserted into the membranes. Another special feature is the ability to vary size of the liposomes by precise control of the conditions of detergent removal. Three methods are applied for the removal of detergent and transition of mixed micelles to concentric bilayered form. They include dialysis, column chromatography and the use of biobeads.

Dialysis

In contrast to phospholipids, detergents are highly soluble in both aqueous and organic media and there is equilibrium between the detergent molecules in the water phase, and in the lipid environment of the micelle. The critical micelle concentration can give an indication to the position of this equilibrium. Upon lowering the concentration of detergent in the bulk aqueous phase, the molecules of detergent can be removed from mixed micelle by dialysis. A higher CMC indicates that the equilibrium is strongly shifted towards the bulk solution, so that removal from the mixed membrane by dialysis becomes relatively easy.

Detergents commonly used for this purpose exhibit reasonably high CMC (~10–20 mM) so that their removal is facilitated. They include the bile salts, sodium cholate and sodium deoxycholate, and synthetic detergents, such as octylglucoside. The treatment of egg PC with sodium cholate (2:1 molar ratio) followed by dialysis results in the formation of vesicles (~100 nm). A commercial version of the dialysis system is available under the trade name LIPOREPTM.

Column Chromatography

Phospholipids in the form of either sonicated vesicles or as a dry film, at a molar ratio of 2:1 with deoxycholate form unilamellar vesicles of approx. 100 nm on removal of deoxycholate by column chromatography. This could be achieved by passing the dispersion over a Sephadex G-25 column presaturated with constitutive lipids and pre-equilibrated with hydrating buffer.

Detergent Adsorption Using Biobeads

Detergent (nonionic)/phospholipid mixtures can form large unilamellar vesicles upon removal of nonionic detergent (Triton X-100) using appropriate adsorbents for the detergent. The ability of biobeads SM-2, to adsorb Triton X-100 selectively and rapidly, makes them a suitable candidate for LUV preparation by detergent solubilization method. On hydration of the casted lipid film with 0.5–1.0 % Triton X-100, washed biobeads are added to the dispersion (0.3 g wet biobeads per ml of dispersion) and rocked for about 2 hours at 4 ±1°C.

Remote (Active) Loading

A general scheme describing various types of liposomes is presented with their preparation methodology. The utilization of liposomes as drug delivery systems is stimulated with the advancements of efficient encapsulation procedures. The membrane from lipid bilayer is in general impermeable to ions and larger hydrophilic molecules. Ions transport can be regulated by the ionophores, while permeation of neutral and weakly hydrophobic molecules can be controlled by concentration gradients. Some weak acids or bases, however, can be transported through the membrane due to various transmembrane gradients, such as electrical, ionic (pH) or specific salt (chemical potential) gradients. Several methods exist for improved loading of the drugs, including remote (active) loading methods, which load drug molecules into preformed liposomes using pH gradients and potential difference across liposomal membranes. A concentration difference in proton concentration across the membrane of liposomes, can drive the loading of amphipathic molecules. Active loading methods have the following advantages over passive encapsulation techniques:

- A high encapsulation efficiency and capacity
- A reduced leakage of the encapsulated compounds.
- 'Bed side' loading of drugs thus limiting loss of retention of drugs by diffusion, or chemical degradation during storage
- Flexibility for the use of constitutive lipids, as drug is loaded after the formation of carrier units.
- Avoidance of biologically active compounds during preparation steps in the dispersion, thus reducing safety hazards.

- The transmembrane pH gradient can be developed using various methods depending upon the nature of the drug to be encapsulated.
- For amphipathic weak bases drug loading could be affected by remote loading procedures, such as using a proton gradient or an ammonium sulfate gradient.
- For amphipathic weak acids drug loading could be affected by using remote loading procedures using a calcium acetate gradient. The weak amphipathic bases tend to accumulate in the aqueous phase of lipid vesicles in response to a difference in pH between the inside and outside of the liposomes (pH-in and pH-out). The pH gradient is created by preparing liposomes with a low pH inside and outside the vesicles, followed by the addition of the base to the extraliposomal medium. Usually, a two-step process generates this pH imbalance and remote loading—first, the vesicles are prepared at a low pH solution, thus generating a low-pH within the liposomal interiors, followed by the addition of the base to the extraliposomal medium. Basic compounds, carrying amino groups are relatively lipophilic at high pH and hydrophilic at low pH. In a two-chambered aqueous system separated by the membrane of liposomes), accumulation occurs at the low-pH side, under dynamic equilibrium conditions. Thus, the unprotonated form of basic drug can diffuse through the bilayer. At the low-pH inside, molecules are predominantly protonated, which lowers the concentration of the drug in the unprotonated form, and thus promotes the diffusion of more drug molecules at the low-pH side of the bilayer. The second step involves the exchange of external medium by gel-exclusion chromatography with a neutral solution. Weak bases like doxorubicin, adriamycin and vincristine, which coexist in aqueous solutions in neutral and charged forms have

been successfully loaded into preformed liposomes via the pH-gradient method. Similarly, short modified peptides and insulin (FITC-insulin), were also loaded successfully in large unilamellar vesicles through pH gradients (inside acidic). Recently, the approach has been further modified using transmembrane differences in salt concentrations, such as ammonium sulfate amine gradient or calcium acetate gradient. This technique takes advantage of the large differences in the permeability coefficients across lipid bilayer of the sulfate anion (P < 10–12 cm/s) and of the ammonia molecule (P = 0.13 cm/s), generated by the dissociation of the ammonium cation. This results into an increase in liposomal internal pH. In addition, the sulfate salt of this molecule has a very low solubility and aggregates inside the liposomes, resulting in even larger encapsulation efficiencies and the stabilization. Figure 11.9 explains a schematic of transmembrane gradient-mediated remote loading of drugs into

LUVs comprising a pH. LUVs were prepared by hydration of dry lipids in 300 mM aqueous amine solution and subsequent extrusion (A). After exchange and equilibration of external amine with 150 mM NaCl or MES/NaCl buffer on a Sephadex G-50 spin column the amine equilibrates leading to a pH (inside acidic) as the neutral form crosses the bilayer (B). The neutral form of externally added drug can cross the bilayer and gets protonated in the process and as a result trapped within vesicle (C).

Similarly, acetate gradient method takes the advantage of the large differences in permeability coefficients across lipid bilayer of the cation and acetic acid molecules, generated on dissociation of the acetate anion. Then this transmembrane pH difference (inside base, outside acid) is used as a driving force for the remote loading of an amphipathic weak acid, since the dissociated part of the acid cannot permeate through the liposomal membrane.

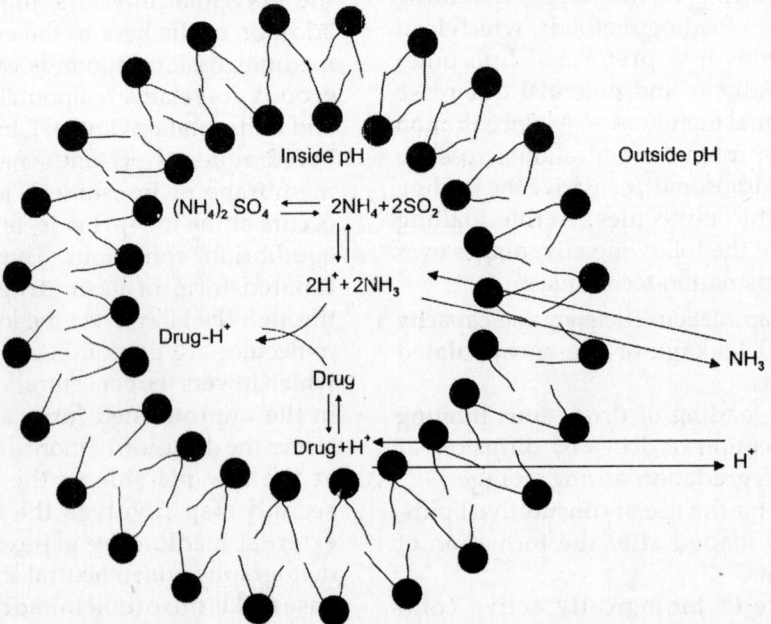

Fig. 11.9: Active loading of a drug into preformed liposomes by a pH gradient, which is obtained by $(NH_4)_2$ SO_4 gradient. Solid arrows indicate the shifts in equilibria resulting in the increased entrapment of the drug

CHARACTERIZATION OF LIPOSOMES

Liposomal formulations after their preparation and processing for a specified purpose are characterized to ensure their predictable *in vitro* and *in vivo* performances. The liposomes produced by different techniques, may have different physicochemical characteristics. These differences do have an impact on their behavior *in vivo* (disposition) and *in vitro*, (e.g. sterilization and shelflife). The characterization parameters for the purpose of evaluation could be classified into three broad categories, which include physical, chemical, and biological parameters. Physical characterization evaluates various parameters, including size, shape, surface features, lamellarity, phase behavior and drug release profile. Chemical characterization includes those studies, which establish the purity and potency of various liposomal constituents. Biological characterization parameters are likewise helpful in establishing the safety and suitability of the formulations for their *in vivo* use or therapeutic applications. Some of the parameters characterized in liposome product development are size and size distribution, surface topology, encapsulation efficiency, capture volume, lamellarity and *in vitro* drug release profile.

Vesicle Size and Size Distribution

The average vesicle size and size distribution are important parameters as far as *in vitro* characterization of the liposomal product is concerned. This is because they influence the physicochemical properties and biological fate of the liposomes and/or entrapped materials following *in vivo* administration. Various techniques are described in the literature for the determination of size and size distribution. These include light microscopy, fluorescent microscopy (if a fluorescent probe is included in either lipid or aqueous domain), electron microscopy (especially transmission electron microscopy and freeze-fracture microscopy), laser light scattering, photon correlation spectroscopy, field flow fractionation, gel permeation and gel exclusion and zetasizer. Most of the methods used in the size, shape and distribution analysis can be grouped into various categories, namely microscopic, diffraction and scattering and hydrodynamic techniques.

Vesicle Shape and Lamellarity

Vesicle shape can be assessed using various electron microscopic techniques, which can also be extended to determine the average size of the vesicles. The lamellarity of MLVs is heterogeneous and usually, it is unilamellar as well as multilamellar.

Surface Charge

Liposomes are usually prepared using charge imparting constituting lipids and hence, it is imperative to study the charge on the vesicle surface. In general two methods are used to assess the charge, namely free-flow electrophoresis and zeta-potential measurement. From the mobility of the liposomal dispersion in a suitable buffer (determined using Helmholtz-Smoluchowski equation), the surface charge on the vesicles can be calculated.

Encapsulation Efficiency and Trapped Volume

Encapsulation efficiency and trapped volume determine the amount and rate of entrapment of water-soluble agents in the aqueous compartment of liposomes.

Encapsulation Efficiency

The encapsulation efficiency describes the percent of the aqueous phase and hence the percent of water-soluble drug that becomes ultimately entrapped during preparation of liposomes and is usually expressed as % entrapment/mg lipid. Encapsulation efficiency is assessed using two techniques including minicolumn centrifugation method and protamine aggregation method.

Minicolumn centrifugation is generally used both as a means of purification and separation of liposomes on a small scale and analysis of a liposomal dispersion to determine encapsulation efficiency. A Sephadex or Sepharose column pre-saturated with the dispersion medium in 1.0 ml disposable syringe is run while applying liposomal dispersion (200 µl) first and saline (250 µl) thereafter and centrifuging the column at 2000 rpm for 3 min and assaying the elutes. Depending upon the different molecular weights of solutes entrapped, various medium and their molecular cut-off point should be chosen. The concentration of free or entrapped material in elutes can be assessed by disrupting liposomes using ethanol (2 ml ethanol for 10 µl of liposomes) or Triton X-100 (10 µl of 10% Triton X-100 for 10 µl of liposomes) and estimating the released contents using standard methods of separation. The lipid concentration can be assessed using Barlett assay.

Protamine aggregation method may be used for neutral and negatively charged liposomes. Liposomal dispersion (~100 µl) can be precipitated with a protamine solution (100 µl, 10 mg µl^{-1}) and subsequent centrifugation at 2000 rpm. By analyzing the material in the supernatant and in the liposome pellet after disrupting liposomal pellet with 0.6 ml of 10% Triton X-100, the encapsulation efficiency of the entrapped material can be estimated.

THERAPEUTIC APPLICATIONS OF LIPOSOMES

Liposomes are used for the following range of therapeutic and pharmaceutical applications:

Liposomes as Drug/Protein Delivery Vehicles

- Controlled and sustained drug release *in situ*
- Enhanced drug solubilization
- Altered pharmacokinetics and biodistribution
- Enzyme replacement therapy and lysosomal storage disorders

Liposomes in Antimicrobial, Antifungal (Lung Therapeutics) and Antiviral (Anti-HIV) Therapy

- Liposomal drugs
- Liposomal biological response modifiers

Liposomes in Tumor Therapy

- Carrier of small cytotoxic molecules
- Vehicle for macromolecules as cytokines or genes

Liposomes in Gene Delivery

- Gene and antisense therapy
- Genetic (DNA) vaccination

Liposomes in Immunology

- Immunoadjuvant
- Immunomodulator
- Immunodiagnosis

Liposomes as Drug Delivery Vehicles

Several modes of drug delivery applications have been proposed for the liposomal systems for some of the opportunistic diseases. The major ones are enhanced drug solubilization (amphotericin B, minoxidil, paclitaxel, cyclosporin), protection of sensitive drug molecules (cytosine arabinose, DNA, RNA, antisense oligonucleotides, ribozymes), enhanced intracellular uptake (anticancer, antiviral and antimicrobial drugs), altered pharmacokinetics and biodistribution (prolonged or sustained release of drugs with short circulatory half-lives). Various advantages are cited for adopting liposomes as versatile delivery systems include:

- The delivery of liposomes could be beneficial for drugs that are rapidly excreted or metabolized.
- An undesirable 'saw-tooth' pattern of circulating drug levels observed in conventional dosage forms can be avoided.
- In common with colloidal carrier systems of other types, liposomes can also provide relatively constant and sustained bloodstream levels of certain types of drugs.

- In contrast to sustained release formulations composed of artificial polymers, liposomes can be injected into the circulation, and thus can serve as an 'intravascular drug depot'.
- The use of liposomal sustained release preparations may be of significant value for drugs with low 'therapeutic windows' or low-water solubility or which require administration by intravenous route.
- Passive macrophage targeting and RES-accumulation can be beneficial in the treatment of ailments caused due to intracellular pathogens using conventional liposomes.

Surface engineered versions of liposomes may effectively circumvent passive uptake by RES-predominant organs and further increase in circulation time and hence effective sustained action than conventional liposomes (active targeting) could be harnessed.

Increased Therapeutic Index

The delivery aspect of liposomes could also be exploited for drugs that have to penetrate the plasma membrane in order to be therapeutically beneficial. The use of liposomal carrier system offers a way of surpassing the membrane barriers (as they structurally mimic natural membrane) and of promoting the non-specific entry of drugs into the cellular interiors. For example, in the case of anti-tumor drug, cytosine arabinoside triphosphate (ara-CTP), the tumor cell population often acquires resistance by reducing the level of deoxycytidine kinase, the first enzyme in the pathway that activates the drug. The drug administration in the liposomal form alleviates the problem of reduced enzyme level. In fact, liposome encapsulation hinders the active transport or passive diffusion (general course of drug uptake of the cells), however, in cases of genetically determined resistance as in the case of tumor cells, the liposomes are of immense value in overcoming the permeability barrier and thus could negotiate the therapeutic effects.

Liposomes in Antimicrobial, Antifungal (Lung Therapeutics) and Antiviral (Anti-HIV) Therapy

Intracellular pathogens (protozoal, bacterial and fungal) reside in the liver and spleen, and offer a targeting opportunity to these organs using liposomes as a carrier system. Due to intrinsic passive vectorization to RES-predominant organs, liposomes offer enormous opportunities to target diseases relating to intracellular pathogens like leishmaniasis, candidiasis, aspergillosis, histoplasmosis, cryptococosis, girardiasis, malaria, and tuberculosis. Liposome-mediated treatment of fungal, viral, bacterial and protozoal infections take the advantage of the passive targeting of liposomes to the RES-predominant organs as well as their 'lysosomotropism' and 'parasitotropism'.

Leishmaniasis infection in human is manifested in three different forms, i.e. visceral leishmaniasis (Kala-azar caused by *L. donovani*), mucocutaneous leishmaniasis (*L. mexicana*) and cutaneous leishmaniasis (*L. tropica*). The drugs of first choice are the pentavalent antimonials, meglumine amtimonate and sodium stilbogluconate whilst the second choice drug, amphotericin B, is dose-compromised because of hepatic, gastrointestinal, cardiac, and renal toxicities. However, on administration of liposomal form of these drugs, exceptional hepatosplenic accumulation of encapsulated drug was observed with minimal toxic side effects. Similarly, the existence of malaria parasite in the hepatocytes and possibly the Kupffer cells in its tissue stage resulted in investigations on use of the liposomes in treatment of malaria. The uptake of liposome entrapped primaquine was shown to occur initially in the Kupffer cells as expected with subsequent intrahepatic redistribution of liposomal contents to the hepatocytes.

The lysomotrophic nature of liposomes also makes them a suitable carrier to target facultative intracellular bacteria (*Brucella, Listeria, Mycobacteria, Legionella, Salmonella, Klebsiella, Escherichia* spp.) with loaded antibiotics. Fusion of liposomes and cell after being uptaken by RES-predominant organs, sustained release of the antibiotic, protection of drug from *in vivo* enzymatic hydrolysis, and increased local concentration of drug are some probable mechanisms considered for better therapeutic effects. The potential for liposomal delivery in bacterial infections at sites other than RES organs is quite vague (except where lipid-based delivery systems reduce the toxicity of the drug and provide a sustained release of the loaded antimicrobial agent). However, in recent years these problems have also been curtailed with the use of ligand-mediated targeting (active targeting) and by applying inverse targeting approaches. These strategies either exploit a recognition port on the target cell, where liposomes get anchored through suitable site-directing ligands and destined to the target sites (active targeting), or provide them a long-circulatory or stealth behavior, which permits targeting to sites other than RES (inverse targeting). Liposomes anchored with glycolipids having terminal galactose residues and liposomes constructed of mannosylated phospholipids (to be recognized by receptors present on Kupffer cells of the liver), were appreciated for active targeting of the entrapped contents to the target site.

Moreover, the most important and commercially successful features of therapeutics are the exploitation of liposomes as a carrier for antifungal agents in the treatment of systemic fungal diseases mainly candidiasis.

Amphotericin B Liposomes

Systemic fungal infections are associated with increasing frequency in the immunocompromised patient. Although, restricted by a variety of side and toxic effects, parenteral amphotericin B (Amp B) is still the drug of choice in most invasive fungal infections. Recent advances are focused on the improvement of its therapeutic index, though reduction of Amp B toxicity by its incorporation in lipid carriers. Several lipid formulations of Amp B are available in the market and include Fungizone (Bristol Myers-Squibb, Woerden, The Netherlands), AmBisome™ (Nexstar, Boulder, CO, USA), ABELECT™ (The Liposome Company, Princeton, NJ, USA), and AMPHOTEC™ (Sequus Pharmaceuticals, Merlo, CA, USA).

Liposomes in Tumor Therapy

Most of the medical applications of liposomes that have reached the preclinical and clinical stages are in cancer treatments. Several clinical studies did not support the use of conventional liposomes in cancer treatment. Although, it is still not clear whether such liposomes (especially the ones which are remote loaded with anthracyclines) can be beneficial in cancer therapy. It has been demonstrated that small and stable liposomes can passively target several different tumors because they can (owing to their biological stability and size) circulate for prolonged times and extravasate (owing to their small size, 50–150 nm) in tissues with an enhanced vascular permeability, which is often the case with tumors. However, recent trends in research predominately opt for specially engineered-long-circulatory liposomes (stealth liposomes) to make certain, the long circulation times and increased probability of their extravasation to the tumor vascular endothelium.

Targeting strategies using liposomes can be designed by following different ways:

- Natural targeting (lysosomotropism) of conventional liposomes (passive vectorization).
- Use of long-circulatory (stealth liposomes).
- Use of ligand mediated targeting (active targeting).
- The use of antireceptor antibodies or antibodies developed against specific-surface antigens on the tumor-vascular endothelium.

- The use of angiogenic peptides and adhesion molecules as ligands against receptors expressed on tumor vascular endothelium.
- Use of stealth liposomes and ligand-mediated targeting in combination.

Sterically-stabilized (Stealth) Liposomes (SSL)

The old dream of site-specific drug targeting requires properly designed and intelligent delivery systems that avoid scavenging through receptor-mediated uptake by mononuclear phagocytic cells of RES-rich organs. Moreover, several targeting strategies require the system to be placed either into tumor cells or extravasation into non-RES cellular lineage. As a matter of fact, recently described approaches which avoid RES-uptake of the drug-carrier composites, lead to the concept of ligand-appended system(s) long circulatory in nature (stealth systems), which resist opsonization and serum protein binding to the surface. Sterically-stabilized liposomes, thus avoid their recognition through RES uptake and this 'stealthing' effect makes them long circulatory in nature (Fig. 11.10).

GM1- and PEG-coated Liposomes

The original research in the field concentrated on the effects of glycolipids and gangliosides, primarily monosialogangiosides GM1 or phosphatidylinositol, in prolonging the circulation half-life and altering the biodistribution of liposomes (categorically known as 'first generation long circulatory liposomes'). However, recent advances in the field of stealth systems have focused on the effect of hydrophilic polymers, such as polyethyleneglycol (PEG) linked by various means to the lipid molecules ('second generation of long circulatory liposomes').

The colloidal basis for this approach is called 'steric stabilization', which due to osmotic and entropic effects of an inert, nonionic, hydrophilic, and flexible polymer coating, increases repulsive forces, which operate on these modified surfaces, resulting in the reduced interaction and adsorption of plasma proteins.

Several attempts have been made to understand the underlying mechanisms. The majority of them however, are based upon the following attributes:

Long circulatory behavior imparted on first-generation long circulatory liposomes could be ascribed to one of the following strategies, either independently or in combinations:

1. Glycocalyx similar to red blood cells (RBC), which is instrumental in providing ability to the surface-modified liposomes to mimic the outer monolayer of RBC.
2. Hypothesis of shielded negative charge that proposes existence of screened negative charge. This leads to increased surface hydrophilicity of the liposomes without imparting a negative charge, binding site at the surface of the liposomes for the liver scavenger systems.
3. Hypothesis of absorption of dysopsonin, the specific recognition of GM1 by a serum protein (dysopsonin) that prevents the attack and recognition of opsonins and hence the phagocytosis.

Similarly, the long circulatory behavior imparted by second generation long circulatory liposomes could be ascribed to one of the following strategies, either independently or in combinations:

1. Hypothesis of steric barrier is based on steric stabilization by the grafted polymer (polymer brush steric hindrance).

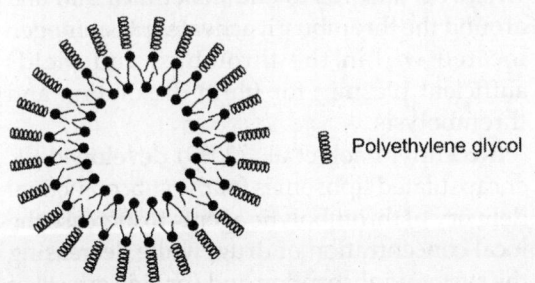

Polyethylene glycol

Fig. 11.10: Sterically stabilized (stealth) liposomes (SSL)

2. Increased surface hydrophilicity that avoids or inhibits specific opsonization of the lipid surface by immunoglobulins.
3. Inhibition of nonspecific adsorption of plasma proteins and lipoproteins.

However, literature is divided upon considering specific mechanisms of stealth and long circulatory behavior to ganglioside GM1 and PEG-grafted liposomes. Increased surface hydrophilicity and steric hindrance, however remain as major mechanisms for long circulation imparted by GM1 and/or PEG-coated liposomal systems. The hydrophilicity contributed by various glycolipids and hydrophilic polymers is supposed to be the central dogma of the stealth behavior of the liposomes and other colloidal systems. Opsonins and/or serum proteins recognize hydrophobic surfaces and scavenge hydrophobic particulates and vesicular systems. However, liposomes coated or appended with hydrophilic polymers possess an opsonin-repelling surface and thus become less susceptible to recognition.

Liposomes in the Thrombolytic Therapy

Among various drug delivery systems, liposomes have been explored by various research groups for the encapsulations of thrombolytic drugs (Holt and Gupta, 2010; Elbayoumi and Torchilin, 2008; Nguyen et al., 1990).

Liposomal encapsulation of plasminogen activators might increase efficacy, improve selectivity, possibly reduce or eliminate antigenic complications, retard systemic deactivation of the agent and effectively lengthen the brief half-lives of the agents (Elbayoumi and Torchilin, 2008). In an *in vitro* experiment, Nguyen et al., (1989) demonstrated ability of liposomes to protect SK in plasma without significant loss of protein activity. Plasminogen activators entrapped in liposomes have shown substantial reductions in the time required to obtain reperfusion and an increased digestion of thrombus as compared to freely infused plasminogen activators. One of the various theories proposed

to increase the effectiveness of the liposomal plasminogen activators is the blocking of channelling by the liposomes, which results in the pressure at the leading edge of the thrombus. To prove this theory, Heeremans et al., (1995b) compared the thrombolytic activity of free t-PA to free t-PA⁺ empty liposomes in a jugular vein model in rabbit. However, it was found that clot lysis activity of free t-PA was nearly equal to that of t-PA⁺ empty liposomes with an equivalent dose. The same results were observed by other investigators also. Thus, on the basis of these studies, it was concluded that increased thrombolytic activity of liposome encapsulated plasminogen activator was not due to pressure created by the blocking of the channels in the thrombus. Moreover, it was suggested that liposomal encapsulation reduces the premature inactivation and prevents degradation of enzymes in the plasma, vis-a-vis releases drug at the site of thrombus by shear stress.

Erdogan et al., (2006) developed three types of vesicular systems, i.e liposomes, niosomes and sphingosomes and evaluated for comparative biodistribution using radiolabeled, SK, they were compared with IV injection of free SK. Results demonstrated detectable amounts of SK from the thrombi in all three types of vesicles, with higher amount at 4 hours than 1hour. Uptake of Tc-99m-labeled SK by the thrombus can be explained by the mechanism of thrombolysis produced by SK. This mechanism involves a series of reactions, where SK adsorbs to and penetrates into and around the thrombus; it activates plasminogen located within the thrombus, and yields sufficient plasmin for fibrin dissolution and thrombolysis.

Recently, Baek et al., (2009) developed SK encapsulated liposomes for the subconjuctival delivery of thrombolytic agents to increase the local concentration of drug, while decreasing the systemic absorption and/or side effects of the drugs. Results of the study demonstrated lower ocular absorption of SK from liposomal formulation as compared to nonliposomal SK. Additionally, no detectable systemic and ocular side effects were observed in animals study. Liposomal formulations also enhanced the rate of subconjunctival hemorrhage (SH) absorption.

Liposomes in Gene Therapy

Recombinant-DNA technology and studies of gene function and gene therapy all depend on the delivery of nucleic acids (genetic materials) into cells *in vitro* and *in vivo*. A variety of physical (e.g. electroporation, microinjection, particle bombardment), chemical (DEAE-dextran, polybrene-dimethyl sulfoxide, calcium phosphate precipitation, liposomes, polylysine conjugates) and biological (e.g. virus) methods are available for transferring genes into cells. The most widely used type of vehicles for gene delivery include viral (e.g. adenovirus, retrovirus and adeno-associated virus) and nonviral (e.g. liposomes and lipid-based systems, polymers and peptides).

Amongst the nonviral vector systems, liposomes and lipid complexes, especially the engineered liposomes such as pH-sensitive liposomes, cationic liposomes, fusogenic liposomes, genosomes, lipoplex, and lipopoly-plex, have extensively been investigated for their potentials in gene delivery.

Lipid based gene delivery is the focus of several specialized high-technology companies, of which Vical (San Diago, CA, USA), Genzyme (Farmington, MA, USA), Gene Medicine (The Woodlands, TX, USA) and Megabios (Burlingame, CA, USA) have products in clinical trials. Some of the engineered liposomal and nonliposomal versions like pH-sensitive cationic and anionic liposomes, pH-sensitive immunoliposomes, fusogenic liposomes, genosomes (DNA-liposomes/lipid complexes), Lipofection™ (lipid-DNA complex) and recently cochleates are investigated as the major gene vectors. However, most of the commercially available nonviral gene vectors used for transfection are cationic liposome-DNA complexes. Some of the widely used cationic liposomes formulations are lipofectin (DOTMA:DOPE:1:1), lipofectamine (DOSPA:DOPE::3:1), trans-fectase (DDAB:DOPE::1:3), cytofectin (DMRIE:DOPE) and transfectam (DOGS).

Liposomes in Antisense Oligonucleotide Therapy

Oligonucleotides are being developed as therapeutic agents to selectively deliver the altered genetic functions, through sequence specific interactions with intracellular RNAs or DNAs. This may occur by involving a variety of mechanisms including antisense, ribozymes, triplex, and decoy. The strategy to halt DNA transcription or messenger RNA translation with code-blocking triplex formation or antisense oligomers. Antisense oligonucleotides interact with specific mRNA sequences, resulting in the reduced synthesis of the proteins those encoded by respective mRNAs encode(s). Liposomal delivery of these agents avoids the drawbacks associated with the other modes of administration including degradation by nucleases, increased toxicity and undesirable interactions with proteins.

Conventional liposomes are useful for the transport of either (a) natural phosphodiester oligonucleotides or (b) modified oligonucleotides, i.e. phosphorothioate, phosphoroamidate, methylphosphonate and C-5 propyne modification) by reducing the administered dose.

Moreover, cationic liposomes, anionic liposomes, pH-sensitive liposomes, antibody coated (immuno-liposomes), fusogenic liposomes or PEG-grafted (sterically stabilized stealth liposomes), are more appropriate in designing an appropriate biodistribution and pharmacokinetic profile (reviewed in Woodle and Leserman, 1998). The encapsulation of oligonucleotides in liposomes is useful for several reasons:

- Protection of oligonucleotides from nucleases degradation
- Enhancement of cellular uptake in several cell types

- Improvement of oligonucleotide potency, especially *in vitro*
- Modification of their intracellular distribution
- Increased retention of oligonucleotides in cells
- Potential for slow release depots for modified oligonucleotides

Immunological Applications of Liposomes

Besides its potential applications in cancer chemotherapy, antifungal therapy, and genetic applications, liposomes as a delivery system have established themselves in the area of immunology and the major areas of interest from a therapeutic point of view are:

- Liposomes as an immunological (vaccine) adjuvant
- Liposomal vaccines
- Liposomes as a carrier of immuno-modulators
- Liposomes as a tool in immuno-diagnostics

Liposomes as an Immunological (Vaccine) Adjuvant

Liposomes have been firmly established as immuno-adjuvants (enhancers of the immunological response), potentiating both cell-mediated (cytotoxic T-lymphocytes) and humoral immunity (antibody production). In recent years, mucosal immuno-adjuvant activity of liposomes involving the induction of strong secretory IGA (s-IGA) responses, while delivering the system in the gastrointestinal or respiratory tracts have been appreciated. Their main advantages as compared to other adjuvants (detoxified cholera toxins, alum etc.) can be summarized as:

- Liposomes are nontoxic, biocompatible and biodegradable
- Nonimmunologically inert in most of the cases and tailor made compositions
- May incorporate other adjuvants to provide strong immune response

- Convert loaded or anchored nonimmunogenic substances into immunogenic ones with small amount of antigen
- Reduce or eliminate the toxicity of toxic antigens and allergic reactions to nontoxic proteins
- Modulate the immune system and may induce cell-mediated immunity.
- Liposomal vaccines produce higher titres of functional antibodies as well as prolonged duration of these antibodies.

Liposomal immuno-adjuvants act by slowly releasing encapsulated antigen after intramuscular injection and also passively accumulating within regional lymph node. Liposomal vaccines can be made by associating microbes, soluble antigens, cytokines or deoxyribonucleic acid with liposomes, the latter stimulating an immune response following processing and presentation of the antigenic protein. Alternatively, antigens can be covalently coupled to liposomal membrane.

Liposomes as Radio-pharmaceutical and Radio-diagnostic Carriers

Liposomes loaded with the appropriate contrast agents have been shown to be suitable for imaging modalities. These imaging modalities are based on different physical principles and capture appropriate signal intensity from an area of interest in order to differentiate certain structures from surrounding tissues. According to the physical principle involved, currently used imaging modalities include:

- γ-scintigraphy (involving the application of emitting radioactive materials)
- Magnetic resonance (MR, phenomenon based on the transition between different energy levels of atomic nuclei under the action of radio-frequency signal)
- Computed tomography (CT, the modality, which utilizes ionizing radiation with the aid of computers to acquire cross-images

of the body and 3-D images of area of interest)

- Ultrasound imaging or ultrasonography (US, the modality using irradiation with ultrasound and based on the different rates at which ultrasound passes through various tissues.

However, the progression from experimental animals to human patients may proceed differently for different liposomal preparations. While liposomes for CT imaging and ultrasonic imaging still are the subject of laboratory research, the advantages of g-scintigraphy and MR imaging with liposomes have been demonstrated in many clinical studies. Liposome-based imaging agents have already been successfully used for MR, CT- and US imaging of tumors. In labeled liposomes for tumor imaging (VenCan, Vester, Inc.) are already in phase II–III clinical trials. Liposomal uptake by RES, which is a useful strategy in localization of contrast agents in RES-rich organs like liver, spleen, and bone marrow, is not useful for localization to non-RES organs. The RES-avoidance/localization of contrast agents can be successfully be achieved using targeted liposomes like immunoliposomes, long circulatory (PEG- and PEG-like polymer coated) liposomes and even by long circulatory immunoliposomes.

SUGGESTED READINGS

1. Adamson AW (1967), *Physical Chemistry of Surface*, II Ed., Interscience, New York, pp. 223
2. Andrieux K, Lesieur S, Ollivon M, Grabielle-Madelmont C (1998), *J. Chromatogr. Biomed. Sci. Appl.* 706, 141–7.
3. Barenholtz Y, Amselem S and Lichtenberg D (1979), *FEBS Lett.*, 99, 210.
4. Barenholz Y and Cromellin DJA (1994), *Encyclopedia of Pharmaceutical Technology* (Swarbrick J., Ed.), Marcel Dekker, pp. 1–39.
5. Barlett GR (1959), *J. Biol. Chem.*, 234–466.
6. Batzri S and Korn ED (1973), *Biochim. Biophys. Acta*, 298, 1015–9.
7. Brooks CJW, MacLachlan J, Cole WJ and Lawrie TDV (1984), *Proceedings of symposium on Analysis of Steroids*, Szeged, Hungary, pp. 349.
8. Buboltz JT and Feigenson GW (1999), *Biochim. Biophys. Acta*, 1417, 232–45.
9. Chapman, D. (1975) Quart. Rev. Biophys. 8, 185-235.
10. Enoch HG, Stritamatter P (1976), *Proc. Natl. Acad. Sci. USA*, 76, 145–9.
11. Fry DW, White C and Goldman DJ (1978), *Anal. Biochem.*, 90, 809.
12. Gregoriadis G, de Silva H and Florence AT (1990), *Int. J. Pharm.*, 65, 235.
13. Gruber HJ, Wilmsen HU, Schurga A, Pilger A and Schindler H (1995), *Biochim. Biophys. Acta* 1240, 266–76.
14. Gunter KK, Gunter TE, Jarkowski A and Rosier, RN (1982), *Anal. Biochem.*, 120, 113.
15. Hamilton RL, Goerke J, Guo LSS, Williams MC and Havel RJ (1980), *J. Lipid Res.*, 21, 981.
16. Hauser H and Gains N (1982), *Proc. Natl. Acad. Sci. USA*, 79, 1683.
17. Hope MJ, Bally MB, Webb G and Culis PR (1985), *Biochim. Biophys. Acta*, 812, 55.
18. Huang C (1969), *Biochemistry*, 8, 344.
19. Jones GR and Cossins AR (1989), Physical methods of study, Liposomes: A practical approach (New, RRC, Ed.), OIRL Press, Oxford, pp. 184–91.
20. Katayama K, Kato Y, Onishi, H, Nagai T, Machida, Y, *Int. J. Pharm.* 248 (2002) 93–9.
21. Kirby C and Gregoriadis G (1984), *Biotechnology*, 2, 979.
22. Kolchens S, Ramaswami V, Birgenheier J, Nett L and O'Brien DF (1993), *Chem. Phys. Lipids*, 65, 1–10.
23. Lasic DD (1998), *Trends in Biotechnology*, 16, 307–21.
24. Lasic DD, Ceh DD, Stuart MCA, Guo L, Frederik, PM and Barenholz Y (1995), *Biochim. Biophys. Acta*, 1239, 145–56.
25. Lesieur S, Grabielle-Madelmont C, Paternostre MT and Ollivon M (1991), *Anal. Biochem.* 192, 334–43.
26. Levy, D. et al., (1990) Biochim. Biopyhs. Acta, 179, 1025.
27. Lopez-Berestein G, Mehta R, Hopffer R, Mills K, Kasi L, Mehta K, Fainstein V, Luna M, Harsh EN and Juliano R (1983), *J. Infect. Dis.*, 147, 939–45.
28. Mandal TK and Downing DT (1993), *Acta Derm. Venereol.*, 73, 12–7.
29. Mayer LD, Hope MJ, Cullis RP and Janoff AS (1985), *Biochim. Biophys. Actu*, 817, 193.
30. Mayhew E, lazo R, Vali WJ, King J and Green AM (1984), *Biochim. Biophys. Acta*, 775, 169.

31. Moon MH and Giddings JC (1993), *J. Pharm. Biomed. Anal.* 11, 911–20.

32. Morgan CG, Thomas EW and Yianni YP (1983), *Biochim. Biophys. Acta,* 728, 356.

33. Nakata T, Sobue K and Hirokawa N (1990), *J. Cell Biol.* 110, 13–25.

34. New RRC (1989), Liposomes: A practical approach, OIRL Press, Oxford, London, pp. 1–30.

35. Ohsawa T, Miura H and Harada K (1985), *Pharm. Bull.,* 33, 2916.

36. Oku N and MacDonald RC (1983), *Biochemistry,* 22, 855.

37. Ostro MJ (1987), Liposomes: From biophysics to therapeutics, Marcel Dekker, New York.

38. Papahadjopoulos D, Vali WJ, Jacobson K and Poste G (1975), *Biochim. Biophys. Acta,* 394, 483.

39. Perkins WR, Minchey SR, Ostro MJ, Taraschi TF and Janoff AS (1988), *Biochim. Biophys. Acta* 943, 103–7.

40. Schmidtgen MC, Drechsler M, Lasch J and Schubert R (1998), *J. Microsc.* 191, 177–86.

41. Stewart JCM (1959), *Anal. Biochem.,* 104, 10

42. Szoka F and Papahadjopoulos D (1978), *Proc. Natl. Acad. Sci. USA,* 75, 4194.

43. Talsma H and Crommelin DJA (1992), Liposomes as Drug Delivery Systems, Part I: Preparation, Pharmaceutical Technology, 16, 96–106.

44. Terao J, Asano I and Matsushito S (1985), *Lipids,* 20, 312.

45. Uster PS and Deamer DW (1981), *Arch. Biochem. Biophys.,* 209, 385.

46. Vyas SP, Katare YK, Mishra V and Sihorkar V (2000), *Int. J. Pharm.,* 210, 1–14

47. Weiner N, Martin F and Riaz M (1989), *Drug Dev. Ind. Phar.,* 15, 1523–54.

48. Wybenga DR, Pileggi VJ, Dirstine PH and Di Giorgio J (1970), *J. Clin. Chem.,* 16, 980.

12

■ Microspheres and Microcapsules

INTRODUCTION

The term microcapsule is defined as a spherical particle with size varying from 50 nm to 2 mm, containing a core substance. Microspheres are, in technical sense, spherical-empty particles. However, the terms microcapsules and microspheres are often used synonymously. In addition, some related terms viz., 'microbeads' and 'beads'. Spheres and spherical particles are also used for microspheres of large size and rigid morphology. The microspheres are characteristically free-flowing powders consisting of proteins or synthetic polymers, which may or may not be biodegradable in nature, and ideally have average particle size less than 200 μm. Solid biodegradable microspheres incorporating a drug dispersed or dissolved throughout particle matrix have the potential for the controlled release of drug. These carriers received much attention not only for prolonged release, but also for the targeting of the anticancer drugs to the tumor.

MATERIAL(S) USED

A number of different substances both biodegradable as well as nonbiodegradable have been investigated for the preparation of microspheres. These materials include the polymers of natural and synthetic origin and also modified natural substances. Synthetic polymers employed as carrier materials are methyl methacrylate, acrolein, lactide, glycolide and their copolymers, ethylene vinyl acetate copolymer, polyanhydrides, etc. The natural polymers used for the purpose include albumin, gelatin, starch, collagen and carrageenan, etc. Some of the commonly used polymers in the preparation of the microspheres are classified and listed in the Table 12.1.

Table 12.1: Classification of polymers
Synthetic polymers
Nonbiodegradable
PMMA
Acrolein
Glycidyl methacrylate
Epoxy polymers
Biodegradable
Lactides and glycolides and their copolymers
Polyalkyl cyanoacrylates
Polyanhydrides
Natural polymers
Proteins
Albumins
Gelatin
Collagen
Carbohydrates
Starch
Agarose

(Contd.)

Table 12.1: Classification of polymers *(Contd.)*

Carrageenan
Chitosan
Chemically-modified carbohydrates
DEAE cellulose
Poly (acryl) dextran
Poly (acryl) starch

PREREQUISITES FOR IDEAL MICROPARTICULATE CARRIERS

The material utilized for the preparation of microparticulates should ideally fulfill the following prerequisites:

- Longer duration of action
- Control of content release
- Increase of therapeutic efficiency
- Protection of drug
- Reduction of toxicity
- Biocompatibility
- Sterilizability
- Relative stability
- Water solubility or dispersability
- Bioresorbability
- Targetability
- Polyvalent

METHODS OF PREPARATION

The microspheres can be prepared by using one of the several techniques discussed in the following sections, but the choice of the technique mainly depends on the nature of the polymer used, the drug, the intended use and the duration of therapy. Moreover, the method of preparation and its choice are equivocally determined by some formulation and technology-related factors as mentioned below:

1. The particle size requirement.
2. The drug or the protein should not be adversely affected by the process.
3. Reproducibility of the release profile and the method.
4. No stability problem.
5. There should be no toxic product(s) associated with the final product.

Synthetic polymers are now materials of choice for the controlled release as well as targeted microparticulate carriers. The initial work was carried-out on the nonbiodegradable polymers, but later on, the interest has been shifted to the biodegradable polymers. Different types of methods are employed for the preparation of the microspheres. These include in situ polymerization, solvent evaporation, coacervation phase separation, spray drying and spray congealing, etc.

Single Emulsion Technique

The microparticulate carriers of natural polymers, i.e. those of proteins and carbohydrates are prepared by single emulsion technique (Fig. 12.1). The natural polymers are dissolved or dispersed in aqueous medium followed by dispersion in the nonaqueous medium, e.g. oil. In the second step of preparation, cross linking of the dispersed globule is carried out. The cross-linking can be achieved either by means of heat or by using the chemical cross-linkers. The chemical cross-linking agents used include glutaraldehyde, formaldehyde, terephthaloyl chloride, diacid chloride, etc. Cross-linking by heat is achieved by adding the dispersion to previously heated oil. Heat denaturation is not suitable for the thermolabile drugs, while the chemical cross-linking has disadvantage of excessive exposure of active ingredient to chemicals, if added at the time of preparation.

Double Emulsion Techniques

Briefly, double emulsion method of microspheres preparation involves the formation of the multiple emulsions or the double emulsion of type W/O/W (Fig. 12.2) and is best suited to the water-soluble drugs such as peptide, protein, and the vaccines. This method can be used with both the natural as well as the synthetic polymers. The aqueous protein solution is dispersed into a lipophilic organic continuous phase. This protein solution may contain the active constituents. The continuous phase consists of the polymer

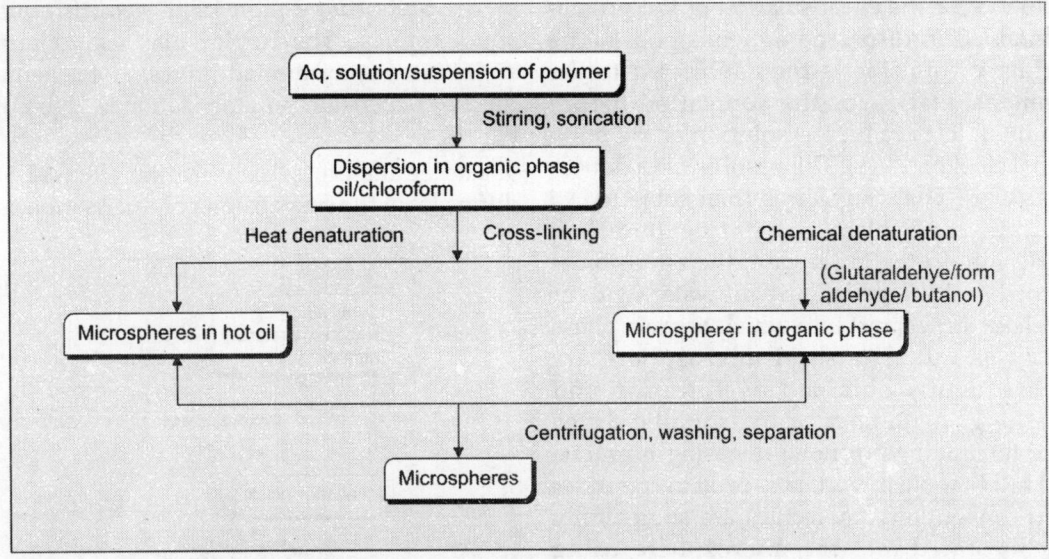

Fig. 12.1: Schematic representing simple emulsion based method of preparation of microspheres

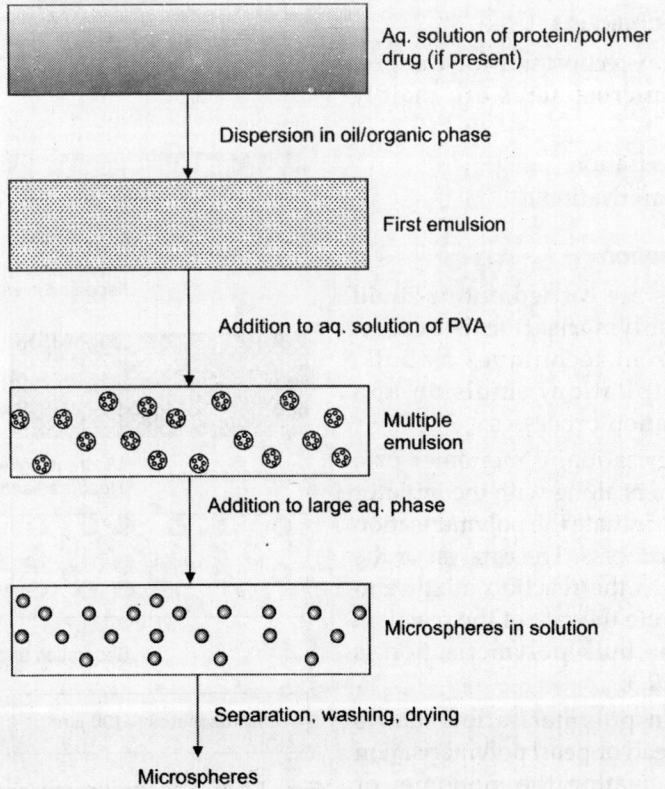

Fig. 12.2: Schematic representing double emulsion method of preparation of microspheres

solution for the encapsulation of the protein contained in dispersed aqueous phase. The primary emulsion is then subjected to the homogenization or the sonication before addition to the aqueous solution of the poly-vinyl alcohol (PVA). This results into a double emulsion. The emulsion is then subjected to solvent removal by solvent evaporation, diffusion. In the latter case, the emulsion is added to the large quantity of water (with or without surfactant) into which organic phase diffuses out. The solid microsphere are subsequently obtained by filtration and washing. A number of hydrophilic drugs like luteinizing-hormone-releasing hormone (LH-RH) agonist, vaccines, protein/peptides and conventional molecules are successfully incorporated into the microsphere using the method of double emulsion solvent evaporation/extraction.

Polymerisation Techniques

The polymerisation techniques for the preparation of the microspheres are mainly classified as:

1. Normal polymerisation
2. Interfacial polymerisation

Normal Polymerisation

The two processes are carried out in liquid phase. Normal polymerisation is accomplished by different techniques as bulk, suspension precipitation, emulsion and micelle polymerisation processes.

In bulk polymerisation, a monomer or a mixture of monomers along with the initiator is usually heated to initiate the polymerisation and carry out the process. The catalyst or the initiator is added to the reaction mixture to facilitate or accelerate the rate of the reaction. The scheme of the bulk polymerisation is presented in Fig. 12.3.

The suspension polymerisation that is referred to as the bead or pearl polymerisation is carried out by heating the monomer or mixture of monomers with active principles

as droplets dispersion in the continuous aqueous phase. The droplets may also contain an initiator and other additives. The scheme for the suspension polymerisation is given in Fig. 12.4.

The emulsion polymerisation (Fig. 12.5) differs from the suspension polymerisation as

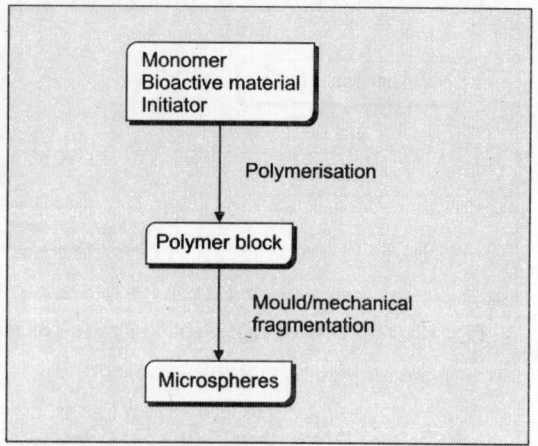

Fig. 12.3: Schematic for bulk polymerisation

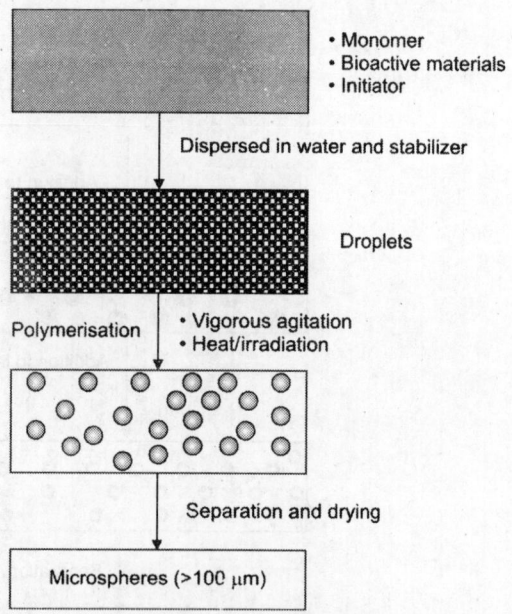

Fig. 12.4: Schematic representing suspension method of microspheres formation

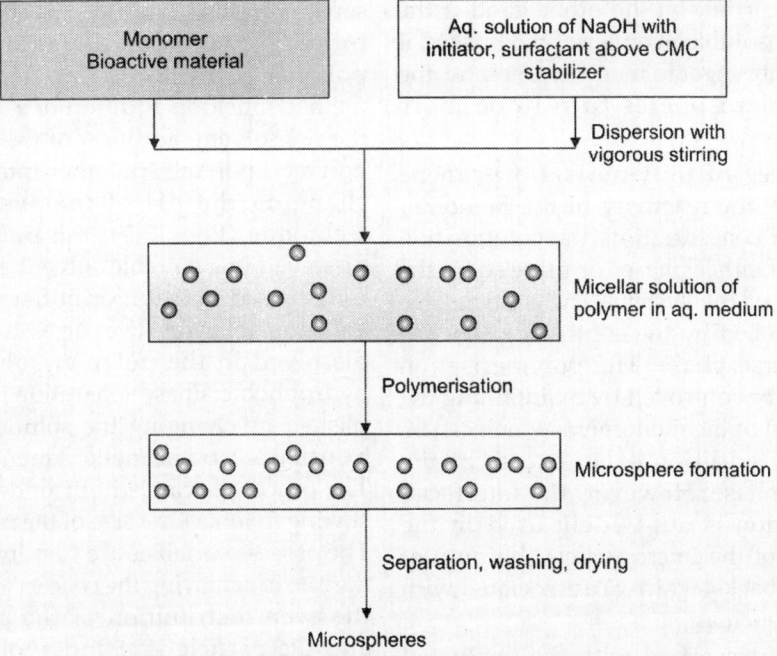

Fig. 12.5: Schematic representation emulsion polymerisation

the initiator present in the aqueous phase, diffuses to the surface of the micelles or the emulsion globules (Fig. 12.6). The bulk polymerisation has an advantage of formation of the pure polymer, but it also has disadvantage, as it is very difficult to dissipate the heat of reaction, which can adversely affect the thermolabile active ingredients. On the other hand the suspension and emulsion polymerisation can be carried out at lower temperature, since continuous external phase is present, through which heat can easily dissipate. The two processes also lead to the formation of the

higher molecular weight polymer at relatively faster rate. The major advantage of suspension and emulsion polymerisation is an intimate association of polymer with the unreacted monomer and other additives.

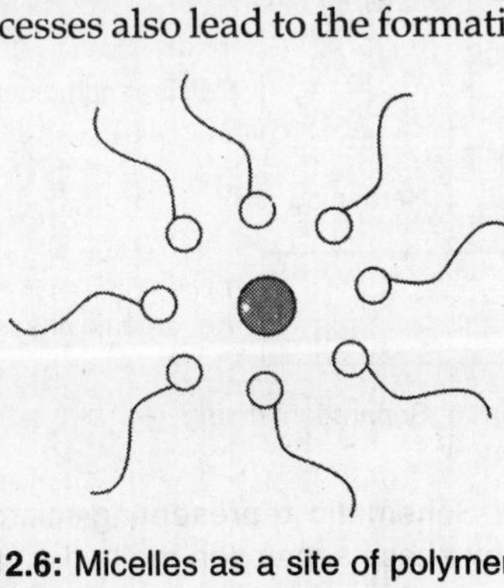

Interfacial Polymerisation

Interfacial polymerisation essentially proceeds involving reaction of various monomers at the interface between the two immiscible liquid phases to form a film of polymer that essentially encapsulates the dispersed phase. In this technique, two reacting monomers are employed; one of which is dissolved in the continuous phase while the other is dispersed in the dispersed phase. The continuous phase is generally aqueous in nature, throughout which the second monomer is emulsified. The monomer present in either phases diffuses rapidly and polymerise rapidly at the interface. Two conditions arise depending upon the solubility of formed polymer in the emulsion droplet. If the polymer is soluble in the droplet it will lead to the formation of the monolithic

Fig. 12.6: Micelles as a site of polymerisation

type of the carrier, on the other hand if the polymer is insoluble in either of the phases; it forms an embryogenic member one and the resultant microspheres turn to be more capsular (reservoir) type.

The degree of polymerisation can be controlled by the reactivity of the monomer chosen, their concentration, the composition of vehicles of either phases or more so by the temperature of the system. The particle size can be controlled by the controlling the size of the disperse phase. The polymerisation reaction can be controlled by maintaining the concentration of the monomers, which can be achieved by addition of an excess of the continuous phase. However, the interfacial polymerisation is not widely used in the preparation of the microparticles because of certain drawbacks, which are associated with the process, such as:

- Toxicity associated with the unreacted monomer
- High permeability of the film
- High degradation of the drug during the polymerisation
- Fragility of microcapsule
- Nonbiodegradability of the microparticle

Phase Separation Coacervation Technique

Phase separation method is especially designed for preparing the reservoir type of the system, i.e. to encapsulate water soluble drugs, e.g. peptides, proteins, however, some of the preparations are of matrix type particularly, when the drug is hydrophobic in nature, e.g. steroids. In matrix type device, the drug or the protein is solublized in the polymer solution. The process is based on the principle of decreasing the solubility of the polymer in the organic phase to achieve the formation of the polymer rich phase called the coacervates. The coacervation can be obtained by addition of the third component to the system, which results in the formation of the two phases, one rich in the polymer, while the other one, i.e. supernatant, depleted of the polymer. Phase separation can be induced by using any of the following methods depending upon the polymer and the reaction conditions. The methods include addition of salt, addition of the nonsolvent, addition of the incompatible polymer, polymer-polymer interaction or by changing the pH of the system. In this technique (Fig. 12.7), the polymer is first dissolved in a suitable solvent and then drug is dispersed in water or buffer to prepare its aqueous solution, if drug is hydrophilic or dissolved in the polymer solution, if it is hydrophobic. Phase separation is then accomplished by changing the solution conditions by using any of the method mentioned above. The process is carried out under continuous stirring to control the size of the microparticles. The process variables are very important since the rate of achieving the coacervate determines the even distribution of the polymer film and the particle size and avoidance of the agglomeration of the formed particles. The agglomeration must be avoided by stirring the suspension using a suitable speed stirrer as the process of microsphere formation begins,

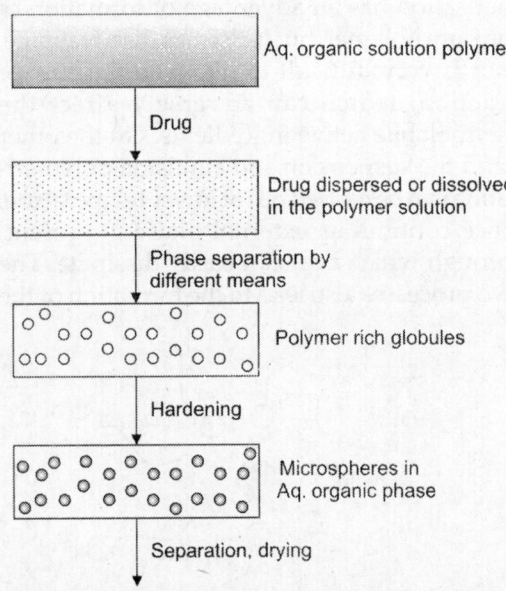

Fig. 12.7: Schematic representing microspheres formation by phase separation method

the formed globules start to stick and tend to form the agglomerates. In this method the process variable are very important, as they control the kinetic of the particles growth and formation.

Spray Drying and Spray Congealing

Spray drying and spray congealing methods are based on the drying of the mist of the polymer and drug in the air. Depending upon the removal of the solvent or the cooling of the solution, the two processes are named spray drying and the spray congealing respectively. The polymer is first dissolved in a suitable volatile organic solvent, such as dichloromethane, acetone, etc. The drug in the solid form is then dispersed in the polymer solution by high-speed homogenization. This dispersion is then atomized in a stream of hot air. The atomization leads to formation of the small droplets or the fine mist from which the solvent evaporates instantaneously leading to the formation of the microspheres of typical size range 1–100 mm. Microparticles are separated from the hot air by means of the cyclone separator, while the traces of solvent are removed by vacuum drying. One of the major advantages of the process is possibility of operation in aseptic conditions. The two processes are rapid and single stage operation, which are suitable for both the batch and bulk manufacturing. These techniques have been used to encapsulate a large number of the drugs. The spray drying process is used to encapsulate various penicillins. Thiamine mononitrate (Koff 1963) and sulphaethyl-thiadizole (John and Becker 1968, Kushimano and Becker 1968) have been successfully encapsulated in a mixture of mono- and di-glycerides of stearic and palmitic acid using spray congealing. The rate of solvent removal by evaporation, strongly influences the characteristics of the formed microspheres. The evaporation further, depends on the temperature, pressure, and the solubility parameters of the polymer, solvent and dispersion media. Very rapid solvent evaporation,

however leads to the formation of porous microparticles.

Solvent Extraction

Solvent extraction is a method of the microparticles preparation, which involves removal of the organic phase by extraction of the organic solvent. The method incorporates water miscible organic solvents, such as isopropanol. Organic phase is removed by extraction with water. This process decreases the hardening time for the microsphere. One variation of the process involves direct addition of the drug or protein to organic polymer solution. The rate of solvent removal by extraction method depends on the temperature of water, ratio of emulsion internal phase volume to the water and the solubility profile of the polymer.

LOADING OF DRUG

The active components are incorporated in the microspheres principally using two methods, i.e. during the preparation of the microsphere or after the formation of the microspheres by incubating them with the drug/protein. The active component can be loaded by means of the physical entrapment, chemical linkage and surface adsorption. The entrapment largely depends on the method of preparation and nature of the drug or polymer (monomer, if used). Maximum loading can be achieved by incorporating the drug during the time of preparation, but it may get affected by many other process variables, such as method of preparation, presence of additives (e.g. cross-linking agent, surfactant stabilizers, etc.) heat of polymerization, agitation intensity, etc. Percent incorporation in preformed microspheres is relatively less, but the major advantage of this loading method is that there is no effect of process variables. The loading is carried out in preformed microspheres by incubating them with high concentration of the drug in a suitable solvent. The drug in these microspheres is loaded via penetration or diffusion of the drug through the pores in the microspheres as well as adsorption on their surface. The solvent is then removed, leaving drug-loaded microsphere. The drugs and protein can also be incorporated by physical or chemical linkage. The adsorption of the drugs/proteins depends on the nature of the polymers. The Freundlich model is applied to determine the adsorption of the drugs.

The Freundlich equation is:

$$X/M = KCP$$

where, K is a constant related to the capacity of the adsorbent for the adsorbate and P is a constant related to the affinity of the adsorbent for the adsorbate. Although, this equation was first employed empirically, it can be derived with the assumption of a continuously varying heat of adsorption. The Freundlich model unfortunately predicts both infinite adsorption at infinite concentration and infinite heat of adsorption at zero coverage.

DRUG RELEASE KINETICS

Release of the active constituent is an important consideration in case of microspheres. Many theoretically possible mechanisms may be considered for the release of drug from the microparticulates.

1. Liberation due to polymer erosion or degradation
2. Self-diffusion through the pore
3. Release from the surface of the polymer
4. Pulsed delivery initiated by the application of an oscillating or sonic field.

In most of the cases, a combination of more than one mechanisms for drug release may operate, therefore, the distinction amongst the mechanisms is not always distinctive and trivial. The release profile from the microspheres depends on the nature of the polymer used in the preparation as well as on the nature of the active drug. The release of drug from both biodegradable as well as non-biodegradable microsphere(s) is influenced by structure or micromorphology of the carrier and the properties of the polymer itself. The drugs could be released through the microspheres by any of the three methods, first is the osmotically driven burst mechanism, second pore diffusion mechanism, and third by erosion or the degradation of the polymer. In osmotically driven burst mechanism, water diffuses into the core through biodegradable or nonbiodegradable coating, creating sufficient pressure that ruptures the membrane. The burst effect is mainly controlled by three factors—the macromolecule/polymer ratio, particle size of the disperse macromolecule, and the particle size of the microspheres. The pore diffusion method is so named because as penetrating waterfront continues to diffuse towards the core. The dispersed protein/drug dissolves creating a water-filled pore network through which the active principle diffuses out in a controlled manner. In case of the biodegradable polymers, the release is controlled by both the erosion as well as diffusion process. The polymer erosion, i.e. loss of polymer is accompanied by accumulation of the polymer in the release medium. The erosion of the polymer begins with the changes in the microstructure of the carrier as water penetrates within it leading to the plasticization of the matrix. This plasticization of the matrix finally leads to the cleavage of the hydrolytic bonds. The cleavage of the bond is also facilitated by the presence of an enzyme (lysozymes) in the surroundings. The erosion of the polymer may be either surfacial or it may be bulk leading to the rapid release of the drug/active components. The rate and extent of water uptake, therefore determines release profile of the system and depends on type of the polymer, porosity of the polymer matrix, protein-drug loading, etc.

Factors affecting the release of the drug from the particulate system in relation to drug, microspheres, and bioenvironment:

1. Drug

• Position in microspheres
• Molecular weight

- Physicochemical properties
- Concentration
- Interaction with matrix

2. Microspheres

- Type and amount of the matrix polymer
- Size and density of the microspheres
- Extent of cross-linking, denaturation or polymerization
- Adjuvants

3. Environment

- pH
- Polarity
- Presence of enzyme

Drug release from the nonbiodegradable type of polymers can be understood by considering the geometry of the carrier. The geometry of the carrier, i.e. whether it is reservoir type, where the drug is present as a core, or matrix type in which drug is dispersed throughout the carrier, governs overall release profile of the drug or active ingredients.

Reservoir Type System

Release from the reservoir type system with rate-controlling membrane proceeds by first penetration of the water through the membrane followed by dissolution of the drug in the penetrating dissolution fluid. The dissolved drug after partitioning through the membrane diffuses across the stagnant diffusion layer. The release is essentially governed by the Fick's first law of diffusion as

$$J = -D(dc/dx) \qquad (12.1)$$

where, J is flux per unit area, D is diffusion coefficient, and dc/dx is concentration gradient.

Diffusion across the membrane determines the effectiveness of the carrier system. The cumulative amount of drug, that is released through the unit area, 'Q_t' at any time 't' is given by equation;

$$Q_t = \frac{C_s K D_m D_d t}{K D_m l_m + D_d l_d} \qquad (12.2)$$

where, C_s represents saturation solubility of drug in dispersion medium, D_m is diffusion coefficient of drug in membrane of thickness l_m, D_d is diffusion coefficient of drug in static diffusion layer of thickness l_d, K is partition coefficient of drug between membrane and reservoir compartments.

The release rate from the carriers can be modified by changing both the composition and the thickness of the polymeric membrane.

Matrix Type System

Release profile of the drug from the matrix type of the device, critically depends on the state of drug, whether it is dissolved or dispersed in the polymer matrix. In the case of the drug dissolved in the polymeric matrix, the amount of drug, and the nature of the polymer (whether hydrophobic or hydrophilic) may affect the release profile. In case, drug is dissolved in the polymeric matrix, the amount of drug appearing in the receptor phase at time 't' is approximated by two separate equations. The first equation determines the initial 60% of the drug release, while the second shows the release profile at later stage.

$$\frac{dM_t}{dt} = 2Mx \, (D/\pi \, l^2 t)^{1/2} \qquad (12.3)$$

$$\frac{dM_t}{dt} = \frac{8DM_x}{l^2} \frac{\exp \pi^2 DT}{l^2} \qquad (12.4)$$

where l is thickness of polymer slab, D is diffusion coefficient, M_x is the total amount of drug present in the matrix and M_t is the amount of drug released in time t. When the drug is dispersed throughout the polymer matrix, then the release profile follows Higuchi's equation, i.e.

$$\frac{dM_t}{dt} = \frac{A}{2} \frac{(2DC_s C_o)_{1/2}}{t} \qquad (12.5)$$

where, A is area of matrix, C_s is solubility of the drug in the matrix and C_o represents total concentration in the matrix. Taking porosity (ε) and tortuosity (τ) of the matrix into the consideration the above equation can be modified as follows:

$$\frac{dM_t}{dt} = \left[\frac{\varepsilon}{\tau}D_m(2C_o - \varepsilon C_s)C_s t\right]^{1/2}$$

CHARACTERIZATION OF MICROPARTICLES

Particle Size and Shape

The most widely used procedures to characterize microparticles are conventional light microscopy (LM) and scanning electron microscopy (SEM) (Fig. 12.8). Both techniques can be used to determine the shape and outer structure (morphology) of the microparticles. Confocal laser scanning microscopy (CLSM) is applied as a nondestructive visualization technique for microparticles, especially within biological system(s).

Degradation Behavior

The surface chemistry of the microspheres, can be determined using the electron spectroscopy for chemical analysis (ESCA). ESCA provides a means to determine the atomic composition of the surface. The spectrum obtained using ESCA reveals the surfacial degradation of the biodegradable microspheres. Similarly, reflectance Fourier transform-infrared spectroscopy (FTIR) is successfully used to determine the degradation of the polymeric matrix of the carrier system.

Attenuated Total Reflectance Fourier Transform-infrared Spectroscopy

FTIR is used to determine the degradation of the polymeric matrix of the carrier system. The

surface of the microspheres is investigated measuring altered total reflectance (ATR). The IR beam passing through the ATR cell reflect many times through the sample to provide IR spectra, mainly of surface material. The ATR-FTIR provides informations about the surface composition of the microspheres.

Density Determination

Density of the microparticles can be measured by using a multivolume pychnometer. Accurately weighed sample in a cup is placed into the multivolume pychnometer. Helium is introduced at a constant pressure in the chamber and allowed to expand. This expansion results in a decrease in pressure within the chamber. Two consecutive readings of reduction in pressure at different initial pressure are noted. From two pressure readings, the volume and hence the density of the microspheres carrier is determined.

Isoelectric Point

The microelectrophoresis is a method that measures the electrophoretic mobility of microspheres from which the isoelectric point can be determined and used for separation and qualitative surface electric property approximation.

Surface Functional Residue

The carboxylic acid functional groups free (residue) are largely measured by using radioactive glycine, whereas surface-associated amino acid residues are determined by the

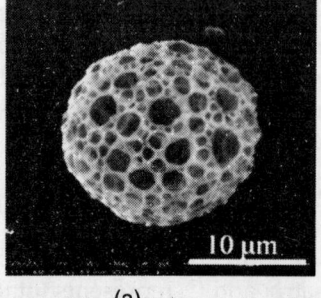
(a)

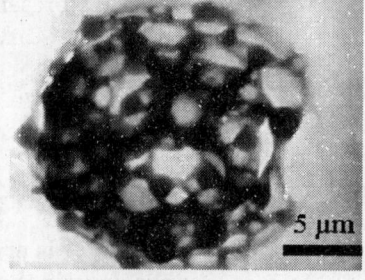
(b)

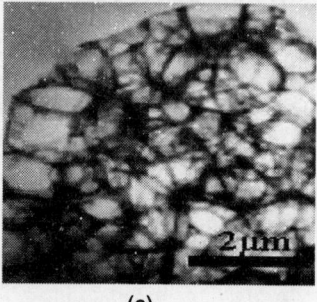
(c)

Fig.12.8: The surface morphology of porous microspheres detected by SEM (a). The inner structure of porous microspheres (b and c)

radioactive 14C-acetic acid conjugate-based radioactive tracers measurement-based techniques.

Capture Efficiency

The capture efficiency of the microspheres or the percent entrapment can be determined by allowing washed-microspheres lysis. The lysate is then subjected to the determination of active constituents as per official monograph drug content requirement. The percent encapsulation efficiency is calculated using following equation:

$$\frac{dM_t}{dt} = \left[\frac{\varepsilon}{\tau}D_m(2C_o - \varepsilon C_s)C_s t\right]^{1/2}$$

Release Studies

Drug release from microspheres is studied in phosphate saline buffer of pH 7.4, using rotating paddle apparatus or by using dialysis method. In the case of the paddle apparatus, the sample is agitated at 100 rpm. The samples are taken at specific time intervals and are replaced by the same amount of saline. Data are treated for cumulative percent drug release; release rate and release kinetics. The active ingredient in the sample withdrawn is analysed as per the monograph requirement and release profile is determined using the plot of amount released as a function of time. The release profile of the drugs or proteins generally depends on the method of formulation, formulation conditions (process variable), and more importantly on the nature of the polymer used for the preparation. Degradation profile of the polymer is another important parameter, which determines, whether the release is sustained, prolonged or burst type. Dialysis is another method used to study the release of the drugs/proteins from the microspheres. The microspheres are kept in a dialysing bag or tube with membrane, while the dialysing media is continuously stirred and samples of dialysate are taken. The withdrawn samples are estimated for drug content. Each time the volume is replaced using fresh buffer solution.

Angle of Contact

The angle of contact is measured to determine the wetting property of a microparticulate carrier. It determines the nature of microspheres in terms of hydrophilicity or hydrophobicity. This thermodynamic property is specific to solid and affected by the presence of the adsorbed component. The angle of contact is measured at the solid/air/water interface. The method for the determination of the angle of contact is given by Nutt, who proposed that the particle floating at interface is subjected to number of forces, such as gravitational, Archimedean thrust, etc. These forces affect the angle of contact. The advancing and receding angle of contact are measured by placing a droplet in a circular cell mounted above objective of inverted microscope. Contact angle is measured at 20°C within a minute of deposition of microspheres.

VARIOUS TYPES OF POLYMERIC MICROSPHERES

Albumin Microspheres

The albumin is a widely distributed natural protein. The particulate or the colloidal form of albumin is considered as the potential carrier of drug/proteins for either site-specific localization or their local application into anatomical discrete sites. Much of earlier use of serum albumin microspheres was limited to the diagnostic purpose as the microspheres of different size range locate themselves differentially at selected sites to facilitate the imaging. Now, because of selected uptake of protein carrier by tumor cells, the microspheres of albumin are being widely used for the targeted drug delivery to the tumor cells (Fig. 12.9). The preparation of the albumin

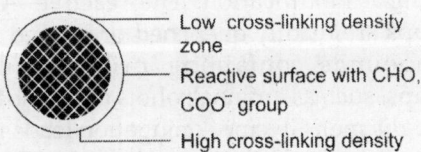

Fig.12.9: Surface cross-linked functional microspheres

microparticles is easy and particles in size range 15 nm to 150 μm diameter could be obtained.

There are numerous methods available for preparation of the albumin microspheres, which involve the drug incorporation either during the preparation or after the formation of the particles. Albumin microparticles are mainly prepared by emulsion polymerization, using either heat denaturation of the particles at elevated temperature (100–180°C) or chemical cross-linking. The albumin microspheres can also be prepared by denaturation of the protein aerosol in gas medium (Przyborowski et al., 1982) or an aerosol step followed by denaturation in oil (Millar et al., 1982).

The microspheres prepared by above methods are hydrophobic in nature, and therefore small amount of surface-active agent is needed to disperse them in parenteral preparation. Hydrophobic microspheres are rapidly cleared from the body. The hydrophilic microspheres are considered to be good carriers as they can carry large amounts of drug. Microspheres with increased hydrophilicity are advantageous because (i) they may exhibit favorable surface-related physical and chemical properties *in vivo*; (ii) they do not require surfactants currently needed to prepare aqueous dispersions, which may influence tissue interaction, drug release, and activity; (iii) hydrophilicity facilitates aqueous chemical modification; and (iv) high concentration of drug can be incorporated after preparation.

The drug release from albumin microspheres depends on the degree of cross-linking. The surface free aldehyde and carboxyl groups (later formed by oxidation) can be used for further surface and bulk chemical modification. The reactive—CHO groups are readily quenched or capped with compounds containing primary amino groups, such as aminoalcohols or aminoacids (e.g. glycine). Glycine conjugation leads to an increased anionic character and hence hydrophilicity. Albumin microspheres loaded with anticancer drug such as mitomycin C, were found to be more effective than the drug alone. Albumin microspheres can also be targeted to the various organ and cell lines and they are found to decrease the toxicity of the incorporated drugs. Intravenous injection can provide efficient targeting of albumin microspheres either to the lung or to the liver. Their ultimate location and accumulation depends on the size range of the microspheres. Microspheres of particle size range 15–30 μm or larger will pass through the heart and deposited in the capillary bed of lung up to 99%. The microspheres of 1–3 μm sizes will pass into reticuloendothelial system, where they deposit with 90% efficiency in the liver. Microspheres with particle size less then 1 μm, when injected intravenously, lead to about 80–90% deposition in lung, about 5–8% in spleen and about 1–2% in bone marrow. The release of drug from heat-stabilized albumin microsphere is more frequently biphasic in character. This biphasic profile is dependent to some extent on the water solubility of the entrapped drug. Highly water-soluble drug exhibits noticeable biphasic release characteristics. Relatively water insoluble drugs, such as steroids, which diffuse relatively slowly from the matrix, exhibit less pronounced biphasic release properties. The concentration of drug incorporated in the microspheres, also plays a major role in governing the biphasic character of the drug release.

Gelatin Microspheres

Gelatin is proteinacious biodegradable polymer obtained from the partial hydrolysis of the collagen derived from the skin, connective tissues and bones of animals. Gelatin microspheres are extensively studied because they are prone to strong opsonization. Figure 12.10 represents the macrophage morphology which on activation of macrophage explicitly translated into multifold protruded membrane as pseudopods. Thus, gelatin microspheres of suitable size range can be used as an efficient carrier system capable of

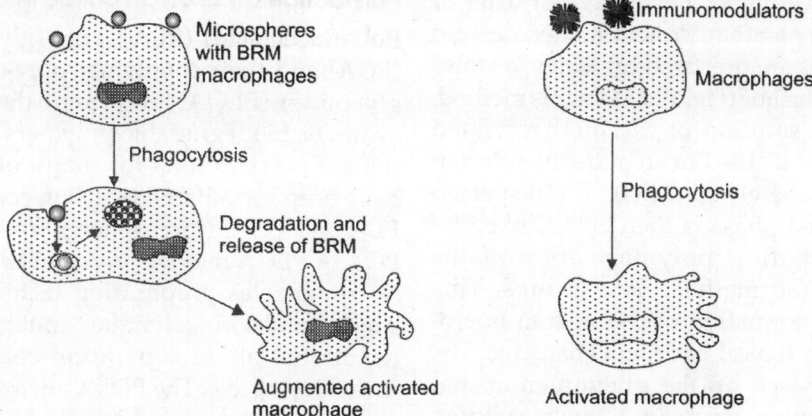

Fig. 12.10: Opsonization of gelatin microspheres by macrophages

delivering the drug or biological response modifiers, such as interferon to the phagocytes (macrophages). Sustained release may be obtained with the glutaraldehyde cross-linked microsphere, while zero-order release has been reported in case of the ethyl cellulose coated microspheres. Gelatin microspheres are reported to be taken up by some of the tumor cells, which do not take albumin.

Gelatin microspheres are prepared by cross-linking gelatin in water-in-oil emulsion with glutaraldehyde. Opsonic gelatin microsphere are also prepared by similar method by dispersing gelatin having IFN-α A/D in oil followed by cross-linking with glutaraldehyde. The shape of the microspheres prepared by this method is spherical and size of the microspheres can be reduced to average diameter of about 1.5 µm by sonicating the emulsion. This size is suitable for macrophagic phagocytosis. The size and the surface characteristics of gelatin microspheres have great influence on their macrophagic uptake. Gelatin microspheres are found to be more opsonic than immunoglobulins and fibronectin, which are serum opsonic proteins. The gelatin microspheres have affinity towards the proteins, so in presence of the serum; the microspheres may get coated by the serum proteins leading to an increased opsonization.

The gelatin microspheres being susceptible for the macrophage recognition, can be used as carrier for the antigens. The antigens from microspheres are released within the macrophages upon their degradation leading to continual processing and presentation for antigen-specific antibodies production and synthesis. Thus, gelatin microspheres can be used as an immunoadjuvants.

Starch Microspheres

Starch is one of the most abundant biodegradable polymers that belongs to carbohydrate class. Starch being a polysaccharide, consists of larger number of the free hydroxyl groups. By means of these free hydroxyl groups a large number of the active ingredients can be incorporated within as well as on surface of microspheres. The starch microspheres when introduced into the body, undergo potential swelling, leading to the development of mucoadhesive character. Therefore, they are not cleared rapidly from the body cavity. Intranasally administered insulin starch microspheres are cleared slowly, thus offer a delivery mode for protein and small molecules.

Dextran Microspheres

Dextran, a carbohydrate is used to prepare hydrogel type of biodegradable and biocompatible systems. It can be chemically modified to provide for higher percentage of drug or proteins incorporation. Protein-loaded dextran microspheres are prepared by water in water emulsion technique (Fig. 12.11). In this method, an aqueous solution of the methacrylated dextran, is emulsified in an aqueous solution of polyethylene glycol (PEG). The dispersed methacrylated phase is then cross-linked by using free radical polymerization of the dextran-bound methacrylate groups. This leads to the formation of the dexran microspheres with typical hydrogel character. The method is based on the phenomenon that phase separation occurs in aqueous solution of the dextran and polyethylene glycol (PEG). By using water and water emulsion technology, it is possible to encapsulate IgG with very high entrapment or loading efficiency (more than 88%).

The release from the hydrogel matrix is dependent on the diffusion of the protein through the hydrogel matrix, if the protein diameter is smaller than the pore size of the matrix; it results in typical first order release. When the protein diameter is larger than the pore diameter, the release tends to be dependent on degradation rate of the gel. The rate of degradation of dextran microspheres depends entirely on the degree of substitution of the dextran and the amount of dextranase enzyme incorporated.

Polylactide and Polyglycolide Microspheres

Poly-(lactic acid) (PLA), poly-(glycolic acid) (PGA) and their copolymer poly-(lactide-co-glycolide) (PLGA), represent the group of synthetic biodegradable polymers. Sustained release preparations for many other drugs have been formulated by using copolymer of PLA and PGA. Microspheres from the PLA, PGA or PLGA may be prepared by any of the microparticles preparation techniques like single emulsion technique, double emulsion technique, phase separation coacervation, spray-drying, etc. The PLGA microspheres are successfully prepared by double emulsion technique and phase separation methods. The phase separation method produces agglomerated microsphere in case of large scale production while the double emulsion method is a lengthy and cumbersome procedure and it is difficult to incorporate the hydrophilic drugs. In contrast to these, spray-drying method is fast and by controlling the different process variable desired type and size of microspheres can be obtained.

Polyanhydride Microspheres

Polyanhydrides are biodegradable and biocompatible polymers. In 1980s, the polyanhydrides were rediscovered, as they can be used for the erosion-controlled devices in the area of drug delivery. Polyanhydride

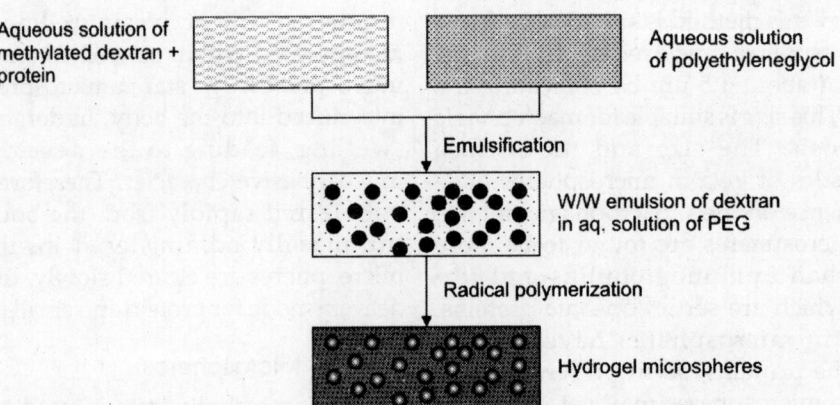

Fig. 12.11: Schematic representing preparation of hydrogel dextran microspheres

microspheres can be prepared by solvent evaporation, solvent extraction, hot melt technique and spray-drying techniques. For the hot melt encapsulation procedure, poly-anhydrides were melted, and drug was dispersed in the melted polymer. This suspension was then transformed into microspheres by addition to or of a nonsolvent, such as silicone or olive oil, at 5°C above the melting point of the polymer. The spheres solidified on subsequent cooling and were washed with petroleum ether. The temperature of the preparation is a limiting step of the method. Apart from these, the double walled poly-anhydride microspheres having two different polymer layers can be prepared using one of the two methods. The first method is based on the partial or complete insolubility of one polymer into other. The cosolution of the two polymers is then added to polyvinyl alcohol (PVA) aqueous solution followed by evaporation of the solvent. On evaporation of the solvent, the polymers separates from each other and finally give rise to core of one polymer while the coat of the other. The second method is based on the modified double emulsion technique. In this method, the microspheres in aqueous phase are dispersed in a polymer solution in organic phase to form W/O emulsion. This is then added to the aqueous PVA solution to form the double-walled microspheres instantaneously.

Polyphosphazene Microspheres

Polyphosphazene polymers have a long chain backbone of alternating nitrogen and phosphorus atoms with two side groups attached to each phosphorus atom (Fig. 12.12). Poly-phosphazene polymers form highly swollen ionotropic gel in the presence of the multi-valent ions in aqueous media, such as calcium. Because of this property, the polyphosphazene microspheres can be prepared in very mild conditions of low temperature and in the absence of the organic solvent. The phosphazene microspheres are prepared by using droplet apparatus, which produces spherical gel particle of size range 0.5–1.5 μm. In this method, the 2.5% phosphazene soltution is added in the form of the droplets to the 7.5% aqueous solution of calcium chloride. The microspheres (1–10 miron) are prepared to target Payer's patch M-cells and sub-epithelial macrophages. In this method the

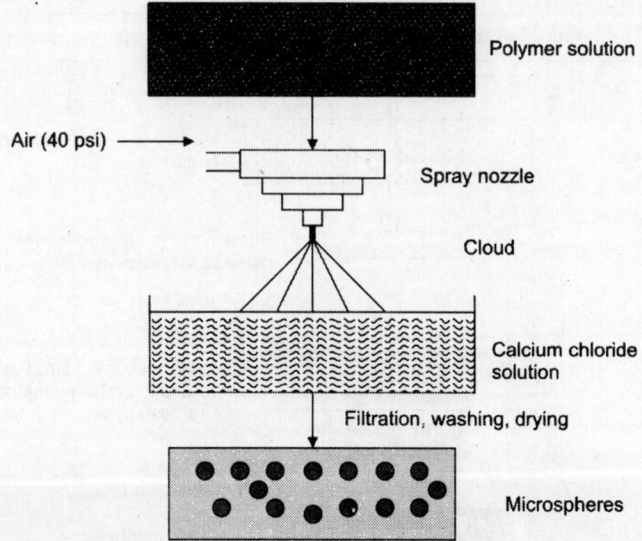

Fig. 12.12: Schematic representing the formation of polyphosphazene microspheres

polyphosphazene polymer solution at pressure (40 psi) is sprayed through an ultrasonic spray nozzle, which produces a spray cloud having the microdroplets of the polymer solution. This cloud when collide with the calcium chloride solution, instantaneously gelled to form the microsphere. The nature of the substrate and the gelation condition determine the encapsulation efficiency and the bioavailability and bioactivity of the substrate.

Chitosan Microspheres

Among polysaccharides, the chitosan is the deacetylated product of chitin and also one of the most useful natural polymers. Chitosan is insoluble at neutral and alkaline pH values, but forms salts with inorganic and organic acids, such as hydrochloric acid. Upon dissolution, the amine groups of chitosan get protonated and the resultant polymer becomes positively charged. Since chitosan exhibits net positive charge, it has been recently introduced in the market as an aid for weight loss and as cholesterol lowering agent. The mechanism behind chitosan may be its effect on lipid transport in the gut, where the positively-charged chitosan can bind to the free fatty acids and bile salt components and

hence disrupts overall lipid absorption. Yao et al., 1995 highlighted the preparation and properties of microcapsules and microspheres of chitosan. Due to attractive properties and wider applications of chitosan-based microcapsules and microspheres, they are used as a carrier for the applications in controlled drug release. Moreover, microcapsules and microspheres have an edge over other forms in regard to their handling and administration.

Carrageenan Microsphere

Carrageenan is an anionic polymer of hemisulfate galactose and 3–4 anhydrogalactose residue alternately linked by α (1–3) and β (1–4) glycosidic linkage. Hemisulfate ester groups impart negative charge to the polymer. Based on the sulfate groups esterification pattern, the polymer is graded as the L, kappa and delta. L-carrageenan has been proved to be a better candidate for the preparation of the microspheres using aqueous microencapsulation process that avoids the use of the organic solvents, which may alter the biological properties. Patil and Speaker, 1997 have described the method for carrageenan microspheres preparation (Fig. 12.13).

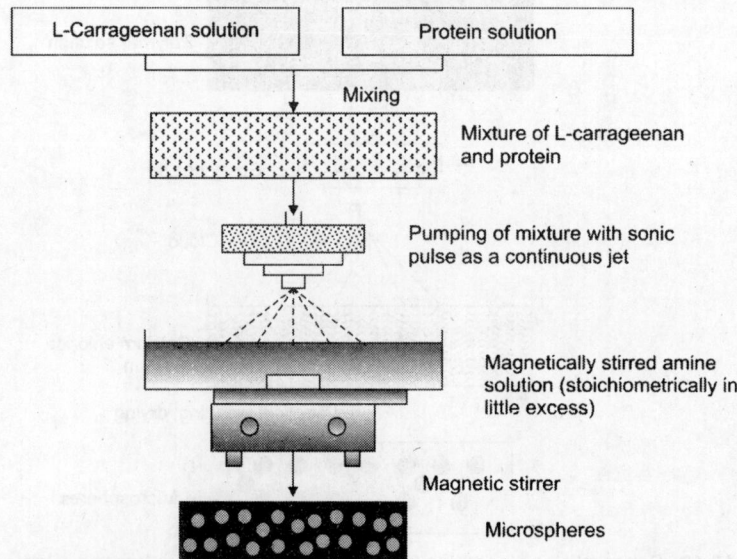

Fig. 12.13: Schematic for preparation of carrageenan microsphere

They pumped a mixture of 0.6 mM L-carrageenan (9 ml) and 1 mg/ml horseradish peroxide at the flow rate of the 1 ml/min through a 76 micron orifice to produce a continuous jet. Against the side of the capillary, sonic pulsing was applied to produce uniform droplets. The formed droplets were allowed to fall into a magnetically-stirred amine solution (15 ml). To establish the correct concentration of the amine, the concentration of amine was varied and tested for stable microspheres. Prepared microspheres were separated by the centrifugation (10,000 g) and washed twice with 10 ml distilled water.

Alginate Microspheres

Many of the present controlled release devices in their preparation involve harsh and hazardous chemicals, such as organic solvents or extreme conditions, such as high temperature, which can adversely affect the drug or the proteins. Alginate microspheres are suggested for such sensitive drugs. Sodium alginate (NaAlg), a water soluble salt of alginic acid, is a natural polysaccharide extracted from marine brown algae. NaAlg has been used as a matrix for entrapment of drugs and macromolecules.

Some of the applications of NaAlg relate to its particular property; it can form hydrophilic gels by interaction with bivalent metal ions. Since, alginate gel can easily be formed by this ionic interaction in aqueous medium, gel beads are commonly obtained by dropping solutions of sodium alginate into solutions of calcium chloride.

The alginate microspheres are usually prepared by suspending the protein in sodium alginate solution and spraying this solution into 1.3% w/v buffered (HEPES buffer) calcium chloride to form cross-linked microcapsules. Poor formation of the capsule occurs due to strong protein alginate interaction. As a result, diffusion technique is employed for the incorporation of the drug and proteins. Protein is then subsequently loaded by allowing its stepwise diffusion from solution of increasing concentration. The drug loaded capsules are coated with a final layer of polycation. In all, three polycation coatings are used, i.e. two prior loading and one after loading. The first coating influences the size, integrity, and loading capacity of the microcapsule. Very low concentration of polycation leads to formation of the capsule with poor integrity and loading while high concentration prevents the loading, of the microcapsules. The first coat also influences duration of the drug release, size, and burst effect. The second coat too influences the drug loading and the release characteristics. The final coat however, has little effect on the drug release.

Poly (Alkyl Cyanoacrylate) Microspheres

Poly (alkyl cyanoacrylate), PAC, is potential colloidal drug carrier for parenteral administration as well as through other alternative routes. The microspheres of the PAC are prepared by simple polymerization techniques. Several polymerization systems can be used for the preparation of the PAC microspheres, which lead to the microspheres production with different particle size ranges. The general method of preparation of PAC microspheres involves addition of the monomer (1% v/v) to the rapidly stirred aqueous phase. The pH of the system is critical in deciding the polymerization rate of the alkyl cyanoacrylate monomers. In body, polyalkyl cyanoacrylate microspheres degrade by reverse Knovenagel reaction resulting in the production of alkyl 2 cyanoacrylate and formaldehyde (Fig. 12.14). The rate of degradation varies with the ester chain length and pH of the media. The choice of the monomer and the polymerization condition also affect the degradation rate of the microspheres. PAC microspheres loaded with anticancerous agents have been extensively studied for the purpose of tumor targeting. PAC microspheres have natural affinity towards the tumors and they also possess inherent antitumor activity. These are found to have higher

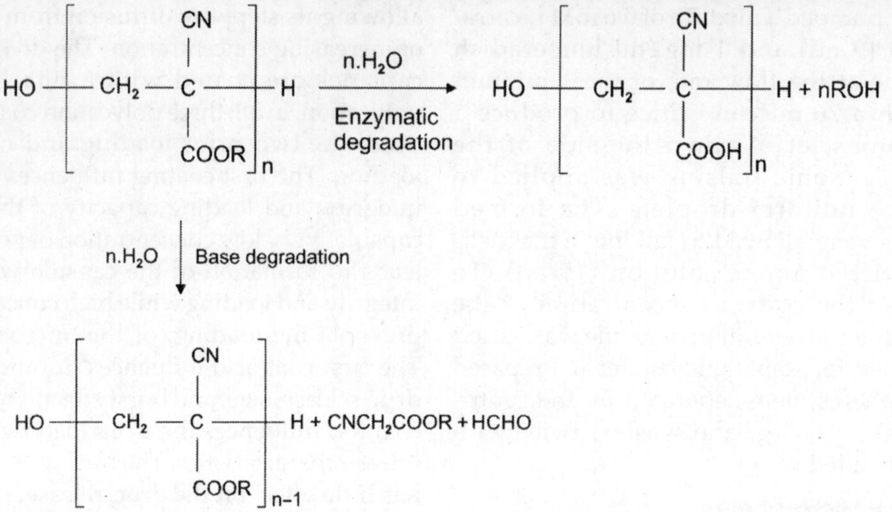

$$HO \left[CH_2 - \underset{\underset{COOR}{|}}{\overset{\overset{CN}{|}}{C}} \right]_n H \xrightarrow[\text{Enzymatic degradation}]{n.H_2O} HO \left[CH_2 - \underset{\underset{COOH}{|}}{\overset{\overset{CN}{|}}{C}} \right]_n H + nROH$$

$$\downarrow n.H_2O \quad \text{Base degradation}$$

$$HO \left[CH_2 - \underset{\underset{COOR}{|}}{\overset{\overset{CN}{|}}{C}} \right]_{n-1} H + CNCH_2COOR + HCHO$$

Fig. 12.14: Degradation pathways of poly (alkyl cyanoacrylate) microspheres

tumor uptake. The studies indicate that anti-tumor effect of cytotoxic drugs increases, when they are administered contained in the PAC microspheres. The PAC microspheres are also used for the targeting of the liver diseases. The tissue toxicity of PAC microspheres decreases with a decrease in the rate of degradation and it increases in a homologous series.

Polyacrolein Microspheres

Polyacrolein microspheres are functional type of the microspheres. These microspheres do not require any activation step, since the surfacial free aldehyde groups over the poly-acrolein can react with amine group of the protein to form Schiff's base. Polyacrolein microspheres remain active for more than a month, when stored at 4°C. The polyacrolein microspheres are prepared by alkaline poly-merization of acrolein monomer (Fig. 12.15) or by copolymerization of acrolein monomer with other monomers. Acrolein microspheres can be prepared by simple radiation polymeri-zation using Cobalt-60. Acrolein molecules have two functionality one is carboxyl while other is vinyl. Polyacrolein microspheres were successfully prepared by aqueous polymeri-zation of acrolein in the presence of an appro-priate surfactant under alkaline condition.

Agarose polyacrolein micro-beads can be prepared by encapsulating polyacrolein microspheres in agarose gel matrix. The cross-linking is affected using divinyl sulfone. This system acts as an efficient immunoadsorbent.

FATE OF MICROSPHERES IN BODY

Microparticulate carrier systems can be administered through different routes to achieve desired activity of either sustained action or targeting or both. Through different

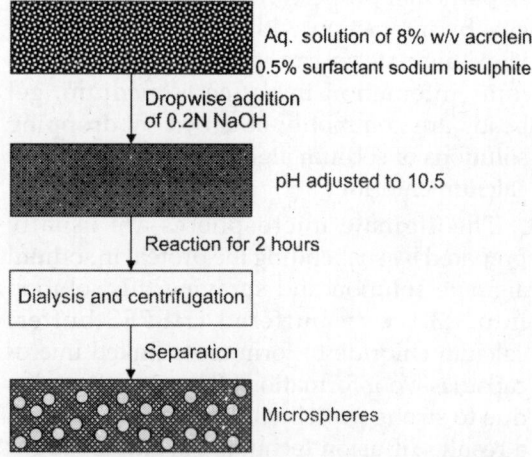

Fig. 12.15: Schematic representation of preparation of polyacrolein microspheres

routes, different mechanisms of uptake, transport and fate of translocated particles have been proposed. Biodegradable microparticulate carriers are of interest for oral delivery of drugs to improve the bioavailability, to enhance drug absorption, to target particular organ and reduce the toxicity, to improve gastric tolerance of gastric irritant to the stomach and as a carrier for antigen. The polystyrene microspheres administered orally are reported to be taken up by Peyer's patch. They are subsequently translocated to discrete anatomical compartments, such as mesenteric lymph vessels, lymph nodes and to a lesser extent in liver and spleen. The particulate matters gain entry into follicle-associated epithelium through Peyer's patches.

After the uptake of the particulate carrier(s) via different mechanism, their fate becomes important (Table 12.2). Some uptake mechanisms avoid the lysosomal system of the enterocytes. The particles following uptake by enterocytes are transported to the mesenteric lymph, then to systemic circulation and are subsequently phagocytosized by the Kupffer cells of liver. However, after uptake by enterocytes, some particulate carriers may be taken up into vacuoles and discharged back into gut lumen. Microspheres can also be designed for the controlled release to the gastrointestinal tract. The release of the drug content depends on the size of microparticles and the drug content within microspheres. The release of the drug could be regulated by selecting an appropriate hydrophilic/lipophilic balance of the matrix, such as in case of matrix of polyglycerol esters of fatty acid. Microparticles of mucoadhesive polymers get attached to the mucous layer in GIT and hence prolong the gastric residence time and functionally offer a sustained drug release. The microspheres of particle size less than 0.87 μm are taken to the general circulation. The fluid environment of the GIT can affect the number and rate of particles translocation. Microspheres given by parenteral route (intravenous) distribute themselves according to their size range. The microparticulate carriers are rapidly cleared from the circulation mainly by means of reticuloendothelial system. After intravenous administration the particulate carriers distribute themselves passively or if suitably designed, then actively. This distribution is referred to as passive mode of the site-specific delivery of the microparticulates.

APPLICATIONS OF MICROSPHERES

Microspheres in Vaccine Delivery

The desirable prerequisite of a vaccine is its ability to offer protection against the microorganism or its toxic product. An ideal vaccine must fulfill the requirement of efficacy, safety, convenience in application and cost. The aspect of safety and minimization of adverse reaction is a complex issue (Fudenberg et al., 1993). The aspect of safety and the degree of production of antibody responses are closely related to the mode of application. Biodegradable delivery systems for vaccines that are given by parenteral route may overcome the shortcomings of the conventional vaccines (Capron et al., 1994, Edelman 1993, Drews 1984). The interest in parenteral (subcutaneous, intramuscular, intradermal) carrier lies since they offer specific advantages including:

1. Improved antigenicity by adjuvant action
2. Modulation of antigen release
3. Stabilization of antigen

Biodegradable polymers constitute a class of polymers of choice for the delivery of the vaccine, since they do not require surgical removal. Apart from biodegradation kinetics, the mode and rate of presentation of antigen, toxicity, tissue compatibility as well as antigen stability are the properties that are critically considered for the selection of an appropriate polymer and method of preparation. Thermoplastic polyesters of poly-(lactic acid), poly (glycolic acid) and their copolymers poly (lactic-co-glycolic acid) (PLGA) are studied extensively as carrier for many antigens.

Stability

Antigen polymer compatibility is a major impediment to be considered in the design of a suitable carrier, because it may lead to the stability problem. The polymer compatibility can be increased by coencapsulating buffer salts and stabilisers for proteins to increase the antigen stability by modifying the internal pH of microspheres and accelerating swelling. The use of triblock (ABA) copolymers having hydrophilic A block (PLA or PLAGA) and hydrophilic B block (polyoxyethylene, PEO) also provides stability to the carrier system by providing more biosoft system.

Microspheres of hydrophilic nature for the delivery of proteins/antigen can be prepared by any of the three methods viz., W/O/W triple emulsion method, spray-drying method and phase separation method. Mostly, antigens are proteins that require of specific three-dimensional configurations for their activity. The factors, which can alter the conformations of proteins (antigens) are listed below:

Factors affecting antigen stability are:

- Polymer
- Moisture
- Lyophilization
- pH
- Shearing
- Temperature
- Hydrophilic/hydrophobic surface
- Salt
- Organic solvent

Microspheres and Immune System

The interaction of the microspheres with macrophages (Fig. 12.16) depends upon the particle size. Microspheres of particle size less than 10 µm are directly taken up by the antigen presenting cells. The microparticles with particle size range greater than 10 µm first undergo degradation or release of antigen, which are then phagocytosed by antigen presenting cells. The antigen presenting cells are responsible for the activation of B- and

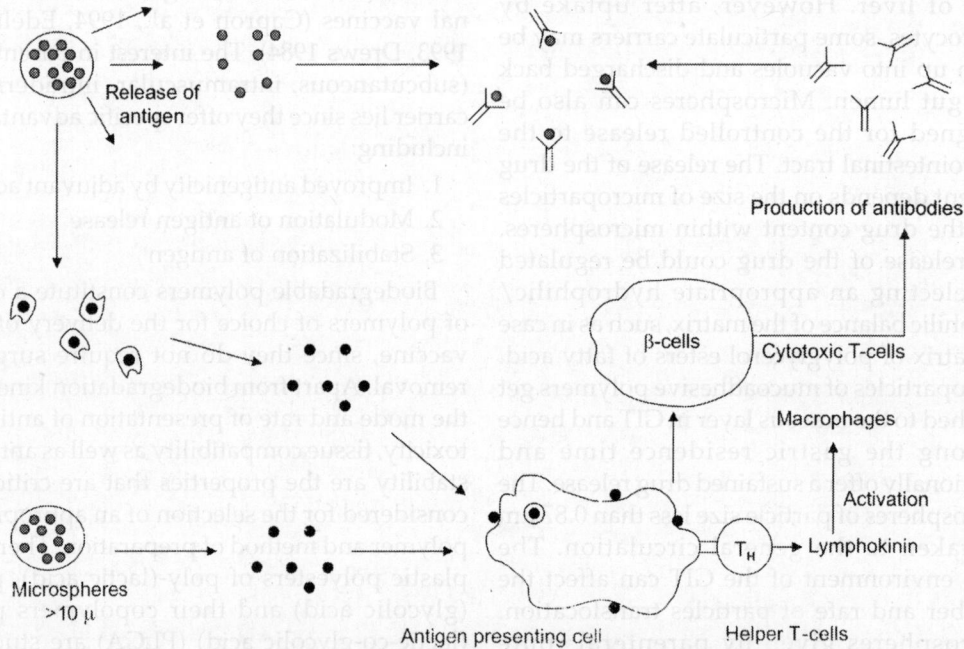

Fig. 12.16: Antigen bearing microspheres interacting with macrophages

T-cells and hence, the immunological consequences. A number of antigens are under investigation for their efficient delivery through the microsphere.

Targeting Using Microparticulate Carriers

The concept of targeting, i.e. site-specific drug delivery is a well-established scientific dogma, which is gaining immense attention. The therapeutic efficacy of the drug relies on its access to and specific interaction of the drug with its candidate receptors.

The ability to leave the blood pool in reproducible, efficient and specific manner a determinant parameter of drug action mediated by use of a carrier system. Placements of the particles in discrete anatomical compartment lead to their retention either because of the physical properties of the environment or biophysical interaction of the particles with the cellular content of the target tissue.

Ocular

The eye and the cornea are easily accessible targets. The washout effect, however presents major difficulties in regard to retention of microparticulate drug carrier in the corneal sac. Gurny has described a novel approach to increase the retention of the microparticulates system by changing them to the gel form in the cul de sac of eye. The rapid conversion of the particulates suspension to gel form reportedly leads to their longer retention in the eye.

Intranasal

The intranasal route is exploited for the delivery of the peptides and proteins. The conventional dosage forms are rapidly cleared from the nasal mucosa. Bioadhesive gels have been proposed to increase the retention of the insulin and calcitonin. The bioadhesive microspheres are used as an alternative to the gel dosage formulations. In comparison to the gel dosage form, the bioadhesive microspheres have shown better control over the surface character and the drug release pattern.

Various improvised therapeutic applications of microspheres in intranasal delivery are widely reported and discussed in the literature.

Oral

Oral route is one of the most convenient routes for the administration of the drug. Thus, a number of the controlled release systems have been developed. Single unit system has disadvantage of being removed with the chyme. Thus, their gastrointestinal transit time is determined by the frequency of the stomach emptying and casual localization in the vicinity of pylorus. In comparison to single unit systems, multiple unit system has marked advantages, as it spreads over a large area and avoids the exposure of high concentration of drug to the mucosa. The risk of dose dumping is considerably low. The drug release is affected by the size of the microspheres as well as the drug content. The smaller size particles and high drug loaded particles show faster release. The faster release from highly loaded microspheres is due to the formation of pores as the drug dissolution proceeds.

Oral route is also suggested for the delivery of the soluble antigens. This as viable alternative of the particles of definite size range, can gain an access to and through the Payer's patches. The particulate carriers are effective for delivery of both the entrapped and adsorbed antigen.

Many drug substances are characterized by poor solubility in aqueous media and thus they impose problems in formulation that is intended specially for oral administration. In spite of promising potentials demonstrated *in vitro*, the development of such substances is often prematurely halted as a consequence of their inadequate oral bioavailability. Besides the use of cosolvents or absorption enhancers, incorporation in carrier systems has been proposed as an alternative to render poorly water-soluble drugs better administrable through oral route. pH-sensitive microparticles are particles composed of polymers, which possess a pH-dependent solubility. While remaining stable at a low pH environment, such as in the stomach, these particles are expected to allow an improved enteric drug delivery. The incorporation of anti-infective agents of weak aqueous solubility into pH-sensitive microparticles provides an efficient oral delivery system.

There is preferential size-dependent deposition of microparticles or nanoparticles in the inflamed tissue in inflammatory bowel disease after oral administration. Such targeted delivery of an entrapped drug reduces side effects. In the inflamed colonic tissue, an increased adherence of particles is observed. This probably results from an increased attachment to the thicker mucus layer at the inflamed regions and an accumulation inside the ulcerated colonic tissue. A size dependency of the deposition was observed. For 10 μm particles only fair deposition was recorded where, 1μm particles showed higher binding. The highest deposition in inflamed tissue was seen in case of 0.1 μm particles. Moreover, attached particles showed a prolonged retention in the inflamed regions for up to 5 days. The size-dependent deposition of particles in the inflamed tissue may allow for designing of carrier systems for the site-specific treatment of inflammatory bowel disease.

The introduction of the drug in the systemic circulation along with the microparticles provides a means to target either to the vasculature or to the extravascular compartments, accessible via capillary endothelium. The intravascular targets are mononuclear phagocytic system, diagnostic imaging, and the blood cells that may be recognized by ligands including antibodies, hormones and simple sugars. These are targeted for various purposes including diagnostic imaging to the delivery of the chemotherapeutics and antigens.

The major objective of drug targeting is to produce localized controlled release of drug(s) within the extravascular compartment of the desired organ or tissue. Efficient transport across microvascular barrier can subsequently be achieved by:

1. Magnetic dragging of the magnetic microparticles (microspheres, nanoparticles) directly through endothelium and basement membrane.
2. Facilitated transport of specific ligand drug conjugates (biochemical targeting) or coated microspheres (bioadhesive targeting) across endothelium, as a result of ligand binding to luminal surface associated antigen or receptors.
3. Transient regional opening of endothelium function combined with vascular infusion of drug carrier that becomes eventually sequestered in the extracellular complex.

The extravascular targets include various tissues and organs which require and utilize carriers especially for selective delivery of drug(s) to tumor sites.

Magnetic Microspheres

Targeting of drug under controlled, burst or modulated release using biophysical approaches is a new way to achieve site-specific drug delivery. These approaches utilize a wide range of modalities, such as hyperthermia, arterial perfusion, arterial chemoembolization, intracavity injection and use of extracorporeal magnetic field. In developing different approaches for drug(s) targeting, it is instructive to observe and consider as to how the body localizes its own biopharmaceuticals in the desired tissues.

Magnetic monitoring has the advantage of being efficient in allowing high local concentration of therapeutic agents. A variety of magnetically responsive carriers have been developed and proposed for chemotherapeutic targeted delivery of agents. These include magnetite containing matrices (microspheres or nanoparticles of the starch, albumin, ethyl cellulose, etc.), ethyl oleate based emulsion and natural cells such as erythrocyte ghosts. Magnetite targeting is most efficient method developed for targeting active agents. Up to 60% of injected dose can be targeted and delivered to the selected non-endothelial organs. Multiple body regions can be accessed using magnetic microspheres, but this must be accomplished sequentially. In order to avoid toxicity due to focal overdosing; hence, a magnet with constant gradient must be used. Magnetic microspheres are prepared by mixing water soluble drugs (for lipophilic drugs, along with the dispersing agents) and 10 nm magnetite (Fe_3O_4) particles in an aqueous solvent of matrix material. This mixture is then emulsified in the oil. Ultrasonication or shearing is applied to produce particles of suitable size range. The matrix is then stabilized by chemical cross-linking or heating. Magnetic microspheres are administered via intra-arterial or intravenous injection. Intra-arterial injection is given to achieve high systemic targeting while intravenous administration helps achieving high pulmonary targeting or medium systemic targeting. Magnetic microspheres in response to extracorporeal magnetic field get captured in small arterioles and capillaries of magnetic target organ.

Monoclonal Antibodies Mediated Microspheres-targeting Immuno-microspheres

Monoclonal antibodies mediated targeting is a method used to achieve selective targeting to the specific sites. Monoclonal antibodies are extremely specific molecules. This extreme specificity of the monoclonal antibodies (MABS) can be utilized to target microspheres loaded bioactive molecules to selected sites. MABS can be directly attached to the microspheres by means of covalent coupling. The free aldehyde groups, amino groups, or hydroxyl groups on the surface of the microspheres can be linked to the antibodies. Microspheres from different material (e.g. Bovine serum albumin and polyacrolein) and prepared using different methods carry different functional groups, which help in the coupling of the antibodies. The MABS can be attached to the microspheres by any of the following methods:

1. Nonspecific adsorption
2. Specific adsorption
3. Direct coupling
4. Coupling via reagents

MABS can be adsorbed nonspecifically on to the surface of the hydrophobic microspheres by physical adsorption, which render them more hydrophilic. Hydrophilic microspheres are more suitable for the cell targeting. Monoclonal antibodies form immunomicrospheres on coupling with the microspheres. Immuno-microspheres are formed nonspecifically by van der Waals–London forces. Mabs can be adsorbed on the surface of polyhexyl cyanoacrylate microparticles by simple incubation of microspheres with excess of antibodies at 40°C in phosphate buffer saline. Specific adsorption can be conducted by means of the ligands, which interacts directly with intact or modified antibodies. Protein A from *Staphylococcus aureus* and avidin biotin are two specific ligands that are used for specific adsorption purpose. *Staphylococcus aureus* protein A binds with Fc portion of the antibodies of subclass IgG. Mabs can be adsorbed by briefly incubating with microspheres carrying protein A at 37°C. Protein A can be incorporated within the microsphere at the time of preparation of the microspheres along with the matrix material. Protein A is used for linking monoclonal antibodies against HLA-BW6 type of carcinoma to human bovine serum albumin microspheres. Biotinylated monoclonal antibodies can be linked to polymethacrylate microspheres bearing acetylated avidin (Fig. 12.17). Specific

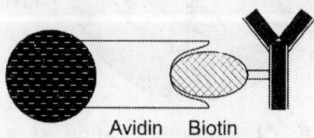

Avidin   Biotin

Fig.12.17: Schematic showing microsphere avidin biotin

adsorption occurs because of natural affinity of some of the natural molecules to their counterparts, e.g. avidin for biotin.

Direct coupling is achieved by means of free functional groups present on the surface of the microspheres. The functional microspheres undergo direct coupling, e.g. polyacrolein microspheres have free functional carboxyl groups, which help them to couple with the monoclonal antibodies.

CHEMOEMBOLIZATION

Chemoembolization is an endovascular therapy, which involves the selective arterial embolization of a tumor together with simultaneous or subsequent local delivery of the chemotherapeutic agent (Fig. 12.18). It is an extension of traditional percutaneous embolization techniques. With chemoembolization, investigators embolize tumors using microparticles soaked with chemotherapeutic agents. The theoretical advantage is that such embolizations will not only provide vascular occlusion, but also will bring about sustained therapeutic levels of chemotherapeutics in the areas of tumor. Generalized ischemia so created would reduce the ability of the cell to relieve itself from the toxicity of chemotherapy. Degradable starch microspheres injected intra-arterially are trapped in an extracapillary network formed in liver metastases. Drug dissolved in the microsphere suspension gets retained in the blood vessels

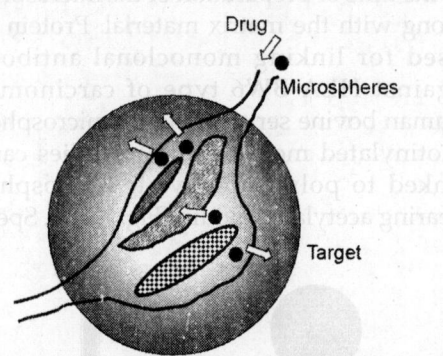

Fig. 12.18: Chemoembolization as a method of targeting

of the target organ, as long as the blood flow remains blocked and then gradually releases, resulting in a longer duration of tumor exposure to the drug. The technique of chemoembolization is a combination of beneficial effect of embolization and local chemotherapy. Intra-arterial injection of the microspheres increases the therapeutic efficacy of the antimitotic drugs by causing temporary embolization. Spherical particles are most useful in achieving distal homogeneous and effective embolism. The kinetics of drug release from the emboli and biodegradation rate of drug carriers are important determinants in determining the bioavailability of the drug in the restricted area. The biodegradable microspheres of starch, PLA or PLGA may be used for the purpose of achieving intended occlusion. The microspheres of size >40 micrometer are injected intra-arterially, it causes blockade of the arteriole at the tumor sites. This blockade of the arterioles and the capillary bed may be beneficial in two ways, first it increases the time of absorption of drugs at the tumor site and second, due to blockade of feeder vessels, it causes ischemia and hence leads to the tumor regression.

Imaging

The microspheres have been extensively studied and used for the targeting purposes. Various cells, cell lines, tissues and organs can be imaged using radio-labeled microspheres. The particle size range of microspheres is an important factor in determining the imaging of particular sites. The particles injected intravenously apart from the portal vein will become entrapped in the capillary bed of the lungs. This phenomenon is exploited for the scintigraphic imaging of the tumor masses in lungs using labeled human serum albumin microspheres.

Surface Modified Microspheres

The objective of drug therapy using carriers is the selective delivery of drug to specific sites in the body. The phagocytosis of colloidal carriers, rapid clearance and passive distribution are frequently encountered common disadvantages of particulate systems. The change in the biophysical behavior of the particle helps to avoid the difficulties in targeting. Different approaches have been utilized to change the surface properties of carriers to protect them against phagocytic clearance and to alter the body distribution pattern. The adsorption of the poloxamer on the surface of the polystyrene, polyester or polymethylmethacrylate microspheres renders them more hydrophilic and hence decreases their MPS uptake. Protein microspheres covalently modified by PEG derivatives show decreased immunogenicity and clearance. Among the most studied surface modifiers are:

1. Antibodies and their fragments
2. Proteins
3. Mono, oligo, and polysaccharides
4. Chelating compounds (EDTA, DTPA or desferroxamine)
5. Synthetic soluble polymers.

The surface of the albumin microspheres can be modified by covalent attachment of polyoxy(C1–4) alkyene chain having terminal ether group. The polyoxyethylene moiety may react with surface amino or carboxyl residues through condensation with an appropriate functional group in the presence of condensing agent, e.g. 1,1-carbonyldi-imidazole and N-(3-dimethyl amino propyl)-N'-ethyl carbodiimide hydrochloride (EDAC). The surface-modified albumin microspheres having terminally linked galactose moiety are used for liver targeting of antitumor agent(s) like 5-flurouracil. Such modifications are provided to the surface of the microspheres in order to achieve the targeting to the discrete organs and to avoid rapid clearance from the body. A list of patents of microsphere is given in Table 12.2.

Table 12.2: List of patents of microspheres

Patent no.	Year	Original assignee/inventor	Title
US5718921	Feb 17, 1998	Edith Mathiowitz, Claudy J.P. Mullon, Abraham J. Domb, Robert S. Langer	Microspheres comprising polymer and drug dispersed there within
US6395302	May 28, 2002	Octoplus B.V., Wilhelmus Everhardus Hennink,Okke Franssen	Method for the preparation of microspheres, which contains colloidal systems
US6905763	Jun 14, 2005	Michael D. Crandall, Terrence E. Cooprider	Microsphere adhesive-coated article for use with coated papers
US7300700	Nov 27, 2007	Andrew J. Callinan, Jason D. Romsos	Cationic microspheres and method of making cationic microspheres
US7374782	May 20, 2008	Larry R. Brown	Production of microspheres
US7815941	Oct 19, 2010	Larry R. Brown, Terrence L. Scott, Debra Lafreniere, Vered Bisker-Leib	Nucleic acid microspheres, production and delivery thereof
US7884085	Feb 8, 2011	Larry R. Brown, Vered Bisker-Leib, Terrence L. Scott, Debra Lafreniere, Jennifer Machen, Nick Giannoukakls	Delivery of AS-oligonucleotide microspheres to induce dendritic cell tolerance for the treatment of autoimmune type 1 diabetes
US7964574	Jun 21, 2011	Larry R. Brown, Nick Giannoukakis, Kimberly A. Gillis, Massimo Trucco	Microspheres-based composition for preventing and/or reversing new-onset autoimmune diabetes.
US7645355	Jan 12, 2010	Lori A. Bilski, Dale O. Bailey, Mark S. Vogel, Frederick J. Gustafson	Method of making a microsphere transfer adhesive

SUGGESTED READINGS

1. Akiyama Y, Yoshioka M, Horibe H, Hirai S, Kitamori N, and Toguchi H, *Journal of controlled release* 26 (1993) 1–10.

2. Albertson AC, Carlfors J and Sturesson C, *J. Appl. Polym. Sci.* 62 (1996) 695–705.

3. Allcock HR and Kwon S, *Macromolecules.* 22(1989) 75–9.

4. Almeida AJ, Alpar HO and Brown MRW, *Proc. Int. Symp. Controlled Release Bioact. Mater.* 20 (1993) 390–401.

5. Alonso MJ, Cohen S, Park TW, Gupta RK, Siber GR and Langer R; *Proc. Int. Symp. Controlled Release Bioact. Mater.* 19 (1992) 120–31.

6. Alpar HO, Field WN, Hyde R and Lewis DA, *J. Pharm. Pharmcol.* 41(1989) 194–6.

7. Anderson JM, *Eur. J. Pharmcol. Biopharm.* 10 (1994) 1–10.

8. Anderson LC, Wise DL and Howes JF, *Contraception* 13 (1976) 375–84.

9. Andrianov AK, Cohen S, Visscher KB, Payne LG, Allcock HR and Langer R, *J. Controlled Release.* 27 (1993) 69–77.

10. Arneodo C, Benoit JP, Thies C, *STP Pharma Sciences.* 2 (1986) 303–306.

11. Aslani P, Kennedy RA, *J Controlled Release.;* 42 (1996) 75–82.

12. Avila JL, *Intersciencia.* 8(1983) 405–17.

13. Axen R, Porath J and Ernback S, *Nature.* 214 (1967) 1302.

14. Badwan AA, Abumalooh A, Sallam E, Abukalaf A, Jawan O, *Drug Dev Ind Pharm.* 11 (1985) 239–56.

15. Barbet J, Machy P and Laserman LD, *J. Supramol. Struct. Cell Biochem.* 16 (1981) 243.

16. Benita S, Benoit JP, Puisieux F, Thies C, *J Pharm Sci.* 73 (1984): 1721–4.

17. Benita S, Benoit JP, Puisieux F and Theis C, *J. Pharm. Sci.* 73 (1984) 1721–4.

18. Benita S, Fickat R, benoit JP, Bonnemain B, Samaille JP and Madoule P, *J. Microencapsulation* 1 (1984) 317–27.

19. Benoit JP, Thies C In: Benita S, *ed. Drugs and the Pharmaceutical Sciences.,* Vol. 73. (1996) New York: Marcel Dekker.

20. Bjork J and Edman P, *Int. J. Pharm.* 47 (1988) 233.

21. Bodmeier R, McGinity J, *J Microencapsul.,* 4 (1987) 279–88.

22. Bodmer D, Kissel T and Traechslin E; *J. Controlled Release.* 21 (1992) 129–134.

23. Bouillot P, Babak V, Dellacherie E. *Pharm Res.,* 16 (1999) 148–54.

24. Bowersock TL, Hogenesch H, Suckow M, et al. *Int J Pharm.* 39 (1996) 209–20.

25. Brasseur F, Couvreur P, Kante B, Deckers-Passau L Roland M Deckers C and Speiser P, *Eur. J. Cancer.* 16(1980) 1441–5.

26. Brown R, Wei CL and Langer R; *J. Pharm. Sci.* 72(1983) 1181–9.

27. Bucher JE and Slade WC, *J. Am. Chem. Soc.* 31 (1990) 1319–21.

28. Burger JJ, Tomlinson E, Mudler EMA and McVie JG, *Int. J. Pharm.* 23 (1985) 333–44.

29. Caponetti G, Hrkach JS, Kriwet B, Poh M, Lotan N, Colombo P, Langer R. *J Pharm Sci;* 88 (1999) 136–41.

30. Capron AC, Locht C and Fracchia GN. Vaccine. 12 (1994) 667–72.

31. Cohen S, Bano MC, Visscher KB, Chaw M, Allcock HR, Langer R; *J. Am. Chem. Soc.* 112 (1990) 7832–3.

32. Cohn ZA, Mononuclear phagocytes. By R van, Blackwell Scientific, Oxford. 1970 pp 121.

33. Couvreur P and Aurby J in "Topics in Pharmaceutical Sciences" DD Breimer ed. Vol II Elsevier Biomedical Press Amsterdam 1984 pp. 305.

34. Cushimano AG and Becker CH, *J. Pharm. Sci.* 57 (1968) 1104–12.

35. Desai MP, Labhasetwar V, Amidon JL and Levy RJ, *Pharmaceutical research* Vol. 13 No. 12 1996 1838–45.

36. Douglas SJ, Illum L and Davis SS, *J. Colloid Interface.* 103(1985a) 154–63.

37. Douglas SJ, Illum L and Davis SS, *J. Controlled Release.* 3 (1986) 15–23.

38. Douglas SJ, Illum L and Holding SR, *J. Br. Polym.* 17 (1985b) 339–42.

39. Ebel JP, *Pharm Res.* 7 (1990) 848–51.

40. Edelman R, Vaccine. 11 (1993) 1361–7.

41. Eldridge JH, Hammond CJ, Meulbroek JA, Staas JK, Gilley RM and Tice TR; *J. Controlled Release.* 11 (1990) 205–14.

42. El-Samaligy MS and Rohdewald P, *Pharm Act. Helv.* 57 (1981) 201–4.

43. Esparza I and Kissel T, *Vaccine.* 10 (1992) 714–720.

44. Franssen O. and Hennink W E.; Int. J. Pharm. 168 (1998) 1–7.

45. Franssen O. Stenekes R J H. and Hennink W E.; J. Cont. Rel. 59 (1999) 219–28.

46. Fudenberg HH, Stites DP, Caldwel JL and Wells JV; Basic and clinical immunology. 2nd ed., Lange Medical, Los Altos CA, 1978.

47. Gohel MC, Sheth MN, Patel MM, Jani GK, and Patel H, *Indian J Pharm Sci*, 56 (1994) 210.

48. Gopferich A, Alonso MJ and langer R, *Pharm Res*. 11 (1994) 1568–74.

49. Grant GT, Morris ER, Rees DA, Smith PJC, Thom D FEBS Lett. 32 (1973) 195–8.

50. Griffin FM, Griffin JA, leider JE and Silverstein SC; *J. Exp. med*. 142 (1975) 1263.

51. Hashida M, Muranishi S, Sezaki H, Tangigawa Nsotomura K and Hikasa Y; *Int. J. Pharm*. 2 (1979) 145–56.

52. Hermann JB, Kelly RJ and Higgins GA; *Arch. Surg*. 100 (1970) 486–90.

53. Hora Ms, Rana RK, Nunberg JH, Tice TR, Gilley RM and Hudson ME, *Pharm. Res*. 7(1990) 1190–94.

54. Ikada Y and Tabata Y; Phagocytosis of bioactive microspheres, *J. Bioact. Compt. Polym*. 1 (1982) 31.

55. Illum L, Davis SS, Muller RH, Mak E and West P, *Life Sci*. 40(1987) 367–74.

56. Illum L, Jones PDE, kreuter J, Baldwin RW and Davis SS, *Int. J. Pharm*. 17(1983) 65–76.

57. Jalil R and Nixon JR, *J. Microecapsulation* 7 (1990) 297–326.

58. Jani P, Halbert GW, Langridge J and Florence A T, *J. Pharm. Pharmacol*. 42 (1990) 821–6.

59. John PM and Becker CH, *J. Pharm. Sci*. 57 (1968) 584–9.

60. Kabanov and Zezin AB, *Sol. Sci. Rev.sec B Chem. Rev*. 4 (1982) 207–82.

61. Kandjia J, Anderson MJD and Muller-Ruchholtz WJ, *Cancer Res. Clin. Oncol*. 101 (1981) 165.

62. Kante B, Couvreur P, Dubois-Krack G, De Meester C, Guoit P, Roland M, Mercier M and Speiser P, *J. Pharm. Sci*. 71(1982) 786–90.

63. Kassab A Ch, Xu K, Denkbas EB, Dou Y, Zhao S, Piskin E, *Journal of Biomat. Sci.: Polymer Edition*, Vol. 8, No. 12, pp. 947–61, 1997.

64. Kikuchi A, Kawabuchi M, Sugihara M, Sakurai Y, Okano T. *Proc Intern Symp Control Rel Bioact Mater*. 23 (1996) 737–8.

65. Kim CK, Lee EJ, *Int J Pharm*. 79 (1992) 11–19.

66. Kreuter J, Berg U, Leihl E, Soliva M and Speiser PP Vaccine. 4 (1986) 125.

67. Kreuter J, Berg U, Leihl E, Soliva M and Speiser PP Vaccine. 4 (1986) 253.

68. Kreuter J, Mills SN, Davis SS, and Wilson CG, *International journal of pharm*. 16 (1983) 105–13.

69. Kreuter J, Nefzger M, Liehl E, Czok R, and Voges R, *J. pharm. Sci*. 72 (1983) 1146–9.

70. Lee TK, Sokoloksi TD and Royer GP, *Science* 213 (1981) 233–5.

71. longo WE, Iwata H, Lindheimer TA and Goldberg EP, *J. Pharm. Sci*. 71 (1982) 1323–8.

72. MacAdam AB, Shafi JB, James SL, Marriott C and Martin GP, *International journal of pharmaceutics* 151 (1997) 47–55.

73. Maincent P, Verge RL, Sado PA, Couvreur P, and Devissaguet JP, *J. Pharm. Sci*. 75 (9186) 955–8.

74. Maincent P, PhD Thesis university of Paris-Sud. 1982.

75. Margel S and Wiesel E, *J Polym. Sci*. 22 (1984) 145–58.

76. Marty JJ, Oppenheim and Speiser PP, *Pharm. Acta. Helv*. 53(1978) 17–23.

77. Millar AM, McMillan L, Hannan WJ, Emmett PC and Aitken RJ, *Int. J. Appl. Radiat*. Isot. 33 (1982), 1423–6.

78. Mumper RJ, Hoffman AS, Poulakkainen PA, Bouchard LS, Gombotz WR, *J. Controlled Release*. 30 (1994), 241–51.

79. Nellore RV, Pande PG, Young D and Bhagat HR, *J. Parent. Sci. Tech*. 46 (1992), 176–180.

80. North RJ, *Endocytosis. Semin. Hematol*. 7 (1970), 161.

81. O'Hagen DT, Palin K and Davis SS, Vaccine. 7(1989a) 213–216.

82. O'Hagen DT, Palin K Davis SS, Artursson P and Sjoholm I, Vaccine. 7(1989b) 421–4.

83. O'Hagen DT, *Advanced drug delivery reviews* 5 (1990), 265–85.

84. Ohya Y and Takei T, *Chem Ind (Jpn.)*, 46 (1993) 798.

85. Oppenheim RC, *Int. J. Pharm*. 8 (1981), 217–34.

86. Patel RP, Lopiekes DV, Brown SP and Price S, *Biopolymers* 5 (1967) 577.

87. Patil RT and Speaker TJ, *J. Micrencapsul*. 14 (1997) 169–74.

88. Patil RT and Speaker TJ, *J. Pharm. Sci*. 89 (2000) 9–15.

89. Rajeev A Jain, *Biomaterial* 21(2000) 2475–2490.

90. Ravi kumar MNV, *J. Pharmaceu. Sci*. 3(2) 2000 234–58.

91. Rembaum A and Dreyer WJ, *Science* 208 (1980) 364–72.

92. Rembaum A US Patent 4, 413 070 (1983).

93. Rembaum A, Margel S and Levy J, *J. Immunol. Methods*. 24 (1978) 239.

94. Richards FM and Knowles JR, *J. Mol. Bio*. 37 (1968) 231.

95. Roitt IM, Brostoff J and Male DK; Kurzes Lehrbuch der Immunologie. George Thieme Verlag. Stuttgart. 1991.

96. Roland M and Speiser P; US Patent. (1982) 329, 332.

97. Rosen HB, Chang J, Wnek GE, Linhardt R J and Langer R, *Biomaterisls* 4 (1983) 131.

98. Rubio MR, Ghaly ES. *Drug Dev Ind Pharm.* 20 (1994) 1239–51.

99. Russel GF, *Pharm. Int.* 4 (1983) 260–63.

100. Sanders E and Ashworth CT, *Exp. Cell Res.* 22 (1961) 137–45.

101. Sefton M, Brown LR and Langer RS, *J. pharm. Sci.* 73 (1984) 1859–61.

102. Shah NH, Railkar AS, Chen FC, Tarantino R, Kumar S, Murjani M, Palmer D Infeld MH and Malick AWJ, *Control Rel.* 27 (1993), 139–47.

103. Shilvey ML, Coonts BA, Renner WD, Southhard H and Benett ATJ, *Control Rel.* 33 (1995) 237–43.

104. Siegel RA and Langer R, *Pharm. Res.* 1 (1984), 1–12.

105. Singh M, Singh A and Talwar GP, *Pharm. Res.* 8 (1991), 958–62.

106. Spier RE, Vaccine. 11 (1993) 1450–54.

107. Tabata Y and Ikada Y Biomaterials 9 (1988), 356.

108. Tabata Y, Nakaoka R, and Ikada Y Vaccine. 13 (1995) 653.

109. Takada S, Uda Y, Toguchi H and Ogawa YJ, *Pharm. Sci. Technol.* 49(4) (1995) 180–84.

110. Tanake N, Takino S and Utsumi I, *J. Pharm. Sci.* 52 (1963) 664–7.

111. Timida H, Mizuo C, Nakamura C, Kiryu, S, *Chem. Pharm Bull.* 41 (1993) 1475–7.

112. Tomlinson E.; *Int. J. Pharm. Tech. Prod. Mfr.* 4 (1983) 49–57.

113. Van Oss CF and Singer JH RES J, *Reticuloendothel. Soc.* 3 (1966) 29.

114. Van Oss CF, Gilman CF and Neumann AW, *"Phagocytic engulfment and cell adhesiveness"* PI dekker, New York, 1975.

115. Van Oss CJ, Phagocytic Engulfment and cell adhesiveness. Marcel Dekker NewYork. 1975.

116. Wakiyama N, Juni K and Nakano M, *Chem. Pharm. Bull,* 29 (1981) 3363–8.

117. Widder KJ, Sanyei AE, Ovadia H. and Paterson PY, *J. Pharm Sci.* 70(1981) 387.

118. Woodland JHR, Yolles S, Blake DA, Helrich M and Meyer FJ; *J. Med. Chem.* 16 (1973) 897–901.

119. Yao K D, Peng T, Yu J J, Xu MX and Goosen M F A, J M S-Rev Macromol Chem Phys, C35 (1995) 155.

120. Yuji YJ, Xu MX, Chen X and Yao KD, Chinese Sci Bull, 41 (1996) 1266.

13

■ Nanoparticles

INTRODUCTION

The colloidal carriers based on biodegradable and biocompatible polymeric systems have largely contributed to the controlled and targeted drug delivery concepts. It was realized that the nanoparticles loaded bioactive element could not only deliver drug(s) to specific organs within the body, but also could control drug delivery rate. The possibilities and potentials further prompted the work and as a result a plethora of informations covering preparation methodologies, characterization, engineering, biofate and toxicology been gathered as well as generated. The understanding that relates to the biodistribution in particular has encouraged and propelled the developments of functionally-designed nanoparticulates.

It is apparent that the polymers, the structural materials of nanoparticulate composites, may be of natural or synthetic origins. Some of them have already been exploited for their biomedical applications. Obviously, the literature is abound relating to their safety, toxicology, and biodegradation consideration.

Nanoparticles are submicrosized colloidal structures composed of synthetic or semi-synthetic polymers. The continual quest and maneuvering towards physical stability improvement of liposomes resulted into

development of solid core nanoparticles in eighties as an alternative drug carrier. The first reported nanoparticles were based on non-biodegradable polymeric systems (polyacrylamide, polymethyl-methacrylate, polystyrene etc.). The possibilities of chronic toxicity due to tissue and immunological response towards nondegradable polymeric burden, their use for systemic administration, however, could not be considered. Soon, the biodegradable polymers were used and nanoparticles based on poly (cyanoacrylate) were prepared and extensively studied. The polymericnano-particles can carry drug(s) or proteinaceous substances, i.e. antigen(s). These bioactives are entrapped in the polymer matrix solid enmeshed or solid solution or may be bound to the particle surface by physical adsorption or chemically. The drug(s) may be added during preparation of nanoparticles or to the preprepared nanoparticles. The term particulate is suggestively general and doesn't account for morphological and structural organization of the system. Thus, they could be nanospheres, nanocapsules, nanocrystals or nanoparticulates. Nanospheres may be defined as solid core spherical particulates, which are nanometric in size. They contain drug embedded within the matrix or adsorbed onto surface; while nanocapsules are vesicular system in which drug is essentially encapsulated within the central core surrounded by an embryonic continuous polymeric sheath. In the later, drug(s) is/are mainly encapsulated in the solution form. The physical chemistry of these systems remains to be the same as of typical colloidal dispersions. The surface charges, dispersibility, density, hydrophobicity and hydrophilicity are some critical factors, which ultimately determine the stability characteristics of a system vis-a-vis its *in vivo* disposition.

PREPARATION TECHNIQUES OF NANOPARTICLES

The selection of the appropriate method for the preparation of nanoparticles depends on the physicochemical characteristics of the polymer and the drug to be loaded. On the contrary, the preparation techniques largely determine the inner structure, *in vitro* release profile and the biological fate of these polymeric delivery systems. Two types of systems with different inner structures are apparently possible including:

- A matrix type system consisting of an entanglement of oligomer or polymer units (nanoparticles/nanospheres)
- A reservoir type of system comprised of an oily core surrounded by an embryonic polymeric shell (nanocapsules)

The drug can either be entrapped within the reservoir or the matrix or otherwise may be adsorbed on the surface of these particulate systems. The polymers are strictly structured to a nanometric size using appropriate methods. These methodologies are conveniently classified as follows:

1. Amphiphilic macromolecule cross-linking
   a. Heat cross-linking
   b. Chemical cross-linking
2. Polymerization based methods
   a. Polymerization of monomers *in situ*
   b. Emulsion (micellar) polymerization
   c. Dispersion polymerization
   d. Interfacial condensation polymerization
   e. Interfacial complexation

3. Polymer precipitation methods
   a. Solvent extraction/evaporation
   b. Solvent displacement (nanoprecipitation)
   c. Salting out

Nanoparticle Preparation by Cross-linking of Amphiphilic Macromolecules

Nanoparticles can be prepared from amphiphilic macromolecules, proteins, and polysaccharides (which have affinity for aqueous and lipid solvents). The technique of their preparation involves firstly, the aggregation of amphiphile(s) followed by further stabilization either by heat denaturation (Gupta et al., 1987a, b) or chemical cross-linking (Widder et al., 1979).

These processes may occur in a biphasic O/W or W/O type dispersed system, which subdivides the amphilic(s) polymers prior to aggregative stabilization. It may also take place in an aqueous amphiphilic solution, where on removal, extraction, or diffusion of solvent, amphiphile(s) are aggregated as tiny particulates, which are subsequently rigidized via chemical cross-linking. The cross-linking generally executed by using dispersed phase solvent extraction, or depletion.

Cross-linking in W/O Emulsion

Kramer (1974) first reported the cross-linking method for the nano-encapsulation of drugs. The method involves the emulsification of bovine serum albumin (BSA)/human serum albumin (HAS) or protein aqueous solution, in oil using high-pressure homogenization (Kramer, 1974) or high frequency sonication (Sugibasayashi et al., 1979). The water-in-oil emulsion so formed is then poured into preheated oil (temperature above 100°C). The suspension in preheated oil maintained above 100°C is held stirred for a specified time in order to denature and aggregate the protein contents of aqueous pool completely and to evaporate the water (Figs 13.1 and 13.2). Proteinaceous subnanoscopic particles are thus formed, where the size of the internal phase globules mainly determines the ultimate size of particulates.

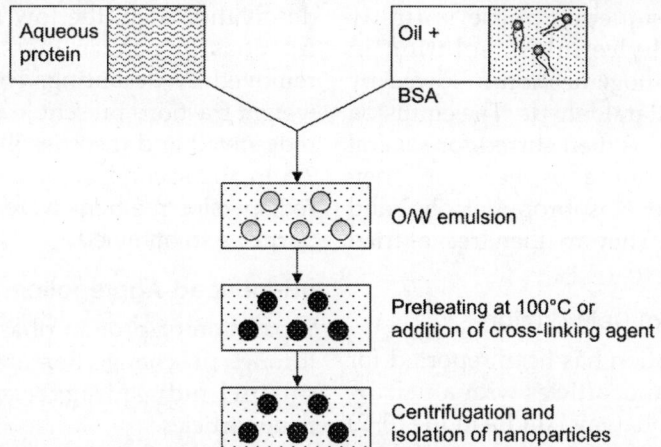

Fig. 13.1: Schematic of macromolecular cross-linking in a water-in-oil (W/O) emulsion technique

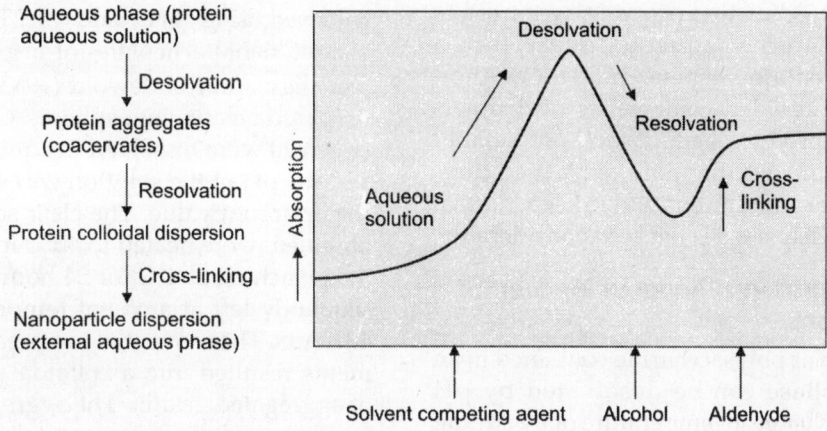

Fig. 13.2: Various steps of solvation and desolvation that leads to the formation of nanoparticles

The particles are finally washed with an organic solvent to remove any adherent or adsorbed oil trace and subsequently collected by centrifugation. The crucial factors, which govern the size and shape of the nanoparticles are mainly emulsification energy and temperature (used for denaturation and aggregation). The high temperature used in the original method (Kramer, 1974) restricts the application of method to temperature-sensitive drugs. As an alternative to heat stabilization, a chemical cross-linking agent, more frequently glutaraldehyde, is incorporated

into the system at a 3% v/v level (Nakagawa et al., 1987). Though the heatborne drawbacks are obviated, yet a need to remove residual cross-linking agent makes the method cumbersome. Further, the aggregation during following emulsification or cross-linking results into variable size of nanoparticles. Gallo and associates (1984) critically analysed the variables, which affect the polydispersity of nanoparticles.

In an interesting modification, albumin containing water droplets are stabilized using cross-linking agent (Roger and Kissel, 1993).

The droplets or aqueous phase is firstly emulsified in ethylcellulose solution in chloroform by homogenization followed by the addition of glutaraldehyde. The emulsion system so obtained is then stirred for several hours. The resultant nanospheres are then washed with toluene, isopropyl alcohol and finally with water. They are then freeze-dried for stability.

Emulsion Chemical Dehydration

Chemical dehydration has been reported for producing BSA nanoparticles with a narrow size distribution. Bhargava and Aindo (1992) suggested a simplified chemical cross-linking method. Hydroxypropyl cellulose solution in chloroform was used as a continuous phase of emulsion, while a chemical dehydrating agent, i.e. 2,2-dimethyl propane, was used to translate internal aqueous phase into a solid particulate suspension. The method reportedly avoided coalescence of droplets and could produce nanoparticles of smaller size (~300 nm). Furthermore, sonication time, required for comminution and to keep internal phase well dispersed is reduced considerably.

Phase Separation in Aqueous Medium (Desolvation)

The protein or polysaccharide contained in an aqueous phase can be desolvated by pH change, or change in temperature or by adding some appropriate counter ions. Cross-linking may be affected simultaneously or subsequently to the desolvation step (Marty et al., 1976; Oppenheim et al., 1982; Krause and Rohdewald, 1985; Oppenheim, 1986).

The method essentially involves three steps, i.e. protein dissolution, protein aggregation and protein deaggregation. In other words, using appropriate levels of desolvation and resolution, the aggregate size could be maintained and finally these nanoparticulates are cross-linked using glutaraldehyde.

Coester and coworkers (2000), reported a two-step desolvation method for manufacturing gelatin nanoparticles. After the first desolvation step, the low molecular gelatin fractions present in the supernatant were removed by decanting. The high molecular weight fractions present in the sediment were redesolved and then desolvated again at pH 2.5 in the second step. Centrifugation and redispersion methods were used to purify the particles so obtained.

pH-induced Aggregation

Separation of protein phase may also occur through pH change. Some workers have used this pH-induced aggregation to prepare nanoparticles.

1. Oppenheim and coworkers (1982) successfully prepared insulin nanospheres. Insulin was firstly precipitated and then redissolved forming nanodroplets, which were hardened using glutar aldehyde. The method yielded nanoparticulates of insulin itself.

2. Samaligy and Rohdewold (1983) similarly prepared gelatin nanospheres. Gelatin and tween 20 were dissolved in aqueous phase and the pH of the solution was adjusted to the optimum value. The clear solutions so obtained, were heated to 40°C followed by its quenching at 4°C for 24 hours and subsequently left at ambient temperature for 48 hours. The sequential temperature treatments resulted into a colloidal dispersion of aggregated gelatin. The aggregates were finally cross-linked using glutaraldehyde as a cross-linking agent. The nanospheres so produced were of 200 nm average size with uniform dispersity. The optimal pH range for ideal and uniform preparation of gelatin nanospheres was 5.5–6.5. Interestingly, pH value below 5.5 produced no aggregation while above 6.5 an uncontrollable aggregation led to the formation of larger nanospheres.

Counter Ion-induced Aggregation

Nanoparticle Preparation using Polymerization-based Methods

The early reports on preparation of polymeric nanoparticles, mainly discuss *in situ* emulsion polymerization. The polymers used for nanosphere preparation include poly (methyl methacrylate), poly (acryl amide), poly (butyl cyanoacrylate), N-N′-methylene-bis-acrylamide, etc. (reviewed by Kreuter, 1991). Two different approaches have been considered for the preparation of nanospheres by in-situ polymerization, depending upon whether the monomer to be polymerized is emulsified in a nonsolvent phase (emulsion polymerization), or dissolved in a solvent that is nonsolvent to the resulting polymer (dispersion polymerization).

Emulsion Polymerization

Emulsion polymerization can be conventional or inverse, depending upon the nature of the continuous phase in the emulsion. In the former case, the continuous phase is aqueous (O/W emulsion), whereas in the latter case it is organic (W/O emulsion). Two different mechanisms were proposed for the emulsion polymerization process, i.e. micellar nucleation and polymerization and homogeneous nucleation and polymerization (Durbin et al., 1979; Kreuter, 1983; Vanderhoff, 1985; Vanderhoff et al., 1988; Kreuter, 1994).

The micellar nucleation and polymerization involves the swollen monomer micelles as the site of nucleation and polymerization. The monomer is emulsified in the nonsolvent phase with surfactant molecules, leading to the formation of monomer-swollen micelles and stabilized monomer droplets. Swollen micelles exhibit sizes in the nanometric range and thus have a much larger surface area in comparison to monomer droplets. The polymerization reaction consisting of a nucleation and a propagation stage takes place in the presence of a chemical or physical initiator. The energy provided by the initiator creates free reactive monomers in the continuous phase, which then collide with surrounding unreactive monomers and initiate the polymerization chain reaction (Fig. 13.3). Being slightly soluble in the surrounding phase, the monomer molecules reach the micelles through diffusion from the monomer droplets through the continuous phase, thus allowing the polymerization within the micelles. So, in this case, monomer droplets would essentially act as monomer reservoirs.

A second mechanism, homogeneous nucleation and polymerization has been proposed to be useful and applicable in cases, where the monomer is sufficiently soluble in the continuous outer phase (Kreuter, 1991; Kreuter, 1994). The nucleation and polymerization stages can exist in this phase, leading to the formation of primary chains called oligomers. In this situation, both the micelles and droplets play a role of monomer reservoirs throughout

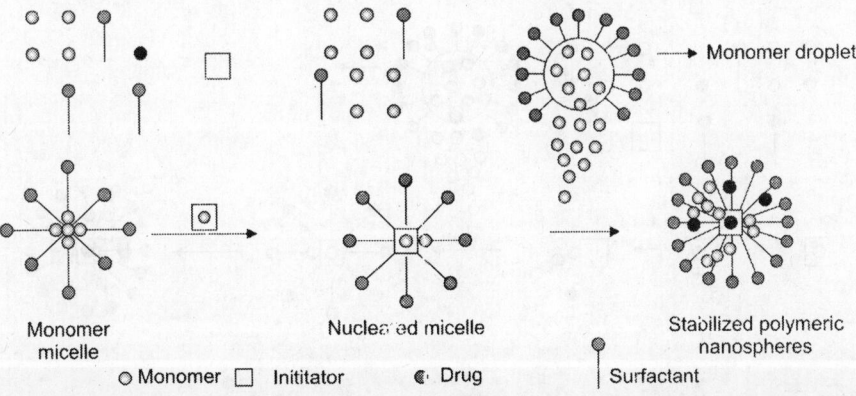

Monomer micelle   Nucleated micelle   Stabilized polymeric nanospheres

○ Monomer   □ Inititator   ◖ Drug | Surfactant

Fig. 13.3: Emulsion polymerization (micellar polymerization mechanism) for nanoparticle preparation. Monomer droplets as reservoir while micelles as site of polymeric particle growth

the polymer chain length. When the oligomers have reached a certain length, they precipitate and form primary particles, which are stabilized by the surfactant molecules provided by the micelles and the droplets. Depending on the bulk conditions and system stability, the end-product nanospheres are formed either by additional monomer input into the primary particles or by fusion of the primary pre-existing particles (Fig. 13.4). Poly (alkylcyanoacrylate) (PACA), a biodegradable polymer has created a great deal of interest in nanoparticulate carriers (Kreuter and Speiser, 1976; Kreuter, 1983; Chiannilkulchai et al., 1989; Couvreur and Vautier, 1991; Alleman et al., 1993a; Verdiere et al., 1997; Soma et al., 2000a). They are essentially prepared by emulsion polymerization. Water insoluble monomer is emulsified in an external active aqueous phase that contains a stabilizer. Monomers polymerize rapidly following anion polymerization mechanism. The polymerization rate is reportedly dependent on the pH of the medium.

Anionic polymerization takes place in micelles after diffusion of monomer molecules through the water phase and is initiated by negatively-charged compound. Thus, at neutral pH the rate of polymerization being extremely fast leads to the formation of aggregates. However, at acidic pH, i.e. pH 2–4, the reaction rate remains well controlled and considerably slow, thus producing uniform nanospheres of relatively high molecular weight. During polymerization, the medium is kept stirred in order to maintain size and dispersibility of phase that is undergoing polymerization. The polymerization is continued for varied time according to monomer, where alkyl chain length serves as determinant, i.e. longer the chain, longer the time of polymerization needed as for ethylcyanoacrylate, it is 2 hours and for hexylcyano acrylate the polymerization is conducted for 10–12 hours. The colloidal suspension on completion of polymerization finally neutralized and lyophilized in the presence of some cryoprotectants, i.e. glucose.

Water-soluble drugs may be associated with PACA nanoparticle either by dissolving the drug in the aqueous phase of polymerization medium or by incubating the blank nanospheres with an aqueous solution of drug. In the former, the drug molecules are entrapped within the polymer matrix and are also adsorbed onto the surface of the nanoparticles. In the latter, the drug molecules are adsorbed only on the surface (Fig. 13.5).

Al-Khouri-Fallouh and coworkers (1985) have discussed the method of polymer based nanocapsule preparation and incorporation/loading of lipophilic drug. The monomers and drug are dissolved in a mixture of polar (methanol/acetone) solvents, or oil (benzyl

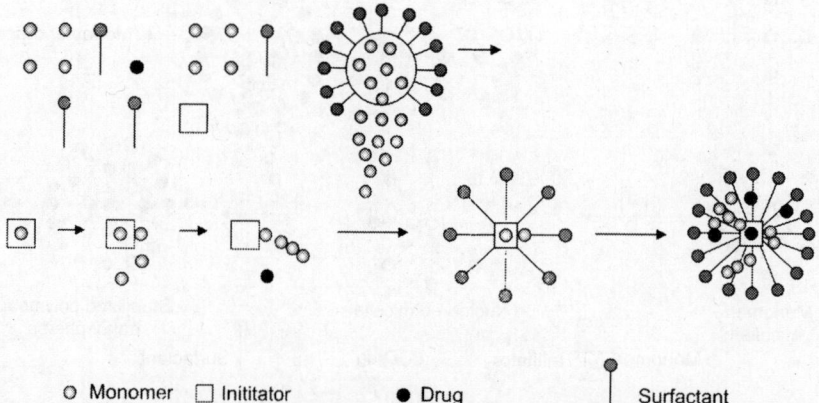

○ Monomer   □ Inititator   ● Drug | Surfactant

Fig. 13.4: Emulsion polymerization (homogeneous polymerization mechanism) for nanoparticle preparation

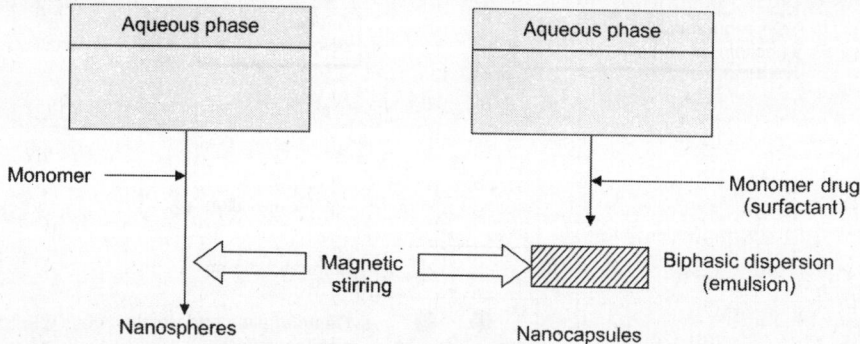

Fig. 13.5: Preparation scheme of PACA nanoparticles using emulsion polymerization process

benzoate, coconut oil) or a lipophilic surfactant, i.e. lecithin. The oil or immescible organic phase is then added to an aqueous phase containing a hydrophilic surfactant. Poloxamer 188 is often used. After oil phase is dispersed into an aqueous phase, critically two processes occur at the oil-water interface, i.e. diffusion of polar solvents from oil phase to the bulk aqueous phase and monomer polymerization at the W/O interface. The polymerization process is catalyzed by OH-ions. Thus, on completion of polymerization a nanocapsular system results, where lipophilic drug dissolved in oil is incorporated in a polymeric sac.

Conversely, a dispersion system, W/O type, where dispersed aqueous phase contains the drug and stabilizer, while organic phase

is typically consisted of an organic solvent (chloroform/n-hexane) and a monomer, can be used to prepare nanocapsules based upon inverse emulsion polymerization mechanism (Vauthier-Holzscherer, 1991; Gasco et al., 1991). The interfacial OH⁻ ions initiated polymerization occurs at W/O interface enveloping aqueous phase with its drug contents in the form of nanocapsules (Fig. 13.6). The inverse polymerization process was rapidly adopted for the preparation of biodegradable poly (alkyl cyanoacrylate) or PACA nanospheres (Gasco and Trotta, 1986; Carpignano et al., 1991) (Fig. 13.7).

In these studies, the drug was dissolved in a small amount of water or hydrophilic solvent (methanol) and emulsified in an organic phase

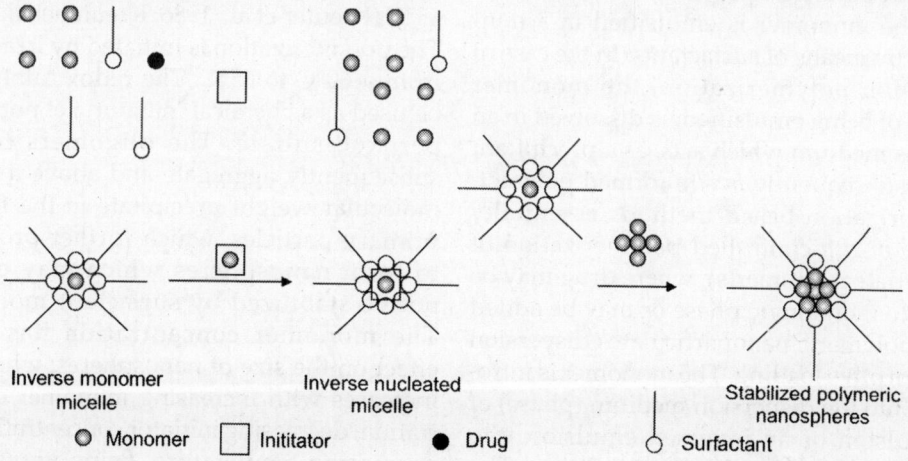

Fig. 13.6: Emulsion polymerization (inverse emulsification polymerization mechanism) for nanoparticle preparation

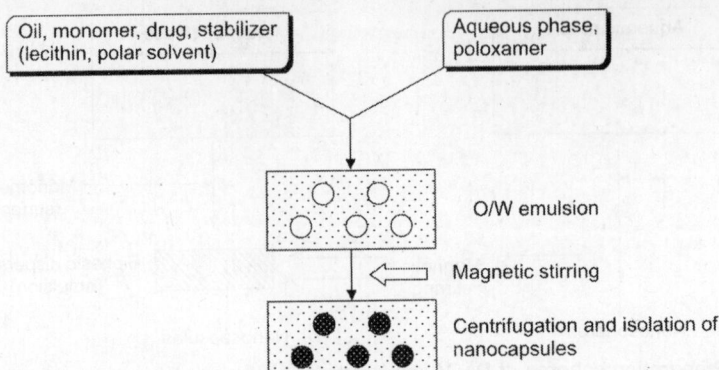

Fig. 13.7: Preparation scheme of PACA nanoparticles using emulsion polymerization process

(i.e. iso-octane, cyclohexane-chloroform, hexane) in the presence of large amounts of surfactants. Alkylcyanoacrylate monomers, were then added directly or dissolved in an organic solvent to the preformed W/O emulsion under stirring. Hydrophilic compounds, such as doxorubicin (Gasco et al., 1991), fluorescein (El-Samaligy et al., 1986) and methylene blue (Gasco and Trotta, 1986) as well as lipophilic compounds, such as triamcinolone acetonide (Krause et al., 1986) were successfully incorporated into PACA nanoparticles using this technique.

Dispersion Polymerization

The term emulsion polymerization is used, when the monomer is emulsified in a non-solvent by means of surfactants. In the case of dispersion polymerization, the monomer instead of being emulsified, is dissolved in an aqueous medium which acts, as a precipitant for the subsequently *in situ* formed polymer. Polymerization based methods essentially involve *in situ*-controlled polymerization of appropriate monomer(s), where drug may be added to monomeric phase or may be added to the polymeric nanoparticulates dispersion for adsorptive loading. The monomer is introduced into the dispersion medium (phase) of an emulsion or an inversed emulsion into nonsolvent based polymeric solution. The polymerization is initiated by adding a

catalyst and proceeds with nucleation phase followed by a growth phase (propagation). The nucleation is directly induced in the aqueous monomer solution and the presence of stabilizer or surfactants is not absolutely necessary for the formation of stable nano-spheres (Fig. 13.8). The method is used to prepare very slowly biodegradable poly-acrylamide and polymethylmethacrylate (PMMA) nanoparticles (Kreuter and Speiser, 1976). The acrylamide or methyl methacrylate monomer is dissolved in aqueous phase and polymerized by irradiation (Kreuter and Speiser, 1976) or by chemical initiation (ammonium or potassium peroxodisulfate) combined with heating to temperature above 65°C (Kreuter et al., 1986; Kreuter et al., 1988). The polymerization is initiated by irradiation from a 60°C to 65°C. The redox catalyst can be used as a chemical initiator, i.e. potassium peroxodisulfate. The oligomers formed subsequently aggregate and above a certain molecular weight precipitate in the form of primary particles, which further propagate to form nanospheres which may or may not be stabilized by surfactant molecules. The monomer concentration has linear effect on the size of nanospheres, where size increases with increasing monomer concentration, decreasing initiator concentration and decreasing temperature. Being very slowly biodegradable and biocompatible, PMMA

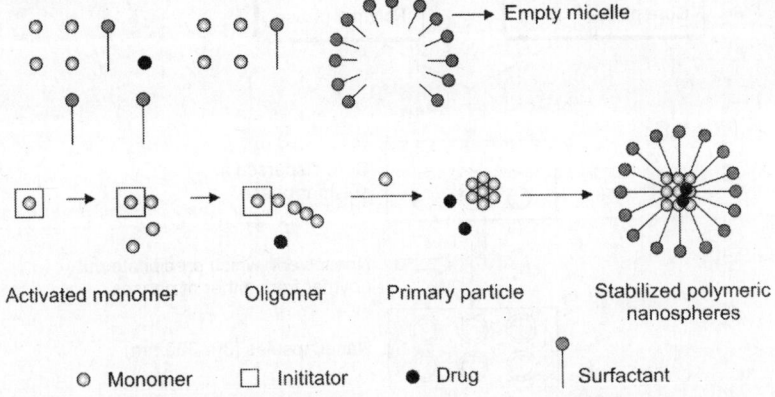

Fig. 13.8: Dispersion polymerization mechanism of nanoparticle preparation

nanoparticles have been appreciated as optimal polymeric systems for vaccination purpose. For this application, initiation by irradiation is useful for the production of PMMA nanoparticles by polymerization in the presence of antigenic material, because it can be carried out at temperatures suitable for these heat-sensitive antigenic materials. The antigenic materials entrapped in PMMA nanoparticles using this technique include influenza virion (Kreuter and Speiser, 1976), influenza subunit antigen (Kreuter et al., 1988), bovine seum albumin (Kreuter et al., 1986), HIV-1 and HIV-2 antigens (Stieneker et al., 1991; Kreuter et al., 1991).

Besides PMMA nanoparticles, copolymer methacrylic nanoparticles are also prepared by dispersion polymerization process using blends of methylmethacrylate with one or several other acrylic acid derivatives (e.g. hydroxyethyl methacrylate, methacrylic acid, ethylene glycol dimethyl acrylate, sulfo-propylmethacrylate) (Rollan et al., 1989; Lukowski et al., 1992; Langer et al., 1996). These copolymers based nanoparticles were developed with an intention of modifying the surface properties of the nanoparticles, namely the hydrophilicity and charge, which are important parameters governing *in vivo* distribution of the particles.

Interfacial Polymer Condensation

In this method, a preformed polymer phase is finally transformed to a embryonic sheath, a phase that eventually becomes core of nano-particle for drug molecules to be loaded are dissolved in a volatile solvent. The solution is then poured into a nonsolvent for both polymer and core phase. The resultant mixture instantaneously turns milky owing to the formation of nanocapsules (Fig. 13.9). The solvent is subsequently removed under vacuum. The size of nanocapsules ranges from 30–300 nm, whereas drug loading efficiency critically depends on drug solubility in core phase. Surfactant in small quantities can be added to stabilize the dispersion.

Interfacial polymerization for encapsula-tion of proteins, enzymes, antibodies and cells was employed and extensively used. Such nanocapsules effectively retain protein macromolecules, such as enzymes at the same time enzyme substrates and reactive products are allowed to permeate. The nanocapsules prepared by interfacial reaction of two monomers are nonimmunogenic in nature. A large assortment of monomer combinations has been studied which react condensing at W/O interface. The method involves the formation of W/O microemulsion as an initial step in which aqueous phase contains

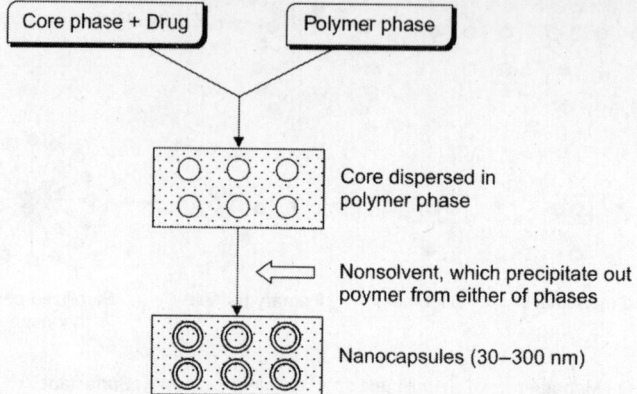

Fig. 13.9: Dual-targeting liposomes for the delivery of anticancer drug

enzymes/protein and water-soluble mono-mer. Second monomer, which is essentially hydrophobic, is added to bulk dispersion phase. The addition of monomer initiates condensation polymerization at the interface (Fig. 13.10). Combination of monomers could yield a variety of polymer systems (Fig. 13.11).

Interfacial Complexation

The method is based on the process of micro-encapsulation introduced by Lin and Sun (1969). In the case of nanoparticle preparation, aqueous polyelectrolyte solution is carefully dissolved in reverse micelles in an apolar bulk phase with the help of an appropriate surface-active agent. Subsequently, competing poly-electrolyte is added to the bulk, which allows a layer of insoluble polyelectrolyte complex to coacervate at the interface.

Nanoparticle Preparation Using Polymer Precipitation Methods

In these methods, the hydrophobic polymer (except dextran, mainly polyesters) and/or a hydrophobic drug is dissolved in a particular organic solvent followed by its dispersion in a continuous aqueous phase, in which the polymer is insoluble. The external phase also contains the stabilizer. Depending upon solvent miscibility techniques, they are designated as solvent extraction/evaporation method (Fig. 13.12). The polymer precipitation

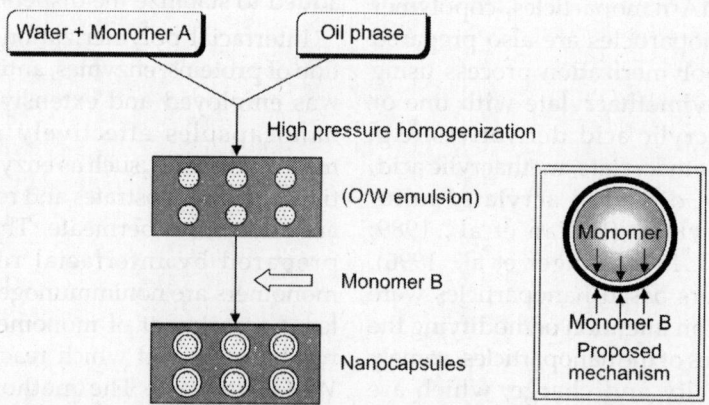

Fig. 13.10: Preparation of nanocapsules using interfacial condensation polymerization

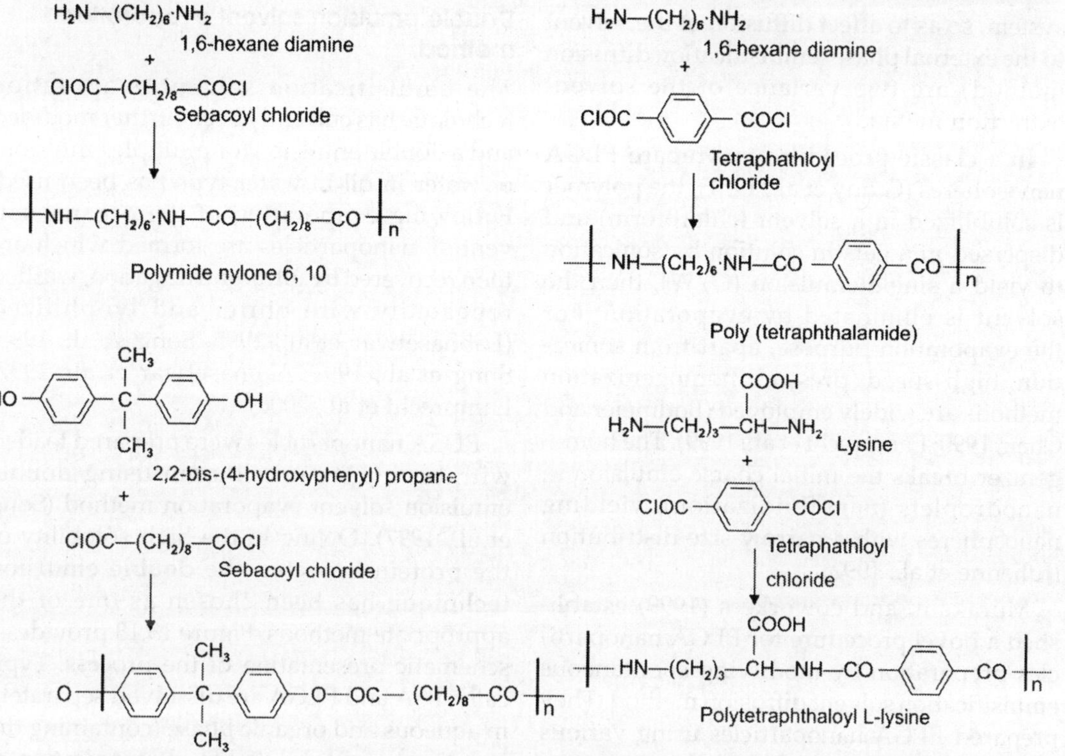

H₂N—(CH₂)₆·NH₂
1,6-hexane diamine

+

ClOC—(CH₂)₈—COCl
Sebacoyl chloride

$$\downarrow$$

—NH—(CH₂)₆·NH—CO—(CH₂)₈—CO—ₙ

Polymide nylone 6, 10

HO—⬡—C(CH₃)(CH₃)—⬡—OH

2,2-bis-(4-hydroxyphenyl) propane

+

ClOC—(CH₂)₈—COCl
Sebacoyl chloride

$$\downarrow$$

O—⬡—C(CH₃)(CH₃)—⬡—O—OC—(CH₂)₈—CO—ₙ

H₂N—(CH₂)₆·NH₂
1,6-hexane diamine

+

ClOC—⬡—COCl
Tetraphathloyl chloride

$$\downarrow$$

—NH—(CH₂)₆·NH—CO—⬡—CO—ₙ

Poly (tetraphthalamide)

H₂N—(CH₂)₃—CH(COOH)—NH₂ **Lysine**

+

ClOC—⬡—COCl
Tetraphathloyl chloride

$$\downarrow$$

—HN—(CH₂)₃—CH(COOH)—NH—CO—⬡—CO—ₙ

Polytetraphthaloyl L-lysine

Fig. 13.11: Various combination of monomers could yield a variety of polymer systems

occurs as a consequence of the solvent extraction or evaporation, which can be brought about using:

1. Increasing the solubility of the organic solvent into the external medium by adding an alcohol (i.e. isopropanol).
2. By incorporating an additional amount of water into the nanoemulsion (to extract or diffuse the solvent).
3. By evaporation of the organic solvent at room temperature or at accelerated temperatures or by using vacuum.
4. Using an organic cosolvent that is completely miscible with the continuous aqueous phase (i.e. acetone) nanoprecipitation.

Solvent Extraction Methods

This method involves the formation of a conventional O/W emulsion between a partially water immiscible solvent containing

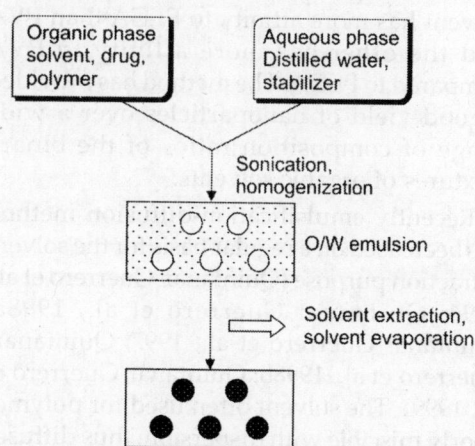

Fig. 13.12: Nanoparticle preparation using emulsion solvent evaporation method

the polymer and the drug, and an aqueous phase containing the stabilizer. The subsequent removal of solvent (solvent evaporation method) or the additions of water to the system, so as to affect diffusion of the solvent to the external phase (emulsification diffusion method) are two variance of the solvent extraction method.

In a classic procedure to prepare PLGA nanospheres (Gumy et al., 1981), the polymer is solubilized in a solvent (chloroform) and dispersed in a gelatin solution by sonication to yield a single emulsion (O/W), then the solvent is eliminated by evaporation. For the evaporation purpose, apart from sonication, high speed/pressure homogenization methods are widely employed (Bodmeier and Chen, 1990; Lamprecht et al., 1999). The homogenizer breaks the initial coarse emulsion in nanodroplets (nanofluidization), yielding nanospheres with a narrow-size distribution (Julienne et al., 1992).

Murakami and coworkers (1999) established a novel procedure for PLGA nanoparticles preparation by modifying spontaneous emulsification solvent diffusion method. They prepared PLGA nanoparticles using various solvent systems consisting of two water-miscible organic solvents, in which one solvent has more affinity to PLGA than PVA and the other has more affinity to PVA compared to PLGA. The method has provided a good yield of nanoparticles over a wide range of composition ratios of the binary mixtures of organic solvents.

Recently emulsification-diffusion method has been used on a regular basis for the solvent extraction purpose (Quintanar-Guerrero et al., 1996; Quintanar-Guerrero et al., 1998a. Quintanar-Guerrero et al., 1997; Quintanar-Guerrero et al., 1998b; Quintanar-Guerrero et al., 1999). The solvent often used for polymer poorly miscible with dispersion, thus diffuses and evaporates out slowly on continual stirring of the system. On the contrary, dispersion medium miscible polymer solvent, i.e. acetone, alcohol, instantaneously diffuses into the aqueous phase and as a result polymer consolidates and precipitates as tiny nanospheres.

Double emulsion solvent evaporation method

The emulsification solvent evaporation technique has currently been further modified and a double emulsion (or multiple emulsion) of water in oil in water type has been used. Following evaporation of the organic solvent(s), nanoparticles are formed which are then recovered by ultracentrifugation, washed repeatedly with buffer and lyophilized (Labhasetwar et al., 1995; Song et al., 1995; Song et al., 1997; Labhasetwar et al., 1997; Lamprecht et al., 2000).

PLGA nanoparticles were prepared loaded with bovine serum albumin using double emulsion solvent evaporation method (Song et al., 1997). Owing to the high solubility of the protein in water, the double emulsion technique has been chosen as one of the appropriate methods. Figure 13.13 provides a schematic presentation of the process. Typically, BSA and PLGA are dissolved separately in aqueous and organic phase (containing the stabilizer) and subjected to ultrasonication to

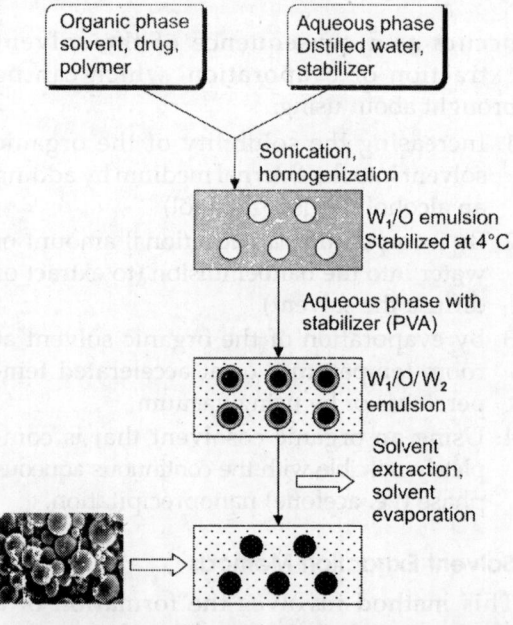

Fig. 13.13: Preparation of nanoparticles using double emulsion solvent evaporation method

yield a water-in-oil emulsion (W_1/O emulsion). This W_1/O was further added to a PVA aqueous solution to yield the (water-in-oil)-in-water (W_1/O/W_2) double emulsion. The organic solvent was allowed to evaporate, while being stirred first at atmospheric pressure for 16 hours and then gradually at reduced pressure (from 100 mmHg to 30 mmHg) to yield nanoparticles (Fig. 13.13).

Solvent Displacement or Nanoprecipitation

This method is based on the interfacial deposition of a polymer following displacement of a semipolar solvent miscible with water from a lipophilic solution (Fessi et al., 1989; Guterres et al., 1995; Chacon et al., 1996; Molpeceres et al., 1996; Govender et al., 1999). Solvent displacement method involves the use of an organic phase, which is completely soluble in the external aqueous phase. The organic solvent diffuses instantaneously into the external aqueous phase, inducing immediate polymer precipitation because of the complete miscibility of both the phases. Consequently neither separation nor extraction of the solvent is required for the polymer precipitation. After nanoparticle preparation, the solvent is eliminated and the free-flowing nanoparticles can be obtained under reduced pressure. This method is particularly useful for drugs that are slightly soluble in water. If the drug is highly hydrophilic, it will diffuse out into the external aqueous phase, whereas if the drug is highly hydrophobic, it may precipitate in the aqueous phase as nanocrystals, which will grow during storage.

In the case of hydrophilic polymer, an aqueous solution of polymer is dispersed/emulsified in oil phase. The precipitation of polymer proceeds on addition of acetone. Using this technique ovalbumin loaded dextran nanospheres of ~1 μm size were prepared (Schroder and Stahl, 1984). The nanospheres were fairly stable and uniform in size.

However, the loading efficiency of lipophilic drugs, such as indomethacin (Fessi et al., 1989), metipranol (Losa et al., 1993), betaxolol (Maincent et al., 1992) in nanoparticles based on PLA, PLGA, and PECL has been increased using a modified solvent displacement method. In this method (Fessi et al., 1987) the drug is dissolved in a small volume of appropriate oil and then diluted in the polar organic solvent (acetone/ethanol/methanol). When the organic solution is dispersed in the aqueous phase, the polymer precipitates around the nanodroplets, forming a reservoir system. Figure 13.14 compares the conventional (nanoparticles) and modified (nanocapsules) solvent displacement methods.

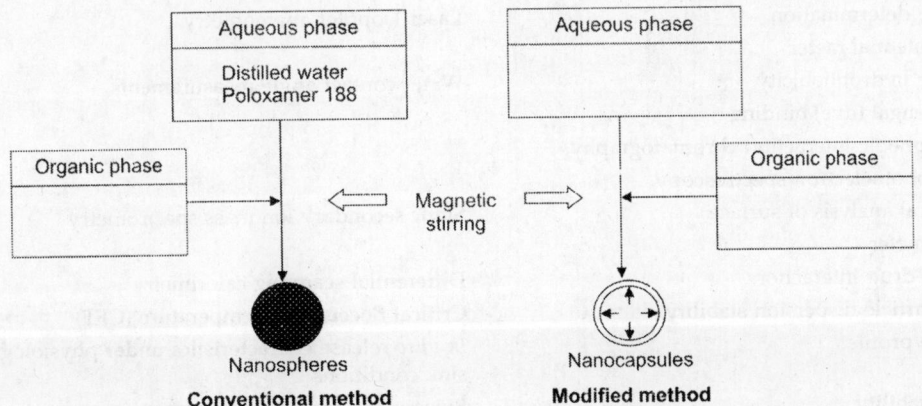

Fig. 13.14: Use of solvent displacement methods to prepare nanoparticles (conventional method) and nanocapsules (modified method)

Salting Out

Salting-out process has been used to prepare nanoparticles by various workers. Salting-out method is based on the incorporation of a saturated aqueous solution of polyvinyl alcohol (PVA) into an acetone solution of the polymer under magnetic stirring to form an O/W emulsion. However, the process differs from technique as in the latter, the polymeric solution (in acetone) was completely miscible with the external aqueous medium. But in the salting-out technique, the miscibility of both the phases is prevented by the saturation of the external aqueous phase with PVA. The precipitation of the polymer occurs when sufficient amount of water is added to external phase to allow complete diffusion of the acetone from internal phase into the aqueous phase. This technique is suitable for drugs and polymers, which are soluble in polar solvents, such as acetone or ethanol (Fig. 13.15).

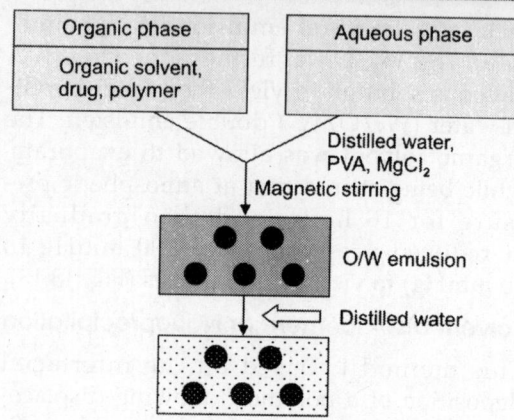

Fig. 13.15: Nanoparticle preparation using salting out of polymer

CHARACTERIZATION OF NANOPARTICLES

The nanoparticles are generally characterized for size, density, electrophoretic mobility, angle of contact and specific surface area (Table 13.1).

Parameter	Characterization method
Particle size and size distribution	Photon correlation spectroscopy (PCS)
Laser defractometry	
Transmission electron microscopy	
Scanning electron microscopy	
Atomic force microscopy	
Mercury porositometry	
Charge determination	Laser Doppler anemometry
Zeta potential meter	
Surface hydrophobicity	Water contact angle measurements
Rose bengal (dye) binding	
Hydrophobic interaction chromatography	
X-ray photoelectron spectroscopy	
Chemical analysis of surface	Static secondary ion mass spectrometry
Sorptometer	
Carrier-drug interaction	Differential scanning calorimetry
Nanoparticle dispersion stability	Critical flocculation temperature (CFT)
Release profile	*In vitro* release characteristics under physiologic and sink conditions
Drug stability	Bioassay of drug extracted from nanoparticles
	Chemical analysis of drug

Table 13.1: Various characterization methods

Size and Morphology

Two main techniques are widely being used to determine the particle size distribution of nanoparticles and include photon correlation spectroscopy (PCS) and electron microscopy (EM). The latter include scanning electron microscopy (SEM), transmission electron microscopy (TEM) and freeze-fracture techniques. A given preparation, when determined for size using different procedures, it was deduced that results coordinate well with better agreement, when freeze-fracturing and photon correlation spectroscopy are quantitatively compared. The freeze-fracturing with poly(methyl methacrylate) is confronted with and interrupted by in process particles aggregation, which only yields a few discrete particles for size measurement or analysis.

Specific Surface

The specific surface area of freeze-dried nanoparticles is generally determined with the help of Sorptometer. The calculation using the equation can be used in the calculation of specific surface area.

$$A = 6/\tau d$$

where, A is the specific surface area, τ is the density, and d is the diameter of the particle.

Surface Charge and Electrophoretic Mobility

The nature and intensity of the surface charge of nanoparticles is very important, as it determines their interaction with the biological environment as well as their electrostatic interaction with bioactive compounds.

The surface charge of colloidal particles in general and nanoparticles in particular, can be determined by measuring the particle velocity in an electric field. Laser light scattering technique, i.e. laser doppler anemometry or velocimetry, has become a fast and high resolution technique for the determination of nanoparticle velocities.

The surface charge of colloidal particles could also be measured as electrophoretic mobility. Generally, the electrophoretic mobility of nanoparticles is determined in phosphate saline buffer (PBS, pH 7.4) and human serum. The zeta potential can be obtained by measuring the electrophoretic mobility applying the Helmholtz-Smoluchowski equation (Hunter, 1983).

Density

In addition to surface scanning electron microscopy, transmission electron microscopy following freeze fracturing could successfully be used in morphological investigation of nanoparticles. Within the interior are continuous or some structural imperfections exist that also provide an indication in regard to density distribution across the matrix. Some polymeric nanoparticles specially polycyanoacrylate and poly (methyl methacrylate) seem to have porous interior, also they exhibit more irregular and rough surface.

The density of nanoparticles is determined with helium or air using a gas pycnometer. The value obtained with air and with helium may differ noticeably from each other. The difference is much more pronounced due to specific surface area and porosity of the structure.

Molecular Weight Measurements of Nanoparticles

Molecular weight of the polymer and its distribution in the matrix can be evaluated by gel permeation chromatography (GPC), using a refractive index detector. Sukuma and co-workers (1997) determined the number average and weight average molecular weight of macromolecules on the polystyrene nanoparticles having surface grafted hydrophilic polymeric chains and correlated these parameters with a good water dispersibility of the system. Using gel permeation chromatography, it was shown that PACA nanoparticles are built by an entanglement of numerous small oligomeric subunits rather than by the rolling up of one or few long polymer chains.

Nanoparticle Recovery and Drug Incorporation Efficiency

The nanoparticle recovery, which is also referred to as nanoparticles yield (Govender et al, 1999). Drug incorporation efficiency has been expressed both as drug content (% w/w), which is also referred as drug loading in the literature (Govender et al., 1999).

In Vitro Release

In vitro release profile can be determined using standard dialysis, diffusion cell or recently introduced modified ultrafiltration technique. *In vitro* drug release from the nanoparticles can be evaluated in phosphate buffer utilizing double chamber diffusion cells on a shaker stand. A Millipore hydrophilic low-protein binding membrane is placed between the two chambers. The donor chamber, is filled with nanoparticulate suspension and the receptor chamber with plain buffer. The receptor compartment is assayed at different time intervals for the released drug using standard procedures.

THERAPEUTIC APPLICATIONS OF NANOPARTICLES

Nanoparticles with different compositions and characteristics have been formulated and investigated for various therapeutic applications (Table 13.2). Several different types of biodegradable polymers including biopolymers (e.g. gelatin, albumin, casein, polysaccharide, lectin etc.) and synthetic

Table 13.2: Various therapeutic applications of nanoparticles/nanocapsules

Application	Material	Purpose
Cancer therapy	Polyalkyl cyanoacrylate nanoparticles with anticancer agents, oligonucleotides	Targeting, reduced toxicity, enhanced uptake of antitumor agents, improved *in vitro* and *in vivo* stability
Intracellular targeting	Polyalkyl cyanoacrylate/polyester nanoparticles with anti-parasitic or antiviral agents	Target reticuloendothelial systems for intracellular infections
Prolonged systemic	Polyesters with adsorbed poly-ethylene glycols or pluronics or derivatized polyesters	Prolong systemic drug effect, avoid uptake by the reticulo-endothelial system
	Polymethyl methacrylate nanoparticles with vaccines (oral and intra-muscular immunization)	Enhances immune response, alternate acceptable adjuvants
Peroral absorption	Polymethyl methacrylate nanoparticles with proteins and therapeutic agents	Enhanced bio-availability, protection from gastrointestinal enzymes
Ocular delivery	Polyalkyl cyanoacrylate nanoparticles with steroids, anti-inflammatory agents, anti-bacterial agents for glucoma	Improved retention of drug/reduced wash out
DNA delivery	DNA-gelatin nanoparticles, DNA-chitosan nanoparticles, PDNA-poly (D,L-lactide-co-glycolide) nanoparticle	Enhanced delivery and significantly higher expression levels
Oligonucleotide delivery	Alginate nanoparticles, poly (D,L) lactic acid nanoparticles	Enhanced delivery of oligonucleotide
Other applications	Polyalkyl cyanoacrylate nanoparticles with peptides	Crosses blood brain barrier
	Polyalkyl cyanoacrylate nanoparticles for transdermal application	Improved absorption and permeation
	Nanoparticles with adsorbed enzymes	Enzyme immunoassays
	Nanoparticles with radioactive or contrast agents	Radio-imaging
	Co-polymerized peptide nanoparticles of n-butyl cyanoacrylate and activated peptides	Oral delivery of peptides

polymers (polycaprolactone, polyesters, polyanhydrides, polycyanoacrylates) with various drug release characteristics ranging from several hours to several months have been used to formulate sustained release nanoparticles. It is the submicron size of this delivery system, which makes it more efficient in certain drug therapy applications, such as in intracellular localization of therapeutic agents. These systems, in addition to sustained drug delivery have been investigated for various therapeutic applications.

Intracellular Targeting

The treatment of infections caused by obligate and facultative intracellular microorganism is difficult because most of the available antibiotics have following limitations:

- Poor intracellular diffusion or reduced activity at the acidic pH of the phagosomes and lysosomes.
- Most intracellular infections are difficult to eradicate because bacteria inside phagosomes are protected from antibiotics.
- Multidrug resistance due to the functional P-glycoprotein pumps.

The nature of antibiotics also determines their fate *in vivo*. Thus, antibiotics with basic character (aminoglycosides) lead to lysosomal overloading, whereas they display a reduced activity in acidic environment. Conversely, acidic antibiotics (-lactams) do not diffuse through the lysosomal membrane because of their ionic character at neutral extracellular or cytoplasmic pH. Finally, certain antibiotics, which permeate the cell more rapidly and to a larger extent (clindamycin) are poorly retained in the cell, as they are effluxed-out fast.

The need for antibiotics with greater intracellular efficacy led to the development of endocytosable drug carriers including nanoparticles, which mimic the entry path of the bacteria by penetrating the cells into phagosomes and lysosomes. Nanoparticles and mostly all nonpolymer coated particles following intravenous administration rapidly accumulate in liver and spleen (MPS rich organs), which are the main organs of reticuloendothelial system.

Nanoparticles in Chemotherapy

The most promising application of nanoparticles is their possible use as carriers for antitumor agents. Enhanced endocytic activity and leaky vasculature of the tumor favors accumulation of intravenously administered nanoparticles. However, to facilitate and optimize the drug targeting to tumor tissues the 'stealth' using polyoxyethylene could contribute to excessive extravasation. Stealth nanoparticles are prepared by coating them with soluble polyoxyethylene, or by using dialkyl polyoxyethylene and phospholipids. Sometimes, the accumulation of nonstealth (conventional) nanoparticles in RES may be exploited for RES prominent organ-specific cancer chemotherapy.

Chemoembolization

One of the approaches, popularly known chemoembolization, makes use of the biodegradable particles administration into the liver tumors, using a catheter that passes directly into an artery of the tumor.

The accumulation of nonstealth mitomycin-C microparticles within the Kupffer cells (liver), has been exploited to target hepatic neoplasm indirectly. This is achieved by providing a depot of drug for killing nearby neoplastic tissues, as the particles (nonstealth), are not actually taken up by the neoplastic tissue. A similar targeting strategy using transcatheter chemoembolization has been reported for cisplatin, doxorubicin, taxol, rifampicin and 5-fluorouracil.

Several studies are reported for prolonged drug retention in tumors, reduction in tumor growth, and prolonged survival of tumor bearing animals using nanoparticle-loaded antitumor agents compared to free drug.

Avoidance of Multidrug Resistance

Multidrug resistance is the main cause of failure of chemotherapeutic agents. This can severely affect the effectiveness of some types of chemotherapy. It is often associated with the overexpression of a cell membrane glycoprotein of 170 kDa molecular weight. The glycoprotein (P-glycoprotein) is a membrane spanning ATPase and located in the plasma membrane. This multidrug transporter could act as an efflux pump and reject positively charged amphipathic drugs from the cells, as shown for bacterial transport proteins. Overexpression of P-glycoprotein in tumor cells can lead to a marked decrease in drug sensitivity. Thus, multidrug resistance is associated with low intracellular accumulation of these drugs. This is more pronounced with drugs, which appear to enter the cell by passive diffusion through the lipid bilayer, e.g. doxorubicin (an anticancer drug).

Upon entering the cell, these drugs bind to P-glycoprotein, which forms transmembrane channels and uses the energy of ATP hydrolysis to pump these compounds out of the cell.

Nanoparticles-loaded drugs has resulted in the effective treatment of a number of chemotherapy refractory cancers, both in animal models and in the clinic. The lysosomal localization of the particulate system protects the loaded drug from the the action of the P-glycoprotein, thus avoiding immediate contact with P-glycoprotein transporter located at the plasma membrane (Fig. 13.16). Along with cell sensitization, nanoparticulate drug delivery may help overcome a broader range of drug resistance due to favorable pharmacokinetics.

Delivery of Anticancer Drugs

The polyalkylcyanoacrylate nanoparticles have been studied in recent years, as a possible means of targeting drugs to specific sites in the body, with particular emphasis in cancer chemotherapy. The small colloidal carriers are biodegradable and drug substances can be incorporated normally by a process of surface adsorption. Some of the anticancer drugs that are either entrapped or adsorbed onto polyalkylcyanoacrylate nanoparticles are doxorubicin polyisohexylcyanoacrylate nanoparticles, mitoxantrone polybutylcyanoacrylate nanoparticles, aclacinomycin. A polyisobutylcyanoacrylate nanoparticle, granulocyte-colony stimulating factor (G-CSF) polyalkylcyanoacrylate nanoparticles, acyclovir polybutylcyanoacrylate nanoparticles, and doxorubicin-loaded polyalkylcyanoacrylate nanoparticles. However, other biodegradable polymers like poly (lactide-co-glycolide) and polyvinylpyrrolidone are also investigated as carrier material for drug delivery in cancer therapy. These include dexamethasone in poly (lactide-co-glycolide) nanoparticles and Taxol in polyvinylpyrrolidone nanoparticles.

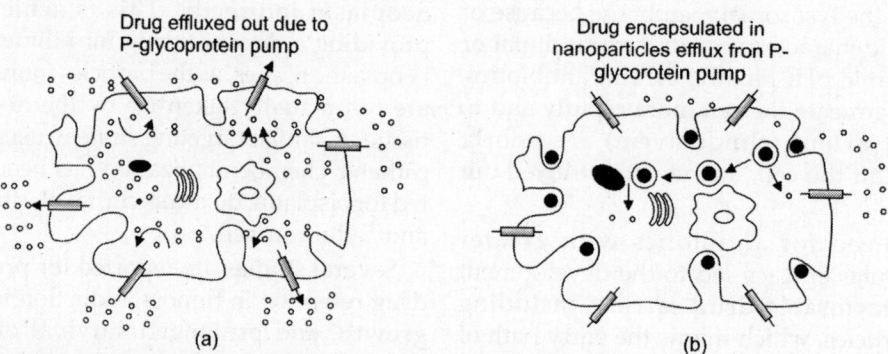

Drug effluxed out due to P-glycoprotein pump

Drug encapsulated in nanoparticles efflux fron P-glycorotein pump

(a)   (b)

Fig. 13.16: Schematic diagram of proposed drug trafficking into multidrug resistant cell of the free drug (a) and of the drug associated with nanoparticles (b)

Adjuvant Effect for Vaccines

An adjuvant effect of the nanoparticles with either matrix-entrapped or surface-adsorbed vaccine has been demonstrated in several studies on subcutaneous or oral administration. The adjuvant effect of nanoparticles could be ascribed to the sustained release of the entrapped antigen or improved uptake and subsequent processing of the nanoparticles bound antigen by the immune system of the body. Kreuter and coworkers have reviewed that polymethylmethacrylate nanoparticles-containing influenza antigen-induced significant antibody response and protected mice against a challenge with mouse-adapted influenza virus to a greater extent than the antigen alone or an alum preparation of the antigen. These workers further demonstrated that a decrease in particle size and an increase in hydrophobicity of the nanoparticles did further increase the adjuvant effect. These nanoparticles were biodegradable after subcutaneous or intramuscular injection.

Oral delivery of antigens with nanoparticles may be an effective means of producing an increased IgA-antibody response. Orally administered nanoparticles-associated antigens are protected from the gastric enzymes and acidic pH and are subsequently taken up by the gut-associated lymphoid tissue. Biodegradable poly(butyl-2-cyanoacrylate) particles have been shown to enhance the secretory immune response after their oral adminitration in association with ovalbumin.

Nanoparticles for Peroral Administration of Proteins and Peptides

Proteins and peptides are increasingly realized as therapeutic drugs. They are quite susceptible to proteolytic degradation and therefore lead to problems of physicochemical and bio-stability coupled with their short biological half-life and inability to pass through most of the biological barriers. For protein/peptide delivery carrier option that possesses both, i.e. carrier as well as adjuvant potential, as a desirable approach, nanoparticles moreover subserves the requirement and offers an attractive oppurtunity. The majority of studies however deal with the stability of the nanoparticles-associated peptides against challenges from the luminal proteases in the gastrointestinal tract. Polyalkyl cyanoacrylate nanoparticles and nanocapsules were developed as peptide carriers for insulin and growth hormone releasing factor. PACA nanoparticles were also proposed as a possible drug delivery system for cyclosporin A, a cyclic oligopeptide possessing a specific immunosuppressive activity. Efforts are directed on delivery of proteins and peptides, especially using biodegradable nanoparticles (PLA/PLG nanoparticles). Nanoparticles of PLGA loaded with amphotericin B, another cyclic peptide have been reported for site-specific delivery with better therapeutic index and low incidences of toxic manifestations.

Insulin encapsulated into nanoparticulate systems, when administered orally was found to induce hypoglycemic effects for several days in fasted and fed diabetic rabbits. Encapsulation protects insulin against proteolytic enzymes. In addition, nanoparticles are known to cross the gut lumen by paracellular pathway and enter the blood circulation, thus demonstrating a systemic drug effect. This strategy is under investigation for an oral administration of other proteins and peptides, and receptor-mediated transport through gut wall, using glycoprotein and glycopeptide-conjugated nanoparticles. Thus, nanoparticles-bound peptides can be used for the sustained oral delivery and also to improve bioavailability.

Nanoparticles for Intra-arterial Applications

Nanoparticles possess several advantages of an ideal carrier system for the intra-arterial localization of therapeutic agents. These advantages include their subcellular size, targeted surface, good suspensibility and uniform dispersity for catheter-based therapy, and an easy penetration into the arterial wall without causing trauma. Nanoparticles could prove to be an effective dosage form for an intra-arterial localization of therapeutic agents for preventing restenosis (Fig. 13.17).

Restenosis may be defined as the process of reobstruction of an artery following interventional procedures such as angioplasty, atherectomy, or stenting and forms the major limitations of these well-established therapies. Nanoparticles are putative drug carriers for the treatment of restenosis, as they localize the therapeutic agents at the site of arterial injury rather than systemic administration. These workers demonstrated that local delivery of drugs like dexamethasone, heparin, and U-86983 (an antiproliferative agent) was facilitated and high-regional concentration could be achieved with prolonged retention, even when used in lower doses and reduced systemic toxicity. These systems possess potentials to be carriers for delivery of genes in restenosis as well as other gene therapy applications.

Nanoparticles for Ocular Delivery

The most significant applications include drug-loaded nanoparticles for ophthalmic delivery in glaucoma therapy, especially effective delivery of cholinergic agonists like pilocarpine. The short elimination half-life of aqueous eyedrops (due probably to lachrymal drainage) can be extended from a very short time (1–3 min) to prolonged time (15–20 min) using biodegradable nanoparticles. These nanoparticles include, polyalkyl cyanoacrylate nanoparticles, polycarolactone, polyester nanoparticles, albumin nanoparticles. In addition, it has been demonstrated that nanoparticles tend to adhere to the inflamed tissue in a more quantitative manner as compared to the healthy tissue, thus these could also be used for targeting of anti-inflammatory drugs to inflamed eyes.

Various advantages of polyalkylcyanoacrylate nanoparticles specially PHCA nanoparticles, are proposed exclusively their biodegradability, tissue adhesion and increased elimination half-life due to their slow clearance. It was found that polyalkylcyanoacrylate nanoparticles could prolong the intraocular pressure reducing effect of the administered drug in rabbits for more than 9 hours as recorded in case of pilocarpine and betaxolol.

Nanoparticles for Brain Delivery

Nanoparticles have been studied for the delivery of drugs in brain. Transport of the hexapeptide dalargin across the blood-brain

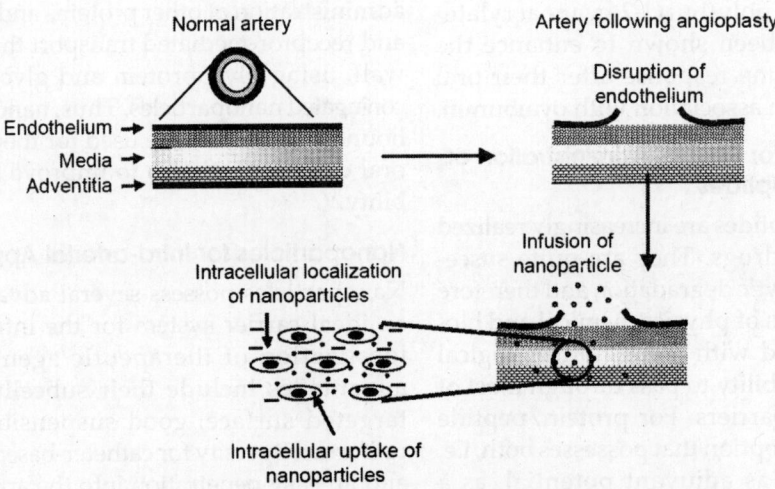

Fig. 13.17: Intra-arterial delivery of nanoparticles for restenosis

barrier using poly (butyl cyanoacrylate) nano-particles, which were coated with polysorbate 80 have been reported. Intravenous injection of polysorbate 80-coated nanoparticles with sorbed drug, resulted in significant analgesic effect in mice model as compared against all controls, including a simple mixture of the three components (drugs, nanoparticles, and surfactant) mixed directly before IV injection. Fluorescent and electron microscopic studies revealed that the passage of the particle-bound drug resulted due to phagocytic uptake of the polysorbate 80-coated nanoparticles by the endothelial cells of brain blood vessel endothelial cells.

Some neuropeptides have also been deli-vered successfully across blood-brain barrier using nanoparticle technology. Leu-enke-phalin dalargin and the Met-enkephalin kyotorphin are neuropeptides that normally do not cross the blood-brain barrier (BBB), when given systemically. To deliver these neuropeptides across the BBB, they were adsorbed onto the surface of poly (butyl cyanoacrylate) nanoparticles, coated with polysorbate 80.

Nanoparticles in Thrombolytic Therapy

Although, liposomal encapsulation has proven to be an effective method for the delivery of thrombolytic drugs, a stability problem exists for such systems. To improve the stability, polymeric carriers have now been used for the delivery of various therapeutic proteins. Encapsulation in polymeric carriers avoided protein deactivation during systemic circula-tion and increased circulation to an acceptable half-life. Leach et al., (2003) developed both types of formulations [liposomal (LESK) and polymeric microcapsules (MESK)] and evalua-ted for various thrombolytic parameters. It was found that both the formulations demonstrated reductions in reperfusion times, residual clot mass and improved return of flow compared to identical dosages of free SK in a thrombosed rabbit carotid, with MESK resulting in comparable or even greater

improvements. Further, the mechanism for increased thrombolysis by MESK was suggested in another experiment, which concluded that MESK resists adsorption to the leading edge of the thrombus, a common limi-tation for the permeation of free plasminogen activators. Thus, by improving the penetration to the interior of clot, a higher thrombolytic activity was recorded (Leach et al., 2004).

Polymeric carriers for the delivery of thrombolytic agents should possess following properties—(i) they should be small enough to circulate without the risk of vascular occlu-sion; (ii) they should possess antiopsonizing properties; (iii) they accumulate at the site of thrombus; and (iv) they must release thrombolytic agents in sufficient concentration to induce clot lysis. To confer these properties Chiellini et al. (2008), synthesized a polymeric material for the development of nanoparticles, which imparts targeting as well as long circulatory property to the colloidal carriers, thus to release fibrinolytic agents in a control-led manner to fibrin clots (Piras et al., 2008), polymer was synthesized by covalently bind-ing PEG moieties and monoclonal antibody antifibrin Fab fragment to the polymer chain. In another study, microspheres of FDA-approved polymers (PLGA and PLA-PEG), were also developed for the delivery of t-PA. It was found that these carriers could retain 5% (w/w) t-PA and released the drug at the site of thrombus at a concentration above 4 g/ml, that is required for the effective clot lysis therapeutically (Xie et al., 2007).

Moreover, size of the particles is a major concerned in systemic drug delivery. Thus, polymeric nanoparticles were developed for the effective delivery of thrombolytic agents to the site of occlusion and subsequently to the interior of the clot. In the case of micro-particles, it was hypothesized that the permeation of particles to the clot may be due to pressure created at the clot. However, in the absence of hydrodynamic pressure, the pores of fibrin clots are highly resistant to the permeation of carriers of size 1 micrometer or larger. Therefore, systems should be developed that permeate through the fibrin network into the interior of the clot for intra-clot lysis in the absence of pressure drop. Surface of the particles should also be modified to increase interaction of particles with the components of the clot, thus increasing penetration to the interior of the clot as well.

Nanoparticle for DNA Delivery

Nanoparticles have been recently used as a delivery vehicle for the transfection of plasmid DNA and to improve their stability in the bio-environment. Truong-Le and coworkers (1998), developed a novel system for gene delivery based on the use of DNA-gelatin nanoparticles (nanospheres) formed by salt-induced complex coacervation of gelatin and plasmid DNA. Nanospheres-DNA incubated in bovine serum were more resistant to nuclease digestion compared to naked DNA (Fig. 13.18). Various bioactive agents could be encapsulated in nanospheres through ionic interaction with their matrix components through, physical entrapment or covalent conjugation.

Oral administration of DNA nanoparticles synthesized by complexing plasmid DNA with chitosan, a natural biocompatible polysaccharide, resulted in transduced gene expression in the intestinal epithelium. Mice receiving nanoparticles containing a dominant peanut allergen gene (pCMVArah2) produced

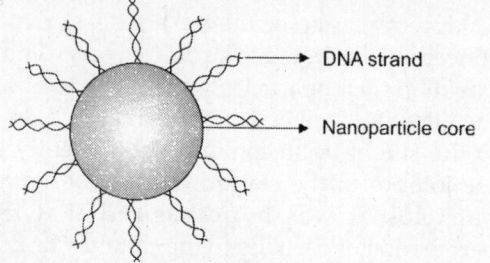

Fig. 13.18: DNA-nanoparticle conjugates used for the transfection of plasmid DNA and to improve their stability in the bioenvironment

secretory IgA and serum IgG2a. Compared with nonimmunized mice or mice treated with 'naked' DNA, mice immunized with nanoparticles showed a substantial reduction in allergen-induced anaphylaxis associated with reduced levels of IgE and plasma histamine.

The ability of colloidal silica particles with covalently attached cationic surface modifications to transfect plasmid DNA *in vitro* has been investigated and the complex was given the name nanoplex.

Biodegradable and biocompatible poly (D,L-lactide-co-glycolide) polymer was used to encapsulate pDNA (alkaline phosphatase, AP a reporter gene) in submicron-size particles. Gene expression mediated by the nanoparticles (NP) was evaluated *in vitro* and *in vivo* and compared with cationic-liposome delivery. Nano size range (600 nm) pDNA-loaded in poly (D,L-lactide-co-glycolide) polymer particles with high encapsulation efficiency (70%) exhibited sustained release of pDNA over a month. The entrapped plasmid maintained its structural and functional integrity. *In vitro* transfection by pDNA-NP resulted in significantly higher expression levels in comparison to naked pDNA.

Nanoparticle for Oligonucleotide Delivery

Antisense therapeutic agents are being investigated *in vitro* and *in vivo* for evaluating their possible use in treating human immuno-deficiency virus infection, hepatitis-B virus infection, herpes simplex virus infection, papilloma virus infection, cancer, restenosis, rheumatoid arthritis, and allergic disorders. A major goal in developing methods of delivering antisense agents is to reduce their susceptibility to nucleases, while retaining their ability to bind to targeted sites. Carrier systems designed to protect the antisense structure and improve passage through the cell membrane include liposomes, water-soluble polymers, and nanoparticles.

Oligonucleotides adsorbed onto poly-alkylcyanoacrylate nanoparticles exhibited enhanced stability against nucleases and ability for specific cellular disposition.

Positively charged nanoparticles prepared from diethylaminoethyl (DEAE)-dextran and polyhexyl cyanoacrylate (PHCA), were evaluated as carriers for ODNs. Oligonucleotides adsorbed onto the surface of the nanoparticles remained protected against endo nuclease DNase I and under *in vitro* cell culture conditions, whereas unprotected ODNs were totally digsted under these conditions.

Recent studies suggest that lipophilic polymethyl methacrylate (PMMA) homopolymer nanoparticles possess a negative surface charge and, therefore, are not suitable for the adsorption of anionic oligonucleotides. However, if the surface charge is changed to positive values by the incorporation of basic monomers, the resultant cationic copolymer (aminoalkyl methacrylate methylmethacrylate copolymer) based nanoparticles containing 30% (w/w) methylaminoethyl-methacrylate (MMAEMC) were found to be optimal in regard to biocompatibility and carrier properties for hydrophilic anionic antisense oligonucleotide entrapment. A significant portion of adsorbed oligonucleotides was protected from enzymatic degradation. The cellular uptake of oligonucleotides *in vitro* in cells was significantly enhanced, when co-incubated with methyl aminoethyl-methacrylate nanoparticles.

Nanoparticles for Theragnostic

Recently, use of nanotechnology in molecular imaging has been appreciated and extended to develop some copolymer based nanoparticles, multifunctional nanoparticles that were able to simultaneously facilitate cancer chemotherapy. Theragnostic nanoparticles show great promise in the emerging field of personalized medicine. because they allow detection as well as monitoring of an individual patient's cancer at an early stage, and delivering anticancer agents over an extended period for enhanced therapeutic efficacy. Moreover, real-time, noninvasive monitoring of the theragnostic nanoparticles revels and this enables clinicians to rapidly decide whether the regimen is effective in an individual patient or not. For these reasons, cancer theragnosis based on multifunctional nanoparticles could be a promising new strategy in cancer treatment. Successful clinical applications of cancer theragnosis require discovery of highly efficient tumor-homing nanoparticles, which can diagnose and deliver targeted therapy.

Cancer researchers have been exploring various tumor targeting nanoparticles made up of lipid-based micelles, natural/synthetic polymeric particles, and inorganic particles for cancer theragnosis. However, the results of tumor targeting have not been as good as one would expect from the targeted delivery. The fact responsible for effective cancer chemotherapy using nanocarriers, yet remains to be unraveled that are not well understood in tumor targeting by nanodelivery systems. Nanoparticles in the size range of 200 nm are known to accumulate at the solid tumor site by the so called menhanced permeation and retention (EPR) effect, resulting in efficient accumulation in solid tumor tissues. Unfortunately, if we examine the reported literature data carefully, *in vivo* studies have shown that the tumor prognosis specificity in the case of nanoparticles based treatment, was relatively better than the controls. Nanoparticles introduced into the circulating blood are quickly removed by the immune system from the body.

Indeed, various nanoparticles preparation with different characteristics (e.g. different surface chemistry, size, surface charge, and molecular weight), were proven unsatisfactory in *in vivo* tests especially with regard to stability, biodistribution, and tumor-targeting specificity. Furthermore, the final *in vivo* destination of nanoparticles has been largely unknown, because it is difficult to acquire direct and noninvasive images on the nanoparticles in animal studies.

MAGNETIC NANOPARTICLES

Engineered magnetic nanoparticles (MNPs) represent a cutting-edge delivery module in medicine because they can be simultaneously functionalized and guided by a magnetic field. Magnetic nanoparticles (MNPs) are a class of nanoparticles, (i.e. engineered particulate materials of 100 nm) that can be manipulated under the influence of an external magnetic field. MNPs are commonly composed of magnetic elements, such as iron, nickel, cobalt and their oxides.

The unique ability of MNPs to be guided by an external magnetic field, has been utilized for magnetic resonance imaging (MRI), targeted drug and gene delivery, tissue engineering, cell tracking and bioseparation. When further 'functionalized' with drugs and bioactive agents, such as peptides and nucleic acids, MNPs form distinct particulate systems could penetrate cell and tissue barriers and therefore, can be organ-specific therapeutic and diagnostic modalities. The ability of MNPs to be functionalized and concurrently responsive to a magnetic field was developed as a useful tool for theragnostics, the fusion of therapeutic and diagnostic technologies, thus lead to the individualize medicine. Through multilayered functionalization, MNPs can simultaneously act as diagnostic molecular imaging agents as well as drug carriers. MNP-based MRI imaging has been already combined with cell replacement therapy, organ-specific gene delivery, intra-operative tumor removal surgery and other applications. However, the resulting variety of MNP composition, shape, size, surface chemistry and state of dispersion, each may infuence their biodistribution and toxic potential.

Hyperthermia is one of the therapeutic stretegies, which may be used in cancer therapy that relies on the localized heating of tumors above 43°C for about 30 min. MNPs can generate heat under alternating magnetic fields due to energy losses in traversing of the magnetic hysteresis loop. Generation of different degrees of heat depends on the magnetization properties of specific MNP formulations and magnetic field parameters. Selectivity to tumors was considerably improved by use of silane coatings and through functionalization approaches. For example, MNPs conjugated with antibodies to cancer specific antigens resulted into improved selectivity of MNP uptake by tumors during hyperthermia therapy. Magnetic hyperthermia using magnetic cationic liposomes has been used in a combination of TNF-α gene therapy and stress-inducible GADD153 promoter. It resulted in a dramatic arrest in tumor growth (Fig. 13.19).

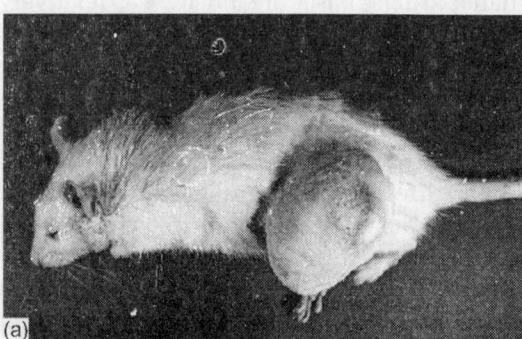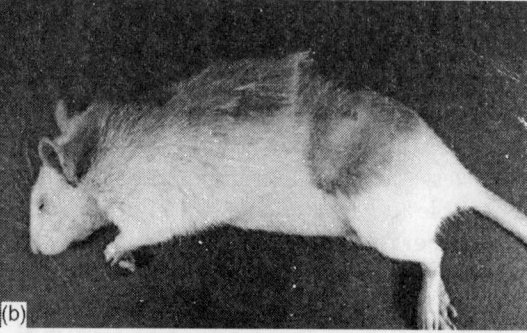

Fig. 13.19: Magnetic hyperthermia based cancer therapy using magnetic cationic liposomes. (a) Rat before treatment, (b) after treatment

SUGGESTED READINGS

1. Alleman E, Gurny R and Doelker E (1993), *Eur. J. Pharmcol. Biopharm.* 39, 173–91.

2. Allemann E, Doelker E and Gurny R (1992), *Eur. J. Pharmacol. Biopharm.*, 39, 13.

3. Allemann E, Gurny R and Doelker E (1992) *Int. J. Pharm.*, 87, 247.

4. Allemann E, Leroux JC, Gurny R and Doelker, E (1993b), *Pharm. Res.* 10, 1732–7.

5. Allen TM (1994), *Adv. Drug Deliv. Rev.*, 13, 285–309.

6. Almeida AJ, Runge S and Muller RH (1997), *Int. J. Pharm.*, 149, 255–65.

7. Alonso MJ, in: Cohen S and Bernstein H (Eds.) Microparticulate systems for the delivery of proteins and vaccines, Marcel Dekker, New York, 1996, pp. 203–42.

8. Ammoury N, Fessi H, Devissaget JP, Puisieux, F and Benita S (1990), *J. Pharm. Sci.*, 79, 763.

9. Arangoa MA, Ponchel G, Orecchioni AM, Renedo MJ, Duchene D and Irache JM (2000), *Eur. J. Pharm. Sci.*, 11, 333–41.

10. Araujo L, Lobenberg R and Kreuter J (1999), *J. Drug Target.*, 6, 373–85.

11. Auvillain M, Cave G, Fessi H and Devissaguet, JP (1989), *STP Pharm. Sci.* 5, 738–44.

12. Aynie I, Vauthier C, Chacun H, Fattal E and Couvreur P (1999), *Antisense Nucleic Acid Drug Dev.*, 9, 301–12.

13. Beck P, Kreuter J, Reszka R and Fichtner I (1993), *J. Microencap.*, 10, 101–14.

14. Bednorz J and Muller A (1986), *Z. Phys.*, B64, 189.

15. Berton M, Allemann E, Stein CA and Gurny R (1999), *Eur. J. Pharm. Sci.*, 9, 163–70.

16. Bhargava K and Aindo HY (1992), *Pharm. Res.* 9, 776.

17. Bindschaedler C, Gurny R and Doelker E (1990), US Patent, 4968, 350.

18. Birrenbach G and Speiser R (1976), *J. Pharm. Sci.*, 65, 1763–6.

19. Bodmeier R and Chen H (1990), *J. Control. Rel.*, 12, 223.

20. Bonduelle S, Foucher C, Leroux JC, Chouinard F, Cadieux C and Linaerts V (1992), *J. Microenacap.*, 9, 173.

21. Breton P et al. (1996), *Eur. J. Pharm. Biopharm.*, 43, 95–103.

22. Carpignano R, Gasco MR, and Morel S (1991), *Pharm. Acta helv.*, 66, 28–32.

23. Carstensen H, Muller BW and Muller RH (1991), *Int. J. Pharm.*, 67, 29–37.

24. Chacon M, Berges L, Molpeceres J, Aberturas, MR and Guzman M (1996), *Int. J. pharm.*, 141, 81–91.

25. Chew CH, Gan LM and Shah DO (1990), *J. Dispers. Sci. Technol.*, 11, 593.

26. Chiannilkulchai N, Driouich Z, Benoit JP, Parodi AL and Couvreur P (1989), *Sel. Cancer Ther.*, 5, 1–11.

27. Coester CJ, Langer K, Briesen HV and Kreuter, J (2000), *J Microencap.* 17, 187–93.

28. Cohen H, Levy, RJ, Gao, J, Fishbein, I., Kousaev, V., Sosnowski, S., Slomkowski, S. and Golomb, G. (2000) Gene Ther., 7, 1896–905.

29. Convreur P and Vauthier C (1991), *J. Control. Rel.*, 17, 187–98.

30. Couvreur P and Vautier C (1991), *J. Control. Rel.* 17, 187.

31. Couvreur P, Grislain L, Linaerts V, Brasseur P, Guiot P and Biernacki A (1986), Biodegradable polymeric nanoparticles as drug carriers for anti-tumor agents, Polymeric nanoparticles as drug carriers for antitumor agents (Guiot P and Couvreur P, Eds.), CRC Press, Boca Raton, FL, pp. 27.

32. Cuvier C, Roblot-Treupel L, Millot JM, Lizard, G Chevillard S, Manfait M, Couvreur P and Poupon MF (1992), *Biochem. Pharmacol.*, 44, 509–17.

33. Darkow R, Groth T, Albrecht W, Lutzow K and Paul D (1999), *Biomaterials*, 20, 1277–83.

34. De Jaeghere F. et al. (1999), *Pharm. Res.*, 16, 864–71.

35. De Verdiere C, Dubernet C, Nemati F, Soma E, Appel M, Ferte J, Bernard S, Puisieux F and Couvreur P (1997), *Br. J. Cancer*, 76, 198–205.

36. de Vringer T and de Ronde H (1995), *J. Pharm. Sci.*, 84, 466–72.

37. Diepold R, Kreuter J, Himber J, Gury R, Lee VHI, Robinson JR, Seattone MF and Schnaudingel O.F (1989), *Archieve Clin. Exp. Opthalmol.*, 227, 188–93.

38. Douglas SJ, Davis SS and Illum L (1986), *Int. J. Pharm.*, 34, 145–52.

39. Douglas SJ, Davis SS and Illum L (1987), *Nanoparticles in drug delivery*, CRC Crit Rev., 3, 233.

40. Durbin DP, El-Aasser MS, Poehlein GW and Vanderhoff JW (1979), *J. Appl. Polym. Sci.*, 24, 703–707.

41. Elghanian R, Storhoff JJ, Mucic RC, Letsinger RL and Mirkin CA (1997), *Science*, 277, 1078.

42. El-Samaligy MS, Rohdewald P and Mahmoud HA (1986), *J. Pharm. Pharmacol.*, 38, 216–8.

43. Endicott JA and Ling V (1989), *Annu. Rev. Biochem.*, 58, 137–71.

44. Ezpeleta I, Arangoa MA, Irache JM, Stainmesse, S, Chabenat C, Popineau Y and Orecchioni AM (1999), *Int. J. Pharm.*, 191, 25–32.

45. Fattal E, Vauthier C, Aynie I, Nakada Y, Lambert G, Malvy C and Couvreur P (1998), *J. Control. Rel.*, 53, 137–43.

46. Fessi H, Puisieux F and Devissaguet JP (1987), *European Patent*, 274 961.

47. Fessi H, Puisieux F, Devissaguet JP, Ammoury, N and Benita S (1989), *Int. J. Pharm.*, 55, R1–R4.

48. Fusai T, Boulard Y, Durand R, Paul M, Bories C, Rivollet D, Astier A, Houin R and Deniau M (1997), *Parasite*, 4, 133–9.

49. Gallo JM, Hung CT and perrier DG (1984), *Int. J. Pharm.* 22, 63.

50. Gasco MR (1993), *European Patent Application*, 9 111 3152.2.

51. Gasco MR and Trotta M (1986), *Int. J. Pharm.*, 29, 267–8.

52. Gasco MR, Morel S and Viano I (1991), *Pharm. Acta helv.*, 66, 47–9.

53. Gaspard R, Preat V, Opperdoes FR and Roland M (1992b), *Pharm. Res.*, 9, 782–7.

54. Gref R, Domb A, Quellec P, Blunk T, Muller RH, Verbavatz JM and Langer R (1995), *Adv. Drug Deliv. Rev.*, 16, 215–33.

55. Gref R, Minimitake Y, Perrachia MT, Trubetskoy V, Torchilin V and Langer R (1994), *Science*, 263, 1600–1603.

56. Guimaraes R, Clement O, Bittoun J, Carnot F and Frija G (1994), *AJR Am. J. Roentgenol.*, 162, 201–207.

57. Gujman L, Labhasetwar V, Song C, Jang Y, Lincoff MA, Levy RJ and Topol EJ (1996), *Circulation*, 92, I–292.

58. Gulyaev AE, Gelperina SE, Skidan IN, Antropov AS, Kivman GY and Kreuter J (1999), *Pharm. Res.*, 16, 1564–9.

59. Gumy R, Peppas NA, Harrington DD and Banker, GS (1981), *Drug Dev. Ind. Pharm.*, 7, 1–7.

60. Gupta PK, Gallo JM, Hung CT and Perrier DG (1987a) *Drug Dev Ind. Pharm.*, 13, 1471.

61. Gupta PK, Hung, CT, Lam FC and Perrier DG (1987b) *Int. J. Pharm.* 43, 167.

62. Guterres SS, Fessi H, Barrat G, Devissaguest JP and Puisiex F (1995), *Int. J. Pharm.*, 113, 57–63.

63. Harper GR, Davies MC, Davis SS, Tadors Th.F., Taylor DC, Irving MP and Waters JA (1991), *Biomaterials*, 12, 695–9.

64. Henry-Micheland MJ, Alonso MJ, Andermout A, Sazueres J and Couvreur P (1987), *Int. J. Pharm.*, 35, 121.

65. Hou MJ and Shah DO (1988), Interfacial phenomenon in biotechnology and materials processing (Attia YA, Moudgil BM and Chander S, Eds.), Elsevier, Amsterdam, p. 443.

66. Hunter, R.J. (1983) Zeta potential in colloidal sciences: principle and applications, Academic Press, London.

67. Hussain N, Jani PU and Florence AT (1997), *Pharm. Res.*, 14, 613–8.

68. Ibrahim H, Bindschaedler C, Doelker E Buri P. and Gurny R (1992), *Int. J. Pharm.*, 87, 239.

69. Illum L and Davis SS (1983), *J. Pharm. Sci.*, 72, 1086–90.

70. Illum L and Davis SS (1984), *FEBS Lett.*, 167, 79–82.

71. Illum L and Davis SS (1986), *Int. J. Pharm.*, 29, 53.

72. Illum L, Davis SS, Muller RH, Mak E and West P (1987), *Life Sci.*, 40, 367–74.

73. Irache JM, Durrer C, Duchene D and Ponchel G (1996), *Pharm. Res.*, 13, 1716–9.

74. Jeon SI and Andrade JD (1991), *J. Colloid Interf. Sci.*, 142, 159–66.

75. Jeon SI, Lee JH, Andrade JD and De Gennes PG (1991a), *J. Colloid Interf. Sci.*, 142, 149–58.

76. Jiang X and Liao G (1995), Hua. His. I. Ko. Ta. Hsueh. Hsueh. Pao., 26, 163–6.

77. Kartner, N. and Ling, V. (1989) Scientific American, 44–51.

78. Kartner, N., Evernden,-Porelle, D., Bradley, G. and Ling, V. (1985) Nature, 316, 820–3.

79. Kassab AC, Xu K, Denkbas EB, Dou Y, Zhao S, Piskin E SOURCE: J Biomater Sci Polym Ed. 1997; 8(12): 947–61.

80. Kattan J, Droz JP, Couvreur P, Marino JP, Bouton-Laroze A, Rougier P, Brauls P, Vranks H, Grognet J, Morge X and Sancho H (1992), Invest. New Drugs, 10, 191.

81. Kneuer C, Sameti M, Bakowsky U, Schiestel T, Schirra H, Schmidt H and Lehr CM (2000), *Bioconjug. Chem.*, 11, 926–32.

82. Kneuer C, Sameti M, Haltner EG, Schiestel T, Schirra H, Schmidt H and Lehr CM (2000), *Int. J. Pharm.*, 196, 257–61.

83. Kramer PA (1974), *J. Pharm. Sci.*, 63, 1647.

84. Krause HJ and Rohdewald P (1985), *Pharm. Res.* 5, 239.

85. Krause HJ, Schwarz, A and Rohdewald P (1986), Drug Dev. *Ind. Pharm.*, 12, 527–52.

86. Kreuter J (1983) *Int. J. Pharm.*, 14, 43–58.

87. Kreuter J (1991), *J. Control. Rel.* 16, 169.

88. Kreuter J (1994), *Eur. J. Drug Metab. Pharmacokinet.*, 19, 253–6.

89. Kreuter J and Speiser P (1976), *J. Pharm. Sci.*, 65, 1624–7.

90. Kreuter J, Alyautdin RN, Kharkevich DA and Ivanov AA (1995), *Brain Res.*, 674, 171–4.

91. Kreuter J, Berg U, Liehl E, Soiva M and Speiser, PP (1986), *Vaccine*, 4, 125–9.

92. Kreuter J, in: Kreuter J (Ed.) Colloidal drug delivery systems, Marcel Dekker, New York, 1994, pp. 219–343.

93. Kreuter J, Liehl E, Berg U, Soiva M and Speiser PP (1988), *Vaccine*, 6, 253–6.

94. Kreuter J, Stieneker F and Lower J (1991), *Proc. Int. Symp. Controlled Release Bioact. Mater.*, 18, 277–8.

95. Labhasetwar V, Song C and Levy RJ (1997), *Adv. Drug Deliv. Rev.*, 24, 63–85.

96. Labhasetwar V, Song CX, Humphery WR, Shebuski RJ and Levy RJ (1995), *Proc. Int. Symp. Control. Release Bioact. Mater.*, 22, 182–3.

97. Lamprecht A, Ubrich N, Hombreiro Perez M, Lehr C, Hoffman M and Maincent P (1999), 184, 97–105.

98. Lamprecht A, Ubrich N, Hombreiro Perez M, Lehr C, Hoffman M. and Maincent P (2000), *Int. J. Pharm.*, 196, 177–82.

99. Langer, K. et al. (1996) Int. J. Pharm., 137, 67–74.

100. Langer K, Seegmullaer E, Zimmer A and Kreuter J (1994), *Int. J. Pharm.*, 110, 21–7.

101. Lewis DH (1990), Controlled release of bioactive agents from lactide/glycolide polymers, Biodegradable polymers as drug carrier systems (Chasin, M. and Langer, R., Eds.), Marcel Dekker, New York, p. 1.

102. Li C, Yang DJ, Nikiforow S, Tansey W, Kuang, LR, Wright KC and Wallace S (1994), *Pharm. Res.*, 11, 1792–29.

103. Li VH, Wood RW, Kreuter J, Harmia T and Robinson JR (1986), *J. Microencap.*, 3, 213–8.

104. Lopez-Quintela MA and Rivas J (1993), *J. Colloid. Interface Sci.*, 158, 446.

105. Lopez-Quintela MA, Quiben-Solla J and Rivas J (1997), Use of microemulsions in the production of nano-structured materials, Industrial applications of micro-emulsions (Solans C and Kunieda H, Eds.), Macel Dekker, Inc., New York pp. 248–65.

106. Losa C, Calvo P, Castro E, Villa JJ and Alonso MJ (1991), *J. Pharm. Pharmacol.*, 43, 548–52.

107. Losa C, Marchal-Heussler L, Orallo F, Vila Jato, JL and Alonso MJ (1993), *Pharm. Res.*, 10, 80.

108. Luck M, Schroder W, Paulke BR, Blunk T and Muller RH (1999), *Biomaterials*, 20, 2063–8.

109. Lukowski G, Muller RH, Muller BW and Dittgen M (1992), *Int. J. Pharm.*, 84, 23–31.

110. Magenheim B, Levy MY and Benita S (1993), *Int. J. Pharm.*, 94, 115–23.

111. Maincent P, Marchal-Heussler L, Sirbat D, Thouvenot P, Hoffman M and Vallet JA (1992), *Proc. Int. Symp. Controlled Release Bioact. Mater.*, 18, 226.

112. Malaiya, A and Vyas SP (1988), *J. Microencaps.*, 5, 243–53.

113. Marchal-Heussler L, Fessi H, Devissaguet JP, Hoffman M and Maincent P (1992), *STP Pharm. Science*, 2, 98–104.

114. Marchal-Heussler L, Maincent P, Hoffman M, Spittler J and Couvreur P (1990), *Int. J. Pharm.*, 58, 115–22.

115. Masson V, Maurin F, Fessi H and Devissaguet JP (1997), *Biomaterials* 18, 327–35.

116. Mirkin CA (2000b), *Inorg. Chem.*, 39, 2258–2272.

117. Mirkin CA, Mucic RC, Letsinger RL, Storhoff JJ, (1996) *Nature*, 382, 607.

118. Moghimi SM and Patel HM (1989), *Biochim. Biophys. Acta*, 984, 379–83.

119. Moghimi SM, Muir IS, Illum L, Davis SS, Kolb-Bachofen V (1993), *Biochim. Biophys. Acta*, 1179, 157–65.

120. Molpeceres J, Guzman M, Aberturas MR, Chacon M and Berges L (1996), *J. Pharm. Sci.*, 85, 206–13.

121. Moore, A., Marecos, E., Bogdanov, A. Jr. and Weissleder, R. (2000) Radiology, 214, 568–74.

122. Muler RH, Wallis KH, Troster SD and Kreuter J (1992), *J. Control. Rel.*, 20, 237–46.

123. Mullaney M, Groth T, Darkow R, Hesse R, Albrecht W, Paul D and von Sengbusch G (1999), *Artif. Organs*, 23, 87–97.

124. Muller RH and Lucks JS (1991), *German Patent Application*, P41 31 562.6.

125. Muller RH and Lucks JS (1996), *European Patent*, 0 605 497 B1.

126. Muller RH, Mehnert W, Lucks JS, Schwarz C, Muhlen A, Weyhers H, Freitas C and Ruhl D (1995), *Eur. J. Pharm. Biopharm.*, 41, 62–9.

127. Muller RH, Schwarz C, Mehnert W and Lucks JS (1993), *Proc. Int. Symp. Controlled Release Bioact. Mater.*, 20, 480–81.

128. Murakami H, Kobayashi, M, Takeuchi H and Kawashima Y (1999), *Int. J. Pharm.* 187, 143–52.

129. Nagy JB (1989), *Colloids Surfaces*, 35, 201.

130. Natsume H, Sugibayashi K, Juni K, Morimoto, Y, Shibata T and Fujimoto S (1990), *Int. J. Pharm.*, 58, 79.

131. Nilsson KG (1989), *J. immunol. Methods*, 122, 273–7.

132. Nishikawa, T., Akiyoshi, K. and Sunamoto, J. (1996) J. Am. Chem. Soc., 118, 6110–15.

133. O'Hagan, D.T., Palin, K. and Davis, K.K. (1989) Vaccine, 7, 213–6.

134. Ogawara K, Yoshida M, Kubo J, Mnishikawa M, Takakura Y, Hashida M, Higaki K and Kimura T (1999), *J. Control. Rel.*, 61, 241–50.

135. Ohki A, Naka K, Ito O and Maeda S (1994), *Chem. Lett.*, 1065.

136. Olivier JC, et al. (1996), *J. Control. Rel.* 40, 157–68.

137. Oppenheim RC (1986), Nanoparticulate drug delivery systems based on gelatin and albumin, Polymeric nanoparticles as drug carriers for antitumor agents (Guiot P and Couvreur P, Eds.), CRC Press, Boca Raton, FL, pp. 27.

138. Oppenheim RC, Stewart NF, Gordon L and Patel HM (1982), *Drug Dev. Ind. Phar.*, 8, 531.

139. Pangburn SH, Trecony PV and Heller J (1984), Partially deacetylated chitin: its use in self-regulated drug delivery system, Chitin, Chitosan and related enzymes (J.P. Ed.), Academic Press, New York, pp. 3.

140. Pappo J, Ermak LH and Steger HJ (1991), Immunol., 73, 277–80.

141. Patel HM (1992), *Crit. Rev. Ther. Drug Carr. Syst.*, 9, 39–90.

142. Pillai V and Shah DO (1997), Microemulsions as nanosize reactors for the synthesis of nanoparticles of advanced materials, Industrial applications of micro-emulsions (Solans C and Kunieda H, Eds.), Macel Dekker, Inc., New York, pp. 227–46.

143. Pitt CG (1990), Poly (-carolactone) and its copolymers, Biodegradable polymers as drug carrier systems (Chasin M and Langer R, Eds.), Marcel Dekker, New York, pp. 71.

144. Ponchel G and Irache J (1998), *Adv. Drug Deliv. Rev.*, 34, 191–219.

145. Putnam DA (1996), *Am. J. Health Syst. Pharm.*, 53, 151–60.

146. Quintanar-Guerrero D, Allemann E, Fessi H and Doelker E (1999), *Int. J. Pharm.*, 188, 155–64.

147. Rajaonaryvony MJ, Vauthier C, Couarraze G, Puisieux F and Couvreur P (1993), *J. Pharm. Sci.* 82, 912.

148. Roger M and Kissel T (1993), *Eur. J. Pharmacol. Biopharm.* 39, 8.

149. Rolland A, Bourel D, Genetet B and Le Verge R (1987), *Int. J. Pharm.* 39, 173–80.

150. Rolland A, Collet B, Le Verge R and Toujas L (1989), *J. Pharm. Sci.*, 78, 481–4.

151. Rolland A, Gibassier D, Sado P and Le Verge R (1986), *J. Pharm. Belg.*, 41, 94–105.

152. Roy K, Mao HQ, Huang SK and Leong KW (1999), *Nat. Med.*, 5, 387–91.

153. Sakai H, Hanawa K and Aoyagi K (1992), *IEEE Trans. Magn.* MAG-28, 3355.

154. Samaligy MS and Rohdewald P (1983), *J. Pharm. Pharmacol.* 35, 537.

155. Sanchez A and Alonso MJ (1995), *Eur. J. Pharmacol. Biopharm.*, 41, 31.

156. Scherer D, Mooren FC, Kinne RK and Kreuter, J (1993), *J. Drug Target.*, 1, 21–7.

157. Scholes PD, Coombes AG, Illum L, Davis SS, Watts JF, Ustariz C, Vert M and Davies MC (1999), *J. Control. Rel.*, 59, 261–78.

158. Schroder U and Sthal A (1984), *J. Immunol. Methods*, 70, 127.

159. Schroeder U, Sommerfeld P, Ulrich S and Sabel, BA (1998), *J. Pharm. Sci.*, 87, 1305–307.

160. Sestier C, Da-Silva MF, Sabolovic D, Roger J and Pons JN (1998), *Electrophoresis*, 19, 1220–26.

161. Shamkhani A, Bhakoo M, Metzger AT and Duncan R (1991), *Proc. Control. Rel. Bioact. Mat.*, Amsterdam, pp. 213–4.

162. Sharma D, Chelvi TP, Kaur J, Chakravorty K, De TK, Maitra A and Ralhan R (1996), *Oncol. Res.*, 8, 281–6.

163. Soma CE, Dubernet C, Barratt G, Benita S and Couvreur P (2000b), *J. Control. Rel.*, 68, 283–9.

164. Soma CE, Dubernet C, Bentolia D, Benita S and Couvreur P (2000a), *Biomaterials*, 21, 1–7.

165. Sommerfeld P, Schroeder U and Sabel BA (1997), *Int. J. Pharm.* 155, 201–207.

166. Song CX, Labhasetwar V, Gujman L, Topol E and Levy RJ (1995), *Proc. Int. Symp. Control. Release Bioact. Mater.*, 22, 444–5.

167. Song CX, Labhasetwar V, Murphy H, Qu X, Humphery WR, Shebuski RJ and Levy RJ (1997), *J. Control. Rel.*, 43, 197–212.

168. Speiser P (1990), European Patent, EP 0 167 825.

169. Stieneker F, Kreuter J and Lower J (1991) *AIDS*, 5, 431–5.

170. Stieneker F, Kreuter J and Lower J (1991), *AIDS*, 5, 431–5.

171. Storhoff JJ and Mirkin CA (1999), *Chem. Rev.*, 99, 1849–62.

172. Sugibasayashi K, Morimotot Y, Nada T, Kato Y, Hasegawa A and Arita T (1979), *Chem. Pharm. Bull.*, 27, 204.

173. Sukuma S, Suzuki N, Kikuchi H, Hiwatari K, Arikawa K, Kishida A and Akashi M (1997), *Int. J.*

174. Tabata Y and Ikada Y (1989), *Pharm. Res.*, 6, 296–301.

175. Tan J, Butterfield D, Voycheck C, Caldwell K and Li J (1993), *Biomaterials*, 14, 823–33.

176. Tiefenauer LX, Tschirky A, Kuhne G and Andres RY (1996), *Magn. Reson. Imaging*, 14, 391–402.

177. Truong-Le VL, August JT and Leong KW (1998), *Hum. Gene Ther.*, 9, 1709–17.

178. Truong-Le VL, Walsh SM, Schweibert E, Mao HQ, Guggino WB, August JT and Leong KW (1999), *Arch. Biochem. Biophys.*, 361, 47–56.

179. Van Snick L, Couvreur P, Vrancks H, Lenarets, V and Ronald M (1985), *Pharm. Res.* 1, 36–41.

180. Vanderhoff JW (1985), *J. Polym. Sci., Polym. Symp.*, 72, 161–98.

181. Vanderhoff JW and El-Aasser MS (1988), *Pharmaceutical dosage forms: Dispersed systems*, Marcel Dekker, New York, pp. 93–149.

182. Vauthier-Holzscherer C (1991), *S.T.P. Pharm. Sci.* 1, 109–16.

183. Verrecchia T, Spenlehauer G and Bazile DV (1995), *J. Control. Rel.* 36, 49–61.

184. Vyas SP and Malaiya A (1989), *J. Microencaps.*, 6, 493–9.

185. Vyas SP and Sihorkar V (2000), *Adv. Drug Deliv. Rev.*, 43, 101–164.

186. Vyas SP, Singh A and Sihorkar V (2001), *Crit. Rev. Ther. Drug Carr. Syst.* (in press).

187. Wang YM, Sato H, Adachi I, Horikoshi I SOURCE: *Chem Pharm Bull* (Tokyo) (1996) Oct; 44 (10): 1935–40.

188. Widder K, Flouret G and Senyei A (1979), *J. Pharm. Sci.*, 68, 79.

189. Zhang Q, Liao G and Yin H (1995), Hua. His. I. Ko. Ta. Hsueh. Hsueh. Pao., 26, 172–6.

190. Zimmer A and Kreuter J (1997), *Adv. Drug Deliv. Rev.*, 16, 61–73.

191. Zimmer A, Mutschler E, Lambrecht G, Mayer, D and Kreuter J (1994), *Pharm. Res.*, 11, 1435–42.

192. Zimmer A, Saettone MF, Zerbe, H and Kreuter, J (1995), *J. Control. Rel.*, 33, 31–46.

193. Zimmer A, Zerbe H and Kreuter J (1994), *J. Control. Rel.*, 32, 57–70.

194. Zobel HP, Junghans M, Maienschein V, Werner, D, Gilbert M, Zimmermann H, Noe C, Kreuter, J and Zimmer A (2000), *Eur. J. Pharm. Biopharm.*, 49, 203–210.

195. Zobel HP, Kreuter J, Werner D, Noe CR, Kumel G and Zimmer A (1997), *Antisense Nucleic Acid Drug Dev*, 7, 483–93.

196. Zobel HP, Stieneker F, Atmaca-Abdel Aziz S, Gilbert M, Werner D, Noe C, Kreuter J and Zimmer A (1999), *Eur. J. Pharm. Biopharm.*, 48, 1–12.

197. Zur Muhlen A, Schwarz C and Mehnert W (1998), *Eur. J. Pharm. Biopharm.*, 45, 149–55.

198. Leach JK, O'Rear EA, Patterson E, Miao Y, Johnson AE (2003), *Thromb. Haemost.* 90, 64–70.

199. Leach JK, Patterson E, O'Rear EA (2004), *J. Thromb. Haemost.* 2, 1548–55.

200. Shubayev VI, Pisanic II TR, Jin S (2009), *Adv Drug Del Rev* 61, 467–77.

14

Resealed Erythrocytes

INTRODUCTION

Red blood cells (RBC, erythrocytes) were discovered in 1658. The developing RBC has the capacity to synthesize hemoglobin; however, adult RBCs do not have this capacity and serve as carriers for hemoglobin. The prime function of these RBCs is to transport gases for respiratory processes. The carrier potential of these cells was first realized in early 1970s. RBC, by their sheer numbers, (5 million/microliter in the circulation totaling 30 trillion in humans), and their long life of 120 days, are uniquely positioned to modulate the properties of blood borne and vascular components. The breadth and diversity of vascular traffic, offer a multitude of opportunities, with a vast clinical potential, for intervening in pathologies involving cellular or humoral components. The idea of using RBCs, as drug carrying containers (erythrocyte encapsulation), whereby biologically active entities can be packaged within the cell and later released, continues to be pursued as a means of drug delivery and targeting.

The desirable properties, which substantiate the suitability of red blood cells (erythrocytes) as drug carriers are:

- The biodegradability and biocompatibility.
- They can circulate throughout the circulatory system.
- Large quantities of material can be encapsulated within small volume of cells.
- They can be utilized for organ targeting within reticuloendothelial system (RES).
- A wide variety of bioactive agents can be encapsulated within them.
- Erythrocytes are biocompatible autologous cells used in patients, hence there is no possibility of triggered immunological response.
- Since cells are in common clinical usage in transfusion much is known about the technique for their collection and storage.
- Easy to prepare.

COMPOSITION OF ERYTHROCYTES

The blood contains about 55% of fluid portion (plasma) and nearly 45% of corpuscles or cellular elements. The fluid portion contains a large number of organic and inorganic substances in solution, which may be diffusible (electrolytes, anabolic, and catabolic substances formed during metabolism) and nondiffusible (proteins). The formed element or cellular portion of the blood is consisted of erythrocytes (red blood cells), leukocytes (white blood cells) and thrombocytes (platelets). The plasma constituents help in maintaining the isotonicity and the morphology of the red blood cells. Manipulation in plasma compositions *ex vivo* could be used to design various delivery systems.

ERYTHROCYTES MORPHOLOGY

Normal blood cells have extensile, elastic, biconcave and non-nucleated configuration with a diameter ranging from 6–9 μm with a mean diameter of 7.5 μm. The thickness is nearly 1μ in the center with an increased thickness (~2 μm) near the periphery. The blood volume of normal human adult male is about 7% of the body weight and about 6.5% in a female. For the blood volume of 5 litres, erythrocytes make up about 40–50% of this volume and there are about 5×10^{12} erthrocytes/litre of the blood. They have a lifespan of about 100–120 days. The erythrocytes are non-nucleated, therefore do not have the machinery to synthesize new carbohydrates, proteins, and lipids and hence replace them with plasma components to rebuild its membrane constituents.

Erythrocytes have a solid content of about 35% (rest 65% being water) most of which is hemoglobin, which remains tightly bound to the stroma of the cell membrane.

Each RBC contains about 280 million hemoglobin molecules. A hemoglobin molecule consists of a protein called globin, composed of four polypeptide chain; a ring like nonprotein pigment called as heme, that is bound to each four chains. The centre of the heme ring combines reversibly with one oxygen molecule, allowing each hemoglobin molecule to bind four oxygen molecules. RBCs include water (63%), lipids (0.5%), gluose (0.8%), mineral (0.7%), nonhemoglobin protein (0.9%), methehemoglobin (0.5%) and hemoglobin (33.67%).

Hemoglobin is determined spectrophotometrically at 540 nm, either directly or after the conversion of hemoglobin to cyanomethyl-hemoglobin using Drabkin's reagent. Most of the remaining solid is represented by proteins and lipids, which form the stroma or framework that concentrates on the cell surface as limiting membrane (cell wall). The phosphate content (50–100 mg/100 gm) of the erythrocytes is higher than that found in the plasma, most of which is organic in nature, i.e. triphosphate, hexosephosphate, ATP, and traces of NAD and NADP. The lipid content of the erythrocytes essentially includes cholesterol, lecithin, and cephaelins.

The electrolyte composition of the erythrocytes is although qualitatively similar to that of plasma, however, quantitatively it differs from that of plasma. The concentration of K^+ and Na^+ differ in that the former is more in erythrocytes and the later in plasma. The osmotic pressure of the interior of the erythrocytes is equal to that of plasma and termed as isotonic (normally equivalent to the osmotic pressure of 0.9% NaCl, commonly known as normal or physiological saline). Changes in the osmotic pressure of the medium surrounding the red blood cells (either *in vivo* or *in vitro*) change and modify the morphology and tonicity of the cells. If the medium is hypotonic, water diffuses into the cells and they get swelled and eventually loose all their hemoglobin content and may burst. On the other hand, if the medium is hypertonic, (i.e. one having a higher osmotic pressure than 0.9% NaCl), they will shrink and become irregular (crenated) in appearance (Figs 14.1 and 14.2). However, 0.9% saline solution lack necessary ions for the functionality of the cells. Balanced ion solutions like Ringer's, Ringer-

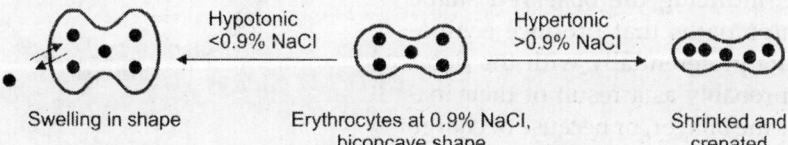

Hypotonic <0.9% NaCl		Hypertonic >0.9% NaCl
Swelling in shape	Erythrocytes at 0.9% NaCl, biconcave shape	Shrinked and crenated

Fig. 14.1: Various shapes and morphology of erythrocytes under different osmotic environments

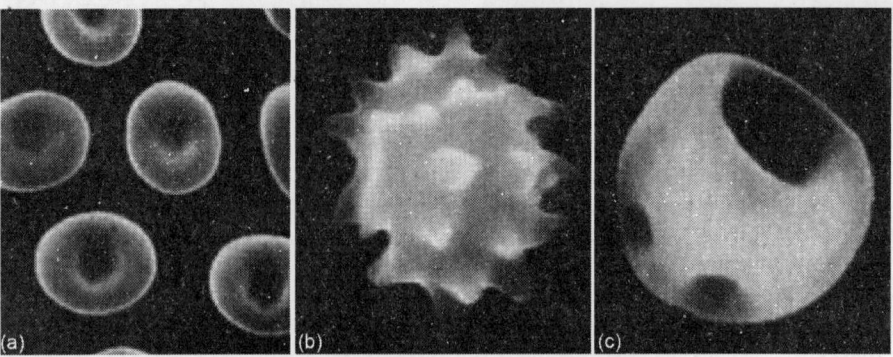

Fig. 14.2: Scanning electron photomicrographs of (a) normal erythrocytes, (b) crenate or echinocytes, (c) cup-shaped or stomatocytes

Loche, and Tyrode's solution, which are not only isotonic, but also contain ions in proper quantity, are used in erythrocyte-related experiments.

Various compounds convert the normal flexible biconcave discoid morphology into other morphologies in suspension, observable with phase contrast microscopy. The sequence of appearance is flexible biconcave disk crenate shape, or a cup shape, or the compound sphere, which is a massively leaking cell ghost geometry. Most compounds, which cause the first morphology change beyond the flexible biconcave disk fall into the classification given by Deuticke. For example, alkylsulfonates cause formation of spiky crenates or echinocytes. Organic cations usually induce smooth cup shapes or stomatocytes. Reversal from the crenate, is often promoted by plasma albumin, which is especially effective in binding organic ions. Sheetz and Singer (1974) proposed that the red cell membrane behaves as a bilayer couple; selective intercalation of the agents into the outer or inner monolayer of the membrane, results in expansion of one monolayer relative to the other, inducing the observed shape changes. Amphipaths that produce echinocytes associate preferentially with the outer monolayer, probably as a result of their inability to cross the bilayer, or because of charge repulsion by negatively charged inner monolayer lipids. Conversely, those compounds that induce stomatocytosis do so by partitioning selectively into the cell inner monolayer, perhaps through association with inner monolayer lipids or proteins.

Several methods can be used to load drugs or other bioactive compounds in erythrocytes, including physical (e.g. electrical pulse method), osmosis-based systems, and chemical methods (e.g. chemical perturbation of the erythrocytes membrane) (Fig. 14.3). Irrespective of the method used, the optimal characteristics for the successful entrapment of the compound require that drug should have a considerable degree of water solubility, resistance against degradation within erythrocytes, lack of physical or chemical interaction with erythrocyte membrane, and well-defined

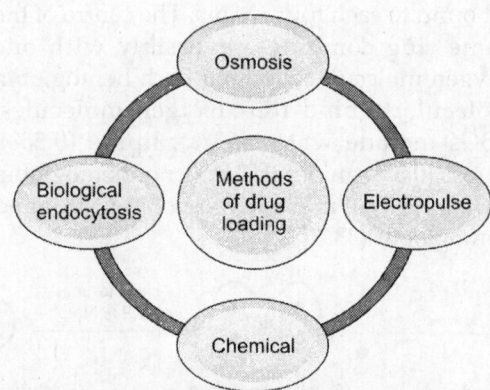

Fig. 14.3: Schematic presentation of different methods of drug loading

pharmacokinetic and pharmacodynamic properties. A comparison of different methods of drug loading is summarized in Table 14.1, and is discussed briefly in the next section.

Hypotonic Hemolysis and Isotonic Resealing Methods

This method is based on the characteristics of erythrocytes to undergo reversible swelling in a hypotonic solution. Erythrocytes have an exceptional capability for reversible shape changes with or without accompanying volume change and for reversible deformation under stress. An increase in volume leads to an initial change in the shape from biconcave to spherical. This change is attributable to the absence of superfluous membrane; hence, the surface area of the cell is fixed.

The cells assume a spherical shape to accommodate additional volume, while keeping the surface area constant. The volume gain is ~25–50%. The cells can maintain their integrity up to a tonicity of ~150 mOsmol/kg, above which the membrane ruptures, releasing the cellular contents. At this point (just before cell lysis), some transient pores of 200–500 Å are generated in the membrane. After cell lysis, cellular contents are depleted. The remnant is called an erythrocyte ghost. The principle of using these ruptured erythrocytes as drug carriers is based on the fact that the ruptured membranes can be resealed by restoring isotonic conditions. Upon incubation, the cells resume their original biconcave shape and recover original impermeability.

Loading by 'Red Cell Loader'

This method has been developed as a novel method for the entrapment of nondiffusible drugs into human erythrocytes. The equipment designed for this method was termed as 'red cell loader'. The method requires as little as 50 ml of blood. By using new apparatus, it is possible to entrap a variety of biological compounds into erythrocytes in as little time as 2 hours at room temperature under blood banking conditions. The method is based on two sequential and controlled hypotonic dilutions of washed red blood cells followed by concentration with a hemofilter. Subsequent isotonic resealing of erythrocytes allow a 35–50% cell recovery with approximate 30% entrapment of added drug.

Dilutional Hemolysis

Erythrocytes when exposed to hypotonic saline solution (0.4% NaCl), swell until they reach a critical value of volume or pressure, where membrane ruptures and becomes permeable to macromolecules and ions, therefore permitting the escape of cellular components. One volume of washed erythrocytes could be treated with 2–20 volumes of materials to be loaded in a hypotonic buffer

Method	% loading	Advantages	Disadvantages
Dilution method	1–8%	Fastest and simplest especially for low molecular wt. drugs	Entrapment efficiency is very less (1–8%).
Dialysis	30–45%	Better *in vivo* survival of erythrocytes; better structural integrity of membrane due to lesser ionic load	Time consuming; heterogeneous size distribution of resealed erythrocytes
Preswell dilution	20–70%	Good retention of cytoplasm constituents and good survival *in vivo*.	
Isotonic osmotic lysis	–	Better *in vivo* surveillance	Impermeable only to large molecules, process is time consuming

Table 14.1: Comparison of various hypo-osmotic lysis methods

at 0°C or 5 min. Further incubation at 25°C in an isotonic solution (0.9% NaCl) reseal them again. In general, the method is rapid and simplest especially for low molecular weight drugs, however the entrapment efficiency remains to be low (1–8%).

Preswell Dilutional Hemolysis

The technique is based upon initial controlled swelling of erythrocytes without lysis by placing them in slightly hypotonic solution followed by centrifugation at low 'g' to take them up to point of lysis. Finally, the addition of small volume of drug solution to obtain drug-loaded resealed erythrocytes.

Isotonic Osmotic Lysis

In order to avoid the potential disadvantages associated with hypotonic hemolysis, efforts were made to prepare resealed erythrocytes under isotonic (and/or isoionic) conditions. Hemolysis in isotonic solutions can be achieved both by chemical and physical means. If erythrocytes are incubated in solutions of a substance with high transerythrocytic membrane permeability, (i.e. small reflection coefficient as defined by the thermodynamics of irreversible processes), the solute will diffuse into the cells due to inwardly directed chemical potential gradient. This will followed by water uptake until osmotic equilibrium is restored. Various methods are based on this mechanism inclu ding, conventional (classical) hemolysis in isotonic urea solutions, polyethylene-induced hemolysis, ammonium chloride-induced hemolysis.

Dialysis

The major limitation of dilution procedure is low entrapment efficiency. It can be improved by carrying-out lysis and resealing within a dialysis tube. Several methods for dialysis based loading of erythrocytes are reported, but all take advantage of the common principle that the semipermeable dialysis membrane maximizes not only the intracellular–

extracellular volume ratio for macromolecules during lysis and resealing, but also allows for free flow of small ions, responsible for lysis and resealing of the erythrocytes. It is this intracellular–extracellular volume ratio during the time that the erythrocyte membrane tends to be permeable affecting the % entrapment of bioactives. It considerably reduces the extra-cellular solution volume that equilibrates with intracellular spaces of erythrocytes during lysis.

Electroinsertion or Electroencapsulation

The erythrocyte membrane could be opened by dielectric breakdown and subsequently the pores can be resealed by incubation at 37°C in an osmotically-balanced medium. The method is based on creating electrically-induced permeability changes at high membrane potential differences. Electric-breakdown is evident, when the membrane is polarized for microseconds using varied voltage values. The components can be entrapped, when an electric pulse of greater than a threshold voltage of 2 kV/cm is applied for 20 μ sec.

Loading by Electric Cell Fusion

In this method, the molecules are first loaded into erythrocyte ghosts. These ghosts are then caused to adhere to target cells. Electric pulses are applied to induce fusion of ghost with target cells with subsequent release of the encapsulated molecule. This loading can be exemplified with the loading of cell specific monoclonal antibody to erythrocyte ghosts. An antibody against a specific surface protein of the target cells can be chemically cross-linked to drug loaded ghosts. The antibody directs these ghosts to target cell for adhesion. Electric cell fusion then allows injection of these drugs into the target cells (Fig. 14.4).

Entrapment by Endocytosis

Endocytosis involves the addition of one volume of washed packed erythrocytes to nine volumes of buffer containing 2.5 mM ATP, 2.5 mM $MgCl_2$, and 1mM $CaCl_2$, followed by incubation for 2 min at room temperature. The

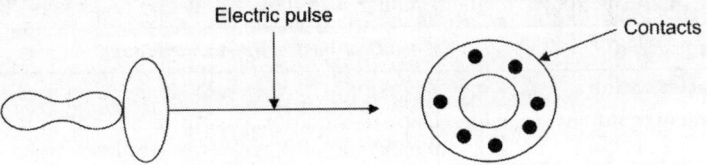

Fig. 14.4: Schematic representing loading by electric cell fusion

pores created by this method are resealed by using 154 mM of NaCl and incubation at 37°C for 2 min. The entrapment of material occurs by endocytosis. The vesicle membrane separates the endocytosed substance from the cytoplasm, which may shelter drugs prone to inactivation in erythrocytes or alternatively protect the erythrocytes from drug. The resulting erythrocytes contain vacuoles and probably have different *in vivo* survival characteristics from resealed cells, prepared using other methods. The swollen ghosts so prepared exhibit larger (>0.5 μ diameter) endocytic vacuoles. The drug substances are trapped in these endocytic vacuoles.

Loading by Chemical Perturbation of Membrane (Drug-mediated Loading)

This method is based upon the observation that the permeability of the erythrocytic membrane is increased, when it is exposed to some chemical agents. This allows the low molecular weight substances to get entrapped. A hemolysis technique in isotonic solution developed by Lin and coworkers, 1975 is based on the use of an anesthetic, halothane, which changes the permeability and selectivity of the membrane (colloid osmotic hemolysis).

Amphotericin-B, a polyene antifungal antibiotic, damages microorganism by increasing permeability of their membranes to metabolites and ions. This feature is utilized for the entrapment of daunomycin in human and mouse erythrocytes. The *in vivo* survival of drug-loaded erythrocytes prepared by using this technique, however was found to be poor. Due to residual membrane defects, they are sequestered from circulation by RES predominant organs.

IN VITRO CHARACTERIZATION

Resealed erythrocytes after loading are characterized for following parameters. These *in vitro* characterizations are pivotal, which help ensure their *in vivo* performance and therapeutic benefits. Table records various parameters often used with their preferred mode of investigations. Some of the routine characterization parameters used to evaluate resealed erythrocytes are described in brief (Table 14.2).

Table 14.2: Erythrocyte characterization with their quality control assays

Characterization parameters	Analytical methods/instrumentation
Physical characterization	
Shape and surface morphology	Transmission electron microscopy, scanning electron microscopy, phase-contrast optical microscopy
Vesicle size and size distribution	Transmission electron microscopy, optical microscopy
Drug release	Diffusion cell/dialysis
% encapsulation [(amount encapsulated/amount added to RBC) × 100]	Deproteinization (using methanol or acetonitrile) of cell membrane and assay for released drug or radio-labeled markers
Electrical surface potential and surface pH	Zeta potential measurements and pH-sensitive probes

Contd.

Table 14.2: Erythrocyte characterization with their quality control assays *(Contd.)*

Characterization parameters	Analytical methods/instrumentation
Cell-related characterization	
% hemoglobin content/volume	Deproteinization (using methanol or acetonitrile) of cell membrane and assay for Hb; laser light scattering for cell volume
Mean corpuscular hemoglobin [hemoglobin (g/100 ml) × 10/ erythrocyte count (per cu mm)]	Laser light scattering
Percent cell recovery (number of intact cells per cubic mm)	Hematological analyzer; Neubeur's chamber
Osmotic fragility	Stepwise incubation with isotonic to hypotonic saline solutions and estimation of drug and Hb
Osmotic shock	Dilution with distilled water and estimation of drug and Hb
Turbulent shock	Passing cell suspension through a 23 gauge needle hypodermic needle (10 ml/min) and estimation of residual drug and Hb
Erythrocyte sedimentation rate	ESR apparatus
Biological characterization	
Sterility	Aerobic or anaerobic cultures
Pyrogenicity	Rabbit fever response test or LAL test
Animal toxicity	

Drug Content

Packed-loaded erythrocytes are first deproteinized and subjected to centrifugation. The clear supernatant is analyzed for the drug content using entrapped drug specific estimation methodology. In case, the resealed erythrocytes are loaded with magnetite to make them magnoresponsive, a horseshoe magnet (1200 G) is placed adjacent to the base of the centrifuge tube in order to retain the entrapped magnetite. The magnetite concentration in drug-loaded erythrocytes could be determined using atomic absorption spectroscopy or some other appropriate procedures.

In Vitro Drug and Hemoglobin Release

Normal and loaded erythrocytes are incubated at 37 ± 2°C in phosphate buffer saline at 50% hematocrit in a metabolic rotating wheel incubator bath. Periodically, the samples are withdrawn with the help of a hypodermic syringe fitted with a 0.8 µm spectropore membrane filter. The samples are then deproteinized with acetonitrile and can be estimated for the amount of drug released. Percent hemoglobin can similarly be calculated at various time-intervals at 540 nm spectrophotometrically (Vyas and Jain, 1994). Percent hemolysis can also be determined by comparing the absorbance of supernatant with the absorbance obtained after complete hydrolysis of same number of cells in distilled water. Laser light scattering may also be used to evaluate hemoglobin content of individual resealed erythrocytes.

Another parameter, that evaluates the hemoglobin disposition after the resealing, is the mean corpuscular hemoglobin. It is the mean concentration of hemoglobin per 100 ml of cells, and is an index, which is independent of the size of the red cell and therefore, it is a true expression of their hemoglobin content. It is expressed as:

$$\text{Mean corpuscular hemoglobin} = \frac{[\text{Hemoglobin (g/100 ml)} \times 100]}{\text{Erythrocytes count (per cu mm)}}$$

Osmotic Fragility

It is the parameter, which simulates and mimics the bioenvironmental stress conditions that are encountered following *in vivo* administration, *in vitro* handling and the effect of loaded contents on the survival rates of the erythrocytes. To evaluate the effects of varying tonicities, drug-loaded erythrocytes are incubated with saline solutions of different tonicities (from isotonic to hypotonic, i.e. 0.9% w/v to 0.1% w/v) at 37 ± 2°C for 10 min. The suspension after centrifugation is assayed for drug and/or hemoglobin release, which should be in the acceptable range for a system to be therapeutically effective.

Osmotic Shock

Osmotic shock describes a sudden (and not tapering) exposure of drug-loaded erythrocytes to an environment, which is far from isotonic to evaluate the ability of resealed erythrocytes to withstand the stress and maintain their integrity as well as appearance.

Turbulence Shock

The parameter indicates the effects of shear force and pressure by which resealed erythrocytes formulations are injected, on the integrity of the loaded cells. Resealing of the erythrocytes makes them sensitive towards turbulence or mechanical agitation and hence an estimation of turbulence shock provides their expected performance *in vivo*.

Morphology and Percent Cellular Recovery

Microscopic methods are used to evaluate the shape, size, and the surface features of the loaded erythrocytes. Percent cell recovery (after loading) can be determined by assessing the number of intact erythrocytes remaining per cubic mm with the help of a hemocytometer.

Shelf and Storage Stability of Resealed Erythrocyte

Storage of resealed erythrocytes places a major challenge in their practical utility as drug delivery system. Under clinical conditions standard blood bags may be used for both, encapsulation and storage. The procedure would be to use Group 'O' (universal donor) cells and by using the preswell or dialysis technique, batches of preparation could be prepared in adequate amounts and stored as normal erythrocytes, which are used in transfusion. Another method utilized for storage has been the cryopreservation of erythrocytes in liquid nitrogen at low temperatures.

IN VIVO SURVIVAL AND IMMUNOLOGICAL CONSEQUENCES

The efficacy of resealed erythrocytes is determined mainly by their survival time in circulation upon reinjection. For the purpose of sustained action, a longer lifespan is required, although for delivery to target specific RES predominant organs, rapid phagocytosis and hence a shorter lifespan is desirable. The lifespan of resealed erythrocytes depends upon its size, shape, and surface electrical charge as well as the extent of hemoglobin and other cell constituents lost during the loading process. The various methods used to deterine *in vivo* survival time include labeling of cells by ^{51}Cr or fluorescent markers such as fluorescein isothiocyanate or entrapment of 14C sucrose or gentamicin.

Erythrocytes loaded using hypotonic hemolysis followed by isotonic resealing, dialysis and electroencapsulaion methods appear to sustain normally the circulation challenges. A bimodal type of survival kinetics is observed—a rapid loss of cells during first 24 hours followed by much slower loss afterwards. The early loss possibly accounts for removal of nearly 15% of total cell population, this represents the cells that are severely damaged during drug-loading procedures. The second phase has a half-life of the orders of weeks for different mammalia erythrocytes. The erythrocyte carriers contructed of red blood cells of mice, cattle, pigs, dogs, sheep, goats, and monkeys exhibit comparable circulaion profile, when compared with unloaded normal erythroytes. On the other hand, resealed erythrocytes prepared from red blood cells of chicken, rats, and rabits exhibit relatively poor circulation profile as compared against unloaded normal erythrocytes. These intra- and inter-species variations from different sources require a critical analysis and use the source before experiment protocol is designed.

There are three general modes of efflux of loaded contents from resealed erythrocytes—phagocytosis, diffusion or specific-transport mechanisms once placed *in vivo*. RBCs are normally removed from circulation by the process of phagocytosis. Phagocytosis occurs within the RES. The degree of cross-linking determines whether liver or spleen will preferentially remove the cells. Similarly, carrier erythrocytes following heat treatment, sulfhydryl treatment, or antibody cross-linking are quickly removed from the circulation by phagocytic cells located mainly in liver and spleen. It is observed that autologous erythrocytes do not elicit immunological consequences.

However, it is customary to realize that during loading process, some antigenic impurities may get entrapped resulting in possible immunological manifestations. Nevertheless, different studies contributed indicate that autologous sources do not generally contribute to undesirable immune responses.

PHARMACOKINETICS OF DRUGS OR PEPTIDES ADMINISTERED IN LOADED ERYTHROCYTES

Erythrocytes loaded with drugs and other substances have different release rates. In *in vitro* studies on release performed with erythrocytes from various animal species loaded with different kinds of substances. revealed a slow release of the encapsulated substance. The studies suggest that the *in vitro*

release of substances from loaded erythrocytes follows a first-order kinetic process, revealing that the substance permeates the erythrocyte membrane by passive diffusion.

However, human carrier erythrocytes containing enalapril have *in vitro*, zero-order release kinetics. The rabbit erythrocytes loaded with insulin have shown that *in vitro* the drug levels in loaded cells droped following a biexponential function relecting the existence of a more complex release process. The treatment of loaded erythrocytes with glutaraldehyde and other substances produces a more delayed *in vitro* release of both the encapsulated substance and the hemoglobin from the loaded erythrocytes. The employment of prodrugs encapulated in erythrocytes permits the use of the red cell as a bioreactor that controls the release rate of the drug.

When the loaded erythrocytes are administered *in vivo*, circulating cells used as drug carriers, may alter the pharmacokinetics of administered drugs. Encapsulation within erythrocytes imparts the drug a clearance that depends on the biological half-life of the erythrocyte, allowing therapeutic levels to be maintained in the blood for longer periods of time, together with the generation of sustained therapeutic effects. *In vivo* survival of human carrier erythrocytes labeled with ^{51}Cr demonstrates a mean cell life and cell half-life of 89 to 131 days and 19 to 29 days, respectively. Various studies *in vivo* with loaded erythrocytes in animals and humans reveal that encapsulation in erythrocytes significantly changes the pharmacokinetic properties of drugs. These changes in the pharmacokinetics when carrier erythrocytes are used involve the prolonged serum half-life of the encapsulated substance in comparison to the free substance, an increase in the area under the curve of serum concentrations and a greater accumulation of the drug in the liver and in the spleen. Enhanced liver accumulation of loaded erythrocytes may likewise be achieved by means of surface treatment with glutaraldehyde and other substances (Fig. 14.5). Changes in the pharmacokinetics may be caused by covalently linking drugs to cell surface proteins of erythrocytes, such as glycophorin-A and band-3. Erythrocyte-anchored drugs present extended half-lives, controlled volumes of distribution, and multivalent interactions. The concept of multivalency previously developed for liposomes targeting, may also be applied to carrier erythrocytes. The multivalent complex between a drug covalently bound to an erythrocyte presents a lower efflux than a univalent complex. The drugs encapsulated in carrier erythrocytes tend to present a pharmacokinetic profile characterised by a sustained-drug concentration over days and weeks, with the ensuing therapeutic advantages. Accordingly, specific mathematical models have been developed to characterise the delivery of drug directly to the macrophages involving phagocytosis of loaded red cells.

APPLICATIONS OF CARRIER RED CELLS

The potential use of red blood cells as a carrier system for the transport and delivery of pharmacological substances (drugs, enzymes, nucleic acids, genes) is well documented. One potential application is the delivery of these substances to the cells responsible for or capable of erythrophagocytosis, which are located primarily in the liver and the spleen. A second potential application, moreover

depends on the ability of loaded cells to survive for substantial periods of time in the circulation after reinfusion (Fig. 14.6).

Erythrocytes as Drug Carriers

Erythrocytes may be used as drug-carriers for a wide range of drugs, such as antineoplastics, antiviral drugs, etc. Different applications of resealed erythrocytes are enlisted in Table 14.3 and list of patents for resealed erythrocytes is given in Table 14.4.

Antineoplastic Drugs

Erythrocytes have been evaluated as carriers of chemotherapeutic agents for targeting the reticuloendothelial system for over 20 years. Antineoplastics constitute a group of drugs that represents the greatest number of studies conducted both *in vitro* and *in vivo* using erythrocytes as carriers. The reticuloendothelial system is the main site for the destruction of abnormal or old erythrocytes. In order to improve the recognition of these cells as carriers, many authors have subjected the loaded erythrocytes to treatments that incorporate some form of structural change on erythrocytes that renders them more readily recognisable by the RES, basically by such organs as the liver and spleen, in a very short period of time. On this basis, the erythrocytes can be used as carriers of drugs to direct them selectively towards these organs, e.g. in the treatment of hepatic tumors.

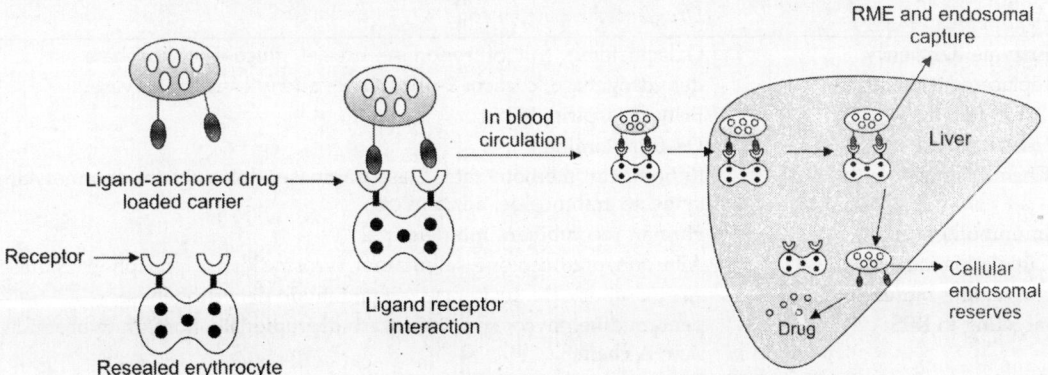

Fig. 14.5: Liver targeting through ligand-anchored carrier system

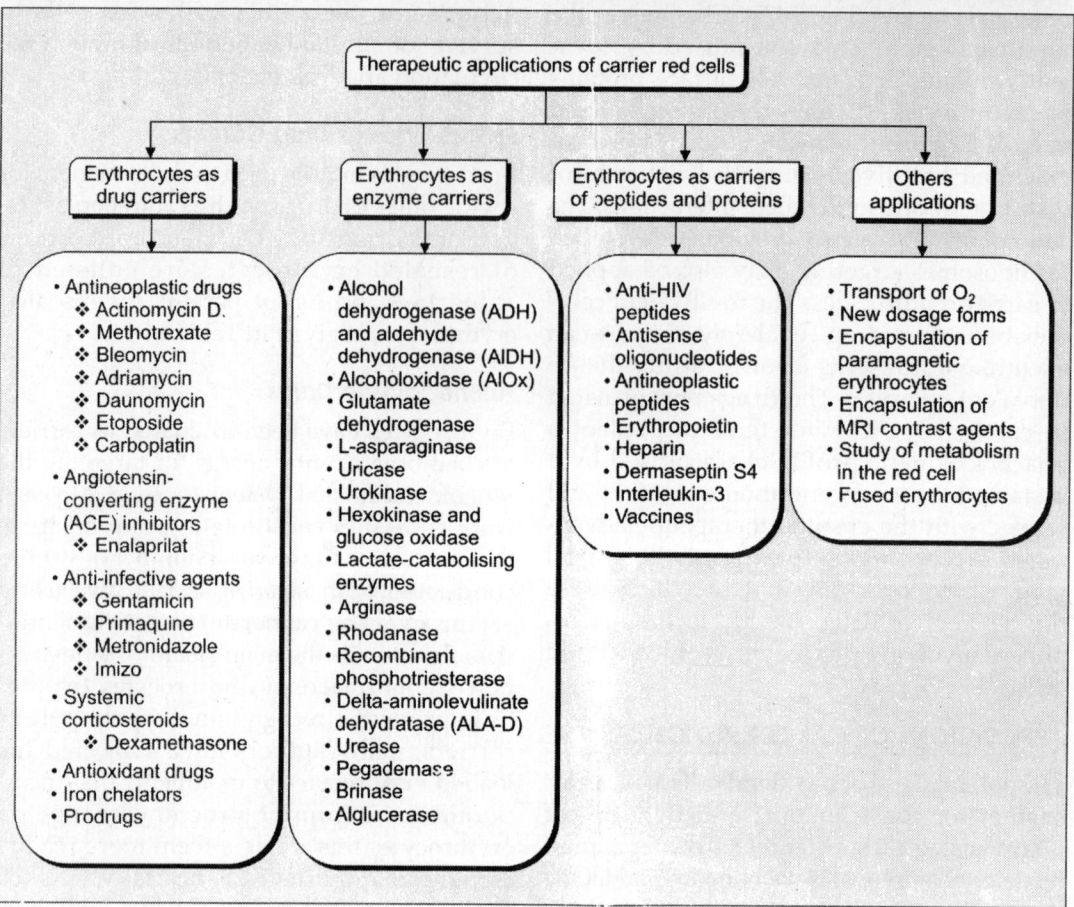

Fig. 14.6: Therapeutic applications of carrier erythrocytes

Table 14.3: Various applications of resealed erythrocytes	
Application	*Drug/enzyme/macromolecules*
Enzyme deficiency, replacement therapy	Galactosidase, fructofuronodase; urease, glucose-6-phosphate dehydrogenase; corticol-2-phosphate; adenylosuccinate lyase
Thrombolytic Activity	Brinase, aspirin, heparin
Iron overload	Desferroxamine
Chemotherapy	Rubomycin, methotrexate, L-asparaginase, doxorubicin, daunomycin, cytosine arabinoside, adriamycin
Immunotherapy	Human recombinant interleukin-2
Circulating carriers	Albumin, prednisolone, salbutamol, tyrosine kinase, phosphotriesterase
Circulating bioreactor	Arginase, uricase, luciferase, acetaldehyde dehydrogenase
targeting to RES	pentamidine, mycotoxin, imidocarb dipropionate, homidium bromide, ricin A chain
Targeting to sites other than RES	Daunomycin, methotrexate, diclofenac sodium

Table 14.4: List of patents for resealed erythrocytes

Patent	Inventor	Title	Publication date
USP 6770478	Crowe, John H et al.	Erythrocytic cells and method for preserving cells	2004
USP 6919208	Levy, Robert J et al.	Methods and compositions for enhancing the delivery of a nucleic acid to a cell	2005
USP 4517080	John R. DeLoach et al.	Apparatus for encapsulating additives in resealed erythrocytes	1985
USP 6139836	Magnani, Mauro et al.	Method of encapsulating biologically active agents within erythrocytes, and apparatus therefore	2000
USP 5328840	Coller, Barry S.	Method for preparing targeted-carrier erythrocytes	1994
USP 20070105220	Crowe, John H	Erythrocytic cells and method for loading solutes	2007
US2010015887	Terman, David Stephen	Sickled erythrocytes with antitumor molecules induce tumoricidal effects	2010
US20100203024	Terman, David S. & Dewhirst, Mark W	Sickled erythrocytes, nucleated precursors and Erythroleukemia cells for targeted delivery of oncolytic viruses, anti-tumor proteins, plasmids, toxins, hemolysins and chemotherapy	2010
US 20080261262	Godfrin, Yann	Lysis/resealing process and device for incorporating an active ingredient, in particular asparaginase or inositol hexaphosphate in erythrocytes	2008
US 20110262415	Grimaldi, Settimio	Erythrocyte-based delivery system, method of preparation and uses thereof	2011
US20100284982	Yang, Victor C.	Erythrocyte-encapsulated L-asparaginase for enhanced acute lymphoblastic leukemia therapy	2010
US 20110098685	Flower, Robert W.	Methods for production and use of substance-loaded erythrocytes (S-Ies) for observation and treatment of microvascular hemodynamics	2011

Actinomycin D

One of the first instances of research with antineoplastics encapsulated in erythrocytes to direct them selectively to the reticuloendothelial system involved actinomycin D. Using a method of hypotonic exchange-loading reaction, a high encapsulation of actinomycin D has been achieved in packed human erythrocytes. The actinomycin D encapsulated in erythrocytes undergoes rapid leakage at 37°C in an isotonic buffer. The rapid leakage of actinomycin D at 37°C occurs through a diffusion process dependent on temperature. However, if the encapsulation of the actinomycin D-DNA is performed, the complex is retained in the cells for longer periods, with up to 50% of the encapsulated drug remaining associated to the membrane of the red cell.

Methotrexate

The pharmacological efficacy of methotrexate-loaded erythrocyte in treating mice bearing hepatoma ascites tumors was recorded to increase average survival time. Numerous methods have been assessed to improve vectorisation of these carriers towards the RES predominant organs. One of these is the exposure of the carrier erythrocytes to agents that stabilise the membrane, basically glutaraldehyde, which acts by reducing the deformability of the erythrocytes. The glutaraldehyde treatment of erythrocytes results in the cross-linking of the membrane proteins and is also reported to target them to the reticuloendothelial system specific. The treated cells are rapidly cleared from circulation by liver and spleen following recognition and are well-accumulated in the liver. The glutaraldehyde treatment of methotrexate canine-loaded canine erythrocytes selectively targeted the drug to the liver. Surface-modified erythrocytes containing methotrexate by attachment with N-hydroxysuccinimide ester of biotin (NHS-biotin) is a new approach for liver specific delivery. The results suggest that recognition of erythrocytes by macrophages *in vitro* and liver-targeting *in vivo* can be further enhanced using biotinylated erythrocytes. Further studies have incorporated other alterations on the surface of the erythrocytes loaded with methotrexate for increasing its uptake by the macrophages and its possible use in the treatment of certain tumors of liver or lungs, by using desialation and hemichrome induction or by treating RBCs with trypsin and phenylhydrazine.

Bleomycin

This glycopeptide antitumor antibiotic, encapsulated in the erythrocytes, was retained in the red cells without any noticeable leakage. It was significantly more effective than the same dose of free drug in suppressing the phagocytic function of the RES in mice.

Adriamycin

The encapsulation of adriamycin (doxorubicin) in human autologous erythrocytes has revealed a limited biotransformation of the drug at intracellular level, a slow release of the unmodified molecule to the medium and an absence of significant erythrocyte damage. The encapsulation in erythrocytes permits a slow release that would increase its antitumor activity and reduce the side effects, largely cardiotoxicity. A new derivative of erythrocyte ghosts-reverse biomembrane

vesicles was developed, loaded with doxorubicin HCl and extensively characterized both *in vivo* and *in vitro*. The plasma clearance data revealed an increase in the half-life and bioavailability of the drug. Further, the tissue concentration data suggest that the liver and spleen remain the major organs involved in clearance, suggesting preferential uptake by the RES. Therefore, this system may provide a further potential application in antineoplastic therapy. As recorded with other antineoplastics, the treatment of erythrocytes with glutaraldehyde has resulted on a slower release of the drug. It has also been shown that the rate of metabolism decreases in canine erythrocytes. The treatment of adriamycin-loaded erythrocytes from mice with 0.1% glutaraldehyde produced a considerable decrease in the *in vitro* leakage of the unmodified drug and a selective liver uptake of the encapsulated drug. No noticeable liver damage resulted. Entrapment of adriamycin within erythrocytes, along with glutaraldehyde treatment of the carrier cells, seems to be a promising therapeutic strategy against liver (and lung) tumors. In experimental tumors in mice, the therapeutic index of adriamycin encapsulated within glutaraldehyde treated erythrocytes increased by more than twofold over that of the free drug. The coating of the carrier cells with IgG or IgM antibodies is another strategy that may be used to modify and enhance selective vectoring. By using an experimental model of canine erythrocytes, the erythrocytes loaded with doxorubicin have been treated with antibodies for their selective vectoring to cytotoxic T-lymphocytes.

Daunomycin

An increase in survival time *in vivo* was obtained, when the erythrocytes with entrapped antileukemic drug, daunomycin, were given to mice bearing L1210 cells. The daunomycin in erythrocytes was entrapped by treating the erythrocytes with amphotericin B, which is a polyene that binds to cholesterol in the plasma membrane of eukaryotic cells and perforates cell membranes. The erythrocytes with entrapped daunomycin may act as a time-release system, as a result cells are exposed to the drug particularly when they enter DNA synthesis phase.

Etoposide

Etoposide is an inhibitor of the topoisomerase, toxic to tumor cells of macrophage origin. Recent studies using peritoneal macrophages from CD1 mice have shown that the encapsulation of etoposide in mouse erythrocytes by hypotonic dialysis with alteration of the membrane involving band-3 cross-linkers produces, *in vitro*, a greater uptake of etoposide by the macrophages mainly by a process of phagocytosis. The macrophage specific toxic effect, determined by the fragmentation of DNA in macrophages, the latter was recorded to be more with encapsulated etoposide than that shown by the free drug.

Carboplatin

The encapsulation of carboplatin was conducted in human erythrocytes *in vitro*. The incubation of the erythrocytes loaded in autologous plasma caused a slow release of the drug from the cells. Furthermore, despite its relatively high stability in aqueous solution, it rapidly transforms into other substances with pharmacological activity within erythrocytes. It has been suggested that hemoglobin and, specifically, divalent iron play a key role in this conversion. The encapsulation of carboplatin in human erythrocytes may represent a therapeutic strategy for increasing the drug concentration in target organs, such as the liver.

Angiotensin-converting Enzyme (ACE) Inhibitors

Enalaprilat

Enalaprilat is an angiotensin-converting enzyme (ACE) inhibitor, widely used as its esterified oral absorbable prodrug, in the management of hypertension and congestive heart failure. Human erythrocytes loaded with enalaprilat using a hypotonic pre-swelling method release the drug *in vitro* following a zero-order kinetics. In a study involving rabbits, the area under the inhibition curve (ACE) versus time over the entire course of study, a measurement parameter, i.e. the extent of the inhibition within the sampled period of time, was measured to be significantly greater following the administration of the drug encapsulated in erythrocytes.

Anti-infective Agents

Gentamicin

The aminoglycoside antibiotic gentamicin was loaded in human erythrocytes and studied as a selective carrier system to the reticuloendothelial system and also as a potential slow release carrier. The antibiotic, being of polar nature, remains inside the cells unless they lyse and this property has been used for the kinetic study of the erythrocytes through the evolution of the levels of the drug. The use of anti-Rh antibody (IgG anti-D)-coated autologous human erythrocytes loaded with gentamicin makes the carrier erythrocytes more recognisable by the macrophages, which permits their increase uptake by the reticuloendothelial system.

Primaquine

The glutaraldehyde-treated erythrocytes appear to be promising carriers of the antimalarial drug primaquine for its hepatic delivery and suggest the possible use of the drug as a slow release system delivery following intravenous administration for the prophylaxis and eradication of malaria. Glutaraldehyde treatment stabilizes the cells, such cells are resistant to osmotic and turbulence shocks. *In vitro* release of drug and hemoglobin was also retarded upon treatment of loaded erythrocytes with glutaraldehyde.

Metronidazole

Tests have also been performed with erythrocytes treated with glutaraldehyde as slow-release systems with other antiparasite drugs, such as metronidazole. The results of dissolution study *in vitro* predict a sustained release following *in vivo* targeting. A slow *in vitro* drug efflux rate was recorded with the trypanocidal drug homidium bromide using bovine carrier erythrocytes. The 24 hours cell survival time was reduced from 80% to 50%, in case of the drug-loaded red cells.

Imizol

Babesiosis is an intraerythrocytic parasitic infection caused by protozoa of the genus Babesia. Erythrocytes have been used as slow release carriers for the delivery of anti-babesia agents for veterinary use. Imidocarb dipropionate (imizol) was encapsulated in murine carrier erythrocytes and injected intraperitoneally in mice, resulting in higher drug levels in blood in animals. The blood levels were sustained after free drug administration with a resultant decrease in parasitemia.

Systemic Corticosteroids

Dexamethasone

Erythrocytes containing dexamethasone have been used *in vivo* in rabbits and humans. Dexamethasone entrapped within rabbit erythrocytes was slowly released from the loaded cells *in vivo*. The encapsulated drug exhibited a much longer half-life than free drug administered intravenously. The rabbits were protected from inflammation caused by histamine for approximately 2 to 5 days after administration. The anti-inflammatory effect recorded reasonably well with the survival of loaded erythrocytes. Encapsulated dexamethasone 21-phosphate administered in patients with chronic obstructive pulmonary disease maintained detectable dexamethasone concentrations in blood for up to 7 days. Dexamethasone 21-phosphate loaded erythrocytes acted as circulating bioreactors, converting the non-diffusible drug into the diffusible dexamethasone. Erythrocytes are promising carriers for corticosteroid analogues and an alternative to oral or inhaled drugs in patients with chronic obstructive pulmonary disease.

Antioxidant Drugs

The cation complexes such as copper(II) complexes were also encapsulated in human erythrocytes to assess their possible use as antioxidant drugs. Encapsulation of copper(II) complexes causes slight oxidative stress, compared to the unloaded and native cells. However, no significant differences were recorded in regard ot major metabolic properties of loaded erythrocytes, with the exception of methahemoglobin levels, which differ depending on the encapsulated complex. The results suggest that methahemoglobin formation can be affected by the type of complex encapsulated, depending on the direct interaction of the complex with the hemoglobin.

Iron Chelators

Erythrocytes carriers for the administration of desferrioxamine and other iron chelators may be useful for improving iron chelation efficiency. The use for iron chelation by desferrioxamine encapsulated in erythrocytes has been studied for the treatment of iron accumulation in patients with thalassemia and other forms of anemia that require regular transfusions. The RES is the main site of destruction of old erythrocytes and, consequently, of iron overaccumulation in these patients. Desferrioxamine is the most widely used chelator. However, the primary and major iron repositories in transfusional siderosis which are reticuloendothelial cells, where iron in these cells does not appear to be directly accessible to desferrioxamine. Accordingly, an encapsulation of desferrioxamine in erythrocytes enables the release and avaialability of the desferrioxamine in the sites storing the iron (in the RES).

Prodrugs

In certain cases, prodrugs have been encapsulated, which are transformed into the active drug following release from the carrier red cells, it therefore resolves some of the problems stemming from the structure and behavior of the drug or due to difficulty in encapsulating the parent drug as such. Erythrocytes have been used for the encapsulation of the new antiopioid prodrugs with increased duration of action. Naltrexone and naloxone are widely used narcotic antagonists but with very short-term effects. Their administration encapsulated in erythrocytes would allow extended active life, however they are not stable within the erythrocytes and are rapidly released. The administration of prodrugs of these narcotic antagonists seems to present undoubted advantages. The triphosphate forms are stable in hemolysed at 37°C and are not released for 24 hours following the incubation of the erythrocytes at 4°C and 37°C. These prodrugs are transformed into an active drug after they are released from erythrocytes.

Erythrocytes as Enzyme Carriers

One of the more widely studied applications has been the encapsulation of enzymes in the erythrocytes. Enzymatic therapeutics are extensively used to treat disorder with enzymatic deficiencies (Gaucher's disease, galactosemia, hyperuricemia) breakdown of toxic compounds in intoxications or for the treatment of specific illnesses. The encapsulation of enzymes in erythrocytes provides unquestionable advantages, as it resolves some of the problems inherent to the therapeutic use of enzymes, including their short half-lives, their tissue toxicity in certain cases, immunological disorders and/or allergies associated with the treatments or the need for repeated administrations. Although, extensive work *in vitro* particularly on the encapsulation of enzymes in erythrocytes is available, the *in vivo* studies are at preclinical level and especially in human beings are limited.

Alcohol Dehydrogenase (ADH) and Aldehyde Dehydrogenase (AlDH)

The erythrocytes encapsulated alcohol dehydrogenase (ADH) and the aldehyde dehydrogenase (AlDH) reduce excessively high levels of alcohol and acetaldehyde in blood due to chronic alcoholism or to genetic causes, through the release of these enzymes into the blood circulation following hemolysis. One of the important paths for the metabolism of alcohol is its oxidation to acetaldehyde by the alcohol dehydrogenase and subsequently to acetate by means of aldehyde dehydrogenase. The acetaldehyde only accumulates in toxicologically significant amounts following the ingestion of ethanol. It has been observed that following the administration of AlDH encapsulated in erythrocytes, the blood levels of acetaldehyde in mice previously treated with a high dose of ethanol, were 35% lower than the level of acetaldehyde in control mice and no significant differences were found in the levels of acetone. Other authors have recorded similar results with concentrations of alcohol in blood, which were approx. 43% lower than the control groups, the clearance values of ethanol from blood in intoxicated mice treated with ADH$^+$ AlDH-RBCs were higher than the control.

Alcohol Oxidase (AlOx)

The enzyme alcohol oxidase show higher affinity for methanol, thus making the loaded erythrocytes useful cellular bioreactors able to catabolise methanol. The use of erythrocytes loaded with AlOx well significantly reduces the levels of methanol in mice. The encapsulation of AlOx in erythrocytes might contribute to detoxification following methanol poisoning.

Glutamate Dehydrogenase

Glutamate dehydrogenase is a mitochondrial enzyme that reversibly catalyses the oxidative desamination of the glutamate to α-ketoglutarate. It is involved in the breakdown of the amino acids. The encapsulation of glutamate dehydrogenase in erythrocytes has reduced the levels of ammonia in mice with induced hyperammonemia. Hyperammonemia is a major disorder caused by different serious and terminal illnesses, such as hepatic encephalopathy and certain neurological complaints. In view of its toxicity, levels of ammonia should be kept low, whereby encapsulation of this enzyme may constitute a potential means for reducing high levels of ammonia in the organism.

L-asparaginase

One of the most widely studied enzymes encapsulated in erythrocytes is L-asparaginase. It is a very clear example that depicts as to how the encapsulation in erythrocytes can improve the nature of a treatment. This enzyme breaks down the amino acid that is vital for neoplastic cells and, accordingly, has been employed for the treatment of certain neoplasias, mainly acute lymphoblastic leukemia, especially in pediatrics. When it is administered as a free enzyme, it presents a very short serum half-life and, its use has been linked to major immunological alterations as it is obtained from plants or bacteria. They include an immune-suppressing activity, intolerance reactions and even toxicity in certain organs and tissues, mainly in the liver and pancreas. Its encapsulation in erythrocytes may attenuate these drawbacks, considerably reducing the immunological reactions and protecting it from plasmatic proteases, thus extending its half-life. Different studies on animals have led to these conclusions. In studies performed on monkeys, guinea-pigs, mice and dogs, it was proven that L-asparaginase loaded into erythrocytes was more effective in eliminating plasma asparagine compared with the same dose of free L-asparaginase, injected in solution. A clinical study performed on humans likewise showed that following the intravenous administering of the encapsulated L-asparaginase, the half-life of the enzyme in circulation is very similar to that of the carrier erythrocytes, 29 and 27 days, respectively, as compared to the 8–24 hours recorded for free enzyme.

Uricase

Uricase enzyme is isolated in mammals; it is responsible for the transformation of uric acid into alantoin. The use of the encapsulation of uricase in erythrocytes as bioreactors for uric acid degradation has been studied. The concentration of the enzyme can be made arbitrarily high and the only rate-limiting step for the uric acid degradation is the rate of substrate entry, so uricase-loaded erythrocytes are potentially capable of removing as much uric acid as the human kidney. By coupling the uricase to the extracellular erythrocyte membrane with a biotin-avidin-biotin-enzyme bridge, Magnani et al. have managed to overcome the low permeation rate of uric acid into erythrocytes and maintain low plasma concentrations of uric acid for several days.

Urokinase

Urokinase is a plasminogen activator that facilitates its conversion into plasmin, which promotes thrombolysis. Urokinase constitutes a useful enzyme in the treatment of recently formed thrombotic or embolic states. Erythrocytes have been proposed as carriers of human urokinase, in the treatment of patients with thrombosis as an alternative to the use of high doses of urokinase. *In vivo* pharmacokinetic studies conducted on rabbits administering free urokinase and urokinase-loaded erythrocytes suggest its uptake in the liver and kidney and the formation of urokinase-proteinase inhibitor complexes. After intravenous administration, the area under the curve of the carrier erythrocytes was estimated to be eight times higher than free urokinase. These results confirm the slow-release of the enzyme from loaded erythrocytes and its protection from plasma inhibitors.

Hexokinase and Glucose Oxidase

Hexokinase is an enzyme that catalyses the ATP-dependent conversion of aldo- and keto-hexose sugars to the hexose-6-phosphate. Glucose oxidase is a specific enzyme that catalyses oxidation of h-D-glucose. Catabolising enzymes such as hexokinase and glucose oxidase encapsulated in erythrocytes may be employed as new therapeutic option for reducing high levels of blood glucose. *In vitro* studies with human erythrocytes encapsulating catabolising enzymes reveal a marked increase in the metabolism of glucose in comparison to normal cells. *In vivo* studies show that a single intraperitoneal administration of hexokinase/glucose oxidase encapsulated erythrocytes in diabetic mice was able to regulate blood glucose at physiological levels for 7 days and injections repeated at intervals of 10 days, were effective in the regulation of glucose levels for several weeks.

Lactate-catabolising Enzymes

Enzymes that metabolise lactate in the presence of oxygen as lactate-2-mono-oxygenase and lactate oxidase, were encapsulated in human and murine erythrocytes separatly and in combination. The coencapsulation of both enzymes results in significant rates of lactate metabolism. The results obtained *in vitro* suggest that the encapsulation of lactate-catabolising enzymes may be useful in the treatment of hyperlactatemia. *In vivo* studies to prove the efficacy of these enzyme-loaded erythrocytes in the removal of blood lactate in mice have failed because of the high aerobic capacity and high lactate metabolism of these animals.

Arginase

Another potential application of encapsulated enzymes for redressing metabolic or enzymatic deficiencies is the encapsulation of arginase for the possible treatment of patients with hyperargininemia. Their capacity for producing urea and catabolising arginine can thus be increased. The results of *in vitro* study on a specific human model show that it is possible to change the metabolic function of a genetically defective erythrocyte by incorporating exogenous human enzyme. The injection into rats of isoionic arginase loaded erythrocytes produces a longer response to arginase, when it is administered to hyperargininemic rats.

Rhodanase

Rhodanase (cyanide sulfur transferase) is a mitochondrial enzyme that converts cyanide into thiocyanate in the presence of sulfur donors. Encapsulated in erythrocytes, it may possibly be used as an antidote in cases of cyanide intoxication. The antidotes used have a short-term effect whereby the encapsulation of this enzyme may provide major advantages by maintaining its action for a sufficient period of time. Previous studies have indicated that resealed mouse erythrocytes containing rhodanase and sodium thiosulfates can rapidly metabolise cyanide, but the potential of this system is restricted because of the limited availability of thiosulfate, due to its poor permeability through across erythrocyte membrane.

Recombinant Phosphotriesterase

The encapsulation of recombinant phosphotriesterase has demonstrated *in vitro* potential use for the treatment of intoxications of organophosphorates. This enzyme has been reported to hydrolyse many organophosphorus compounds, including paraoxon, a potent cholinesterase inhibitor. Paraoxon is rapidly hydrolysed by this enzyme to p-nitrophenol and diethylphosphate. The addition of paraoxon to reaction mixtures containing resealed murine erythrocytes loaded with phosphotriesterase resulted in the rapid hydrolysis of paraoxon.

Delta-aminolevulinate Dehydratase (ALA-D)

The toxicity of lead causes a reduction in the intraerythrocytic concentration of the enzyme delta-aminolevulinate dehydratase (ALA-D), which leads to the accumulation of delta aminolevulinic acid in tissues, blood and urine, which is manifested as acute porphyria and alterations of the SNC. The administration of ALA-D encapsulated in erythrocytes in normal mice, does not produce any significant changes in the enzyme activity in blood, liver, spleen or kidney. However, the administration of ALA-D encapsulated in erythrocytes in lead-intoxicated mice produces an immediate and permanent recovery in erythrocytic enzyme activity. The entrapped ALA-D was stabilized to allow retention both in circulation and phagocytized red cells.

Urease

Urease is an enzyme that catalyses the hydrolysis of urea into carbon dioxide and ammonia. Alaninedehydrogenase (AlaDH) catalyse the reversible oxidative deamination of L-alanine to pyruvate and ammonium. Urease/AlaDH has been encapsulated in human erythrocytes *in vitro*. With this encapsulated system, urea is broken down into ammonia and bicarbonate. The released ammonia is converted into alanine by reacting with pyruvate under the catalytic action of AlaDH. The results *in vitro* suggest the potential application of such system in the treatment of high blood levels of urea in patients with chronic renal failure.

Pegademase

Pegademase (polyethylene glycol-conjugated adenosine deaminase) is a modified enzyme used in enzyme replacement therapy in the treatment of severe combined immuno-deficiency disease (SCID) associated with a deficiency of adenosine deaminase. The studies in humans using pegademase encapsulated in erythrocytes, reveal a significant increase in the half-life of this enzyme, whilst maintaining therapeutic blood levels.

Brinase

Brinase is a fibrinolytic enzyme produced by *Aspergillus orzae*. Brinase has been encapsulated *in vitro* in rabbit erythrocytes with potential use in thrombolytic therapy since the inclusion of this loaded system into clotting blood revealed almost complete lysis of the clot.

Alglucerase

Gaucher's disease is a rare hereditary disorder in which the enzyme, h-glucocerebrosidase is deficient. This results in the accumulation of the lipid, glucocerebroside, within macro-phages that become very enlarged and known as Gaucher's cells. This disease leads to a progressive hematological, skeletal and neurological dysfunction. Alglucerase is a modified form of the enzyme, h-glucocerebro-sidase, and is a unique form of replacement therapy in patients with a confirmed diagnosis of Gaucher's disease. Studies have been performed *in vitro* using different concen-trations of alglucerase as a sustained delivery system to the macrophages of the RES using human carrier erythrocytes using hypo-osmotic dialysis. High concentrations of alglucerase in the formulation and an exten-ded dialysis time favor the encapsulation of the enzyme.

Erythrocytes as Carriers of Peptides and Proteins

Erythrocytes are potential vectors for releasing peptides, modified oligonucleotides and even genes, and direct them selectively to their site of action.

Anti-HIV Peptides

The use of carrier erythrocytes containing anti-HIV peptides constitutes one of the more promising therapeutic applications of these biological carriers.

It is a well-known fact that the infectivity and replication of immunodeficiency viruses are inhibited by certain analogues of nucleo-sides following their intracellular trans-formation into triphosphate derivatives. Furthermore, the monocyte macrophage system plays a key role in infection by HIV-1. These cells become infected immediately after exposure to HIV; they are relatively resistant to virus attack and constitute an important reservoir for the virus.

Both AZT, which is an analogue of thymidine, and DDI, which is a nucleoside analogue, is reverse transcriptase inhibitors and both are prescribed as anti-human immunodeficiency virus (HIV) drugs. One strategy is based on protecting the macrophages from infection by HIV-1 using AZT + DDI encapsulated in erythrocytes using a murine AIDS model. Mice treated with AZT + DDI GSH-loaded erythrocytes presented a proviral DNA content in macrophages that was significantly lower than in mice treated with AZT + DDI.

Efficient protection of the macrophages was also obtained in a murine AIDS model, alternating the administering of AZT encapsulated in GSH-loaded erythrocytes to protect lymphocytes and macrophages not yet infected and the lymphocytic drug fludarabine to eliminate the infected cells. Similar results have been obtained with AZT prodrugs, such as AZTp2AZT, a new homodimer of AZT, AZTp2ACV, a new heterodinucleotide of AZT, and acyclovir, using carrier erythrocytes in a murine AIDS model.

Disseminated infection with *Mycobacterium avium* complex (MAC) is one of the most common serious opportunistic infections in patients with AIDS. MAC is not killed by any standard antituberculous drug except ethambutol at concentrations achievable in plasma. For *in vivo* killing, the drug must penetrate macrophages as well as the MAC cell wall. In practice, there is a need for therapeutic strategies to be able to inhibit HIV and Mycobacterium replication that permit reduced toxicity and prolonged administration.

Dermaseptin-S4

Some peptides, derivatives of dermaseptin-S4, have a high antimicrobial activity with reduced hemolytic activity. The dermaseptin derivative K4-S4 has affinity for the plasma membrane of erythrocyes, but under certain conditions, the peptide leaves its position and transfers to another cell for which it has a greater affinity, such as bacteria, yeast and protozoan target cells. A study has been conducted, where dermaseptin-S4 was attached to the membrane of erythrocytes and evaluated for ability to target the bacterial membrane.

Interleukin-3

Interleukin-3 is a cytokine that regulates blood-cell production by controlling the production, differentiation, and function of granulocytes and macrophages. *In vitro* studies have been performed on the encapsulation of interleukin-3 in mouse erythrocytes; and also the effect of chemical cross-linking with band-3 reagents on incorporation of cytokine into peritoneal mouse erythrocytes was studied. The performance of the encapsulation of interleukin-3 mouse carrier erythrocytes was higher, when the erythrocytes were loaded hypotonically as opposed to the isotonic incubation method. The treatment of mouse erythrocytes containing interleukin-3 with band-3 cross-linking reagents increases the recognition of carrier erythrocytes by macrophages *in vitro*.

Vaccines

Erythrocytes may be of interest in the field of vaccines as natural carriers and adjuvants of antigens. Several attempts have been made accordingly, thus Polvani et al. have encapsulated three bacterial toxoids. A mutation of the diphtheria toxin, the tetanus toxoid and a double mutant of the pertussin toxin, were encapsulated in murine erythrocytes by a hypotonic dialysis method. A comparative study was performed *in vivo* administering mice multiple intravenous injections of the different toxoids encapsulated in carrier erythrocytes compared to the same doses of toxoids administered in a saline solution. Titers in sera of specific antibodies against each antigen and neutralizing antibodies were tested. Titers of both antibodies against diphtheria toxin and tetanus toxoid were higher upon immunisation using toxoid loaded erythrocytes in comparison with free toxoids.

OTHER APPLICATIONS

Transport of O_2

Inositol hexaphosphate is an allosteric effector of hemoglobin that has a limited capacity for penetration in the erythrocytes. The incorporation of inositol hexaphosphate in erythrocytes produces a modification of the hemoglobin-oxygen affinity, increased O_2 release and reduces cardiac output. Encapsulated in red cells, it is irreversibly joined to the intracellular hemoglobin and as a result of its action it increases the transport of O_2 and CO_2 between lung and tissues. This effect is particularly important for different therapeutic applications, such as ischemic pathologies in myocardium, brain and other tissues. Some authors have studied the consequences of a substantial and long-term increase of the *in vivo* partial pressure of oxygen in piglets after exchange transfusion with inositol hexaphosphate enriched erythrocytes. The physiological modifications, such as reduced cardiac output in the absence of any other effects detectable, suggest the possible use of these inositol hexaphosphate-loaded erythrocytes to restore normal oxygenation in case of impaired blood flow.

New Dosage Forms

Tests have been performed involving new methods of administering drugs encapsulated in erythrocytes, such as the buccal administration of insulin encapsulated in erythrocytes in rats or propranolol encapsulated in erythrocytes as bioadhesive system for nasal administering in rats, where *in vivo* studies revealed a sustained release of the drug.

Encapsulation of MRI Contrast Agents

Further applications of the carrier erythrocytes are their possible use as contrast agents of MRI. Gadolinium-DTPA dimeglumine was encapsulated in human and rat erythrocytes. Comparative studies *in vivo* of gadolinium-DTPA encapsulated erythrocytes and in free form indicate a more prolonged tissue enhancement of carrier erythrocytes. Increased longitudinal and transverse relaxation rate constants were recorded using human and rat loaded red cells. Similar studies have been undertaken with encapsulated gadolinium-DOTA in human, mice and dog erythrocytes. Changes in the pharmacokinetic behavior of gadolinium-DOTA loaded erythrocytes in dogs, characterised by a significant increase in gadolinium-DOTA half-life, were observed.

Study of Metabolism in the Red Cell

Attempts have been made to encapsulate substances to study their metabolism in the erythrocyte or to observe the effect of said substances on a normal cell. Accordingly, various studies have been performed with human erythrocytes loaded with glucose-1, 6-biphosphate to study the metabolic influence of this molecule on red blood cells. Encapsulation has also been made in erythrocytes of enzymes, such as hexokinase and glucokinase in order to study the role, they play in the metabolism particularly erythrocytes, when there are enzymatic deficiencies. Glucose oxidase of *Aspergillus niger* has been encapsulated in human erythrocytes as a model system for cytotoxicity studies.

Fused Erythrocytes

Another interesting application, though less developed, is as 'fused cells', which is a method that permits the delivery of substances into the cytoplasmic compartment of tissue culture cells using loaded erythrocytes. In this procedure, the erythrocyte membrane merges with that of the host eukaryotic cell by means of the fusogenic agent and the content of the erythrocyte, including the substance previously encapsulated, is transferred to the host cell. This method has been tested *in vitro* with arginase, fragments of DNA, nucleic acids, ferritine, albumin, thymidin kinase with different types of eukaryotic cells.

Erythrosomes

Erythrosomes are novel class of cellular carriers in which chemically cross-linked human erythrocyte cytoskeletons are used as a support, upon which a lipid bilayer is coated. The lipid coating is affected by the reverse phase evaporation procedure normally used in REV preparation. These proteoliposomes, which we term erythrosomes, are of large size (an average diameter of 3 μm) and extremely uniform in size distribution. They are mechanically stable and easily prepared in large quantities. The protein content of erythrosomes is well defined, essentially being that of the erythrocyte cytoskeleton. The erythrosomes can be made from well-defined exogenous lipids. They contain less than 4% of erythrocyte lipids. The encapsulation efficiency of the erythrosomes is at least 4 times greater than that of typical REV and 200 times greater than that of SUVs. The erythrosomes possess a diffusion barrier to many ions and noncharged molecules as tight as those of SUV and REV. These carriers may serve as a useful carrier system for drug delivery.

Nanoerythrosomes

These are prepared by extrusion of erythrocyte ghosts to produce small vesicles with an average diameter of 100 nm.

SUGGESTED READINGS

1. Milanick MA, Ritter S, Meissner K (2011), *Blood Cells Mol Dis*, 47(2), 100–6.
2. Shavi GV, Doijad RC, Deshpande PB, Manvi FV, Meka SR, Udupa N, Omprakash R, Dhirendra K (2010), *Pak J Pharm Sci*, 23(2), 194–200.
3. Yamagata K, Kawasaki E, Kawarai H, Iino M (2008), *Ultrasound Med Biol*, 34(12): 1924–33.
4. Patel PD and N Hirlekar, RS, Kadam, VJ (2008), *Curr Pharm Des.*; 14(1): 63–70.
5. Hamidi M, Zarrin A, Foroozesh M, Mohammadi-Samani S (2007), *J Control Release*, 118(2), 145–60.

6. Annese V, Latiano A, Rossi L, Lombardi G, Dallapiccola B, Serafini S, Damonte G, Andriulli A, Magnani M (2005), *Am J Gastroenterol*, 100(6), 1370–5.
7. Lizano C, Pérez MT, Pinilla M (2001), *Life Sci*, 68(17), 2001–16.
8. RS Hillman, CA Finch, Red Cell Manual, FA Davis, Philadelphia, 1996.
9. JB West, Physiological Basis of Medicine Practice, Panamericana, Buenos Aires, 1995.
10. HF Bunn, Erythrocyte destruction and hemoglobin catabolism, Semin. Hematol. 9 (1972) 317.
11. U Sprandel, L Way (Eds.), Erythrocytes as Drug Carriers in Medicine, Plenum Press, New York and London, 1997.
12. "JR Deloach, JL Way (Eds.), Carrier and Bioreactor Red Blood Cells for Drug Delivery and Targeting, Elsevier, Tarry-town, NY, 1994.
13. M Magnani, JR Deloach, The Use of Resealed Erythrocytes as Carriers and Bioreactors, Plenum, New York, 1992.
14. N Talwar, NK Jain, Drug Dev. Ind. Pharm. 18(16) (1992), 1799–812.
15. S Grimaldi, A Lisi, D Pozzi, N Santoro, Res Virol. 148 (1997), 177–80.
16. L Chiarantini, RE Droleskey JR DeLoach, in: M Magnani, JR DeLoach (Eds.), dvances in Experimental Medicine and Biology, vol. 326, 1992, pp. 269–77.
17. M Magnani, L Rossi, A Fraternale, M Bianchi, A. Antonelli, R. Crinelli, L. Chiarantini, Gene Ther. 9 (11) (2002) 749–51.
18. M Hamidi, H Tajerzadeh, Drug Deliv. 10 (2003) 9–20.
19. E Zocchi, M Tonetti, C Polvani, L Guida, U Benatti, A De Flora, *Proc. Natl. Acad. Sci.* USA 86 (1989) 2040–4.
20. Gasparini L, Chiarantini H, Kirch JR, DeLoach, in: M Magnani, JR DeLoach (Eds.), *Adv Exp Med Biology*, vol. 326, 1992, pp. 291–7.
21. HG Eichler, S Gasic, K Bauer, A Korn, S Bacher, *Clin. Pharmacol. Ther.* 40(3) (1986), 300–303.
22. S Noel-Hocquet, S Jabbouri, S Lazar, JC Maunier, G Guillaumet, C Ropars, in: M Magnani, JR DeLoach (Eds.), *T Adv in Exp Med and Biology*, vol. 326, 1992, pp. 215–21.
23. BE Bax, MD Bain, PJ Talbot, EJ Parker-Williams, RA *Chalmers, Clin. Sci.* (Lond.) 96 (2) (1999) 171–8.
24. WE Lynch, GP Sartiano, A. Am. J. Hematol. 9(3) (1980) 249–59.

25. Jain NK Jain, *Indian J. Pharm. Sci.* 59 (1997) 275–81.

26. HA Moss, SE Tebbs, MH Faroqui, T Herbst, JL Isaac, J Brown, TS Elliott. *Eur. J. Anaesthesiol.* 17(11) (2000) 680–7.

27. M Valbonesi, R Bruni, G Florio, A Zanella, H Bunkens, *Transfus. Apher. Sci.* 24 (2001) 91–4.

28. Y Sugai, K Sugai, A Fuse, CTransfus. *Apher. Sci.* 24 (2001), 255–9.

29. FE A. lvarez, B. Lichtiger, Med. 3 (3) (1995).

30. M Magnani, L Rossi, MD'ascenzo, I Panzani, L Bigi, A Zanella. *Appl. Biochem.* 28 (1998) 1–6.

31. PR Mishra, NK Jain, *Int. J. Pharm.* 231 (2) (2002), 145–53.

32. P. Kravtzoff, C Ropars, M Laguerre, JP Muh, M, *J. Pharm. Pharmacol.* 42(7) (1990) 473–6.

33. M Hamidi, H Tajerzadeh, AR Dehpour, S Ejtemaee-Mehr, *I. J. Pharm. Pharmacol.* 53 (9) (2001) 1281–6.

34. M Tonetti, AB Astroff, W Satterfield, A De Flora, U Benatti, JR DeLoach, *Am. J. Vet. Res.* 52 (1991) 1630–35.

35. R Green, KJ Widder (Eds.), *Methods in Enzymology*, vol. 149, Academic Press, San Diego, 1987, pp. 221–9.

36. JR DeLoach, G Ihler, Biochim. Biophys. Acta 496 (1977) 136–45.

37. MA el-Kalay, Z Koochaki, PW Schutz, JD Gaylor, Efficient continuous flow washing of red blood cells for exogenous agent loading using a hollow fiber plasma separator, Artif. Organs 13 (6) (1989) 515–24.

38. GM Ihler, RH Glew, FW Schunure, Enzyme loading of erythrocytes, Proc. Natl. Acad. Sci. USA 70 (1973) 2663–6.

39. G Dale, in: R Green, KJ Widder (Eds.), *Methods in Enzymology*, vol. 149, Academic Press, San Diego, 1987, pp. 229–34.

40. M Magnani, L Rossi, G Brandi, GF Schiavano, M Montroni, G Piedimonte, *Proc. Natl. Acad. Sci. USA.* 89 (14) (1992) 6477–81.

41. G Dale, D Villacorte E Beutler, *Biochem. Med.* 18 (1977) 220–25.

42. Tamura N, Tominaga T, Sato T, Fujii, Yakuzai-gaku 48 (1988) 86–91.

43. Y Ito, T Ogiso, M Iwaki, I Yoneda Y Okuda, *J. Pharmacobio-Dyn.* 12 (1989) 201–207.

44. DJ Jenner, DA Lewis, E Pitt, RA Offord, *Br J. Pharmacol.* 73 (1981) 212–3.

45. Mosca R, Paleari V, Russo E, Rosti R, Nano A, Boicelli S, Villa A, Zanella, in: M Magnani, JR DeLoach (Eds.), vol. 326, 1992, pp. 19–26.

46. Ropars M, Chassaigne MC, Villereal G, Avenard C, Hurel C, Nicolau, in: JR DeLoach, U. Sprandel (Eds.), Karger, Basel, (1985), pp. 82–91.

47. R Green, J Miller, W Crosby, Blood 57(5) (1981), 866–72.

48. MG Ihler, H Chi-Wan Tsang, in: R Green, KJ Widder (Eds.), *Methods in Enzymology*, vol. 149, Academic Press, San Diego, 1987, pp. 221–9.

49. FJ A ´ lvarez, JA Jordan, A Herra´ez, JC. D?´ez, C Tejedor, *J. Biochem.* 123 (1998) 233–9.

50. JR DeLoach, in: R Green, KJ Widder (Eds.), vol. 149, *Academic Press, San Diego,* (1987), pp. 235–42.

51. JR DeLoach, S Peters, O Pinkard, R Glew, G Ihle, Effect of glutaraldehyde on enzyme-loaded erythrocytes, Biochim. Biophys. Acta 496 (1977), 507–15.

52. S Sanz, C Lizano, J Luque, M Pinilla, *Life Sci.* 65(26) (1999) 2781–9.

53. P Franchetti, GA Sheikha, L Cappellacci, S Marchetti, M Grifantini, E Balestra, CF Perno, U Benatti, G Brandi, L Rossi, M Magnani, *Antivir. Res.* 47 (2000). 149–58.

54. CF Perno, N Santoro, E Balestra, S Aquaro A. Cenci, G Lazzarino, D Di Pierro, B Tavazzi, J Balzarini, E Garaci, S.

55. Grimaldi R, *Calio, Antivir. Res.* 33 (3) (1997) 153–64.

56. Ropars G, Avenard M, Chassaigne, in: R Green, KJ Widder (Eds.), *Methods in Enzymology*, vol. 149, Academic Press, San Diego, 1987, pp. 242–8.

57. Corsi L, Galluzzi R, Crinelli M, Magnani J, *Biol. Chem.* 270 (15) (1995) 8928–35.

58. EI Sinauridze, VM Vitvitsky, AV Pichugin, AM Zhabotinsky, FI Ataullakhanov, in: M Magnani, JR DeLoach (Eds.), T vol. 326, 1992, pp. 203–206.

59. J Luque, MI Gar?´n, S Sanz, P Ropero, M Pinilla, in: M Magnani, JR DeLoach (Eds.), vol. 326, 1992, pp. 81–9.

60. M Tonetti, E Zocchi, L Guida, C Polvani, U Benatti, P Biassoni, F Romei, A Guglielmi, C Aschele, A Sobrero, A De Flora, in: M Magnani, JR DeLoach (Eds.), vol. 326, 1992, pp. 307–17.

61. RS Franco, M Weiner, K Wagner, OJ Martelo, *Life Sci.* 32 (1983) 2763–8.

62. NC Santos, J Figueira-Coelho, C Saldanha, *J. Martins-Silva,* 31(4) (2002) 183–8.

63. MI Garin, RM Lo´pez, S Sanz, M Pinilla, J Luque, Erythrocytes as carriers for recombinant human erythropoietin, Pharm. Res. 13 (6) (1996) 869–74.

64. JR DeLoach, U Sprandel, Red Blood Cells as Carriers for Drugs, Karger, Basel, 1985.

65. TY Tsong, Biophys J 60 (1991), 297–306.

66. Lizano S, Sanz J, Luque M. Pinilla, Biochim. Biophys. Acta 1425 (2) (1998), 328–36.

67. Lizano MT, Perez M Pinilla, *Life Sci.* 68 (2001), 2001–2016.

68. Q Dong, W Jin, *Electrophoresis* 22 (13) (2001) 2786–92.

69. M Haritou, D Yova, D Koutsouris, S Loukas, *Clin. Hemorheol. Microcirc.* 19(3) (1988) 205–17.

70. PC Mangal, A Kaur, *Indian J. Biochem. Biophys.* 28 (3) (1991) 219–21.

71. Ben-Bassat, KG Bensch, SL Schrier, *J. Clin. Invest.* 51 (7) (1972) 1833–44.

72. LM Matovcik, IG Junga, SL Schrier, Blood 65 (5) (1985) 1056–63.

73. SL Schrier, A Zachowski, PF Devaux, Blood 79 (3) (1992) 782–6.

15

Transfersomes and Ethosomes

INTRODUCTION

The topical administration of drugs for the local treatment of skin diseases, has been used for a long time, but the use of transdermal delivery for the systemic action is relatively new area. Delivery via the transdermal route is an interesting option being convenient and safe. Figure 15.1 gives a comparison between

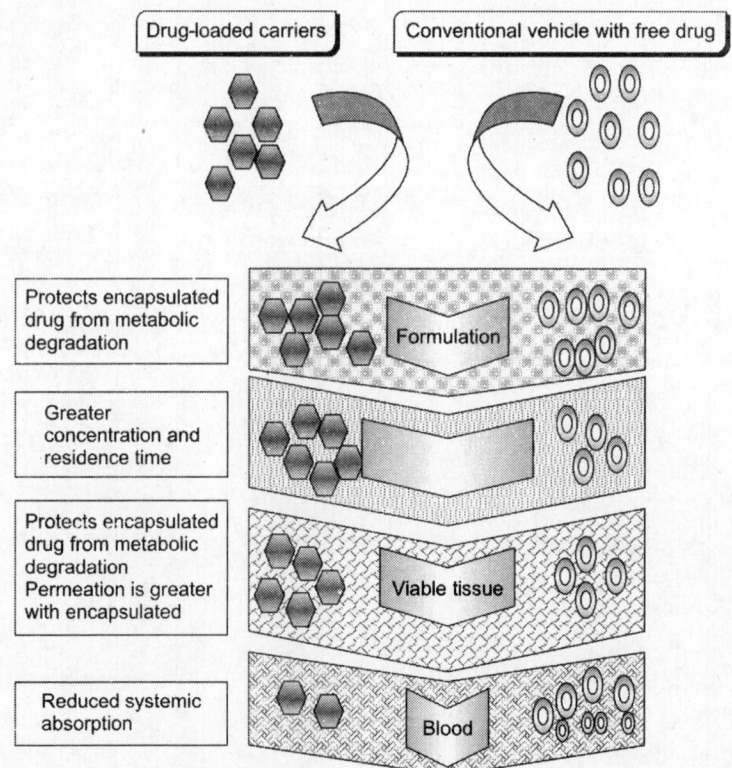

Fig. 15.1: A schematic representation of drug transport through the skin and benefits of a carrier system

conventional therapy and drug carriers. The rapid development of transdermal delivery formulations in the last years, is due to certain advantages of transdermal administration compared to the conventional oral route—it circumvents the fluctuations, which appear on gastrointestinal absorption; it increases the bioavailability of drugs because using the transdermal delivery the active principle passes directly into the circulatory system, bypassing the hepatic route; it can give a constant, controlled drug input while decreasing the variations in drug plasma levels; it increases the patient compliance by providing a simplified way of administration, with a minimum risk of trauma or any other injury of tissue.

SKIN

In order to design a drug for transdermal administration, certain problems are needed to be resolved. The major difficulty is the penetration of skin that acts as a two ways barrier, controlling the loss of water, electrolytes and other constituents. The skin is one of the most extensive and readily accessible organs of the human body. It receives about one-third of the blood circulation through the body (Fig. 15.2). It serves as a barrier against physical and chemical attacks and shields the body from invasion by microorganisms. The skin is a membranous, flexible, protecting cover, mainly formed by two major layers, i.e. an external, unvascularized one (epidermis) and an internal, vascularized one (dermis). The skin barrier properties reside in outermost layer, the stratum corneum. The stratum corneum is effectively a 10-15 μm thick matrix of dehydrated, dead keratinocytes (coenocytes) embedded in a lipid matrix. There are two important layers in the skin, the dermis and epidermis. The outermost layer, the epidermis, is approximately 100–150 μm thick, has no blood flow and includes a layer within it, known as the stratum corneum.

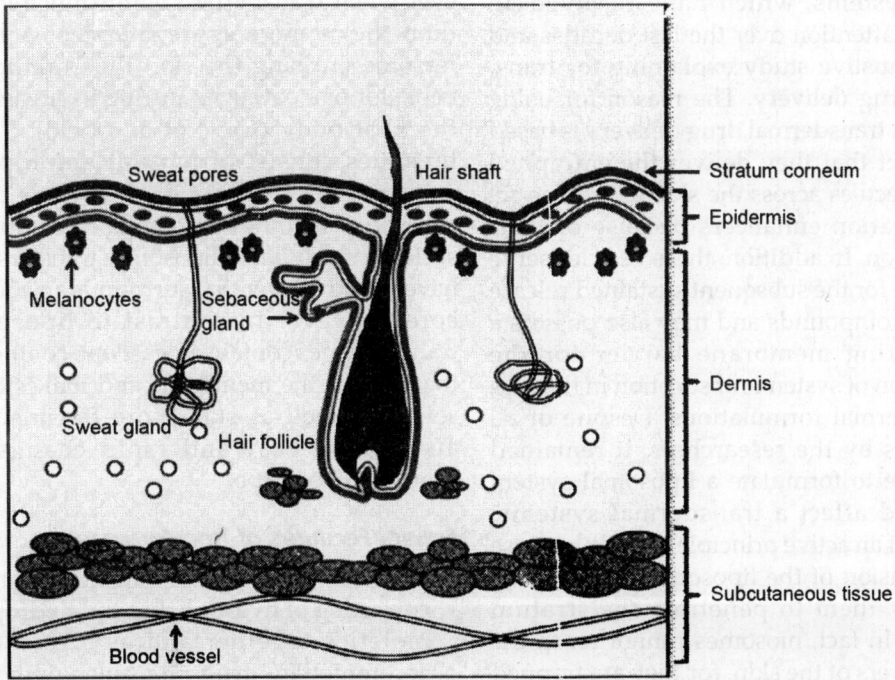

Fig. 15.2: Diagrammatic representation of cross-section of human skin showing the different cell layers and appendages

Beneath the epidermis, the dermis contains the system of capillaries that transport blood throughout the body. If the drug is able to penetrate the stratum corneum, then it can enter the blood stream and the process is referred to as passive diffusion.

In order to increase the permeability of the skin for transdermal delivery of drugs, several passive as well as active techniques have been proposed including penetration enhancers, supersaturated systems, iontophoresis, electroporation, phonophoresis, microneedles, jet injectors, etc. More recently the drug carrier systems, such as lipid vesicles (liposomes and proliposomes) and nonionic surfactant vesicles (niosomes and proniosomes), have been utilized for transdermal delivery. A novel, vesicular system relatively the newer elastic, highly deformable vesicles (trans-ferosomes and ethosomes) have emerged as a promising module effective for delivering a wide variety of materials across the skin.

Liposomes and niosomes are the vesicular carrier systems, which have received an intensive attention over the last decades and with exhaustive study explaining for trans-dermal drug delivery. The reason for using vesicles in transdermal drug delivery is based on the fact that they deliver the entrapped drug molecules across the skin as well as act as penetration enhancers because of their composition. In addition, these vesicles serve as a depot for the subsequent sustained release of active compounds and may also possess a rate-limiting membrane barrier for the modulation of systemic absorption in the case of transdermal formulations. Despite of all the efforts by the researchers, it remained impossible to formulate a liposomal system that could affect a transdermal systemic delivery of an active principle, mainly because the dimension of the liposomes, which does not allow them to penetrate the stratum corneum. In fact, niosomes cannot reach the deeper layers of the skin, for they are trapped in the superior layers of stratum corneum.

To overcome this problem, the subsequent researchers introduced a novel generation of vesicular elastic systems, transfersomes (ultradeformable vesicles consisting of phosphatidylcholine and an edge activator) and ethosomes (ultradeformable vesicles with high alcohol content). The main advantage of these ultradeformable vesicular systems, is the elasticity of their bilayer, imported by the surfactant molecules in the case of transfersomes and ethanol in the case of ethosomes; this elasticity effectively allows them to squeeze through the channels in the stratum corneum that are less than one-tenth the diameter of the vesicles.

TRANSFERSOMES

Transfersomes are complex, most often, vesicular aggregates optimized to attain extremely flexible and self-regulating membrane; this makes the vesicle flexibly deformable. Transfersome vesicles, therefore, can cross microporous barrier very efficiently, even when available passage are much smaller than the average aggregate size. A trans-fersome crossing the skin thus mimics the behavior of a pathogen during its invasion of the host body (Cevc et al., 1998). Trans-fersomes consist of natural amphipathic compounds suspended in a water-based solution, sometimes containing biocompatible surfactant. Similar to liposomes transfersomes have a lipid bilayer that surrounds an aqueous core, however in contrast to liposomes, transfersomes contain at least one component that softens the membrane and makes them-selves as well as skin more flexible. This also allows easy and rapid changes on transfersome shape.

Salient Features of Transfersomes

• Transfersomes possess an infrastructure consisting of hydrophobic and hydrophilic moieties together and as a result can accommodate drug molecules with wide range of solubility.

- Transfersomes can deform and pass through narrow constriction (from 5 to 10 times less than their own diameter) without measurable loss of entrapped contents.
- The high deformability affects better penetration of intact vesicles.
- They can act as a carrier for low as well as high molecular weight drugs, e.g. analgesic, anesthetic, corticosteroids, sex hormone, anticancer, insulin, gap-junction protein, and albumin.
- They are biocompatible and biodegradable, as they are made up of natural phospholipids similar to liposomes.
- They have high entrapment efficiency, in case of lipophilic drug, it approximates to 90%.
- They protect the encapsulated drug from metabolic degradation.
- They act as depot, releasing their contents slowly and gradually.
- They can be used for both systemic as well as topical delivery of drug.
- Easy to scale up, as procedure is simple, do not involve lengthy and complicated operations and unnecessary use or pharmaceutically unacceptable additives. Some additives used are listed in Table 15.1.

Limitations of Transfersomes

- Transfersomes are chemically unstable because of their constituting contents are predisposted to oxidative degradation.
- Purity of natural phospholipids is another criteria against the adoption of transfersomes as drug delivery vehicles.
- Transfersomes formulations are relatively expensive.

Mechanism of Penetration

Transfersomes when applied under suitable condition, can transfer 0.1 mg to 0.5 mg of lipid per hour, per cm^2 area across the intact skin. This value is substantially higher than that which is typically driven by the transdermal concentration gradients. The reason for this high flux rate is naturally occurring 'transdermal osmotic gradients', i.e. another much more prominent gradient is available across the skin (Gompper and Kroll, 1995). This osmotic gradient is developed due to the skin penetration barrier, prevents water loss through the skin and maintains a water activity difference in the part of the epidermis (75% water content) and nearly completely dry stratum corneum, near to the skin surface (15% water content) (Warner et al., 1988). The gradient is very stable because ambient air is a perfect sink for the water molecule, even when the transdermal water loss is nonprecedentially high. All polar lipids attract some water; this is due to the energetically favorable interaction between the hydrophilic lipid residues and their proximal water. Most lipid bilayers thus; spontaneously resist an induced dehydration (Rand and Porsegian, 1990; Cevc and Marsh, 1987). Consequently all polar lipid based vesicles move from rather dry location to the sites with a sufficiently high water concentration. So, when a lipid suspension (transfersomes) is placed on the skin surface, that is partly dehydrated by the water evaporation loss and under 'osmotic gradient' tend to move and try to escape complete drying by moving along this gradient (Schatzlein and Cevc, 1995), so that complete drying could be avoided. They can only achieve this, if they are sufficiently deformable to pass through the narrow pores in the skin, because transfersomes composed of surfactant have more suitable rheologic and hydration properties that contribute to their greater deformability. Less deformable vesicles including standard liposomes are confined to the skin surface, where they dehydrate completely and fuse, so they have less penetration ability than transfersomes. Transfersomes are optimized in this respect and thus attain maximum flexibility, so they respond to the transepidermal osmotic gradient (water concentration gradient) (Cevc and Blume, 1992), with a resultant penetration of epidermis. The transfersomes vesicles penetration through skin and their deformability were represented in different stages by Cevc et al., 1996. Vesicle larger than the narrow pore segment is first pressed against the pore entry, where it fluctuates until it deforms enough to fit into the constriction. Upon complete elongation, it squeezes through the pore surpassing further resistance (Fig. 15.3).

Transfersomes Versus Other Carrier Systems

At a glance, transfersomes appear to be distantly related to lipid bilayers vesicle, liposomes. However, in functional terms, transfersomes differ vastly from commonly used liposomes in that they are much more flexible and adaptable. Extremely high flexibility of their membrane permits transfersomes to squeeze themselves even through pores much smaller than their own diameter. This is due to high flexibility of the transfersomes membrane and is achieved by judicious combination of two lipophilic/amphiphilic components (phospholipids plus biosurfactant) with sufficiently different packing characteristics into a single bilayer. The high resultant deformability permits transfersomes to penetrate the skin spontaneously. This tendency is supported by the

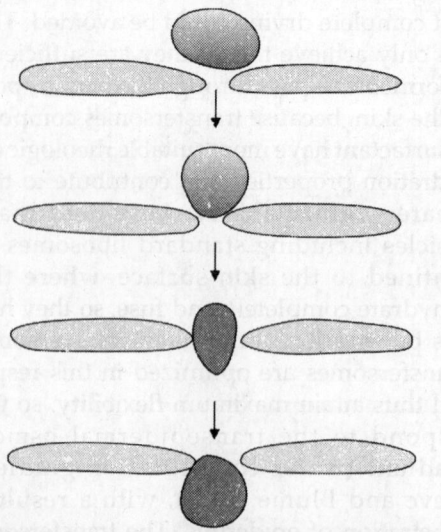

Fig. 15.3: Mechanism of penetration of transfersomes

higher surface hydrophilicity of transferosomes that enforces the search for surrounding hydrous bioenvironment.

It is almost certain that the high penetration potential of the transfersomes is not primarily a consequence of stratum corneum fluidization by the surfactant because micellar suspension contains much more surfactant than transfersomes yet it has shown limited penetration, (PC/sodium cholate 65/35 w/w %, respectively). Thus, if the penetration enhancement via the solubilization of the skin lipids is the reason for the superior penetration capability of transfersomes, one would expect an even better penetration performance of the micelles. In contrast to this postulate, the higher surfactant concentration in the mixed micelles does not improve the efficacy of material transport into or across the skin. On the contrary, mixed micelles stay confined to the upper part of the stratum corneum even they are applied nonocclusively (Chapman et al., 1998). The reason for this is that mixed micelles are much less sensitive to the trans-epidermal water activity gradient than transfersomes. Transfersomes differ in at least two basic features from the mixed micelles, first a transfersome is normally by one to two orders of magnitude greater in size than standard lipid micelles. Secondly and more importantly, each vesicular transfersome contains a water filled core, whereas a micelle is just a simple fatty droplet. Transfersomes thus carry water as well as fat-soluble agent in comparison to micelles that can only incorporate lipoidal substances (Gompper et al., 1995, Wearner et al., 1988).

To differentiate the penetration ability of all these carrier systems, Rand et al., 1989 proposed the distribution profiles of fluorescently labeled mixed lipid micelles, liposomes and transfersomes as measured by the confocal scanning laser microscopy (CSLM) in the intact murine skin. In all these vesicles the highly deformable transfersomes traversed the stratum corneum and entered into the viable epidermis in significant quantity.

Chapman and Walsh (Cevc et al., 1997) also showed that the former two types of aggregates are confined to the outer half of the horny layer, where the cellular packing and intercellular seals are already compromised by the desquamation process. Pure lipid vesicles or micelles seem to have access to the low-resistance pathway only and thus very seldom reach the lower stratum corneum or even get into the viable part of the skin in significant quantities.

Method of Preparation

All the methods of preparation of transfersomes are comprised of two steps. First, a thin film is prepared, hydrated and then brought to the desired size by sonication; and secondly, sonicated vesicles are homogenized by extrusion through a polycarbonate membrane. Figures 15.4 and 15.5 presents a schematic representation of mechanism of formation of transfersomes, for more detailed discussion the reader is suggested to refer to

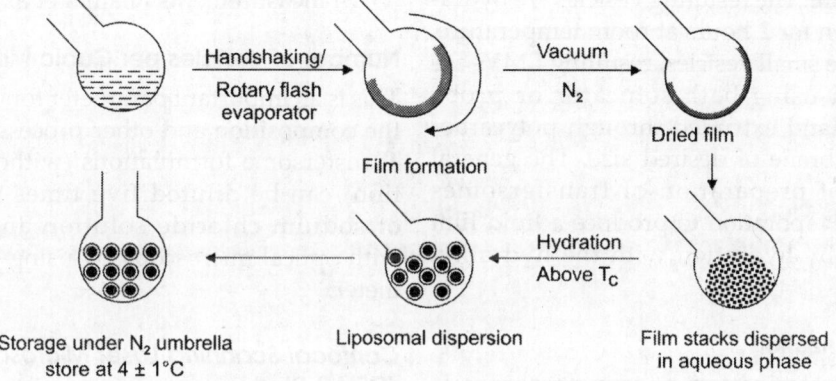

Fig. 15.4: Mechanism of transfersomes formation

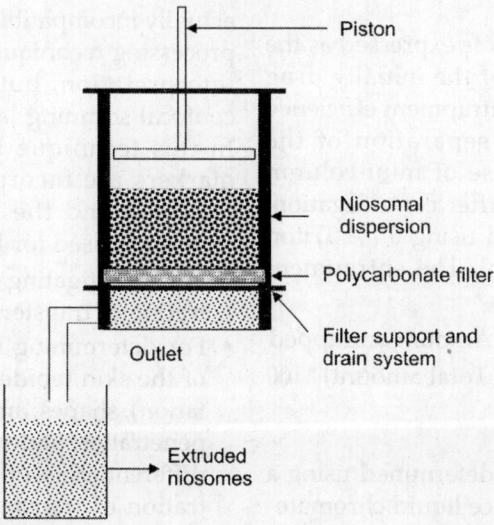

Fig. 15.5: Transfersomes preparation using extrusion technique based on polycarbonate filters

the chapters on liposomes and niosomes. The mixture of vesicles forming ingredients, i.e. phospholipids and surfactant are dissolved in volatile organic solvent, organic solvent is then evaporated above the lipid transition temperature (room temperature for pure PC vesicles, or 50°C for dipalmitoyl phosphatidyl choline) using rotary evaporator. Final traces of solvent are removed under vacuum for overnight. The deposited lipid films are then hydrated with buffer (pH 6.5) by rotation at 60 rpm min^{-1} for 1 hour at the corresponding temperature. The resulting vesicles are hydrated swollen for 2 hours at room temperature. To prepare small vesicles, resulting LMVs are sonicated using bath sonicator or probe sonicated and extruded through polycarbonate membrane of desired size. The general method of preparation of transfersomes involves evaporation to produce a lipid film followed by hydration with the hydration medium.

Characterization

The characterization of transfersomes is generally similar to liposomes, niosomes, and micelles. Transfersomes are generally characterized for following parameters:

Entrapment Efficiency

The entrapment efficiency is expressed as the percentage entrapment of the initially drug added for entrapment. Entrapment efficiency is determined by first separation of the unentrapped drug by use of mini-column centrifugation method. After centrifugation, the vesicles are disrupted using 0.1% Triton X-100 or 50% n-propanol. The entrapment efficiency is calculated as:

Entrapment efficiency = (Amount entrapped / Total amount) *100

Drug Content

The drug content can be determined using a modified high performance liquid chromatography method (HPLC) method using a UV detector, column oven, auto sample, pump, and computerized analysis program.

Vesicle Diameter

Vesicle diameter is generally determined using photon correlation spectroscopy or dynamic light scattering (DLS) method. Samples are prepared in distilled water, filtered through a 0.2 μm membrane filter and diluted with filtered saline and then size is measured by using photon correlation spectroscopy or dynamic light scattering (DLS) measurements (Gamal et al., 1999).

Number of Vesicles per Cubic Millimeter

This is an important parameter for optimizing the composition and other process variables. Transfersome formulations (without sonication) can be diluted five times with 0.9% of sodium chloride solution and studied with optical microscopy by using hemocytometer.

Confocal Scanning Laser Microscopy (CSLM) Study

Conventional light microscopy and electron microscopy both face problem of fixation, sectioning, and staining of the skin samples. Often the structures to be examined are actually incompatible with the corresponding processing techniques; these give rise to mis interpretation, but can be minimized by confocal scanning laser microscopy (CSLM). In this technique lipophilic fluorescence markers are incorporated into the transfersomes and the light emitted by these markers is used for following purpose:

- For investigating the mechanism of penetration of transfersomes across the skin.
- For determining histological organization of the skin (epidermal columns, interdigitation), shapes, and architecture of the skin penetration pathways for comparison and differentiation of the mechanism of penetration of transfersomes with liposomes, niosomes and micelles.

Different fluorescence markers used in CSLM study are:

i. Fluorescein-DHPE [1, 2-dihexadecanoyl-sn-glycero-3-phosphoethanolamine-N-(5-fluorecein-5-thiocarbamoyl denthiocarbamoyl), triethylammonium salt].

ii. Rhodamine-DHPE [1, 2-dihexadecanoyl-sn-glycero-3-phosphoethanolamine triethylammonium salt (Lissamine™ rhodamine B)]

iii. NBD-PE [1,2-dipalmitoyl-sn-glycero-3-phosphoethanolamine-N-(7-nitro-2-1, 3-benzoxadiazol-4-yl)]

iv. Nile red.

Degree of Deformability or Permeability Measurement

In case of transfersomes, the permeability study is one of the important and unique parameter is used for characterization. The deformability study is conducted against the pure water as standard. Transfersomes preparation is passed through a large number of pores of known size (through a sandwich of different microporous filters, with pore diameter between 50 nm and 400 nm, depending on the starting transfersomes suspension). Particle size and size distributions are noted after each pass by dynamic light scattering (DLS) measurements.

Occlusion Effect

Occlusion of skin is considered to be helpful for permeation of drug in case of traditional topical preparations. But the same proves to be detrimental for elastic vesicles. Hydrotaxis (movement in the direction) of water is the major driving force for permeation of vesicles through the skin, from its relatively dry surface to water rich deeper regions. Occlusion affects the hydration forces, as it prevents evaporation of water from skin.

Penetration Ability

Penetration ability of transfersomes can be evaluated using fluorescence microscopy.

In vitro drug release

In vitro drug release study is performed for determining the availability of drug for the permeation. Time needed to attain steady state permeation and the permeation flux at steady state and the information from *in-vitro* studies are used to optimize the formulation before more expensive *in vivo* studies are performed. For determining drug release, transfersomes suspension is incubated at 32°C. The samples are taken at different times and the free drug is separated by mini-column centrifugation (Fry et al., 1978). The amount of drug released

Table 15.1: Different additives used in formulation of transfersomes

Class	Example	Uses
Phospholipids	Soya phosphatidyl choline	Vesicles forming component
	Dipalmitoyl phosphatidyl choline	
	Distearoyl phoshatidyl choline	
Surfactant	Sod. cholate	For providing flexibility
	Sod. deoxycholate	
	Tween-80	
	Span-80	
Alcohal	Ethanol, methanol	As a solvent
Dye	Rhodamine-123	For CSLM study
Rhodamine-DHPE		
Fluorescein-DHPE		
Nile-red		
Buffering agent	Saline phosphate buffer (pH 6.4)	As a hydrating medium

is then calculated indirectly from the amount of drug content at zero times as the initial amount (considering 100% entrapped and 0% released).

Applications

Transferosomes have been widely studied as a carrier for the transport of proteins and peptides. Proteins and peptides are large biogenic molecules, which are difficult to transport into the body, when given orally they are completely degraded in the GI tract. Therefore, these are the reasons why these peptides and proteins are introduced into the body through injections. Various approaches have been developed to improve these situations.

Delivery of Insulin

Very large molecules which cannot diffuse intact across the skin can be transported across the skin with the help of transfersomes. For example, insulin, interferon can be delivered through intact mammalian skin. Delivery of insulin by transfersomes could be the successful means of noninvasive therapeutic use of such large molecular weight, i.e. proteineous compound. Insulin is generally administered by subcutaneous route that is inconvenient and also painful. Encapsulation of insulin into transfersomes (transfersulinR) may overcome the problems of inconvenience.

Carrier for Interferons and Interleukin

Transfersomes have also been studied as a carrier for interferons like leukocytic derived interferon-gamma is a naturally occurring protein having antiviral, antiproliferative and some immunomodulatory effects.

Transfersomes as drug delivery systems have the potential for providing controlled release of the administred drug and increasing the stability of labile drugs. List of drugs used for transfersomes is shown in Table 15.2. Hafer et al. studied the formulations of interleukin-2 and interferon-gamma containing transfersomes for potential transdermal application. They reported delivery of IL-2 and INF-gamma entrapped in transfersomes in concentration sufficient for immunotherapy.

Carrier for Other Proteins and Peptides

Transfersomes have been widely used as a carrier for the transport of other proteins and peptides. Various approaches have been developed to improve these situations. The bioavaibility obtained from transfersomes is somewhat comparable to that resulting from subcutaneous injection of the same protein suspension. Human serum albumin or gap junction proteins were found to be effective in producing the immune response, when delivered by transdermal route encapsulated in transfersomes. Transport of certain drug molecules that have physicochemical channels, which otherwise prevent them from diffusing across stratum corneum, can be successfully transported.

Peripheral Drug Targeting

The ability of transfersomes to target peripheral subcutaneous tissues is due to minimum carrier-associated drug clearance through blood vessels in the subcutaneous tissue. These blood vessels are nonfenestrated and also possess tight junctions between endothelial cells, thus do not allow vesicles to enter directly into the blood stream. This automatically increases drug concentration locally along with the probability of drug to enter peripheral tissues.

Transdermal Immunization

Since ultradeformable vesicles have the capability of delivering the large molecules, they can be used to deliver vaccines topically. Transfersomes containing proteins like integral membrane protein, human serum albumin, gap junction protein are used for this purpose. Advantages of this approach are injecting the protein, can be avoided and higher IgA levels are attained. Transcutaneous hepatitis-B vaccine has given encouraging results. A 12 times higher AUC was obtained for zidovudine as compared to normal control administration. Selective accumulation in RES (which is the usual site for residence of HIV) was also increased.

Delivery of NSAIDS

NSAIDS are associated with number of GI side effects. These can be overcome by their transdermal delivery using ultradeformable vesicles. Studies have been carried out on diclofenac and ketotifen. Ketoprofen in a transfersome formulation gained marketing approval by the Swiss regulatory agency (SwissMedic) in 2007; the product is expected to be marketed under the trademark Diractin. Further therapeutic products based on the transfersome technology, according to IDEA AG, are in clinical development.

Delivery of Steroidal Hormones and Peptides

Transfersomes have also been used for the delivery of corticosteroids. Transfersomes improve the site specificity and overall drug safety of corticosteroid delivery into skin by optimizing the epicutaneously administered drug dose. Transfersomes containing cortiosteroids are biologically active at dose several times lower than the currently used formulation for the treatment of skin diseases. Flexible vesicles of ethinylestradiol showed significant antiovulatory effects as compared to plain drug given orally and traditional liposomes given topically. Extensive work has been carried out on other drugs including hormones and peptides, viz. estradiol, low molecular-weight heparin, retinol, melatonin, etc.

Delivery of Anesthetics

Transfersome based formulations of local anesthetics-lidocaine and tetracaine showed permeation equivalent to subcutaneous injections. Maximum resulting pain insensitivity is nearly as strong (80%) as of a subcutaneous bolus injection, moreover the effect of transferosomal anesthetics last for longer.

Delivery of Anticancer Drugs

Anticancer drugs like methotrexate 5-fluorouracil were tried for transdermal delivery using transfersome technology. The results were favorable. This provided a new lead for treatment especially, skin cancer.

Delivery of Herbal Drugs

Transfersomes can penetrate through stratum corneum and subsequently can supply the nutrients locally to maintain skin functions. Transfersomes of capsaicin have been prepared by Xiao-Ying et al. which showed the better topical absorption in comparison to pure capsaicin.

ETHOSOMES

Ethosomes are essentially lipid based vesicles containing phospholipids, alcohol (ethanol and isopropylalcohol) in relatively high concentration and water. Ethosomes are slightly modified liposomes. Ethosomes are soft vesicles made of phospholipids and ethanol (in higher quantity) and water. The size range of ethosomes may vary from tens of nanometers to microns. Ethosomes permeate through the skin layers more rapidly and possess significantly higher transdermal flux in comparison to conventional liposomes. Although, the exact mechanism of permeation and accmulation of drug into deeper skin layers using ethosomes is still not clear. The synergistic effects of combination of phospholipids and high concentration of ethanol in vesicular formulations have been suggested to be responsible for deeper penetration followed by lipid exchange with the skin lipid bilyers. The high concentration of ethanol makes ethosomes unique in character. The ethanol in ethosomes causes disturbance of skin lipid bilayer organization, when incorporated into a vesicle membrane, it enhances the activity of vesicles to penetrate the stratum corneum. Also, because of their high ethanol concentration, the lipid membrane is packed less tightly than conventional vesicles, but has equivalent stability, allowing a more malleable structure with improved drug distribution ability.

- Ethosomes are mainly used for the delivery of drugs through transdermal route. Unlike classic liposomes that are known mainly to deliver drugs to the outer layers of skin, ethosomes can enhance permeation through the stratum corneum barrier. Ethosomes can entrap drug molecule with various physicochemical characteristics, i.e. of hydrophilic, lipophilic, or amphiphilic. Enhanced permeation of ethosomal drug through skin has been recorded.
- Delivery of large molecules (peptides, protein molecules) is possible.
- It contains nontoxic raw material in formulation.
- High patient compliance—the ethosomal drug is administrated in semisolid form (gel or cream) hence ensures high patient compliance.
- Ethosomal transdermal drug delivery is noninvasive and delivers the drug to the deep skin layers and subsequentlly to the systemic circulation. They are composed mainly of phospholipids, (phosphatidyl choline, phosphatidylserine, phosphatidic acid), high concentration of ethanol and water. Some of the advantages of ethosomes over other vesicular systems are:

- The ethosomal system is passive, non-invasive and is available for immediate commercialization.
- Ethosomal drug delivery system, can be applied widely in pharmaceutical, veterinary, cosmetic fields.
- Simple method for drug delivery in comparison to iontophoresis and phonophoresis and other complicated methods.

Mechanism of Drug Penetration

The main advantage of ethosomes over liposomes is an enhanced trans-skin permeation of the drug. The mechanism of the drug absorption from ethosomes is not clear. The drug absorption probably occurs in following two phases:

1. **Ethanol effect:** Ethanol acts as a penetration enhancer through the skin. The mechanism of its penetration enhancing effect is well known. Ethanol penetrates into intercellular

Table 15.2: List of drugs used for transfersomes

Drugs	Inference
Norgesterol, tamoxifen, oestradiol	Improved transdermal flux
Topical analgesic and anesthetic agent (Tetracaine, lignocain)	Suitable means for the non invasive treatment of local pain on direct topical drug application.
Corticosteroids	Improved site specificity and overall drug safety.
Hydrocortosone	Biologically active at dose several times lower than currently used formulation.
Triamcinolone acetonide	Used for both local and systemic delivery.
Soluble proteins	Permits noninvasive immunization through normal skin.
Human serum albumin	Antibody titer is similar or even slightly higher
Integralmembrane protein	than subcutaneous injection.
Interferon-α	Efficient delivery means (because delivery other route is
Interleukin-2	difficult). Controlled release. Overcome stability problem.
Insulin	High encapsulation efficiency. Transfer across the skin with an efficiency of >50%. Provide noninvasive means of therapeutic use.
Capsaicin, colchicine	Increase skin penetration
Vincristine	Increase entrapment efficiency and skin permeation

lipids and increases the fluidity of cell membrane through lipids solublization and decrease the density of lipid multilayer of cell membrane. Furthermore, due to high ethanol concentrations ethosomal lipid membrane tends to be packed less tightly than conventional vesicles; however, it possesses an equivalent stability. This allowed a softer and malleable structure giving more freedom and stability to the membrane, which could squeeze through small openings created in the disturbed lipids.

2. **Ethosomes effect:** Increased cell membrane lipid fluidity caused by the effect of ethanol of ethosomes results into an increased skin permeability. Thus the ethosomes permeate easily through the deep skin layers, where it is fused with skin lipids and releases the drugs into deep layer of skin.

Composition

The ethosomes are vesicular carriers comprised of hydroalcoholic or hydro/alcoholic/glycolic phospholipid in which the concentration of alcohols or their combination is relatively high. Typically, ethosomes may contain phospholipids with various chemical structures like phosphatidylcholine (PC), hydrogenated PC, phosphatidic acid (PA), phosphatidylserine (PS), phosphatidylethanolamine (PE), phosphatidylglycerol (PPG), phosphatidylinositol (PI), hydrogenated PC, alcohol (ethanol or isopropyl alcohol), water and propylene glycol (or other glycols). Such a composition enables delivery of high concentration of active ingredients through skin. Drug delivery can be modulated by altering alcohol-water or alcohol-polyol-water ratio. Some preferred phospholipids are soya phospholipids, such as phospholipon 90 (PL-90). It is usually employed in a range of 0.5–10% w/w. Cholesterol at concentrations ranging between 0.1–1% can also be added to the preparation. The alcohols, which can be used, include ethanol and isopropyl alcohol, propylene glycol and transcutol. In addition, nonionic surfactants (PEG-alkyl ethers) can be combined with the phospholipids in these preparations. Cationic lipids like cocoamide, POE alkyl amines, dodecylamine, cetrimide etc. can be added too. The concentration of alcohol in the final product may range from 20–50%. The concentration of the nonaqueous phase methods commonly being used for the formulation of ethosomes. (alcohol and glycol combination) may range between 22 and 70% (Table 15.3).

Method of Preparation

The methods used for the preparation of ethosomes are very simple and convenient and do not involve any sophiscated techniques or instrumentation. There are two methods commonly being used for the formulation of ethosomes.

Table 15.3: Different additives employed in formulation of ethosomes

Class	Example	Uses
Phospholipid	Soya phosphatidyl choline	Vesicles-forming component
	Egg phosphatidyl choline	
	Dipalmityl phosphatidyl choline	
	Distearyl phosphatidyl choline	
Polyglycol	Propylene glycol	As a skin penetration enhancer
	Transcutol RTM	
Alcohol	Ethanol	For providing the softness for vesicle membrane
	Isopropyl alcohol	As a penetration enhancer
Cholesterol	Cholesterol	For providing the stability to vesicle membrane
Vehicle	Carbopol 934	As a gel former

Cold Method

This is the most common method utilized for the preparation of ethosomal formulation. In this method phospholipid, drug and other lipid materials are dissolved in ethanol in a closed vessel at room temperature by applying vigorous stirring. Propylene glycol or other polyols are added under stirring. This mixture is heated to 30°C on a water bath. The water heated to 30°C in a separate vessel is then added to the mixture, which is then stirred for 5 min in a covered vessel. The vesicle size of ethosomal formulation can be reduced to desired extend using sonication or extrusion method. Finally, the formulation is stored under refrigeration.

Hot Method

In this method phospholipid is dispersed in water by heating in a water bath at 40°C until a colloidal solution is obtained. In a separate vessel, ethanol and propylene glycol are mixed and heated to 40°C. Once both the mixtures reach 40°C, the organic phase is added to the aqueous phase. The drug is dissolved in water or ethanol depending on its hydrophilic/hydrophobic properties.

The vesicle size of ethosomal formulation can be reduced to the desired extent using probe sonication or extrusion method.

Characterization

The characterization parameters for ethosomes are similar to that of transferosomes and are already discussed in detail in the previous section of this chapter. Parameters and methods used in their determination are enlisted in Table 15.4.

Applications of Ethosomes

Applications of Delivery of Anti-Parkinsonism Agent

Dayan and Touitou prepared ethosomal formulation of psychoactive drug trihexyphenidyl hydrochloride (THP) and compared its delivery with classical liposomal formulation. THP is a M1 muscarinic receptors antagonist and used in the treatment of Parkinson disease. The results indicated better skin permeation potential of ethosomal-THP formulation and its use for better management of Parkinson disease.

Table 15.4: Methods for the characterization of ethosomal formulation

Parameters	Methods
Vesicle shape (morphology)	Transmission electron microscopy
	Scanning electron microscopy
Entrapment efficiency	Mini-column centrifugation method
	Fluorescence spectrophotometry
Vesicle size and size distribution	Dynamic light-scattering method
Vesicle-skin interaction study	Confocal laser-scanning microscopy
	Fluorescence microscopy
	Transmission electron microscopy
	Eosin-hematoxylin staining
Phospholipid-ethanol interaction	^{31}P NMR differential-scanning calorimeter
Degree of deformability	Extrusion method
Zeta potential	Zeta meter
Turbidity	Nephalometer
In vitro drug release study	Franz's diffusion cell with artificial or biological membrane, dialysis bag diffusion
Drug deposition study	Franz's diffusion cell

Delivery of Antiarthritis Drug

Topical delivery of antiarthritis drug is a better option for its site-specific localized delivery that overcomes the problem associated with conventional oral therapy. Cannabidol (CBD) is a recently developed drug candidate for treating rheumatoid arthritis. Lodzki et al. prepared CBD-ethosomal formulation for transdermal delivery. Results shown significantly increased biological anti-inflammatory activity of CBD-ethosomal formulation, when tested using carrageenan induced rat paw edema model. It was concluded that encapsulation of CBD in ethosomes significantly increased its skin permeation, accumulation and hence its biological activity.

Delivery of Antiviral Drugs

Zidovudine is a potent antiviral agent acting on acquired immunodeficiency virus. Oral administration of zidovudine is associated with strong side effects. Therefore, an adequate zero order delivery of zidovudine is desired to maintain its expected effect. Jain et al. concluded that ethosomes could increase the transdermal flux, prolong the release and present an attractive route for sustained delivery of zidovudine (Tables 15.5 and 15.6)

Table 15.5: Examples of ethosomes as a drug carrier

Drug	Purpose of ethosomal delivery	Application
Azelaic acid	Improves the sustained release	Treatment of acne
Diclofenac	Selective targeting of the cells	NSAIDS
Testosterone topical formulation	Low oral bioavailability, dose-dependent side effects	Steroidal hormone
Trihexyphenidyl hydrochloride	4.5-times higher than that from liposome	Treatment of Parkinson disease
Zidovudine and lamivudine	Better cellular uptake	Anti-HIV
Bacitracin	Better cellular uptake	Antibacterial
Erythromycin	Better cellular uptake	Antimicrobial
DNA	Expression into skin cells	Treatment of genetic disorders
Acyclovir	To overcome poor skin permeation	Treatment of herpes labialis
Insulin	Noninvasive delivery as it suffers GIT degradation	Treatment of diabetes
Cyclosporin	GIT degradation Poor oral	Treatment of inflammatory skin disease
Ammonium glycyrrhizinate	Poor skin permeation and poor oral bioavailability	Treatment of inflammatory-based skin diseases
Salbutamol	Enhanced drug delivery through skin with ethosomes	Antiasthmatic
Minoxidil	Pilocebaceous targeting Accumulation in skin increased	Treatment of baldness
Proteins and peptides	Large molecules; has limited skin permeation, to enhance skin permeation	Overcoming the problems associated with oral delivery
Enalapril maleate	Low oral bioavailability	Treatment of hypertension
Cannabidol	Major side effects in oral delivery low bioavailability • first pass metabolism • GIT degradation • Encapsulation of CBD in ethosomes significantly increased its skin permeation, accumulation and hence its biological activity.	Treatment of rheumatoid arthiritis

Table 15.6: Commercial products based on ethosomal technique

Name of the product	Uses	Manufacturer
Nanominox	First minoxidil containing product which uses ethosomes. Containing 4% minoxidil, well known hair growth promoter, that must be metabolided by sulfation to the active compound.	Sinera, Germany
Supravir cream	For the treatment of herpes virus, formulation of acyclovir drug has a long shelflife with no stability problems, stable for at least 3 years, at 25°C. Skin permeation experiments showed that the cream retained its initial penetration enhancing properties even after 3 years.	Trima, Israel
Cellulite EF	Topical cellulite cream, contains a powerful combination of ingredients to increase metabolism and breakdown of fat.	Hampden Health, USA
Decorin cream	Antiaging cream, treating, repairing, and delaying the visible aging signs of the skin including wrinkle lines, sagging, age spots, loss of elasticity, and hyperpigmentation	Genome Cosmetics, Pennsylvania, U.S.
Noicellex	Topical anticellulite cream	Novel Therapeutic Technologies, Israel
Skin genuity	Powerful cellulite buster, reduces orange peel	Physonics, Nottingham, UK

shows some marketed products available in the market. Acyclovir is another antiviral drug that is widely used topically for treatment of herpes labialis. The conventional marketed acyclovir external formulation is associated with poor skin penetration of hydrophilic acyclovir to dermal layer resulting in weak therapeutic efficiency. It is reported that the replication of virus takes place at the basal dermis. To overcome this problem associated with conventional topical preparation of acyclovir, Horwitz et al. formulated acyclovir ethosomal formulation for dermal delivery. The results showed faster healing time and higher percentage of abortive lesions was observed, when acyclovir applied loaded into ethosomes.

Transcellular Delivery

Touitou et al. in their study demonstrated better intracellular uptake of bacitracin, DNA and erythromycin as using CLSM and FACS techniques in different cell lines. Better cellular uptake of anti-HIV drug zidovudine and lamivudine in MT-2 cell line from ethosomes

as compared to the marketed formulation suggested ethosomes to be an attractive clinical alternative for anti-HIV therapy.

Pilosebaceous Targeting

Hair follicles and sebaceous glands are increasingly recognized as significant elements in the percutaneous drug delivery. Touitou et al. compared the skin permeation potential of testosterone delivered in ethosomes exploiting the follicles as transport shunts for systemic drug delivery.

Transdermal Delivery of Hormones

Oral administration of hormones is associated with problems like high first pass metabolism, low oral bioavailability and several dose-dependent side effects. The risk of failure of treatment is known to increase with each missed pill. Skin permeation potential of Testosome across rabbit pinna skin with marketed transdermal patch of testosterone (Testoderm® patch, ALZA). They observed nearly 30-times higher skin permeation of testosterone from ethosomal formulation as compared to marketed formulation.

Topical Delivery of DNA

Many environmental pathogens attempt to enter the body through the skin. Skin therefore, has evolved into an excellent protective barrier, which is also immunologically active and able to express the gene. On the basis of above facts, another important application of ethosomes is to use them for topical delivery of DNA molecules to express genes in skin cells. Touitou et al. in their study encapsulated the GFP-CMV-driven transfecting construct into ethosomal formulation. They applied this formulation to the dorsal skin of 5-week old male CD-1 nude mice for 48 hours. After 48 hours, treated skin was removed and penetration DNA corresponding to green fluorescent protein (GFP) formulation was observed by CLSM. It was observed that topically applied ethosomes-GFP-CMV-driven transfecting construct enabled efficient delivery and expression of genes in skin cells. It was suggested that ethosomes could be used as carriers for gene therapy applications that require transient expression of genes. These results also showed the possibility of using ethosomes for effective transdermal immunization. Gupta et al. recently reported immunization potential using transfersomal formulation. Hence, better skin permeation ability of ethosomes opens the possibility of using these dosage forms for delivery of antigens.

Delivery of Problematic Drug Molecules

The oral delivery of large biogenic molecules such as peptides or proteins is difficult because they are completely degraded in the GI tract. Noninvasive delivery of proteins is a better option for overcoming the problems associated with oral delivery. Dkeidek and Touitou investigated the effect of ethosomal insulin delivery in lowering blood glucose levels (BGL) *in vivo* in normal and diabetic SDI rats. In this study, a Hill Top patch containing insulin ethosomes was applied on the abdominal area of an overnight fasted rat. The results showed that insulin delivered from this patch produced a significant decrease (up to 60%) in blood glucose levels in both normal and diabetic rat; while insulin application from a controlled release formulation was unable to reduce the blood glucose levels.

Delivery of Antibiotics

Topical delivery of antibiotics using ethosomes could be a better choice for increasing the therapeutic efficacy of these agents. The ethosomes essentially deliver an appreciable fraction of drugs into the deeper layer of skin and supress deep rooted infections. With this aim in mind Godin and Touitou prepared bacitracin and erythromycin-loaded ethosomal formulations for dermal and intracellular delivery. The results of this study showed that the ethosomal formulation of antibiotic was highly efficient and could overcome the problems associated with conventional therapy.

SUGGESTED READINGS

1. Ainbinder D, Paolino D, Fresta M, Touitou E, (2010), *J. Biomed. Nanotechnol.*, 6(5), 558–68.
2. Ainbinder D, Touitou, E (2005), *Drug. Deliv.*, 12(5), 297–303.
3. Akhtar N, Pathak, K (2012), *AAPS Pharm Sci Tech*, 13(1), 344–55.
4. Barupal AK, Gupta V, Ramteke S (2010), *Ind. J. Pharm Sci.*, 72(5), 582–6.
5. Bhalaria MK, Naik S, Misra AN (2009), *Indian J. Exp Biol* 47(5), 368–75.
6. Celia C, Cilurzo F, Trapasso E, Cosco D, Fresta, M, Paolino, D Biomed (2012) *Microdevices*, 14(1), 119–30.
7. Celia C, Trapasso E, Cosco D, Paolino D, Fresta M, (2009) *Colloids Surf B Biointerfaces*, 72(1), 155–60.
8. Chen JG, Liu, YF, Gao TW, *J. Liposome Res* 2010 Dec; 20(4): 297–303 Epub 2010 Jan. 27.
9. AN Ravani, L Esposito, EJ (2010), *Liposome Res* 20(4), 277–85.
10. Cortesi R, Ravani L, Zaid, AN, Menegatti, E, Romagnoli, R, Drechsler, M, Esposito, E (2010), *Pharmazie*, 65(10), 743–9
11. Dayan N Touitou, E (2000), *Biomaterials* 21(18), 1879–85.

12. Dubey V, Mishra D, Dutta T, Nahar M, Saraf D K, Jain NK (2007), *J Control Release*, 123(2), 148–54.

13. Dubey V, Mishra D, Jain NK (2007), *Eur. J. Pharm. Biopharm.*, 67(2), 398–405.

14. Elsayed MM, Abdallah OY, Naggar, VF, Khalafallah NM, (2007) *Pharmazie*, 62(2), 133–7.

15. Elsayed MM, Abdallah OY, Naggar VF, Khalafallah NM, (2006) *Int. J. Pharm.*, 322 (1–2), 60–6.

16. Esposito E, Menegatti E, Cortesi R (2004), *J. Cosmet. Sci.*, 55(3), 253–64.

17. Fang YP, Huang YB, Wu PC, Tsai YH (2009), *Eur. J. Pharm. Biopharm*, 73(3), 391–8.

18. Fang YP, Tsai YH, Wu PC, Huang YB, *Int. J. Pharm.* (2008), May 22; 356 (1–2): 144–52.

19. Fireman S, Toledano O, Neimann K, Loboda N, Dayan, N (2011), *Dermatol. Ther.*, 24(5), 477–88.

20. Godin B, Touitou E (2003), *Crit Rev Ther Drug Carrier Syst*, 20(1), 63–102.

21. Godin B, Touitou E (2004), *J. Contr. Rel.*, 94 (2–3), 365–79.

22. Jain, S , Tiwary, A K , Sapra, B , Jain, N K (2007) AAPS Pharm Sci Tech 21, 8(4), E111.

23. Liu X, Liu H, Liu J, He Z, Ding C, Huang G, Zhou, W, Zhou, L Int J (2011) *Nanomedicine*, 6, 241–7.

24. Madsen JT, Vogel S, Karlberg, AT, Simonsson C, Johansen JD, Andersen KE (2010), *Acta Derm Venereol*, 90(4), 374–8.

25. Madsen JT, Vogel S, Johansen JD, Andersen, KE (2011), *Cutan. Ocul. Toxicol.*, 30(2), 116–23.

26. Madsen JT, Vogel S, Johansen JD, Sørensen JA , Andersen KE, Nielsen JB (2011), *Cutan. Ocul. Toxicol.*, 30(1), 38–44.

27. Madsen JT, Vogel S, Karlberg AT, Simonsson C, Johansen JD, Andersen KE (2010), *Contact Dermatitis*, 63(4), 209–14.

28. Maestrelli F, Capasso G, González-Rodríguez ML, Rabasco AM, Ghelardini C, Mura P (2009), *J. Lipo. Res.* 19(4): 253–60.

29. Mao X, Wo Y, He, R, Qian, Y, Zhang, Y, Cui, D (2010), *J. Nanosci Nanotechnol*, 10(7), 4178–83.

30. Mishra D, Mishra PK, Dabadghao S, Dubey V, Nahar M, Jain NK Nanomedicine 2010; 6(1): 110–8 (2009), 14.

31. Nanda A, Nanda S, Ghilzai NM (2006), *Curr Drug Deliv*, 3(3), 233–42.

32. Nounou MI, El-Khordagui LK, Khalafallah NA, Khalil SA Recent Pat Drug Deliv Formul 2008; 2(1): 9–18.

33. Paolino D, Lucania G , Mardente D, Alhaique F, Fresta M (2005), *J Control Release*, 106 (1–2), 99–110.

34. Rajan R, Jose S, Mukund VP, Vasudevan DT (2011), *J Adv Pharm Technol Res*; 2(3): 138–43.

35. Rajera R, Nagpal K, Singh SK, Mishra DN (2011), *Biol Pharm Bull*, 34(7), 945–53.

36. Rao Y, Zheng F, Zhang X, Gao J, Liang W, *AAPS Pharm. Sci. Tech* 2008; 9(3): 860–5.

37. Song YK, Hyun SY, Kim HT, Kim CK, Oh JM, *J Microencapsul* 2011; 28(3):151–8.

38. Song CK, Balakrishnan P, Shim CK, Chung SJ, Chong S, Kim DD (2012), *Colloids Surf B Bioint*; 92: 299–304.

39. Touitou E, Dayan N, Bergelson L, Godin B , Eliaz M (2000), *J. Control Release*, 65(3), 403–18.

40. Touitou E, Godin B, Dayan N, Weiss C, Piliponsky A, Levi-Schaffer, F (2001), *Biomaterials*, 22(22), 3053–9.

41. Verma P, Pathak K, (2010), *J Adv Pharm Technol Res*, 1(3), 274–82.

42. Wo Y, Zhang Z, Zhang Y, Wang D, Pu, Z , Su, W, Qian, Y, Li, Y, Cui, D (2011), *J. Nanosci Nanotechnol* 11(9), 7840–7.

43. Xing XJ, Yang L, You, Y, Zhong BY, Song, QH , Deng J, Hao F, (2011) *Exp Dermatol*, 20(11), 945–7.

44. Xu DH, Zhang Q, Feng X, Xu X, Liang WQ (2007), *Pharmazie*, 62(4), 316–8.

45. Zhang JP, Wei YH, Zhou Y, Li, YQ, Wu, XA (2012), *Arch Pharm Res*, 35(1), 109–17.

46. Zhaowu Z, Xiaoli W, Yangde Z, Nianfeng L (2009), *J Liposome Res*, 19(2), 155–62.

47. Zhou Y, Wei YH, Zhang GQ, Wu, XA (2010), *Arch Pharm Res*, 33(4), 567–7.

16 ■ Organogels

INTRODUCTION

Gels are considered as materials which are 'easier to recognize than define.' There are various definitions proposed orginal to gels, they include; (1) gel has a continuous structure of macroscopic dimensions that are permanent over the time-span of an experiment and (2) it is soiid-like in its rheological behavior, to the more basic descriptions stating that if it looks like 'Jell-O', it must be a gel. It is now generally accepted that a gel is a semi-solid material composed of low concentrations (~15%) of gelator molecules that, in the presence of an appropriate solvent, self-assembles via physical or chemical interactions into massive mesh network preventing solvent flow as a result of surface tension. A simple working definition of the term 'gel' is a soft, solid or solid-like material, which contains both solid and liquid components, where the solid component (the gelator) is usually present as a mesh/network of aggregates, which immobilizes the liquid component. The solid network prevents the liquid from flowing, primarily via surface tension. The gel is said to be a hydrogel or an organogel depending on the nature of the liquid component, viz. water in hydrogels and an organic solvent in case of organogels. Gels can also be classified according to the bonds present in the gelator network; physical gels are held by weaker

physical forces of attraction, such as van der Waals' interactions and hydrogen bonds, whereas chemical gels are held by covalent bonds.

Hydrogels (composed of water held by a three-dimensional polymeric network), have been extensively studied as vehicles for a wide range of drugs. They have been fabricated in a variety of different shapes (e.g. rods, disks, films and microparticles), depending on the intended applications and sites of administration. In addition, some thermoresponsive gels can be administered parenterally as a liquid, which forms a gel in situ at body temperature. In contrast to hydrogels, research into organogels for drug delivery began fairly recently and interest in physical organogels increased dramatically, with the (often, serendipitous) discovery and synthesis of a very large number of diverse molecules which are able to gel, a range of organic solvents at low concentrations (typically a few weight percent). Examples of gellable organic solvents include aliphatic and aromatic hydrocarbons, alcohols, silicone oil, dimethyl sulfoxide and vegetable oils.

Organogels can be distinguished from hydrogels by their predominantly organic continuous phase and can then be further subdivided based on the nature of the gelling molecule—polymeric or low molecular weight

(LMW) organogelators. Polymers immobilize the organic solvent by forming a network of either cross-linked or entangled chains for chemical and physical gels, respectively. The latter is possibly further stabilized by weak inter-chain interactions, such as hydrogen bonding, van der Waals' forces, and π-π stacking. Likewise, the self-assembly of LMW organogelators depends on physical interactions for the formation of aggregates sufficiently long to overlap and induce solvent gelation. Depending on the kinetic properties of aggregates, an important distinction amongst LMW organogels is made between those which are composed of solid (or strong) versus fluid (or weak) fiber networks.

ORGANOGELATORS

Despite the numerous trends in gelling processes, as well as the impressive variety of gelators identified, it remains difficult to predict the molecular structure of a potential gelator, as well as one cannot readily foresee preferentially-gelled solvents. Today still, the discovery of gelators remains serendipitous and is usually followed by investigative screening of different solvent systems potentially compatible with gelation. Prediction of gelation potential of a given molecule might seem possible by investigation of its propensity towards chemical or physical intermolecular interactions, however no generalizations are so far possible. Many factors such as steric effects, rigidity, and polarity can counter the aggregating tendency of molecules. Control over the gelation process as well as the conception of new gelling molecules are important challenges remain to be faced in the quest of new organogelators.

The simplest organogelators are n-alkanes (C = 24, 28, 32, 36), which gel other relatively short chain n-alkanes, such as hexadecane and other organic liquids. Other examples of organogelators include substituted fatty acids (e.g. 12-hydroxyoctadecanoic acid); 1,3:2,4-di-O-benzylidene-d-sorbitol (D-DBS); sorbitan

monostearate, a nonionic surfactant; steroids and their derivatives; anthryl derivatives (e.g. 2,3-bis-n-decyloxyanthracene); macrocyclic gelators (e.g. calixarenes); ALS compounds (an aromatic moiety attached to a steroidal group by a linker segment); cyclodipeptides; bisurea compounds; bisamides; bolaform amides derived from amino acids; n-alkyl perfluoroalkanamides; carbohydrate derivatives; perfluoroalkanes, which gel liquid carbon dioxide, a mixture of highly reactive methyl 2,6-di-isocyanatohexanoate and alkylamines in an organic solvent, which react when mixed to form a product that gels the organic solvent; primary alkyl amines, which gel organic solvents following the uptake of CO_2, NO_2, SO_2 or CS_2; the light-responsive gelators, which produce gels, whose sol-to-gel transition may be switched by irradiation with UV and visible light; oxadiazole-based benzene 1,3,5-tricarboxamide, a nonfluorescent gelator, which produces highly fluorescent organogel; cobalt(II) triazole complexes, which, unlike most organogels, form gels at high temperatures and solutions at low tempratures; and fatty acid derivative of L-alanine, which selectively gels the organic solvent, but not the aqueous phase when added to an oil/water mixture. Certain compounds can only gel organic solvents in the presence of other compounds, e.g. aminopyrimidine and dialkylbarbituric acid gel cyclohexane when present at 1:1 molar mixtures. The chemical structures of some of these gelators are shown in Table 16.1, stating organogelators are diverse in nature and it is not possible, so far, to predict whether a molecule will gel the organic solvents. As mentioned earlier, the ability of many of these compounds to gel organic liquids was discovered by chance. Subsequently, many more compounds related to the organogelators have been synthesized to produce libraries of gelators in an attempt to understand the chemical moieties needed for gelation, and the forces of attraction involved in gelation as well as the mechanisms of gelation.

Table. 16.1: Chemical structure of few organogelators used in drug delivery

Sorbitan monostearate	
2,3-bis-n-decyloxyanthracene	
12-hydroxyoctadecanoic acid	
1,3:2,4-di-O-benzylidene-d-sorbitol	
n-alkane (C=26)	
Lecithin	
N-lauroyl-l-glutamic acid di-n-butylamide	
Poly(ethylene)	
Sorbitan monostearate (SMS) or molaureate	$R = (CH_2)_{16} CH_3$ or $(CH_2)_{10} CH_3$
N-stearoyl-L-alanine methyl or ethyl ester	$R = CH_3$ or $CH_2 CH_3$
P(MAA-co-MMA)	
P(MAA-co-MMA) and cPAA	

Gel preparation

Most organogels are prepared by heating a mixture of the gelator and the liquid component to form an organic solution/dispersion, followed by cooling of the latter, which sets into a gel (Fig. 16.1). Heating allows dissolution of the gelator in the liquid, whereas following cooling, the solubility of the gelator in the liquid phase decreases, and gelator-solvent interactions are reduced, which results in the gelator molecules 'coming out' of solution. Gelator-gelator interactions lead to gelator self assembly into well-defined aggregates, such as tubules, rods and fibres. Entanglement of the aggregates and connections among them, result in the formation of a three-dimensional network, which immobilizes the fluid phase, (i.e. a gel is formed). The three-dimensional network acts as the gel skeleton and confers strength and resilience to the gel. Interconnections among gelator aggregates are important for gel formation; in their absence, the gel state may be lost even if numerous gelator aggregates are present.

The physical organogels, held together by noncovalent forces, are thermoreversible, i.e. following heating, the gel melts to the sol phase as the gelator aggregates dissolve in the organic liquid, whereas on cooling the hot sol phase results in gelation.

One can appreciate the requirement for gelator solubility in the liquid at high temperature, but insolubility at lower temperatures, for gelation. The temperature at which the sol-to-gel or gel-to-sol transition occurs is called the gelation temperature (T_g). The latter is usually broad, over a few degrees Celcius, as a number of events occur at the transition, e.g. the breakup of the connections between gelator aggregates and the dissolution of individual aggregates. Different methods have been used to measure T_g, e.g. differential-scanning calorimetry, rheological measurements, melting point apparatus, hot-stage light microscopy (when gelator aggregates are large enough to be visible with light microscopy) and 'falling drop' method. These methods often give slightly different

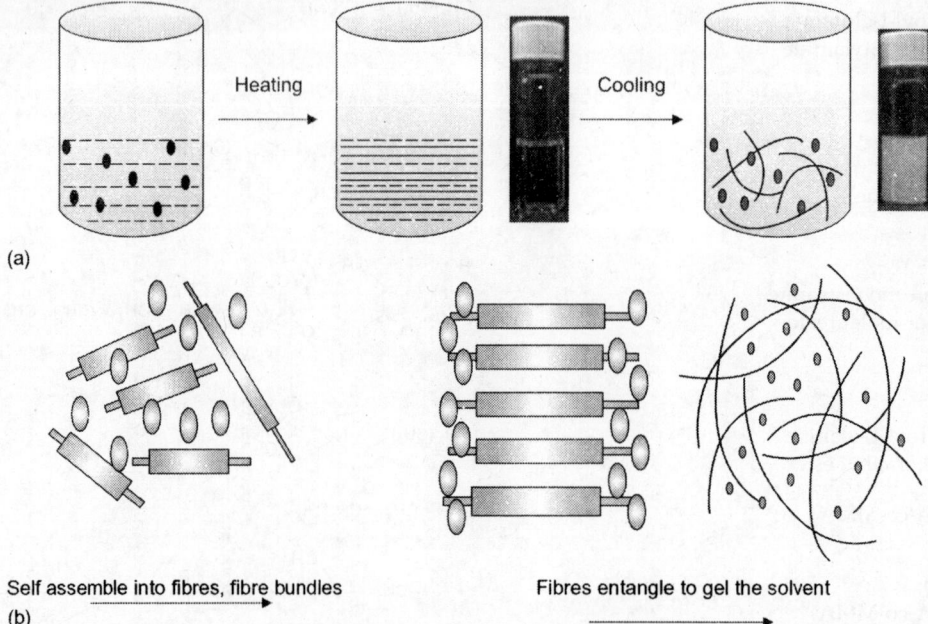

(a)

Self assemble into fibres, fibre bundles

(b)

Fig. 16.1: (a) Method of preparation of organogel, (b) Organogel where gelator self assemble as fibres

values for T_g because different events are monitored. For example, when the melting point apparatus or 'falling drop' method is used, the temperature at which the gel flows is measured; gelator aggregates and aggregate-aggregate interactions may still exist. In contrast, when the hot-stage light microscopy is used, the operator may record the temperature at which all the gelator aggregates have disappeared. In addition, the T_g found by heating the gel to the sol phase or cooling the sol to the gel state differ slightly. The gel T_g is usually lower than the melting point of the gelator, e.g. the T_g of a 10% weight-to-volume (w/v) sorbitan monostearate/hexadecane gel was found to be 41–44°C, compared with melting point 51°C recorded for sorbitan monostearate.

In contrast to the gel preparation described above, a number of organogels are prepared by the addition of a third component to an organic solution (Fig. 16.2), e.g. an organic solution of bis-(2-ethylhexyl) sodium sulfosuccinate (AOT) can be gelled by the addition of phenolic species. Solutions of lecithin in an organic solvent, such as iso-octane can be gelled by the addition of trace amounts of a polar substance, e.g. water, glycerol, ethylene glycol or formamide. Complex organogels have also been pre-pared by the gelation of water-in-oil (W/O) micro-emulsion using gelatin, a hydrogelator. A simple visual test to determine whether gelation has taken place involves inverting the reaction vessel; gelation is said to have occurred, if the sample does not flow. Rheological measurements provide a more objective diagnosis of gelation. The gels formed can be characterized in terms of the concentration of gelator required to immobilize the liquid, the rheology of gel, lifetime (the period of time that gels can remain intact when stored in sealed containers at room temperature) and its micro- and ultra-structures. The manner in which the gelator molecules are self-assembled into aggregates and the aggregate-aggregate interactions are especially interesting. A variety of techniques have been used to elucidate the nature of gelator self-assemblies.

Gelator Self-assembly

A variety of gelator aggregates, such as platelets, tubules, fibres, rods, worm-like chains, ribbons and fan-like structures have been reported. Aggregate thickness ranges from a fraction of a nanometre (e.g. when an aggregate consists of one gelator molecule per cross-section area) to microns; although, the diameter along the length of fibres seems to be fairly uniform, which may reflect unidimensional aggregate growth.

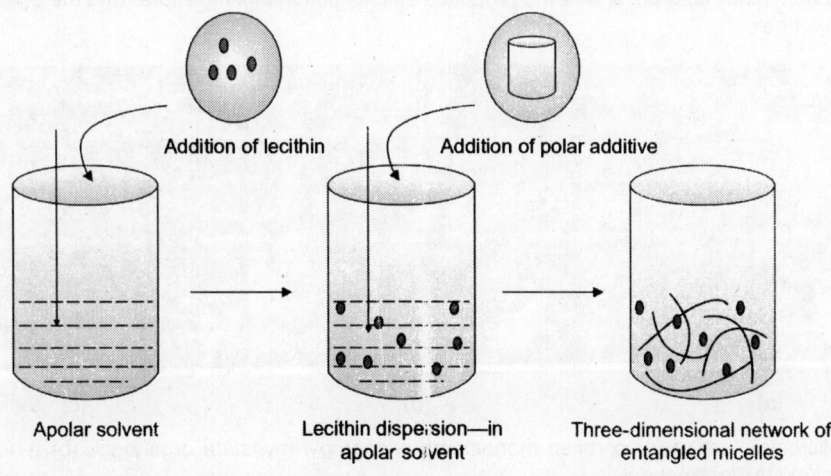

Fig. 16.2: Method of preparation of organogel by addition of third component for gel formation

The manner in which gelator molecules self-assemble and the nature of the gelator aggregate depends to a large extent on the gelator, whose component groups dictate the forces of interactions involved in gelator self-assembly. For example, molecules of the non-ionic surfactant sorbitan monostearate are thought to assemble into bilayers, which are then organized into tubules (Fig. 16.3). A bilayer arrangement is indicated from freeze-fracture microscopy and X-ray diffraction studies. AOT/phenol gelator assemblies are consisted of stacks of phenol molecules, stabilized by π–π interactions between pre-formed tubules joining at a central point rather they grew as an independent and discrete entity. The action of polysorbate 20 was solvent-specific; that is in short chain alkane (C <14) gels, inclusion of polysorbate 20 decreases the solubility of the gelator in the liquid and the stability of the resulting gel. Figure 16.4 illustrates microstructures of gels with different organogelators.

The cooling rate of the sol phase also influences gelation, e.g. alkane-in-alkane gels were prepared by cooling the sol phases under a stream of cold water, as slower cooling produced gels which were less stable. The dimensions of the container, where gelation proceeds also have an impact on the gel network. Furman and Weiss reported that if the size of the container was smaller

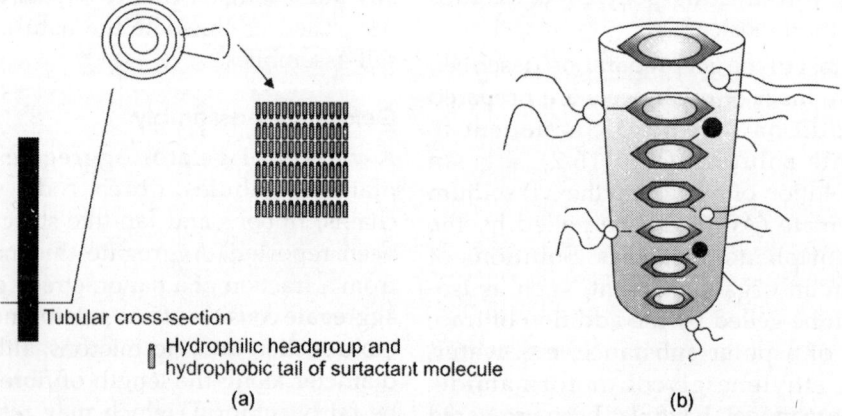

Tubular cross-section

Hydrophilic headgroup and hydrophobic tail of surtactant molecule

(a)

(b)

Fig. 16.3: (a) Schematic diagram shows the possible arrangement of bilayers within sorbitan monostearate tubules. (b) Schematic diagram shows the proposed stacking of phenol molecules and the position of AOT in AOT/phenol gels

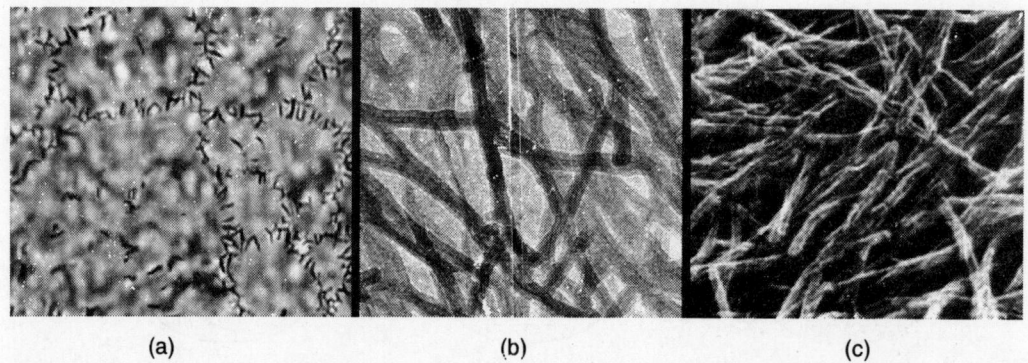

(a)

(b)

(c)

Fig. 16.4: Microstructure of (a) sorbitan monostearate/isopropyl myristate organogel, (b) d-homosteroidal nitroxide gel, (c) CAB/octanol gel

than the mesh size of a particular gel network, gelation was either inhibited or a different type of gel network (mesh) is formed.

PROPERTIES OF ORGANOGELATORS

Viscoelasticity

Viscoelasticity is a term, which is associated with the materials having both viscous and elastic properties. The organogels seem to follow Maxwell model of viscoelasticity. As discussed above, organogels are the three-dimensional structures, which are formed due to the physical interactions amongst the gelator molecules. The organogels behave like a solid at lower shear rates and hence show an elastic property. As the shear stress increases, the physical interacting points amongst the fiber structures start getting weakened until the shear stress is high enough to disrupt the interactions amongst the fiber structures, and the organogels starts flowing. This behavior is in accordance with the plastic flow.

The flow property of the organogels can also be understood by monitoring the rheological properties of the gelator solution in apolar solvents during the preparation of the organogels. Let us first take up the case of fluid-fiber containing organogels. It has been observed that, when the trace amounts of water is added to the gelator solution in apolar solvents; there is a subsequent exponential increase in the viscosity, which may be attributed to the formation of rigid structure due to the entanglement of the fluid-fiber structures (tubular reverse micelles).

A typical example includes the formation of organogels in the presence of lecithin, where there is an increase in the viscosity by a factor of 10^4–10^6 (approx.) occurs on the addition of water to the apolar solution of lecithin. In case of solid-fiber containing organogels, the gelators are dissolved in the apolar solvents at a higher temperature. With the subsequent decrease in the temperature, there is an increase in the viscosity of the solution, which can be attributed to the precipitation of

organogelators and subsequent physical interactions amongst the same, resulting in the formation of the organogels.

Nonbirefringence

The organogels, when viewed under polarized light appear as a dark matrix. This can be accounted to the isotropic nature of the organogels, which does not allow the polarized light to pass through the matrix. This property of the organogels not allowing the polarized light to pass through its matrix, is regarded as nonbirefringent.

Thermoreversibility

As the organogels are heated up above a critical temperature, the organogels loss their solid matrix-like structure and start flowing. This has been attributed to the disruption in the physical interactions amongst the gelator molecules due to the increase in the thermal energy within the organogels. However, as the heated organogels systems are subsequently cooled down, the physical interaction amongst the organogelators prevails and the organogels revert back to the more stable configuration.

Thermostability

The organogels are thermostable in nature. The stability of the organogels, may be attributed to the ability of the gelators to undergo self-assembly, under suitable conditions, so as to form organogels. As a gelator undergoes self-assembly, it results in the decrease in the total free energy of the system and thus renders the organogels to be a low-energy thermostable system. Due to the inherent thermostability of the organogels, they have been proposed as a delivery vehicle for bioactive agents and for cosmetic applications, where a longer shelflife is desirable.

Optical Clarity

Depending on the composition of the organogels, the organogels may be transparent or opaque in nature. The lecithin organogels are generally transparent in nature, while the sorbitan monostearate organogels are opaque.

Chirality Effects

Chirality is neither necessary nor sufficient for gelation; however, despite not being a gelling force in itself, chirality seems to be intimately related to the growth and stability of the self-assembled fibrillar networks of LMW physical gels. Although, exact explanation remains yet to be unravelled, a general empirical rule suggests that a molecule has a better chance of being a good gelator if it is chiral. Thermoreversibility of the gels formed due to the formation of the self-assembled solid-fiber network has also been associated with the chirality. In general, it has been found that a good solid-fiber gelator possesses a chiral center, whereas chirality as such does not have any effect on fluid-fiber gelators. The presence of chiral centers within the gelators helps in the formation of a compact molecular packing, which provides a thermodynamic and kinetic stability to the system.

Molecular chirality is most often transferred to the morphology of self-assembled fibers.

Crown ether phthalocyanine organogels, composed of supercoiled helical fibers, are the excellent example of chiral organogels. Initial molecular packing which is driven by π-π stacking between aromatic substituent rings, imparts molecular chirality to individual fibers (Fig. 16.5). The fibres further twist around each other, to maximize van der Waals' interactions, thus forming helical super structures. As opposed to flat aggregates, the contact area between such twisted structures is reduced due to their curvature, which makes them less prone to uncontrolled aggregation and resulting precipitation. This increases the favors of gelation by such chiral molecules.

Biocompatibility- initially, organogels were developed using various nonbiocompatible organogels. Moreover, of late, research on organogels using various biocompatible constituents has opened up new dimensions of their use in various biomedical applications.

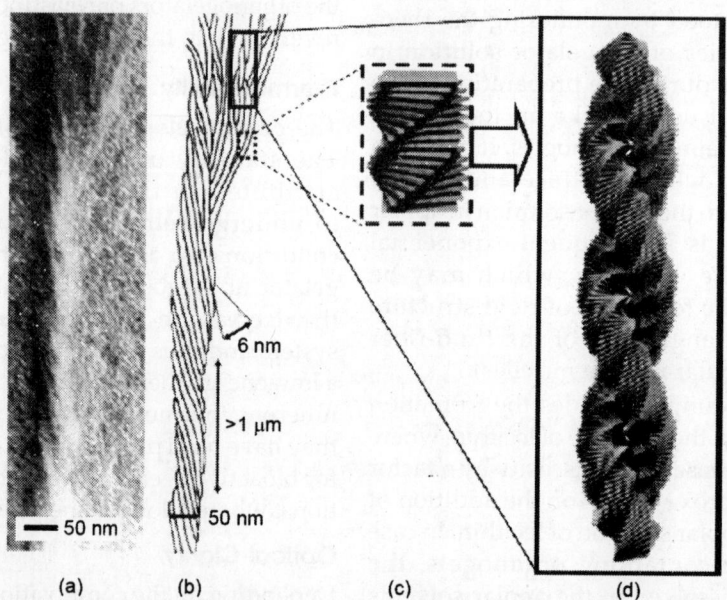

Fig. 16.5: (a) Transmission electron micrograph of organogel of a crown ether phthalocyanine in chloroform, showing a left-handed coil. (b) Schematic representation of helical fibers in (a). (c) The helical aggregates are formed by the stacking of crown ether rings with a staggering angle, constant in magnitude and direction. (d) Supercoiled structure is obtained from side-on aggregation of individual fibers. Reproduced from Engelkamp et al., 1999

LOW MOLECULAR WEIGHT ORGANOGELATORS

Amongst LMW organogels, a subtle but crucial distinction is made between those composed of entangled networks of solid versus fluid fibers. The solid fibers, of which most organogels are composed, are generally produced following a drop in temperature below the gelator's solubility limit. Consequently, a fast partial precipitation of gelator molecules in the organic medium results in the formation of aggregates via co-operative intermolecular interactions. On the other hand, fluid matrices are formed upon the incorporation of polar solvents to organic solutions of surfactants, owing to the reorganization of surfactant molecules into mono- or bilayer cylindrical aggregates that immobilize the solvent. The key distinction between the two systems is the kinetic stability of the networks constituting the gel state. Strong gels are formed of permanent, most often crystalline networks, in which junction points are relatively large (pseudo)crystalline microdomains. Conversely, weak gels are formed of transient networks, characterized by the continuous process of breaking and recombination of the constituent rods, as in the case of reverse cylindrical micelles. Similarly, aggregates undergo dynamic exchange of individual gelator molecules with the bulk liquid. Junction points in these fluid networks are simple chain entanglements, equally transient in nature.

The distinction between solid and fluid fibers is not much emphasized in the literature, although it is of great importance from a physicochemical point of view. Indeed, physical properties of organogels vary with the nature of their networks. Solid matrix gels are more robust, as demonstrated by rheological studies. This may be at least partially due to the fact that, fluid fibers do not aggregate into higher-order structures, whereas solid fibers are generally aligned in bundles as a result of their rigidity, they are likely to contribute robustness to the gel. Similarly, while molecular and supramolecular chirality plays a great role in the formation and stability of solid fibers, its effect is rare in fluid networks (Table 16.2).

Solid-matrix Organogels

Solid-matrix gels are prepared by dissolving the gelator in the heated solvent, at concentrations typically near or below 15%; very low concentrations even less than 0.1% have been reported in the case of sugar-derived 'supergelators'. Upon cooling, the affinity between organogelator and solvent molecules decreases and the former self-assembles into solid aggregates held together by intermolecular physical interactions. The remaining solvent-aggregate affinity stabilizes the system by preventing complete phase separation. Aggregates most often unidimensionally grow into fibers with high aspect (length-to-width) ratios, generally measuring a few tens of nanometers in width and up to several micrometers in length. One such example is of L-alanine fatty acid derivatives which form opaque gels in pharmaceutical oils as a result of hydrogen bonding and van der Waals' interactions. Although less common, examples exist of two-dimensional growth patterns, as in the case of hexatriacontane, a 36-carbon n

Table 16.2: Bioactive agents successfully incorporated within various organogels	
Type of organogels	*Bioactive agents incorporated*
Lecithin organogels	Broxaterol, scopolamine, nicardipine
PLO organogels	Methimazole, dexamethasone
Premium lecithin organogels	Methimazole
MBG organogels	Propranolol hydrochloride, ketorolac tromethamine
Sorbitan organogels	Antigens, sumatriptan, doxorubicin
Poly (ethylene) organogels	Leuprolide

alkane (C36), which reportedly forms micro-platelets arrangements (Fig. 16.6a).

Irrespective of the one- or two-dimensional morphology of aggregates, these structures are frequently crystalline in nature. The crystalline arrangement can be the same in the gel and the plain solid, as in the case of C36 molecules, of which the gel microplatelets arrangements are free of liquid molecules in the inter-lamellar spaces. However, more often, the crystalline packing differs between the gel and the neat solid. Irrespective of the one- or two-dimensional morphology of aggregates, these structures are frequently crystalline in nature. The crystalline arrange-ment can be the same in the gel and the plain solid, as in the case of C36 molecules, of which the gel microplatelets arrangements are free of liquid molecules in the inter-lamellar spaces. However, more often, the crystalline packing differs between the gel and the neat solid.

Macroscopically, organogels range from white opaque to translucent systems, depen-ding on aggregate size and ability of gel to scatter incoming light. Sometimes, a gel system changes upon small variations in composition. While hydrophobic attractions are a major driving force for aggregation in water, the phenomenon is of secondary importance in the case of organogels. In non-aqueous liquids, the attractive forces involved are mainly hydrogen bonding, van der Waals' interactions, p-stacking, and metal-coordina-tion bonds. Because of the strength and high directionality of their hydrogen bonds, numerous emerging organogelators are derivatized peptides, sugars, and bis-urea-based compounds. These are particularly efficient organogelators because of their well defined hydrogen-bonding core that provides a gelling scaffold, which can be functionalized with extended versatility.

Organogels obtained by long n-alkanes (chain length varying from 24 to 36 carbon atoms), are capable of gelling short-chain n-alkanes and a variety of other organic liquids, and have proven to be of particular interest in demonstrating the mechanisms of gelation. They represent not only rare exam-ples in which hydrogen bonding does not play a role in gel formation, but are even more unusual in regard to van der Waals' forces which alone lead to gelation. As a consequence of gelling solely through these weak physical interactions, such gels are not stable over long periods, eventually phases tend to separate due to transitions towards thermodynami-cally-favored packing arrangements. Not surprisingly, it was noted that gel shelflife increased with gelator chain length as a result of involvement of extended van der Waals' interactions, going from under a day to several months for C24 and C36, respectively.

A recent study conducted with a family of 3,5-diaminobenzoate derivatives demon-strated, although not for the first time, the

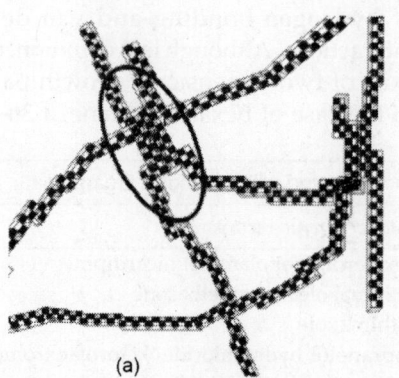

(a)

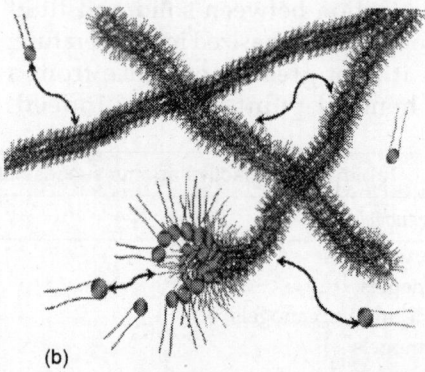

(b)

Fig. 16.6: (a) Solid matrix organogels, (b) fluid matrix organogels. Adapted from Terech and Weiss, 1997

implication and importance of aromatic stacking in the process of gelation. Indeed, increasingly stronger gels were formed upon incorporation of additional aromatic substituents to gelator molecules. Another interesting gelators involving p-p interactions, are cholesterol-derivatized molecules. These can be suitable for the design of functionalized organogelators because of their remarkably high synthetic tunability.

The cholesterol group induces unidirectional self-association, though van der Waals' interactions, while functional groups added onto the cholesterol backbone stabilize the fiber via hydrogen bonding and/or p-interactions. The hydroxyl group at the C3 position of the cholesterol molecule is crucial to gelation, likely due to its participation in hydrogen bonding. Alternatively, ALS compounds are known to form stable organogels. These gelators are prepared by functionalizing the steroidal moiety (S) at the C3 position with anthraquinone (A) via a linker (L) of varying length. The fused aromatic rings of the anthraquinone group stabilize gel fibers through p-stacking.

Overall, it is generally the interplay of different physical interactions that leads to the formation of the gelling matrix. The only constant in the gelation mechanism is the balance needed between the gelator's solubility and insolubility in a given solvent, so as to ensure fiber formation while preventing phase separation.

Fluid Matrix Organogels

Fluid fibers gel in the organic solvents in the same way as solid fibers—aggregate size increases and the eventual entanglement of these structures immobilizes the solvent as a result of surface tension. Just as strong gels, fluid-matrix systems are thermoreversible and can be transparent or opaque. The critical difference arises in the kinetic behavior of the two types of matrices. While solid matrices have a robust and permanent morphology over the entire lifespan of gel, fluid matrices are transient structures under constant continuous dynamic remodeling. Owing to the aggregate fluidity and the transience of junction points, these structures are also referred to as 'worm-like' or 'polymer-like' networks. This section presents two such systems, lecithin and sorbitan monostearate (SMS)/sorbitan monopalmitate organogels, which are of interest in pharmaceutical science.

Poly (ethylene) organogels (PO) are commonly used as ointment bases and are composed of 5% low molecular weight poly (ethylene) in mineral oil (Plastibase®). The polymer is dissolved in the oil at about 130°C and 'shock cooled'. This leads to the partial precipitation of the polymer chains and the formation of a colorless organogel. They are also of common application in pharmaceutics. Some of them are copolymers of methacrylic acid (MAA) and methyl methacrylate (MMA) in 1:1 (Eudragit L®) and 1:2 (Eudragit S®) molar ratios. These can be used in the preparation of organogels that have been evaluated as vehicle for rectal sustained release of drug(s).

Typically, these gels are consisted of the model drug dissolved in propylene glycol containing high concentrations of the gelling polymer [30 and 40% for 1:1 and 1:2 P(MAA-co-MMA), respectively]. Basic drugs weaken the gel's structure more prominently than acidic drugs, a phenomenon attributed to an increased disturbance of the hydrogen-bond interactions between polymer and propylene glycol molecules by the former.

Recently, Jones et al. presented the preparation of star-shaped alkylated poly (glycerol methacrylate) amphiphiles, capable of forming polymeric micelles in pharmaceutically acceptable apolar solvents, such as ethyl oleate. It was found that organogel formation occurred at high polymer concentrations (10%), when the latter was derivatized with medium length C12 and C14 alkyl chains. On the other hand, gelation occurred at much lower concentrations (1%) in the case of

C18-derivatized polymers, showing the importance of intermolecular van der Waals' interactions in the gelation mechanism. Hydrogen bonding via the hydroxyl groups of the core polymers was suggested to be a driving force for gelation. The systems were shown to increase the solubility of hydrophilic compounds in oils making them potentially useful for the preparation of anhydrous peptide formulations. Potential drug delivery from these organogels remains an interesting option to be explored (Fig. 16.6b).

ORGANOGELS AS DRUG DELIVERY VEHICLES

The growing research on organogelators and their gels, has a range of potential industrial applications. This includes immobilization of enzymes for biocatalysis, synthesis and transformation of toxic wastes, separation technology, temperature sensors, flatbed displays, recovery of oil spills and templates for the creation of inorganic structures. Only a few organogels have been investigated for drug delivery. Reasons for this may be due to the fact that most organogels are composed of pharmaceutically unacceptable (or untested) gelators and organic solvents. Organogels that have been studied for drug delivery, however include in situ forming organogels from L-alanine derivatives, Eudragit gels, lecithin gels, microemulsion-based gels (MBGs) and sorbitan monostearate gels. The latter are the only organogels that have been investigated for vaccine delivery. Pluronic lecithin or-ganogels (PLOs) are not strictly speaking organogels but are included in this section. Organogels have mainly been investigated for transdermal drug delivery, although oral, rectal and parenteral routes have been studied, however to a limited extent. Drugs may be incorporated into the gels during gel formation or may be mixed in preformed gels. Most of the drugs studied have been hydrophobic molecules, which are dissolved in the organic liquid phase. Hydrophilic entities (such as vaccines) are generally dissolved in small volumes of an aqueous medium, which is then incorporated into the organogel. The different organogels are discussed in more detail below.

Sorbitan Monostearate Organogels and Amphiphilogels

Sorbitan Monostearate Organogels

Sorbitan monostearate (Span 60) and sorbitan monopalmitate (Span 40) have been found to gel a number of organic solvents at low concentrations. Span 60 gels were found more stable than Span 40 gels and have been investigated in greater depth. The thermoreversible gels are prepared by heating the gelator/liquid mixture in a water bath at 60°C (which results in dispersion of the gelator in the liquid medium) and cooling of the resulting suspension, following which the latter sets to an opaque, white, semisolid gel. Cooling results in reduced affinities between the solvent and the gelator molecules, allow-ing them to self-assemble into tubules. X-ray diffraction and freeze-fracture studies indicate that sorbitan monostearate molecules are arranged in inverted bilayers within the tubules. The tubules form a three-dimensional network, which immobilizes the liquid, and hence a gel is formed. For an organic liquid to be gelled by sorbitan monostearate, the liquid must provide the desirable solubility (following heating) and insolubility (following cooling the sol phase) towards the gelator. Sorbitan monostearate gels alkanes (C > 5), such as hexane, cyclohexane, octane, cis- and trans-decalins, hexadecane, the alkene squalene, vegetable oils (e.g. corn oil, olive oil) and the long-chain synthetic esters, isopropyl myri-state, ethyl oleate and ethyl myristate. The ungellable solvents include relatively more polar alkanols, ethanol, 2-propanol and buta-nol, and chloroform and dichloromethane, which dissolve sorbitan monostearate upon heating but from which the sorbitan mono-stearate precipitates out on cooling. Benzene and toluene are good solvents for sorbitan monostearate and cannot be gelled, because on cooling the sol phase, the sorbitan monostearate remains dissolved in the solvent.

Sorbitan monostearate gels have been investigated as delivery vehicles for hydrophilic vaccines. It was hypothesised that a W/O gel containing a hydrophilic vaccine may act as a depot for the vaccine following intramuscular administration *in vivo*, as the organic phase imposes barriers to the diffusion of the hydrophilic vaccine. The organic medium in the gel delayed the absorption of BSA into the systemic circulation and clearance from the injection site. The depot effect was of a short duration, thus, the study suggested that sorbitan monostearate organogels could not be used as long-term sustained release implants, but could have applications, where a short-term depot is required. Multi-compartment sorbitan monostearate organogels are resulted, when an aqueous vesicle suspension (niosome) is incorporated into organogels (Fig. 16.7).

Sorbitan Monostearate Amphiphilogels

The nonionic surfactants, sorbitan monostearate and sorbitan monopalmitate, also gel other nonionic surfactants, such as liquid sorbitan esters (e.g. sorbitan mono-oleate and polysorbates). Based on the amphiphilic nature of the liquid component of these gels, the latter were termed 'amphiphilogels'. The amphiphilogels can be hydrophilic, when the liquid phase is a hydrophilic polysorbate or hydrophobic when the liquid is a hydrophobic sorbitan ester. These gels are prepared in the same way as sorbitan ester organogels, have similar microstructures and are stable for 2 years, when kept in a sealed container at room temperature. The amphiphilogels can solubilize certain poorly water-soluble drugs, such as cyclosporin, ibuprofen, aspirin and paracetamol. Drug solubilization in the gel alters the T_g (it can increase or decrease, depending on the nature of the drug) and the gel microstructure. The amphiphilogels have been investigated as oral vehicles for cyclosporin.

Water-soluble active agents, e.g. proteins and antigens can be incorporated into hydro-philic amphiphilogels. Protein stability seems to be maintained following incorporation into the gel, and amphiphilogels containing a model antigen, ovalbumin, were studied as vehicles for topical vaccination. Topical application of ovalbumin in gels did not result in the generation of ovalbumin-specific antibodies. This shows that vaccine permeation into the skin did not occur to a sufficient extent. This may be related to the fact that the gels did not disrupt the stratum corneum sufficiently.

In Situ Formed Organogel of L-alanine Derivative

N-lauroyl-L-alanine methyl ester (LAM) gels the pharmaceutically acceptable organic solvents, soybean oil and medium-chain triglycerides. Normally, the system exists in the gel state at room temperature. However, the addition of ethanol to a gelator/solvent solution inhibits gelation because ethanol disrupts the formation of hydrogen bonds (essential for gelator self-assembly into aggregates) between the gelator molecules. This means that a solution of LAM in an organic solvent can remain in the sol phase at room temperature, when some ethanol is added to the mixture. When such a sol phase (20% LAM + 14% ethanol in soybean oil) was

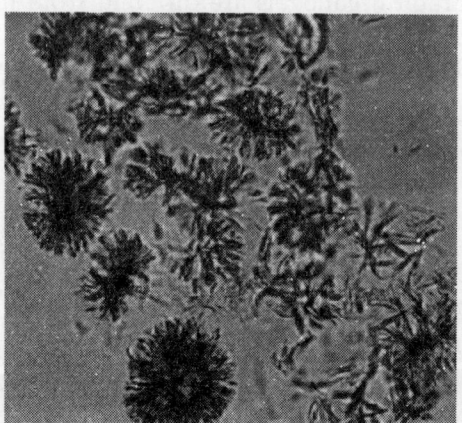

Fig. 16.7: Sorbitan gel microstructure consists of clusters of tubules in the presence of small amounts of polysorbate 20

placed in phosphate buffered saline at 37°C, it turned into a opaque gel within 2 min, as the hydrophilic ethanol diffused away into the aqueous buffer, and as gelator-gelator hydrogen bonds are formed. Thus, theoretically, such a LAM/ethanol/soybean oil solution could form gels in situ following its subcutaneous injection, due to ethanol diffusion from the formulation, into the surrounding tissues; in situ gel formation in rats was investigated. The main advantage of in situ forming gels is their injectability at room temperature. Once a drug-containing gel is formed in situ, it could act as a sustained-release implant. Various L-alanine derivates, viz. N-stearoyl-L-alanine (m) ethyl esters (Fig. 16.8), may be used to immobilize vegetable and synthetic oil in the presence of a hydrophilic solvent. These gels are thermo-reversible in nature. The gel-to-sol transition of the L-alanine based organogels was dependent on the concentration of the gelator and the nature of the solvent. Experimental results indicate that the organogels system, when injected subcutaneously in rats, releases the bioactive agents (e.g. leuprolide) over a period of 14–25 days with subsequent degradation of the gelled structure.

Eudragit Organogels

Eudragit organogels are different from the organogels described in the introduction section, as they are really the mixtures of Eudragit (L or S) and polyhydric alcohols, such as glycerol, propylene glycol and liquid polyethylene glycol, containing high concentrations (30 or 40% w/w) of Eudragit. Drug-containing gels were prepared by dissolving the drug (salicylic acid, sodium salicylate, procain or ketoprofen) in propylene glycol, pouring the resulting solution into Eudragit powder (contained in a mortar), and immediately mixing with a pestle for 1 min. Gel viscosity increases with increasing concentrations of Eudragit and tends to decrease with increasing drug content. The inclusion of the drug procaine reduces gel rigidity, which is due to the influence of the drug molecules on the intermolecular forces (e.g. hydrogen bonds) between Eudragit and propylene glycol. The release of model drugs salicylic acid, sodium salicylate and ketoprofen from Eudragit L and S organogels has been investigated *in vitro* by the rotating disk method. Interestingly, the mechanisms of salicylic acid release from Eudragit L and S organogels into a phosphate buffer, are reportedly different. Release was due to surface erosion of the Eudragit L organogel, while it was following diffusion in the case of Eudragit S gel matrix. Drug release from Eudragit S organogel, thus increased with increasing temperature and agitation rate of the release medium. Eudragit L organogels were evaluated as rectal sustained release preparations in rabbits.

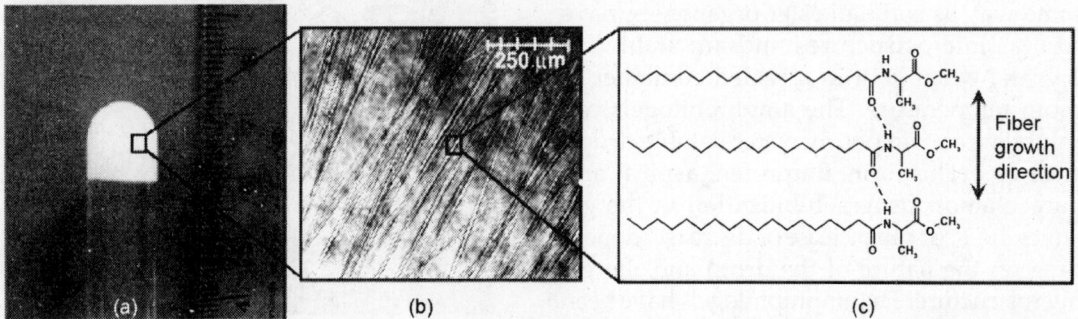

Fig.16.8: (a) Photograph depicting the opaque N-stearoyl-L-alanine methyl ester organogel. (b) Optical micrograph showing the fibrous aggregates responsible for gelation. (c) Molecular packing within fibers. Adapted from Vintiloiu et al., 2008

Microemulsion Based Gels

Microemulsion-based gels (MBGs) are also different from most organogels in that the gelator, gelatin, is a hydrophilic polymer, which gels water (Fig. 16.9). MBGs were initially prepared by dissolving solid gelatin in a hot water-in-oil microemulsion (which was composed of water, AOT and iso-octane) followed by cooling. The whole microemulsion gelled into a transparent semisolid with a high viscosity and a high electro-conductivity. A w/o microemulsion comprising 80–90% oil phase (iso-octane + AOT) had been gelled by a relatively small amount (7–11% w/v) of gelatin; a hydrophilic polymer that would be present mainly in the water phase of the system. Such MBGs have also been prepared by the addition of an aqueous gelatin solution to a micellar solution of AOT in an organic solvent. The T_g of the thermoreversible gel, measured by differential scanning calorimetry, was found to be in the region of 34–38°C, which is close to the transition temperature of gelatin hydrogels. MBG microstructure is thought to be consisted of an extensive network of rigid rods of water and gelatin (surrounded by a shell of AOT surfactants) coexisting with microemulsion water droplets, although other similar structures may also exist.

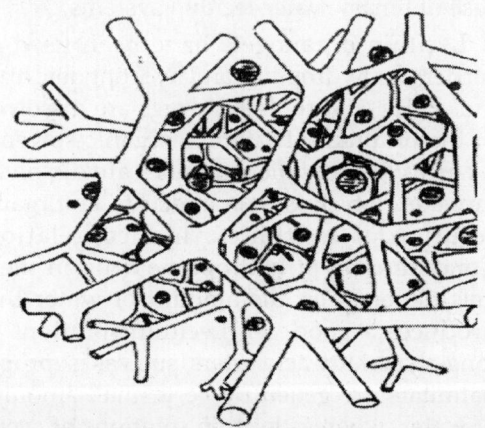

Fig. 16.9: A proposed structure of MBG; an extensive network of rigid rods of water and gelatin coexisting with microemulsion water droplets

One of the first applications of MBGs has been the entrapment of enzymes, especially lipases, for esterification and catalysis. For drug delivery applications, MBGs have been formulated with pharmaceutically acceptable oil (e.g. isopropyl myristate) and by replacing ~85% of the anionic AOT with the more acceptable nonionic surfactants such as Tween 21, 81 and 85. The resulting MBGs possessed an appropriate viscosity for topical application to the skin. They were electro-conducting and were, therefore, investigated as vehicles for iontophoretic transdermal drug delivery. The model water-soluble drug (sodium salicylate) was entrapped within MBG. The advantage of the gel over the aqueous drug solution was said to be its higher viscosity, making it suitable for topical application, and its resistance to microbial contamination due to the large apolar oil component. When an electrical current was applied to the MBG or to the control aqueous drug solution, the drug flux through the porcine skin was enhanced due to iontophoresis of the drug. The system has shown promise as a vehicle for iontophoretic transdermal drug delivery. MBGs have also been investigated for transdermal delivery of piroxicam and it was found that MBGs did not cause any sensitisation, when applied to the shaved back of rabbits for a period of 3 days.

Lecithin Organogels

A lecithin organogel is formed when small amounts of water or other polar substances, such as glycerol, ethylene glycol or formamide, are added to a nonaqueous solution of lecithin (Table 16.3).

The molar ratio of water to lecithin is typically 2:10 and depends on the nature of the organic solvent. Excess water leads to destabilisation of the gel and phase separation. A wide range of nonaqueous solvents, such as linear, branched and cyclic alkanes, ethers and esters, fatty acids and amines containing lecithin have been gelled following the addition of small amounts of water. Gel

---

Table 16.3: Salient features of lecithin organogels

- LOs provide opportunities for incorporation of a wide range of substances with diverse physicochemical characters (e.g. chemical nature, solubility, molecular weight, size)
- Spontaneity of organogel formation, by virtue of self-assembled supramolecular arrangement of surfactant molecules, makes the process very simple and easy to handle
- Being thermodynamically stable, the structural integrity of LOs is maintained for longer time periods
- LOs are moisture insensitive, and being organic in character, they also resist microbial contamination
- Being well balanced in hydrophilic and lipophilic character, they can efficiently partition with the skin and therefore, enhance the skin penetration and transport of the molecules
- LOs also provide the desired hydration of skin in a lipid-enriched environment, so as to maintain the bioactive state of skin
- Use of biocompatible, biodegradable, and nonimmunogenic materials makes them safe for long-term applications

---

formation is thought to be due to changes in the structure of the lecithin micelles in the non-aqueous medium; before the addition of water (or glycerol, ethylene glycol or formamide), the surface active lecithin molecules are present as spherical reverse micelles in the nonaqueous medium. The addition of water is thought to cause uniaxial growth of the micelles into giant cylindrical micelles, which overlap and entangle, and form a three-dimensional network; an increase in viscosity and gel formation is resulted. There is some controversy to this widely accepted theory. Conversion of the spherical micelles into giant cylindrical ones is thought to occur when the added molecules of water (or formamide, ethylene glycol or glycerol) form hydrogen bonded 'bridges' between the phosphate head groups of neighboring lecithin molecules, allowing their assembly into tubular aggregates.

From a drug delivery standpoint, lecithin organogels (LO) represents interesting systems, owing to their biocompatibility, their amphiphilic nature, facilitating dissolution of various drug classes, as well as their permeation enhancement properties. Lecithin, or phosphatidylcholine, is the most abundant phospholipid in biological systems and is typically purified from soy beans and egg yolk. Due to its amphiphilic structure, lecithin can assume many different forms, such as

mono- and bi-molecular films, vesicles, liquid crystals, emulsions. When mixed to organic solvents, lecithin yields isotropic reverse-micelle solutions. Upon the addition of small amounts of polar solvents, cylindrical reverse micelles start to grow until they entangle into a gelling network (Fig. 16.10). Despite having been termed 'weak' organogels, LO present very high viscosities, in several cases higher than that of gelatin. However, the LO's fluid nature is a dependence between their rheology and the relaxation time for micellar breaking and recombination. The rise in the systems' viscosity is indeed due to the growth and overlap of reverse tubular micelles and not to any form of liquid crystalline order, as in the case of binary water-lecithin systems.

Lecithin organogels have been used as carriers for hydrophilic and hydrophobic drug molecules. Hydrophobic drugs are dissolved in the oil phase (lecithin + organic solvent), whereas hydrophilic molecules are dissolved in water, which is then added to an organic solution of lecithin to induce gelation. Concentration of hydrophilic drug in these gels depends on the amount of water that produces a good gel. Lecithin solutions of long-chain fatty acid esters, such as isopropyl palmitate are gelled by very small amounts of water, whereas lecithin solutions of cyclo-octane can incorporate much larger amounts of water. To increase the amount of (and hence

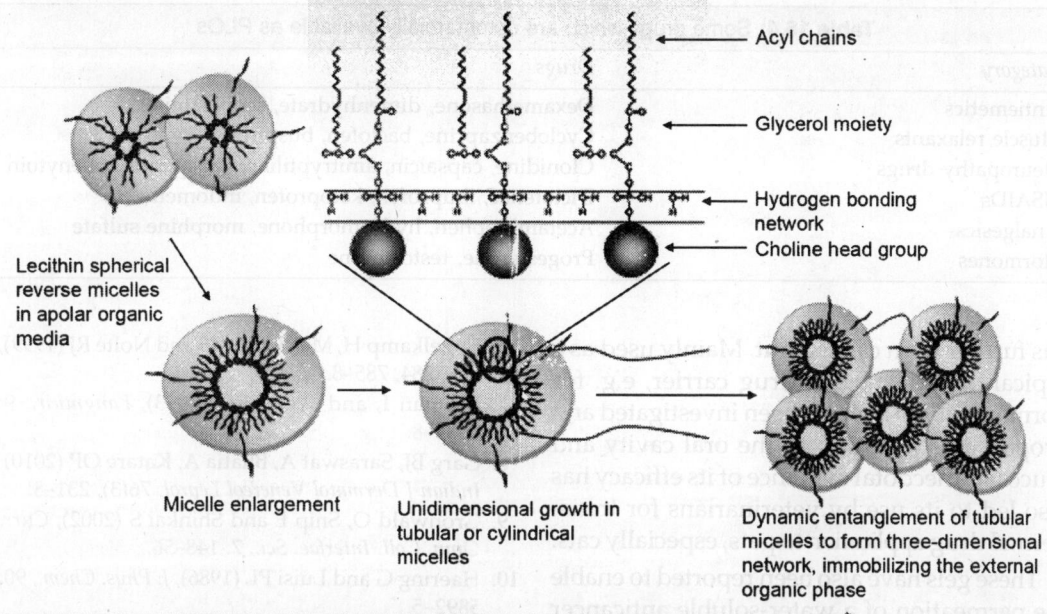

Fig.16.10: Formation of a three-dimensional network of reverse cylindrical micelles in lecithin organogels

the amount of hydrophilic drug) incorporated water in the gels, mixtures of organic solvents, e.g. isopropyl myristate and short-chain esters, such as ethyl or propyl acetate can be used. Drug incorporation into lecithin organogels has effects on the drug as well as on the gels. The solubility of certain drugs, such as broxaterol and nifedipine, was enhanced compared with solubility in the pure solvent. Drug incorporation may reduce gel viscosity, sometimes to a small extent only but at other times the gel can be destroyed, e.g. by the addition of high concentrations of indomethacin or diclofenac.

Lecithin Gels as Transdermal Drug Delivery Vehicles

Isopropyl palmitate/lecithin organogels were tested as matrices for transdermal drug delivery. Isopropyl palmitate was used as the oil component because of its pharmaceutical acceptability. Gels were prepared of drugs such as scopolamine or broxaterol. Incorporation of scopolamine into lecithin gel resulted

in 10 times higher skin permeation as compared to an aqueous scopolamine solution. Lecithin/isopropyl myristate organogels have also been tested as transdermal delivery vehicles for piroxicam to reduce the drug's adverse effects and to avoid its first pass metabolism when administered orally.

Pluronic Lecithin Organogels

An opaque, yellow gel, PLO is composed of isopropyl palmitate, soy lecithin, water and the hydrophilic polymer, Pluronic F127. The difference between PLO and its precursor, lecithin gels, is the presence of Pluronic F127 (a hydrophilic polymer that gels water) and the greater amount of water compared with the oil. Pluronic F127 was added to the original lecithin organogel in order to stabilize the gel formulation (Table 16.4).

The incorporation of many different drugs, such as nonsteroid, anti-inflammatory, haloperidol, prochlor perazine and secretin for patient use and to anecdotal evidence of its efficacy as a transdermal drug delivery vehicle,

Table 16.4: Some drugs which are commercially available as PLOs

Category	Drugs
Antiemetics	Dexamethasone, dimenhydrate, scopolamine
Muscle relaxants	Cyclobenzaprine, baclofen, buspirone
Neuropathy drugs	Clonidine, capsaicin, amitryptiline, gabapentin, phenytoin
NSAIDs	Diclofenac, ibuprofen, ketoprofen, indomethacin
Analgesics	Acetaminophen, hydromorphone, morphine sulfate
Hormones	Progesterone, testosterone

has further been carried out. Mainly used as a topical or transdermal drug carrier, e.g. for hormones, PLO has also been investigated and proposed as a vehicle to the oral cavity and mucosa. Anecdotal evidence of its efficacy has also led to its use by veterinarians for transdermal drug application to pets, especially cats.

These gels have also been reported to enable the permeation of a water-soluble anticancer agent, the bromo derivative of tetra-p-amidinophenoxy neopentane (TAPP-Br), through the skin to act locally on a subcutaneous tumor. Tumor growth was arrested only when drug-containing lecithin gel was applied onto the skin directly around the tumor site. Absence of tumor growth arrest when the drug containing lecithin gel was topically applied away from the tumor site suggests that the drug was not absorbed into the systemic circulation. Absorption of the anticancer agent into the skin shows that lecithin gels could be used as vehicles for the treatment of skin tumors.

SUGGESTED READING

1. Abdallah DJ, and Weiss RG (2000), *Langmuir.*, 16: 352–55.
2. Agrawal V, Gupta V, Ramteke S Trivedi P (2010), *AAPS Pharm Sci Tech,* 11(4): 1718–25.
3. Ajayaghosh A, Praveen VK, Vijayakumar C. (2008), *Chem Soc Rev,* 37(1): 109–22.
4. Amaike M, Kobayashi H and Shinkai S (2000), *Bull. Chem. Soc. Jpn.,* 73: 2553–8.
5. Bastiat G, Plourde F, Motulsky A, Furtos A, Dumont Y, Quirion R, Fuhrmann G, Leroux JC (2010), *Biomaterials,* 23, 6031–8.
6. Engelkamp H, Middelbeek S and Nolte RJ (1999), *Sci.,* 284, 785–8.
7. Furman I, and Weiss RG (1993), *Langmuir.,* 9: 2084–8.
8. Garg BJ, Saraswat A, Bhatia A, Katare OP (2010), *Indian J Dermatol Venereol Leprol,* 76(3), 231–8.
9. Gronwald O, Snip E and Shinkai S (2002), *Curr. Opin. Coll. Interfac. Sci.,* 7: 148–56.
10. Haering G and Luisi PL (1986), *J. Phys. Chem.,* 90: 5892–5.
11. Hinze Wl, Uemasu I, Dai F and Braun JM (1996), *Curr. Opin. Coll. Interfac. Sci.,* 1: 502–13.
12. Iwanaga K, Sumizawa T, Miyazaki M, Kakemi, M (2010), *Int J Pharm.* 388 (1–2): 123–8.
13. Jones DS, Muldoon BC, Woolfson AD, Sanderson, FD (2007), *J Pharm Sci,* 96(10), 2632–46.
14. John G, Shankar BV, Jadhav SR, Vemula PK (2010), *Langmuir,* 26(23), 17843–51.
15. Kantaria S, Rees GD and Lawrence MJ (2003), *Int. J. Pharm.,* 250: 65–83.
16. Kuang GC, Teng MJ, Jia XR, Chen EQ, Wei Y. (2011), *Chem Asian J,* 6(5), 1163–70.
17. Jadhav KR, Kadam VJ, Pisal SS (2009), *Curr Drug Deliv,* 6(2), 174–83.
18. Liu H, Wang Y, Han F, Yao H, Li S (2007), *J. Pharm Sci,* 96(11), 3000–9.
19. Lin Y, Kachar B and Weiss RG (1989), *J. Am. Chem. Soc.,* 111: 5542–51.
20. Morales ME, Gallardo V, Clarés B, García MB, Ruiz MA (2009), *J Cosmet Sci,* 60(6), 627–36.
21. Murdan S, (2005), *Expert Opin. Drug Deliv.,* 2, 3.
22. Murdan S, Gregoriadis G, and Florence AT (1999), *Int. J. Pharm.,* 180: 211–4.
23. Pal K, Banthia AK and Majumdar DK (2009), *Polymers.,* 38; 12: 197–220.
24. Palui G, Garai A, Nanda J, Nandi AK, Banerjee, A (2010), *J Phys Chem B,* 28,114(3), 1249–56.
25. Pierre T and Richard GW Chem Rev, 1997, 97 (8), 3133–60.

26. Scartazzini R and Luisi Pl (1994), *J. Phys. Chem.*, 92 (3), 829–33.

27. Shchipunov YA and Shumilina EV (1996), *J. Colloid* 58(1): 117–25.

28. Shchipunov YA (1995), *J. Colloid*, 57: 556–60.

29. Suzuki M and Hanabusa K (2010), *Chem. Soc. Rev.*, 39, 455–63.

30. Tata M, John VT, Waguespack YY and Mcpherson Gl (1994), *J. Phys. Chem.*, 98: 3809–17.

31. Terech P (1992), *J. Phys II France.* 2: 2181–95.

32. Toro-Vazquez J, et al. (2007), *J. Am. Oil Chem. Soc.*, 84(11), 989–1000.

33. Vanesch Jh, Feringa Bl, (2000), New functional materials based on selfassembling organogels: from serendipity towards design. *Angew. Chem. Int. Ed.* 39(13), 2263–6.

34. Vintiloiu A, Leroux JC (2008), *J Control Release*, 125(3), 179–92.

35. Vintiloiu A and Leroux JC (2008), *J. Contr Rel.*, 125(3): 179–92.

36. Wade RH, Terech P, Hewat EA, Ramasseul R, Volino F, (1986), *J. Coll. Interface Sci.*, 114: 442–51.

37. Wang K, Jia Q, Han F, Liu H, Li S (2010), *Drug Dev Ind Pharm.*; 36(12): 1511–21.

38. Wang K, Jia Q, Yuan J, Li S. (2011), *Int J Pharm*, 404 (1–2), 176–9.

39. Wright A and Marangoni A (2006), *J. Am. Oil Chem. Soc.*, 83(6), 497–503.

40. Yang M, Zhang Z, Yuan F, Wang W, Hess S, Lienkamp K, Lieberwirth I, Wegner G (2008), *Chemistry*, 14(11): 3330–7.

17

▪ Dendrimers

INTRODUCTION

Dendritic polymers have tree-like structures and consist of hyperbranched polymers commonly referred to as dendrigrafts, dendrons, and dendrimers. Each of these four classes reflects the structural features of these complex macromolecular architectures. Dendrimers, which belong to the most extensively investigated class, are highly branched symmetrical macromolecules of nano-sized dimensions, have well-defined molecular mass and geometry consist of a central core, repeating units and terminal functional groups. They are prepared under complex experimental conditions and therefore, for this reason, they are expensive. However, because of their diverse properties, they have attracted significant scientific and technological interest. Dendrimers are monodispersed macromolecules with a regular and highly branched three-dimensional architecture. They are produced in an iterative sequence of reaction steps, in which each repetition leads to a higher generation. Despite the term dendrimer was proposed and coined in early 1980s, dendritic architecture can be traced back to 1978. These synthetic macromolecules distinguish themselves from normal polymer in two critical aspects. First, they are constructed from AB_n monomer (n usually denotes 2 or 3) rather than standard

AB monomers, which produce linear polymers. Thus, they contain hyperbranched structures; secondly, they are synthesized in an iterative fashion.

Dendritic architectures have immense potential over the other carrier systems, particularly in the field of drug delivery because of their unique properties, such as structural uniformity, high purity, efficient membrane transport, high drug pay load, targeting potential, and good colloidal, biological, and shelf stability. They offer a precise control and predictability of modifications that is required for modern drug delivery and targeting; almost all aspects of the dendrimers can be modified to fit the needs, which include its chemical nature, molecular weight, size, structure, and dimensions. They can shield the drugs within the core, thus prevent their biodegradation, and improve the solubility of hydrophobic molecules. By varying the central core and peripheral groups, as well as modifying the attached molecules, dendrimers can be customized for specific therapeutic needs. Despite their diverse applicability in different areas, the inherent cytotoxicity, reticuloendothelial system (RES) uptake and accumulation, drug leakage, immunogenicity, and hemolytic toxicity restrict their use in clinical applications, which is primarily associated with cationic charge on the periphery due to amine groups. To overcome the toxic effects of dendrimers, some nontoxic, biocompatible, and biodegradable dendrimers have been developed (e.g. polyester dendrimer, citric acid dendrimer, arginine dendrimer, carbohydrate dendrimers, etc.). The surface engineering of parent dendrimers is interestingly a convenient strategy, which not only shields or masks the positive charge to make this carrier more biomimetic but also improves the physicochemical and biological behavior of parent dendrimers. Thus, surface modification chemistry of parent dendrimers as such holds promise in these modification for pharmaceutical applications (such as solubilization, improved drug encapsulation, enhanced gene transfection, sustained and controlled drug release, intracellular targeting) and also in the diagnostics field. Development of multifunctional dendrimer holds greater promise toward the biomedical applications because a number of targeting ligands could determine the specificity in the manner as other type of groups would ensure them stability in biological milieu for prolonged circulation, while yet others may facilitate their transport through cell membranes (Fig. 17.1).

The drug carrying capacity of a dendrimer mainly depends on its generation, which refers to the number of repeated branching cycles used in its synthesis. For example, if branching reactions are performed thrice during synthesis, then the dendrimer is considered to be of third generation. Each successive layer creates a generation with double number of active sites (known as end groups), and a molecular weight of approximately twice that of the previous generation. Higher generations display larger particle sizes and internal cavities, and more rigid structure. The multiple numbers of functional groups on the surface thus attribute to their binding ability to cells, owing to the so-called multivalent effect, as more than one of the cell receptors can be accessed simultaneously by a single dendritic polymer.

ORIGIN OF DENDRIMERS

The term dendrimer is derived from Greek word 'Dendron' for tree/branches, due to its resemblance with a tree and 'Meros' meaning part. Dendrimers possess three distinguishable components—an initiator core, interior layers

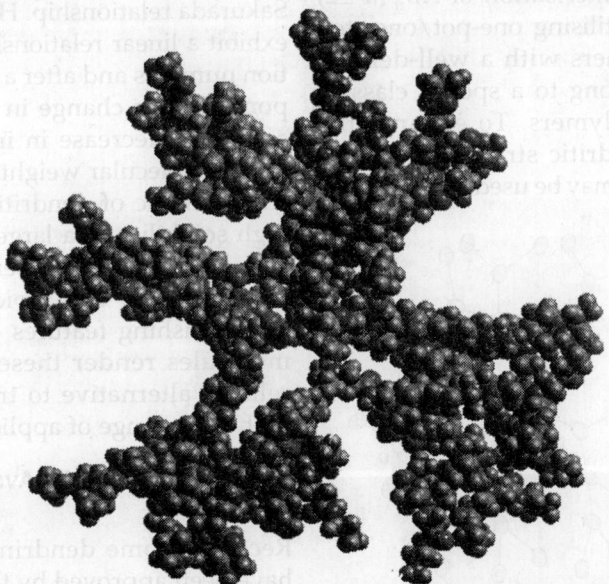

Fig. 17.1: Molecular model of dendrimer (www.umich/edu/~bhgroup/dendrimer/dendrimers.html)

(generations) that are formed by repeating units radially attached to the interior core and exterior or terminal functionality (Fig. 17.2).

DENDRIMERS AND POLYMERS: A COMPARISON

A comparison of the features of dendrimers with those of linear polymers shows that the dendritic architecture can provide several advantages for drug delivery applications. For example, the multivalency of dendrimers can be used to attach several drug molecules, targeting groups, and solubilizing groups to the periphery of the dendrimers in a well-chemically defined manner.

In addition, the low polydispersity of dendrimers should provide reproducible pharmacokinetic behavior in contrast to that of some linear polymers containing fractions with vastly different molecular weight within a given sample. Furthermore, the more globular shape of dendrimers, as opposed to the random coil structure of most of the linear polymers, could affect their biological properties.

The term hyperbranched polymer describes a major class of polymers mostly synthesized by incoherent polymerisation of AB_n ($n \geq 2$) monomers, often utilising one-pot/one step reactions. Dendrimers with a well-defined finite structure belong to a special class of hyperbranched polymers. To enhance the availability of dendritic structures, hyperbranched polymers may be used as dendrimer

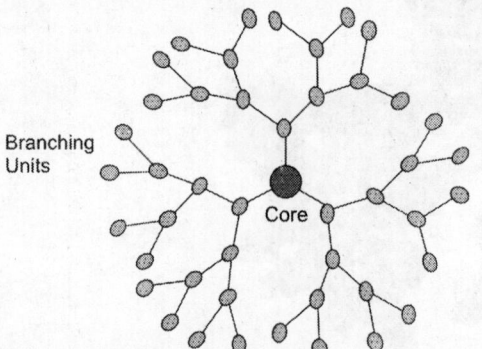

Branching Units

Core

Fig. 17.2: A typical dendrimer

'mimics', because of their more facile synthesis. However, being polydisperse, these dendrimers structure analogs are not suitable to study chemical phenomena, which generally require a well-defined chemical pattern enabling the scientist to analyze the chemical events. The physicochemical properties of the undefined hyperbranched polymers are at large intermediate to dendrimers and linear polymers.

When a dendrimer reaches a specific generation (a variable factor according to the dendritic structure but in general equal to or greater than 4) a significant conformational change occurs, and the structure assumes a densely packed globular shape. This change in conformation correlates with a decrease in chain entanglements and molecular aspect ratio, therefore conferring different solution and bulk properties to dendrimers, when compared with their linear analogues. An important area, where linear and dendritic polymers exhibit diverse characteristics, is their viscosity behavior. It is well known that the intrinsic viscosity of a linear polymer increases with an increase in molecular weight (MW), according to the Mark-Houwink-Sakurada relationship. However, dendrimers exhibit a linear relationship at lower generation numbers and after a maximum, it corresponds to the change in shape, followed by a smooth decrease in intrinsic viscosity at higher molecular weight. Another important characteristic of dendritic molecules is their high solubility in a large number of organic solvents, potentially offering better processability property and rapid dissolution. These distinguishing features of dendritic macromolecules render these novel materials a reliable alternative to traditional polymers with wide range of applications.

Some Commercially Available Dendrimer Products

Recently, some dendrimer-based products have been approved by the FDA. VivaGel ™ (Starpharma) has been designed as a topical microbicide to prevent the transmission of HIV and other sexually transmitted diseases. SuperFect®, developed by Qiagen, is used for gene transfection of a broad range of cell lines. US Army Research Laboratory has developed Alert Ticket™ for anthrax detection. Stratus® CS, for cardiac marker diagnostic, commercialized by Dade Behring, is also based a dendrimer.

PROPERTIES OF DENDRIMERS

1. Theoretically, dendrimers are monodispersed molecules. Due to minor defect during synthesis process, polydispersity index is about 1.001.
2. All molecules have exactly the same molecular weight and structure.
3. Dendrimers having globular shape and the presence of internal cavities provide the possibility to encapsulate guest molecules within the macromolecule.
4. A multivalent surface, with a high number of functionalities, dependent on the dendrimer generation, the surface may act as a borderline shielding barrier of the dendrimer interior from the surroundings. This increasingly 'closed' surface structure may result in reduced diffusion of solvent molecules into the dendrimer interior.
5. The core, which as the dendrimer generation increases, gets increasingly shielded off from the surroundings by the dendritic wedges. The interior of the dendrimer creates a microenvironment, which may have very different properties compared to the surroundings. For example, water-soluble dendrimers with an apolar interior have been constructed to carry hydrophobic drugs in the bloodstream.

FEATURED ADVANTAGES OF DENDRIMERS AS DRUG CARRIER

- Well-defined globular structure, predictable molecule weight, and monodispersity of dendrimers ensure reproducible pharmacokinetics.

- Controllable size (generation-dependent) of dendrimers satisfies various biomedical purposes.
- High penetration abilities of dendrimers through the cell membrane result in an increased cellular uptake level of the drugs complexed or conjugated to them.
- The lack of comparative immunogenicity of dendrimers makes them much safer choices than synthetic peptidal carriers and natural protein carriers.
- Enhanced penetration and retention (EPR) further offers preferential accumulation of the dendrimers by or in the cancer tissues.
- Well-established methodologies proposed to construct nanodevices with various functional moieties based on dendrimers provide miscellaneous biomedical applications of these promising materials, including targeted cancer chemotherapy, magnetic response imaging, photodynamic therapy, neutron capture therapy.
- Perfectly programmed release of drugs or other bioactives from dendrimers leads to reduced toxicity, increased bioavailability and simplified dosing schedule. Generally, the size, shape, and surface properties of the polymeric carriers greatly influence the pharmacodynamic (PD) and pharmacokinetic (PK) behaviors of drugs encapsulated in/complexed or conjugated to the carrier.

CLASSIFICATION OF DENDRIMERS

Dendrimers have been classified on the basis of chemical structure and physical characteristics:

Chemical Classification

1. PAMAM dendrimers (Fig. 17.3a)
2. PPI dendrimers (Fig. 17.3b)
3. L-lysine-based dendrimers
4. Poly ether dendrimers
5. Phenyl acetylene dendrimers

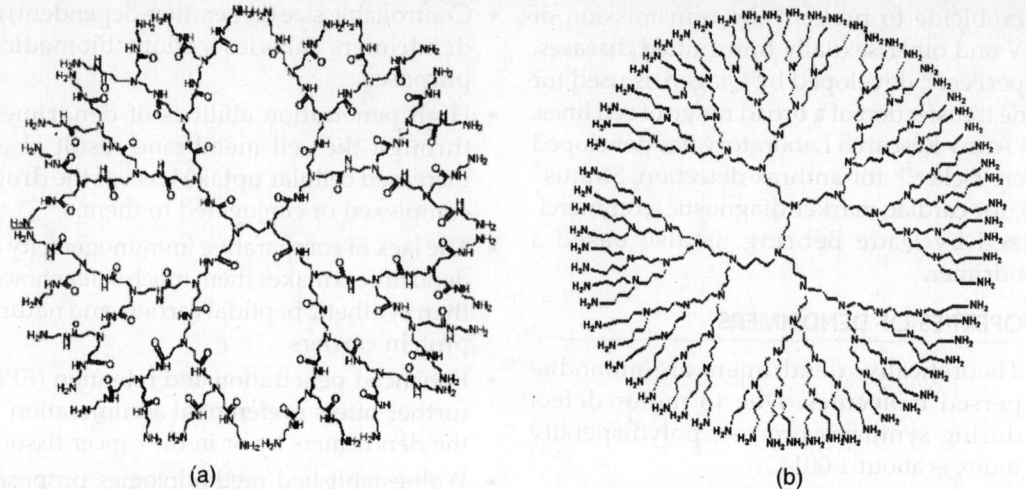

Fig. 17.3: (a) Typical structure of a PAMAM dendrimer (3.0 G), (b) 5.0 G polypropylene imine dendrimer

6. Tetra-thio fulvalene (TTF) glycol dendrimers
7. Penta porphyrin dendrimers
8. Aryl ester monodispersed dendrimers

Physical Classification

1. Simple dendrimers
2. Liquid crystalline dendrimers
3. Chiral dendrimers
4. Micellar dendrimers
5. Hybrid dendrimers
6. Amphiphilic dendrimers
7. Metallo dendrimer

SYNTHESIS AND DESIGNING OF DENDRIMERS

Dendrimers can be prepared by controlled branched chemistry. There are two main strategies for the synthesis of dendrimers: divergent and convergent. Fundamentally, different methods have been developed for stepwise synthesis. The choice of growth dictates the way in which the branching is introduced into the dendrimer.

Divergent Dendrimer Growth

In this approach the dendrimer grows outward from the core, diverging into space. The reaction steps can be repeated to provide subsequent generation of dendrimer (Fig. 17.4).

In the divergent approach, the synthesis of the dendrimer takes place in a stepwise manner starting from the core and building up the molecule towards the periphery using two basic operations—(1) coupling of the monomer, and (2) deprotection or transformation of the monomer end-group to create a new alternative reactive functionality (which was protected during earlier steps) and then coupling of a new monomer etc., in a manner, somewhat similar to that known from solid-phase synthesis of peptides or oligonucleotides. Each step must be taken to completion to avoid the formation of trailing generations, in which some branches are shorter than the others. Such deformations can impair the functionality of the dendrimer, and are extremely difficult to eliminate because the relative size difference between 'pure' and 'impure' dendrimers is miniscule.

Convergent Dendrimer Growth

Convergent synthesis involves independent production and eventual combining of fragment. Growth begins at what will end up being the surface of dendrimer, and works inwards by gradually linking surface units together with more monomers (Fig.17.5). It suffers from low yields particularly in synthesis of large structures. In contrast to the

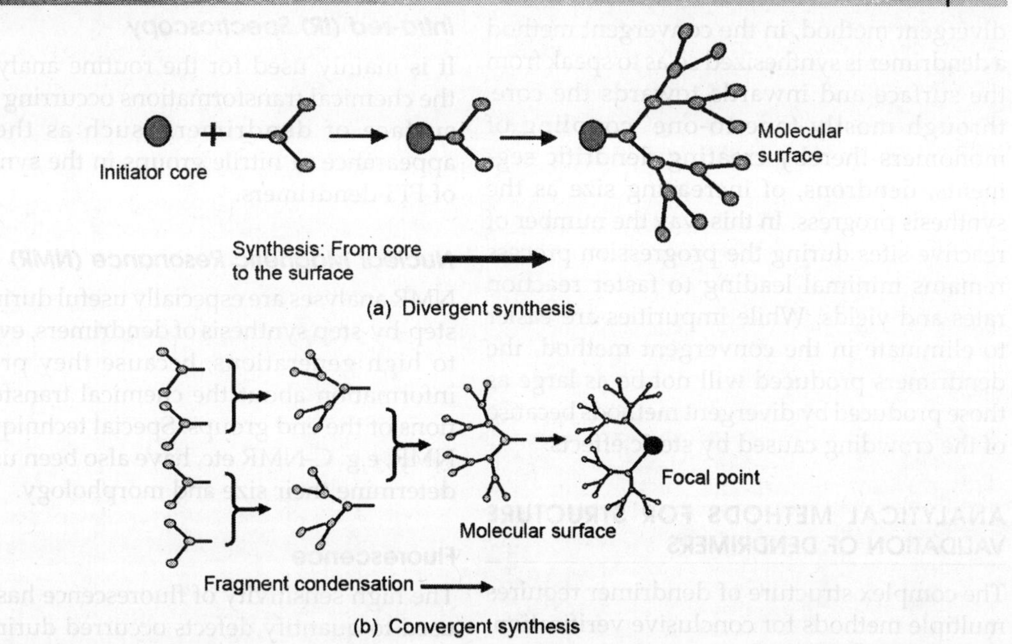

Fig. 17.4: (a) Synthesis of dendrimers by divergent method, (b) convergent synthesis method

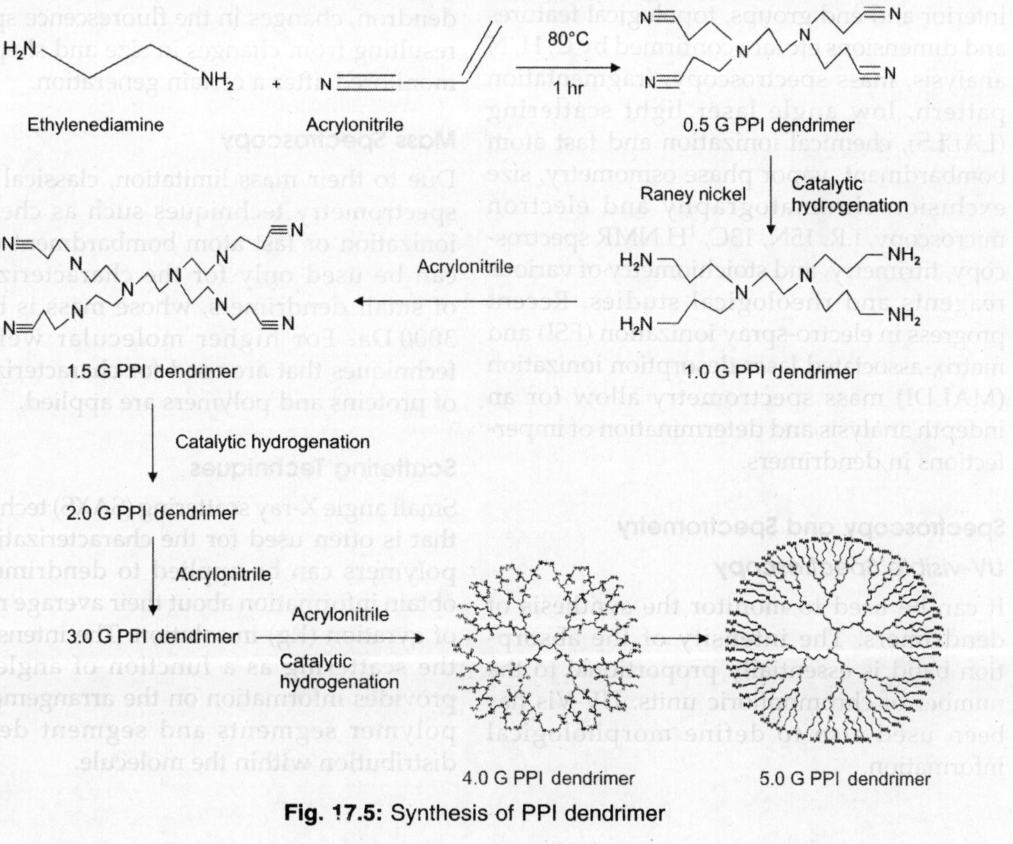

Fig. 17.5: Synthesis of PPI dendrimer

divergent method, in the convergent method a dendrimer is synthesized so as to speak from the surface and inwards towards the core, through mostly 'one-to-one' coupling of monomers thereby creating dendritic segments, dendrons, of increasing size as the synthesis progress. In this way the number of reactive sites during the progression process remains minimal leading to faster reaction rates and yields. While impurities are easier to eliminate in the convergent method, the dendrimers produced will not be as large as those produced by divergent methods because of the crowding caused by steric effects.

ANALYTICAL METHODS FOR STRUCTURE VALIDATION OF DENDRIMERS

The complex structure of dendrimer requires multiple methods for conclusive verification. The structural subtleties like elemental composition, molecular weight homogeneity, interior and end groups, topological features and dimensions etc. are confirmed by C, H, N analysis, mass spectroscopy, fragmentation pattern, low angle laser light scattering (LALLS), chemical ionization and fast atom bombardmant, vapor phase osmometry, size exclusion chromatography and electron microscopy, I.R, 15N, 13C, ^{1}H NMR spectroscopy, titrimetry, and stoichiometry of various reagents and rheological studies. Recent progress in electro-spray ionization (ESI) and matrix-associated laser desorption ionization (MALDI) mass spectrometry allow for an indepth analysis and determination of imperfections in dendrimers.

Spectroscopy and Spectrometry

UV-visible Spectroscopy

It can be used to monitor the synthesis of dendrimers. The intensity of the absorption band is essentially proportional to the number of chromophoric units. UV-Vis has been used also to define morphological information.

Infra-red (IR) Spectroscopy

It is mainly used for the routine analysis of the chemical transformations occurring at the surface of dendrimers, such as the disappearance of nitrile groups in the synthesis of PPI dendrimers.

Nuclear Magnetic Resonance (NMR)

NMR analyses are especially useful during the step-by-step synthesis of dendrimers, even up to high generations, because they provide information about the chemical transformations of the end groups. Special techniques of NMR, e.g. C-NMR etc. have also been used to determine their size and morphology.

Fluorescence

The high sensitivity of fluorescence has been used to quantify defects occurred during the synthesis of dendrimers. When a fluorescent unit is attached to the core of a dendrimer or dendron, changes in the fluorescence spectra resulting from changes in size and shape are monitored after a certain generation.

Mass Spectroscopy

Due to their mass limitation, classical mass spectrometry techniques such as chemical ionization or fast atom bombardment (FAB) can be used only for the characterization of small dendrimers, whose mass is below 3000 Da. For higher molecular weights, techniques that are used for characterization of proteins and polymers are applied.

Scattering Techniques

Small angle X-ray scattering (SAXS) technique that is often used for the characterization of polymers can be applied to dendrimers to obtain information about their average radius of gyration (Rg) in solution. The intensity of the scattering as a function of angle also provides information on the arrangement of polymer segments and segment density distribution within the molecule.

Microscopy

Two types of microscopy have been used for imaging dendrimers. In transmission electron microscopy, electrons or light amplified images are produced, with a resolution ultimately limited by the wavelength of the source. In scanning microscopy, such as atomic force microscopy (AFM), the images are produced by touch contact Q at a few angstroms of a sensitive cantilever arm with the sample. Visualizing single molecules by optical microscopy has been successfully carried out for dendrimers those possess a fluorescent core.

Size Exclusion Chromatography

Size exclusion (or gel permeation) chromatography allows the separation of molecules in accordance with the size. A detector such as a differential refractive index or a LLS detector is connected to the size exclusion chromatography (SEC) apparatus for the determination of the polydispersity, which is generally very close to unity. Most of the dendrimers have been characterized by SEC, including even self-assembled dendrimers.

Electrical Techniques
Electron Paramagnetic

Electron paramagnetic resonance is used for the quantitative determination of the substitutions on the surface of PAMAM dendrimers. It can also detect interactions between the end groups of large PPI dendrimers.

Electrophoresis

Gel electrophoresis is widely used in biology for the routine analysis and separation of biopolymers such as proteins and nucleic acids. This technique is used for the assessment of purity and homogeneity of several types of water-soluble dendrimers, such as PAMAM dendrimers with NH_3^+ or COO^- end groups. Gel electrophoresis is also used for studying the interaction between positively charged dendrimers and DNA to assess the transfectivity in transfection experiments. It was found that complex formation depends both upon the generation (size), and the charge ratio of PAMAM dendrimers.

Rheology
Intrinsic Viscosity

Rheology and particularly dilute solution viscosimetry studies can be used as analytical probe for the determination of morphological structure of dendrimers. Dendrimers in general exhibit a dependence of the intrinsic viscosity (g) on generation, because the volume grows faster with generation than the molecular weight for the first generations, whereas, subsequently an inverse relation has been observed after a certain number of generations.

Differential Scanning Calorimetry

The differential scanning calorimetry (DSC) technique is generally used to detect the glass transition temperature (T_g), which depends on the molecular weight, entanglement and chain-end composition of polymers. The T_g is affected by the end-group substitutions, and molecular mass. DSC and temperature modulated calorimetry (TMC) can be used to detect physical aging of dendrimers.

DENDRIMER TOXICITY

Dendrimers have brought some remarkable advances in the field of drug delivery, however because of nanometric size, i.e. 1–100 nm they may interact effectively and specifically with the components of cell, such as plasma membranes, cell organelles (endosomes, mitochondria, nucleus) and proteins such as enzyme etc., as all of these cellular components are also nanometeric in size. Regardless of the extensive pharmaceutical and biomedical applications of dendrimers, toxicity associated due to terminal-NH_2 groups and multiple cationic charge, limits their clinical applications. Dendrimers like PPI, PAMAM, and PLL exert significant *in vitro* cytotoxicity due to their surface associated cationic groups. The cytotoxicity is found to be concentration and generation-dependent (free amine groups present at their periphery). Not only dendrimers, but also cationic macromolecules in general cause destabilization of the cell membrane resulting into cell lysis. Dendrimers are also responsible for hemolysis of RBCs. The free cationic terminal groups of dendrimers interact with RBCs and this polycationic nature of dendrimers causes RBC hemolysis. The hemolytic toxicity of dendrimers is determined by mixing dendrimers and RBC suspension followed by incubation for definite time intervals at 37°C, centrifugation at 3000 rpm for 15 min followed by analysis of hemoglobin in the supernatant at 540 nm spectrophotometrically against a blank (in normal saline). Higher generation dendrimers may have greater hemolytic toxicity, which may be ascribed to the greater overall cationic charge. Dendrimers also influence other hematological parameters including white blood corpuscles (WBCs), red blood corpuscles (RBCs), hemoglobin (Hb), hematocrit (HCT) and mean corpuscular hemoglobin (MCH). A significant decrease in RBC count, a substantial increase in WBC count, decrease in Hb content and MCH value, and a considerable difference in HCT value are reported.

Membrane Interaction

The fast developing field of nanotechnology is apprehended to emerge out as another source of potential toxicity to human health through inhalation, skin uptake, and injection of engineered nanomaterials. Toxicity of nanocarriers disposed off has physiological, physiochemical molecular consideration. Regardless of potential application in diagnosis, imaging and therapy, there are also controversies generated relating to the possible toxic effects of nanoparticles and this has raised an urgent need for evaluation of safety and potential hazards of engineered nanostructures and nanodevices. Polymer size

and modulation of cell membrane by cationic dendrimers play an important role in the transepithelial transport of dendrimers. Interaction with these dendritic carriers increases the permeability and decreases the integrity of biological membrane. This leads to the leakage of cytosolic proteins such as lactate dehydrogenase (LDH) and luciferase (Luc.) etc., and finally membrane disruption and cell lysis. Dendrimers with surface cationic charges interact with negatively charged biological membrane because of their positive charge. This interaction induces the formation of nanoholes or membrane thinning or erosion leading to membrane disruption that is responsible for the toxicity of dendrimers.

Biodegradable/Biocompatible Dendrimers

The chemical and physical properties of a dendrimers can be optimized by systematically changing the monomer(s). The dendrimers can be made to degrade into biodendrimers, which subsequently degrade to biocompatible building blocks *in vivo*. Development of some less toxic dendrimers with a biodegradable core and branching units may be an alternative approach to decrease the toxicity of dendrimers. Use of monomers in the synthesis of dendrimers, which are metabolic products of various biological pathways enables the synthesis of biodegradable dendrimers. Biodegradable/biocompatible carriers in the development of a drug delivery system can deliver the drug at a rate dictated by the needs of the body over a specified period of treatment. Suitable monomers for biodendrimers include α-hydroxy acids, sugars, amino acids, fatty acids, poly (ethylene glycol) (PEG), poly (caproic acid) (PCL), and poly (trimethylene carbonate). Factors affecting the degradation rate include (1) the strength of the chemical bond between the monomers, (2) the hydrophobicity of the dendrimer, (3) the generation and molecular weight of the dendrimer, and (4) the chemical reactivity of the macromolecule.

Surface Engineered Dendrimers

Surface engineering appears to be one of the best strategies for abatement of dendrimer toxicity. The presence of multiple surface helps attachment of moieties of various functionalities onto the surface through covalent or noncovalent bonding. Surface modification of dendrimers leads to the protection of surface amine groups and reduces the inherent cytotoxicity of dendrimers (Fig. 17.6).

Apart from reduction in inherent toxicity of dendrimers, functionalization also imparts some other properties beneficial for their use as drug delivery system. They include improvement in drug encapsulation efficiency, biodistribution and pharmacokinetic properties, and increase in solubility, targeting to specific site, better transfection efficiency, sustained and controlled drug release. The improvement in stability profile, also improves the therapeutic potential as antiviral, antibacterial activity, which are otherwise poorly bioavailable.

PEGylation

Modification of the surface amine/cationic groups with neutral or anionic moieties is one of the most important steps used to reduce the cytotoxicity and hemolytic toxicity of dendrimers. Prevention of electrostatic interactions of dendrimers with cellular membranes, actually is a necessary step toward minimizing the toxicity of delivery vehicles to the endothelium. PEGylation, i.e. linking or conjugation of dendrimers with PEG is another important strategy effective in reduction of toxicity of dendrimers. In addition to reduction of cytotoxicity PEGylation reportedly proven to improve other limitations associated with dendrimers, such as RES uptake, drug leakage, immunogenicity, stability and hence may contribute to the improvement in drug therapy. Various purposes of PEGylation of dendrimers include improved biodistribution and pharmacokinetics, increase in solubility of dendrimers, shielding of peripheral cationic groups to reduce toxicity (cytotoxicity and hemolytic toxicity), increase in drug loading to prepare a sustained drug delivery system.

Dendrimer Drug Conjugate

There are two main methods which are based on conventional linear polymers as drug carriers. The first involves the polymers as matrices in which the drug is embedded and

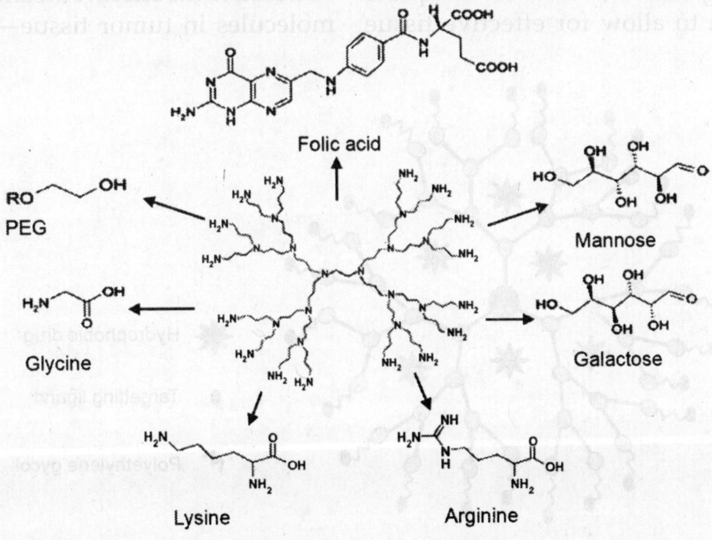

Fig. 17.6: Some surface modification strategies for dendrimer

then released by physical and chemical modifications, such as swelling of the polymer, diffusion or chemical erosion of the polymeric matrix.

The main advantage of this method is the conservation of the chemical integrity and pharmacological properties. The second method involves drug-conjugation to an appropriate polymeric carrier. In this case, the drug is covalently bound to the polymer and released via chemical or enzymatic cleavage of hydrolytically labile bonds. The main advantage of this method is that the drug-polymer conjugate diffuses more slowly than the free drug and can be absorbed on specific interfaces, therefore allow tissue targeting and controlled delivery. Dendritic systems are perfect drug delivery systems as their low polydispersity can assure reproducibility of the pharmacokinetic behavior. Futhermore, the presence of modifiable end groups allows improved water solubility and nonstatistical attachment of drug molecules. The covalent scaffold also provides a stable structure for the internal encapsulation of a drug, which is independent of thermodynamics and physical factors. An ideal dendritic drug-carrier must be nontoxic, nonimmunogenic, and preferably biodegradable; with an adequate biodistribution to allow for effective tissue targeting. Drug molecules can be either chemically conjugated to the dendrimer surface or physically entrapped within a dendrimer core (Fig. 17.7). For chemical conjugations, a good coupling efficiency may be achieved, if functional groups are activated prior to coupling. Hydroxyl (OH), carboxyl (COOH), primary amine (NH_2), thiol (SH) and guanidino are commonly found functional groups in drug molecules as well as in polymers. Hydroxyl groups can be converted to active intermediates that favor nucleophilic reactions. For example, coupling hydroxyl groups with primary amine groups causes primary amine groups to form secondary amines or stable carbamate bonds. Amides are relatively stable in basic, acidic and enzymatic conditions. In some cases, direct coupling may lead to the deactivation of drugs, so that the conjugated drugs, (i.e. prodrugs) will not have any pharmaceutical effect until they are cleaved of from the bonding.

Dendritic carriers can also facilitate the passive targeting of drugs to the solid tumors. This targeting is possible because of the increased permeability of tumor vasculature to macromolecules and also because of limited lymphatic drainage. These factors in combination lead to the selective accumulation of macromolecules in tumor tissue—a phenomenon

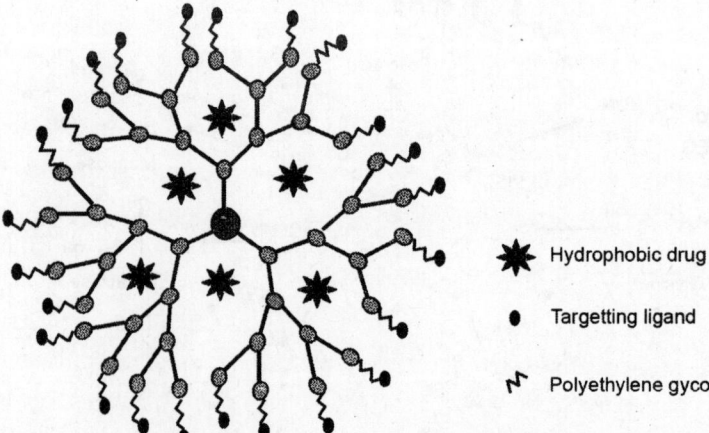

Hydrophobic drug

Targetting ligand

Polyethylene gycol

Fig. 17.7: Dendrimer encapsulating hydrophobic drug with targeting ligand on the surface

termed as 'enhanced permeation and retention' (EPR) effect. The unique properties of dendrimers make them interesting candidates for the development of delivery systems particularly for anticancer drug for their site specific delivery. To improve the drug delivery effectiveness, these polymers have been functionalized on their surface with a diverse class of active groups imparting multifunctional characters. Each type of external group plays a specific function. Thus, as is the case with other targeted nanoparticles, specificity for certain cells has been achieved by attaching targeting ligands on the surface of dendritic polymers. Dendrimers can be used as coating agents to protect or deliver drugs to specific sites in the body or as time-release vehicles for biologically active agents. Well-defined macromolecular structures of dendrimers offer the polyvalent characteristic. Through polyvalent interactions with receptors and binding sites, dendrimers may be designed to achieve higher activity compared to small molecules. In addition, dendrimers may be constructed and modified to have relatively long duration of action, reduced side effects and improved other beneficial effects as compared with currently available pharmaceuticals.

Transdermal Delivery of Drugs

Transdermal route is evolving as a non-invasive option to systemic delivery and also to improve pharmacokinetics of drug(s) using novel drug delivery modules. There are many approaches for delivering bioactives via the routes, amongst them dendrimers gained an immense attention. Encapsulation and conjugation of bioactives with these nanocarriers have shown great promises with possibilities for delivery of hydrophobic and G.I. labile drugs. Their transport from layers of skin depends upon dendrimer characteristics. These characteristics include generation size, molecular weight, surface charge, incubation time and concentration (Table 17.1).

Permeation of anti-inflammatory drugs like ketoprofen and diflunisal was reportedly enhanced into the skin as compared to conventional systems such as pure drug gels. Dendrimers facilitate the diffusion of drugs into and across the skin. Wang et al., 2003 conjectured that the PAMAM dendrimers itself does not voyage in the interior of the skin; however, it takes steps as polymeric skin permeation enhancer by altering the macroscopic constitution of water in the skin as well as in formulation.

Solubility Enhancer

The hydrophobicity of a new chemical entity is a major limitation frequently encountered during its product development and, hence, it is a major hindrance in achieving satisfactory bioavailability. The use of dendrimers as solubilizing agent has attracted the attention

Table 17.1: List of drugs administered via different routes using dendrimers

Administration route	Drug
Intravenous	Flurbiprofen, chloroquine phosphate, doxorubicin, fluorouracil, primaquine
Transdermal	Tamsulosin, indomethacin, ketoprofen, diflunisal
Oral	5-ASA, camptothecin, naproxen, propanolol, ibuprofen
Intramuscular	Aretemether
Ocular Pilocarpine,	Tropicamide
Subcutaneous	Cisplatin
Intranasal	Methylprednisolone
Topical Ketoprofen,	Naproxen
Intraperitoneal	Methotrexate

of many scientists especially due to its characteristic static micelle-like properties, which are different from conventional micelles. A range of dendrimers in their original or modified form considered to be the most common vector for gene delivery; however the risks associated with them are currently necessiating the search for safe and effective alternative synthetic DNA or gene delivery systems. Dendrimers can act as carrier, commonly referred as vectors, in gene therapy. Vectors transfer the target genes through the cell membrane into the nucleus. Currently, liposomes and genetically engineered viruses have been implicated as vector for gene delivery. Dendrimers are under investigation as an alternative module for the delivery of DNA and small molecules and drugs, especially for cancer chemotherapy. PAMAM and PPI dendrimers have been studied thoroughly as vectors for gene delivery, and reported as efficient transfectants of DNA. It is noteworthy that dendrimers of high structural flexibility belonging to partially degraded high-generation dendrimers, (i.e. hyperbranched architectures) appear to be better suited for gene delivery operations than intact high-generation symmetrical dendrimers. Perhaps, this is due to their enhanced flexibility, which allows the formation of more compact complexes with DNA.

Dendrimer as Imaging Agents

Macromolecular contrast agents have become very important tools in modern diagnostic medicine. Dendrimers provide multiple binding sites on the periphery, allowing many magnetic resonance imaging (MRI) contrasting agent complexation. One dendrimer molecule can host up to 24 contrasting agents as complexes (depending on generation), thereby attaining a higher signal to noise ratio.

Dendrimers in Boron Neutron Capture Therapy

A very interesting application of PAMAM dendrimer-antibody immunoconjugates has been demonstrated in a boron delivery system developed for use in neutron capture therapy. Boron neutron capture therapy is a special treatment given to the patients suffering from cancer. This therapy is based on the nuclear capture reaction that occurs when boron-10, a stable isotope, is irradiated by low energy or thermal neutrons to liberate α-particles and lithium-7. The liberated particles are able to kill the cancerous cells. In order to achieve the desired effects, the boron-10 species need to be delivered selectively to the cancer cells in a concentration approximately 10^9 atoms per tumor cell. The required level of boron could, however be delivered to the target provided a high number of boron atoms are loaded or attached to each antibody and also if the antibodies interact with a very high density antigenic receptors. Although several approaches examining the benefits of peptides and linear polymers as feasible boron-delivery systems have been reported, nevertheless none have been reportedly satisfactory.

Dendritic Boxes as Drug Delivery Systems

The internal architecture of dendrimers is well suited for the host-guest interactions and encapsulation of drug as guest molecules or biological actives or hydrophobes (Fig. 17.8). The acid-base reaction between the dendrimer(s) and the guest(s) with subsequent Coulombic attractions pull the guest molecules within the dendrimers architecture, whereas the hydrogen bonding keeps the guest bound to the host. Such an interaction was reported initially for some dyes, such as pyrene and Bengal Rose. However, it should be noted that the guest molecules are retained within the dendritic branching clefts through weak ionic interactions with internal protonated groups. This interaction of insoluble drug molecules results in higher percentage of drug loading in a single nanoscopic molecule. This reduces the dose and sometimes provides stability to the encapsulated drug by protecting it from external environment, which, in turn, enhances the bioavailability of the drugs. The

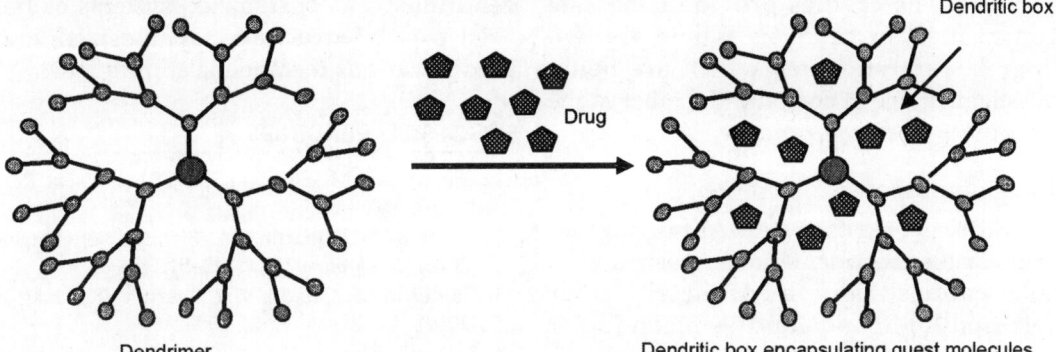

Fig. 17.8: A typical dendritic box

use of dendritic macromolecules as drug containers offers the potential advantages of prolonging the residence time of the drug in the blood circulatory tissue, thereby offering ample opportunities for carrier target cell interaction and home as a consequence targeting of contained ligand. Dendritic architecture offers opportunity for various biological actives, drugs and guest molecules to form complexes, both covalently and noncovalently. List of patents related to dendrimers is given in Table 17.2.

Dendrimers as Biomimetic Artificial Proteins

Based on their dimensional length scaling, narrow size distribution, and other biomimetic properties, dendrimers are often referred to as artificial proteins. Within the PAMAM family, dendrimers closely match the sizes and contours of many important proteins and bioassemblies.

Miscellaneous

Catalysis and Reaction Sites

Dendrimers have nanoscopic cavities, which provide a microenvironment for molecular

Table 17.2: List of some of the patents related to dendrimers

Cited patent	Issue date	Original assignee	Title
US4568737	1986	The Dow Chemical Company	Dense star polymers and dendrimers
US4737550	1988	The Dow Chemical Company	Bridged dense star polymers
US4713975	1987	The Dow Chemical Company	Dense star polymers for calibrating/ characterizing submicron apertures
US5387617	1995	The Dow Chemical Company	Small cell foams and blends and a process for their preparation
US5393795	1995	The Dow Chemical Company	Polymer blend containing a modified dense star polymer or dendrimer and a matrix polymer
US5393797	1995	The Dow Chemical Company	Smal¹ cell foams containing a modified dense star polymer or dendrimer as a nucleating agent
US5560929	1996	The Dow Chemical Company	Structured copolymers and their use as absorbents, gels and carriers of metal ions
US5739218	1998	Dow Corning Corporation	Radially layered copoly (amidoamine-Michigan Molecular Institute organosilicon) dendrimers

reactions. The cavities provide nanoscale reactor sites for catalysis. There are two possible catalytic sites which are being investigated; one at core and the other at the surface.

Nanocomposites

It was discovered that PAMAM dendrimer forms stable interior nanocomposites with metal cations, zero valent metals, other electrophilic ligands and semiconductor particles. These materials are actively being explored and investigated for their applications in electronics and optoelectronics.

Nanodevices

Multifunctionality of dendrimer-based nanodevices is a crucial determinant that plays an important role in the development of targeted drug delivery. Multifunctional cancer therapeutic nanodevices have been designed and synthesized using the PAMAM dendrimer as a carrier.

Cross-linking Agent

Dendritic macromolecules may act as ideal cross-linking agents. Newly emerging dendritic cross-linked hydrogels can be made by using multifunctional dendrimers as cross-linking agents. The number and hence the density of crosslinks junctions can be controlled by varying the generation of the

dendrimer. The customized systems as per need may be structured, synthesized, and used in various therapeutic applications.

SUGGESTED READINGS

1. Bronstein LM, Shifrina ZB (2011), *Chem Rev*, 111(9), 5301–44.
2. Calderón M, Quadir MA, Strumia M, Haag R (2010), *Biochimie* 92(9), 1242–51.
3. Calderón M, Quadir MA, Sharma SK, Haag R (2010), *Adv Mater*, 22(2), 190–218.
4. Cheng Y, Zhao L, Li Y, Xu T (2011), *Chem Soc Rev*, 40(5), 2673–703.
5. Hayder M, Fruchon S, Fournié JJ, Poupot M, Poupot R (2011), *Scientific World Journal*, 11, 1367–82.
6. Kaminskas LM, Porter CJ (2011), *Adv Drug Deliv Rev*, 63(10–11): 890–900.
7. Kesharwani P, Gajbhiye V, Tekade RK, Jain, NK (2011), *Curr Drug Targets*, 12(10), 1478–97.
8. McNerny DQ, Leroueil PR, Baker JR (2010), *Wiley Interdiscip Rev Nanomed Nanobiotechnol.* 2(3), 249–59.
9. Paleos CM, Tsiourvas D, Sideratou Z, Tziveleka LA (2010). *Expert Opin Drug Deliv*, 7(12), 1387–98.
10. Sebestik J, Niederhafne P, Jezek J (2011), *Amino Acids*, 40(2), 301–70.
11. Soliman GM, Sharma A, Maysinger D, Kakkar A (2011), *Chem, Commun*, 47(34), 9572–87.
12. Troiber C, Wagner E (2011), *Bioconjug Chem*, 22(9), 1737–52.
13. Tsai HC, Imae T (2011), *Prog Mol Biol Transl Sci*, 104, 101–40.
14. Wang Z, Itoh Y, Hosak AY, Kobayashi I, Nokano Y, Maeda I (2003), *J. Biosci Bioeng* 95, 541–3.

18

Niosomes

INTRODUCTION

The self assembly of nonionic surfactants into vesicles was first reported in the seventies by researchers in the cosmetic industry. Since then a number of groups worldwide have studied nonionic surfactant vesicles (niosomes) with a view to evaluate their potential as drug carriers. Niosomes or NSVs are now widely studied as an alternative to liposomes (Baillie et al., 1985). Nonionic surfactant vesicle results from the self-assembly of hydrated surfactant monomers. Nonionic surfactants of a wide structural variation have been found to be useful alternatives to phospholipids in the fabrication of vesicular systems (Florence, 1993). Though the terminology suggests that distinctions exist between niosomes and liposomes of which the former is having chemical differences in the monomer units, niosomes possess physical properties, which are similar to liposomes, which are formed from phospholipids. As the name indicated, generally, nonionic surfactant vesicles are prepared by incorporation of components containing nonionic surfactants.

However, they may also be prepared with various ionic amphiphiles, such as dicetylphosphate, stearylamine, etc., in order to achieve a stable vesicular suspension. The chemical stability as well as relatively low cost of the materials used to prepare niosomes makes this vesicle more attractive than liposomes for industrial productions both for pharmaceutical and cosmetic applications. A schematic diagram of a niosome, formed with nonionic surfactant and cholesterol is shown in Fig. 18.1. Nonionic surfactants form a variety of aggregates from micelles to large vesicles, which can be used as vehicles for drug delivery. They include, drug carriers in oncology, for delivery of antiparasitic agents, cosmetic formulations, topical vehicles and as potential diagnostic devices.

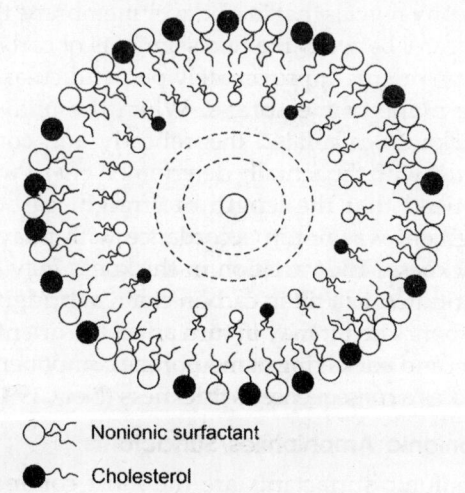

⟠⟋ Nonionic surfactant

●⟋ Cholesterol

Fig.18.1: Schematic representation of nonionic surfactant vesicle (niosome)

FORMULATION ASPECTS

It seems desirable to understand the role of the basic structural components of niosomes before their preparation. These components include nonionic amphiphiles/surfactants and the hydration medium.

Niosomes Bilayer

Like lipids, the nonionic surfactants also orient in an aqueous medium as planner bilayer lattices, wherein polar or hydrophilic heads align facing aqueous bulk (media) while hydrocarbon segments align in such a way that their interaction with aqueous media is minimized. Every bilayer for thermodynamic reasons folds over itself to be a continuous membrane, i.e. forms a vesicle so that hydrocarbon/water interface remains no more exposed. Obviously, every liquid compartment exists isolated from continuous phase. The alignment of amphiphiles in bilayer is mainly attributed to hydrophobic interaction in order to avoid or minimize unfavorbale thermodynamic state resulted due to the exposure of hydrocarbon segments to an aqueous bulk. Such interactions could be avoided effectively in closed/sealed vesicular shape as compared to planner bilayer orientation. An understanding of X-ray crystallography reveals that in a bilayer membrane the glycerol between the two segments of carbon chain orients approximately perpendicular to the plane of membrane. When the bilayer thickness calculated theoretically and compared with the actually determined one, it was noticed that the length of straight carbon segment was not in accordance with bilayer thickness. The variation in thickness may be attributed to a tilt in carbon chain at bridging carbon. The tilt may in turn affect the orientation and packaging of membrane components and as a consequence its thickness (New, 1990).

Nonionic Amphiphiles/Surfactants

Nonionic surfactants are the most common type of surface active agent used in preparing vesicles due to the superior benefits, they impart stability, compatibility, and toxicity compared to their anionic, amphoteric or cationic counterparts. They are generally less toxic, less hemolytic and less irritating to cellular surfaces and tend to maintain near physiological pH in solution. They have many functions including acting as solubilizers, wetting agents, emulsifiers and permeability enhancers. They are also strong P-glycoprotein inhibitors, a property useful for enhancing drug effect by addressing MDR and for drug targeting to specific tissues. Nonionic surfactants are comprised of polar and nonpolar segments and possess high interfacial activity. The formation of bilayer vesicles instead of micelles is dependent on the hydrophilic-lipophilic balance (HLB) of the surfactant, the chemical structure of the components and the critical packing parameter (CPP). On the basis of the CPP of a surfactant, the type of vesicle, which it will form, can be predicted as shown in Fig. 18.2. A CPP of between 0.5 and 1, indicates that the surfactant is likely to form vesicles. A CPP of below 0.5 (indicating a large contribution from the hydrophilic head group area), is said to give spherical micelles and a CPP of above 1 (indicating a large contribution from the hydrophobic group volume), should produce inverted micelles, the latter presumably formed only in an oil phase, otherwise in aqueous phase precipitation would occur.

The HLB value of a surfactant plays a key role in controlling drug entrapment of the vesicle it forms. A surfactant with a HLB value in the range 14–17 is not suitable to produce niosomes, whereas one with a HLB value of 8.6 gives niosomes with the highest entrapment efficiency. Entrapment efficiency decreases as the HLB value decreases from 8.6 to 1.7. For HLB > 6, cholesterol must be added to the surfactant in order to form a stable bilayered vesicle and also for lower HLB values, cholesterol enhances stability of vesicles. It is also seen that the addition of cholesterol enables more hydrophobic surfactants to form vesicles, suppresses the tendency of the

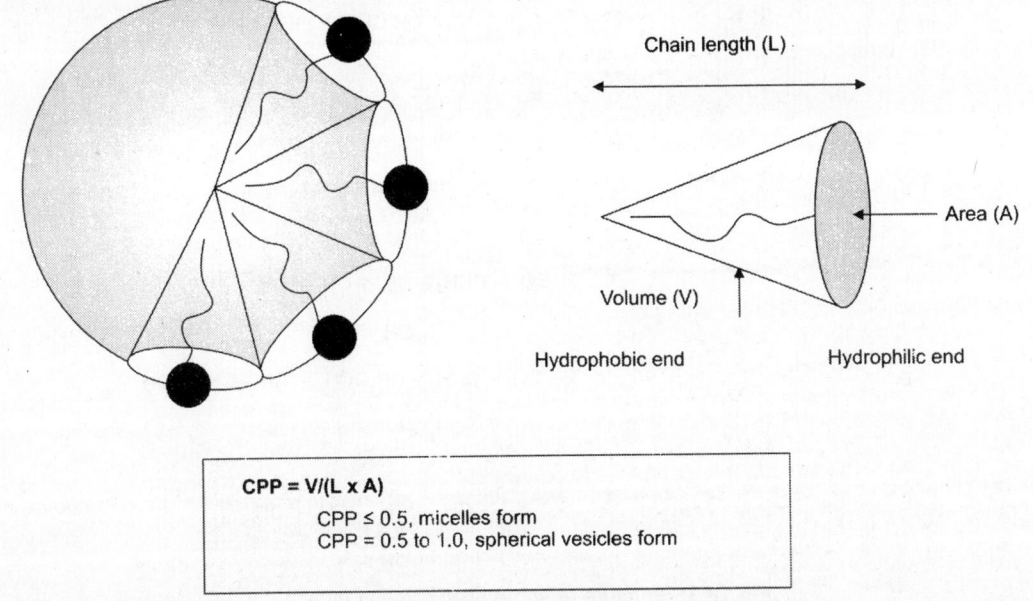

$$CPP = V/(L \times A)$$

CPP ≤ 0.5, micelles form
CPP = 0.5 to 1.0, spherical vesicles form

Fig. 18.2: Critical packing parameter (CPP) of an amphiphile where V is the hydrophobic group volume, L the critical hydrophobic group length and A the area of the hydrophilic head group

surfactant to form aggregates, and provides greater stability to the lipid bilayer by promoting and favoring the gel liquid transition temperature of the vesicle. The entrapment efficiency is affected by the phase transition temperature (T_c) of the surfactant. Thus, Span 60 with a high T_c exhibits the highest entrapment efficiency.

Principal among vesicle forming nonionic compounds are the alkyl ether lipids. These can be broadly divided into two classes, based on the nature of their hydrophilic head group—alkyl ethers in which the hydrophilic head group consists of repeat glycerol subunits, related isomers or larger sugar molecules and those in which the hydrophilic head group consists of repeat ethylene oxide subunits. In addition, alkyl esters, amides and fatty acids, and amino acid compounds also form vesicles.

Alkyl Ethers

Alkyl ethers are good vesicle forming nonionic surfactants. They are stable, relatively nonirritant to the skin and compatible with other surfactants. Due to their high stability they can be used to encapsulate proteins and peptides although it, was shown that their encapsulation capacity decreases, when combined with cholesterol. Alkyl glycerol ethers synthesized at L'Oreal, France (Vanlerberghe et al., 1972) were the first compounds reported to form NSVs (Fig. 18.3). L'Oreal nonionic surfactants have been explored for a wide variety of drug delivery applications. Apart from the alkyl glycerol their analogues, alkyl glycosides have also been studied as drug carriers. In addition, a group of alkyl ethers bearing polyhydroxyl head groups is also reported as vesicle forming surfactants. The second group of alkyl ether amphiphiles in which the hydrophilic head group consists of ethylene oxide units have also received considerable attention.

Brij 52, 56 and 58 are cetyl derivatives of polyoxyethylene with vesicle forming properties. Among them, Brij 58 has got special importance due to its ability to form inverted

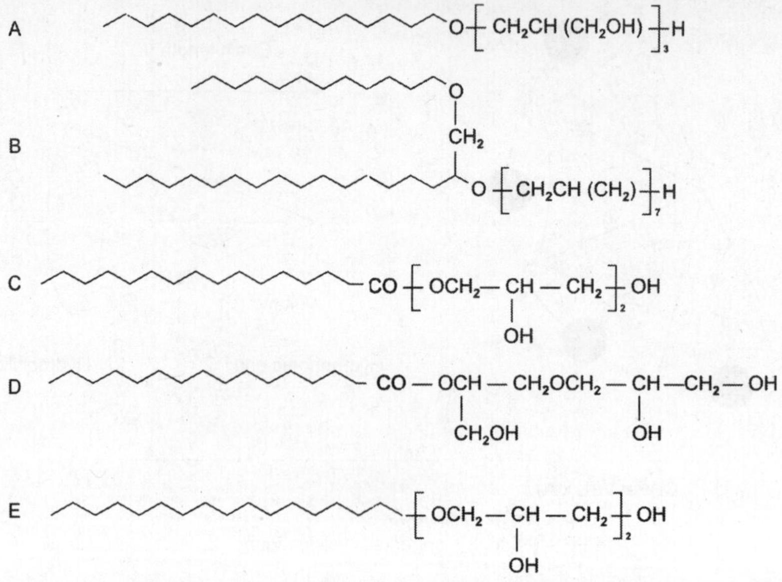

Fig.18.3: Structure of some alkyl glyceryl ethers

vesicles, which are useful for studying ion-pumping activity (H+-ATPase and Ca2+-ATPase) at the plasma membrane. This ability is the result of 'nondetergent behavior' associated with its large head group (E20–23). Brij 58 is commercially available under a variety of trade names including poly (oxyethylene) cetyl ether, Brij W1, polyethylene oxide hexadecyl ether, polyethylene glycol cetyl ether, Brij 38, Brij 52, poly (oxyethylene) palmityl ether, Brij 56, Atlas G3802, cetocire, cetyl alcohol ethoxylate, Nikkol BC40, etc.

Polyoxyethylene stearyl ethers (Brij 72 and 76) are stearyl derivatives of polyoxyethylene ether with good vesicle forming properties. In particular, Brij 72 forms multilamellar vesicles with a high encapsulation efficiency.

Alkyl Esters

The widely used alkyl esters in food industry, the sorbitan esters (Fig. 18.4), have been studied as a principal constituents of NSVs. Esters of plain (non-PEGylated) sorbitan with fatty acids are usually referred to as Spans. Their gel transition temperature increases as the length of the acyl chain increases. Thus,

sorbitan monolaurate (Span 20) with a C9 chain is liquid at room temperature; sorbitan monopalmitate (Span 40) with a C13 chain has a gel transition temperature of 46–470°C; sorbitan monostearate (Span 60) with a C15 chain has a gel transition temperature of 56–580°C. Vesicles made with these higher

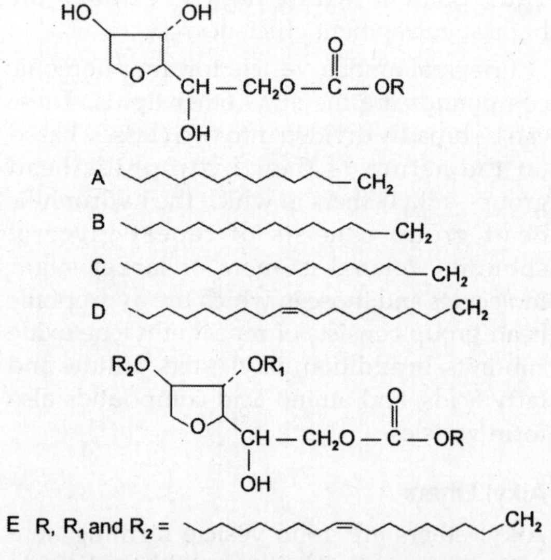

Fig.18.4: Structure of some sorbitan esters

molecular weight Spans are less leaky and more stable to osmotic stresses.

Alkyl Amides

Alkyl galactosides and glucosides incorporating amino acid spacers have also been found to produce vesicles (Zarif et al., 1993; Guedj et al., 1994; Gtiener et al., 1993). While as a general rule, the alkyl groups in all vesicle-forming amphiphiles consist of fully or partially saturated C12 to C22 hydrocarbons, certain novel amide compounds bearing fluorocarbon chains also form vesicles and small disk shaped structures.

Fatty Acids and Amino Acid Compounds

Amino acid moieties, when made suitably amphiphilic by the addition of hydrophobic alkyl side chains, form vesicles (Neumann and Ringsdor, 1986). Peptide liposomes were prepared using these amino acid vesicles in the presence of a water soluble carbodi-imide condensing agent. Long chain fatty acids also form 'Ufasomes', closed vesicles formed from fatty acid bilayers (Gebicki and Hick, 1976).

Cholesterol

Steroids are important components of bio-cell membrane and their presence in membrane brings about discernible changes in regard to bilayer fluidity and permeability. Cholesterol can be incorporated in bilayers at significantly higher molar ratio, however, by itself, it does not form bilayers. Thus, it could be used to ameliorate and manipulate the bilayer characteristics being co-component of bilayer.

Further, being amphiphile in nature cholesterol aligns itself in such a way that its OH group orients towards aqueous phase, while aliphatic chain aligns parallel to the hydrocarbon chain of surfactant. Interestingly, in a mixed molecular bilayer, it occupies an alternate position. Thus, 3B hydroxyl group could be positioned with polar glycerol and hydroxyl group of surfactant molecules allowing very little verticle movements. The presence of rigid steroidal skeleton alongside the carbon chain of surfactant could possibly restrict the freedom of movements of the carbons of hydrocarbon segment, thus providing an absolute rigidization. The free space occupation of cholesterol minimizes the amphiphile carbon segment tilt and provides rigidization to the bilayer (New, 1990). As in the case of liposomes hydrophilicity, lipophilicity, temperature of hydration and T_c are of importance similarly for nonionic surfactants, the hydrophilic-hydrophobic segments and a balance between them are of paramount importance.

The amount of cholesterol to be added, depends on the HLB value of the surfactants. As the HLB value increases above 10, it is necessary to relatively increase the amount of cholesterol to be added in order to compensate for the larger head groups. Higher entrapment of minoxidil occurred in Brij 76 niosomes in the presence of a higher content of cholesterol, whereas no significant increase in entrapment efficiency recorded in Brij 52 (HLB 5.3) based niosomes. In fact, above a certain level of cholesterol, entrapment efficiency tends to decrease possibly due to a decrease in volume diameter and its resulting effect on CPP (CPP < 0.05).

Encapsulated Drug/Bioactive

Another factor to be considered is the nature of the drug to be encapsulated (Fig.18.5). When doxorubicin is encapsulated in niosomes, aggregation occurred that was overcome by the addition of a steric stabilizer. The increase in encapsulation of a drug that occurs when more drug is added to the medium could be the result of saturation of the medium. This suggests that the solubility of certain poorly soluble drugs can be increased by formulation in niosomes, but only up to a certain limit, above which drug precipitation will occur. An increase in the encapsulation of flurbiprofen due to saturation of drug in the hydration medium has been reported. However, when niosomes were prepared using higher amounts of minoxidil, optical

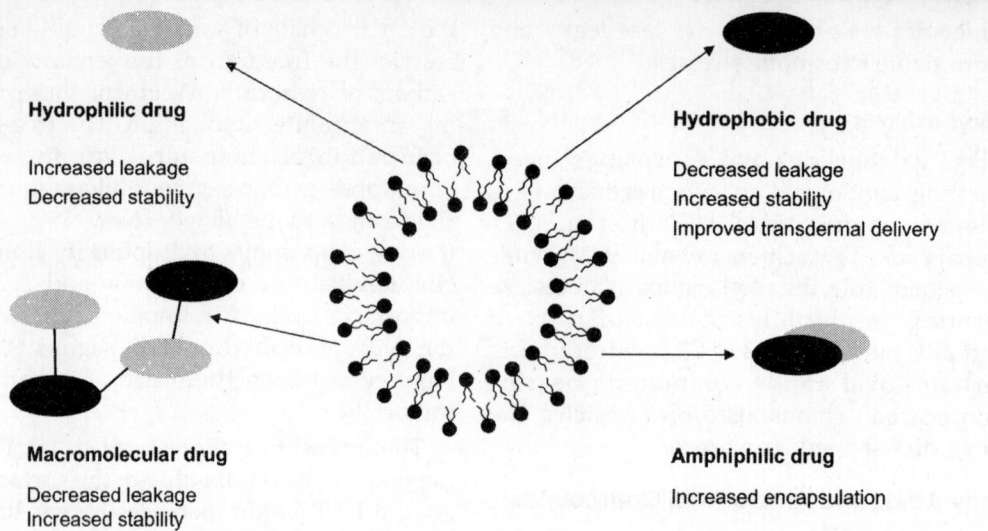

Hydrophilic drug

Increased leakage
Decreased stability

Hydrophobic drug

Decreased leakage
Increased stability
Improved transdermal delivery

Macromolecular drug

Decreased leakage
Increased stability

Amphiphilic drug

Increased encapsulation

Fig. 18.5: The effect of the nature of the encapsulated drug on the properties of the niosome dispersion

microscopy appearance and measure revealed minoxidil crystals dispersed in between the niosomal particles.

The encapsulated solute and the solute retention capacity of the encapsulating membrane, together with the stability of both the surfactant and the vesicle structure, all together contribute to the stability of the formulation. Encapsulation efficiency is governed by the method of loading, nature of solute, and hydration temperature. Vesicles loaded by transmembrane ion gradient method show higher entrapment efficiency than those loaded using conventional film hydration method. As a general rule, larger niosomes show higher entrapment efficiencies than smaller vesicles. Encapsulation of water soluble solutes results in an increased vesicle size, which can be attributed to the interaction of solutes with the amphiphile head groups.

Investigations over the years have shown that cholesterol plays an important role encapsulation efficiency of a formulation and in turn governs the stability of the vesicles. The synthetic alkyl glycosides are capable of forming vesicles without the inclusion of cholesterol. However, a threefold increase in

encapsulation efficiency of C16-glucoside vesicles was measured after incorporation of 29 mole % cholesterol. Similarly, 50–100% increase in encapsulation efficiency was measured with vesicles formed using synthetic polyhydroxyl lipids with 20 mole % cholesterol content up to 50 mole % was reported with a series of sorbitan monoesters.

CPP of a potential niosomes system must take into account the presence of amphipathic or hydrophobic drugs as both of these substances will get incorporated into the vesicle membrane. Nonionic surfactant vesicles prepared using surfactants with identical alkyl groups, but different hydrophilic groups (epoxy *vs* glycerol moieties) revealed that the glycerol moieties had lower head group area compared to ethoxy group. This gives an increased mobility to the polyethoxylated alkyl chains, which as a result increases the fluidity of the corresponding bilayers and ultimately leading to leaky membranes as compared to alkylglycerol derivatives. The change from a poly-5-oxyethylene to a diglycerol head group resulted in twofold increase in the encapsulation efficiency of a macromolecular prodrug.

Temperature and pH of the Hydration Medium

Temperature of the hydration medium plays a major role in the formation of vesicles and affects their shape and size. The temperature should always be above the gel to liquid phase transition temperature of the system. Temperature affects the assembly of surfactants into vesicles and also induces changes in vesicle shape. For example, polyhedral vesicles formed by C16-solulan C24 (91:9) at 250°C transformed into spherical vesicles upon heating to 480°C, but on cooling from 550°C, formed a cluster of smaller spherical niosomes at 490°C and changed to a polyhedral structure at 350°C. In contrast, vesicles formed by C16-cholesterol-solulan C24 (49:49:2) showed no shape transformations on heating or cooling. Volume of the hydration medium and duration of hydration of the lipid film also affect vesicle structure and yield.

Entrapment efficiency of niosomes is greatly affected by the pH of the hydration medium. High entrapment of flurbiprofen was reported at acidic pH with a maximum encapsulation efficiency of 94.6% at pH 5.5. The fraction of flurbiprofen encapsulated increased to 1.5 times as pH decreased from 8 to 5.5 and decreased significantly at pH >6.8. The lowest entrapment of flurbiprofen recorded at pH 7.4 and 8 with no significant difference between them. The increase in encapsulation efficiency of flurbiprofen at lower pH is presumably due to its ionizable carboxylic acid group. At lower pH, the proportion of unionized flurbiprofen increases and partitions more readily into the lipid bilayer than the ionized species. At lower pH, niosomes formulations should be examined by optical microscopy for the presence of drug precipitates both before and after centrifugation and washing. This helps to determine the concentration of drug in the hydration medium giving optimum encapsulation in niosomes.

Surface Charge

The presence of surface charge in vesicular dispersions is critical. It has been found that aggregation of vesicles in isotonic saline solution occurs when the vesicles were prepared without the inclusion of a charged molecule in the bilayer (Haran et al., 1993). Aggregation is attributed to the shielding of the vesicle surface charge by ions in solution and thereby reducing the electrostatic repulsion. However, a reduction in the formation of aggregates was observed when a charged molecule like dicetylphosphate was incorporated in CnEOm bilayer vesicles (Cable, 1989).

METHODS OF PREPARATION

The general method of preparation of niosomes involves evaporation to produce a lipid film followed by hydration with the hydration medium (Fig. 18.6). However, there are variants of this method that are described here in detail (Figs 18.7–18.9). The various methods of preparation of niosomes are similar to those discussed for liposomes.

Handshaking Method

Surfactant and cholesterol mixture are dissolved in diethylether in a round bottomed flask. The ether is evaporated under vacuum at room temperature in a rotary evaporator. Upon hydration the dry film nonionic surfactant(s) swells and is peeled off the support into a film, like lipids in lipid-based film. Swollen bilayer of amphiphiles eventually fold on itself to form vesicles. The liquid volume entrapped in vesicles appears to be small, i.e. 5–10%. The entrapable volume seems to be unsuitable for water soluble solute(s), although the absolute yield/ml of solution/gram of lipid/surfactant may be satisfactory for practical purposes.

Sonication

Niosomes using sonication method were prepared by dispersing surfactant-cholesterol

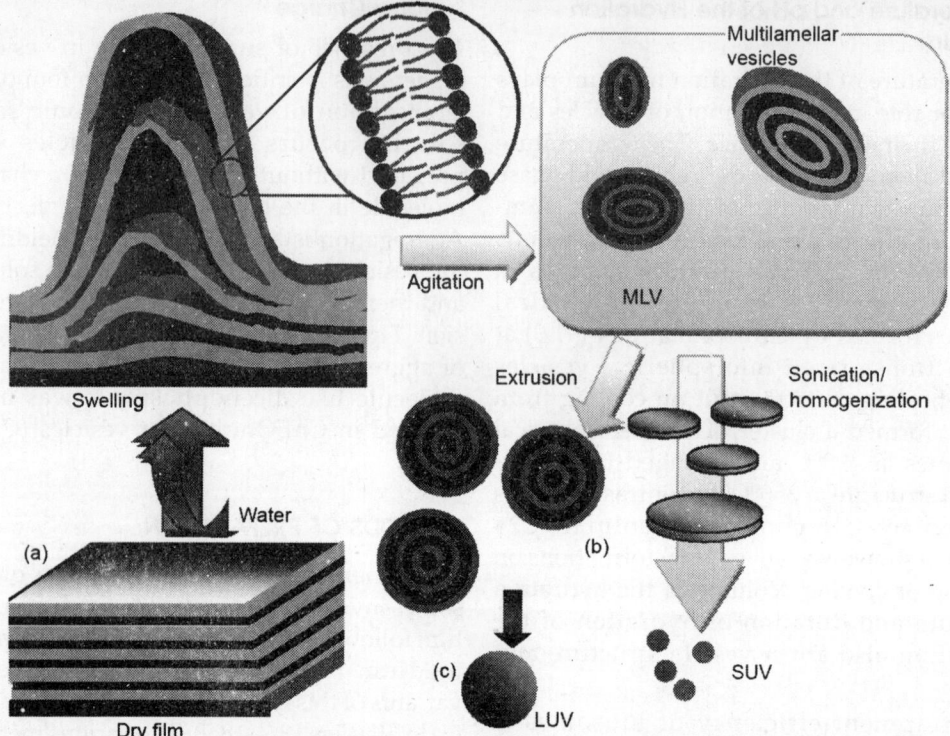

Fig. 18.6: Mechanism of niosome formation and subsequent processing to get various types of vesicles

mixture in 2 ml of aquoues phase in a vial. The dispersion was probe sonicated at 60°C. Essentially, the method involves the formation of MLVs, which are subsequently subjected to ultrasonic vibrations. The sonication may be accomplished using probe sonicator, where sample size is a small volume. However, for larger sample volume bath sonicator is considered to be suitable. The vesicles are unilamellar in shape. Great care must be taken while working with a temperature sensitive solute.

Ether Injection

The ether injection method is essentially based on slow injection of surfactant-cholesterol solution in ether through a 14 gauge needle at rate approximately 0.25 ml/min into a preheated aqueous phase maintained at 60°C. The mechanism whereby relatively larger unilamellar vesicles are formed, however is not understood, presumably it could be ascribed to the slow vaporization of solvent resulting into a ether gradient extending across the interfacial lipid/surfactant mono-layer at ether-water interface. The later subsequently may result into the formation of a bilayer sheet, which eventually folds on itself to form sealed vesicles. Fluorinated hydrocarbons evaporating at much lower temperature could substitute ether in cases, where drug(s) to be incorporated are highly susceptible to temperature. The variation in vesicular size in aqueous phase may be varied via varying the volume of ether in etherial solution of surfactants whilst effective volume of aqueous phase remains to be constant.

Reverse Phase Evaporation

Surface active agents are dissolved in chloro-form and 0.25 volume of phosphate saline buffer is emulsified to get W/O emulsion. The mixture is then sonicated and subsequently chloroform is evaporated under reduced pressure. The lipid or surfactant forms a gel first and subsequently hydrates to form vesicles. Free drug (unentrapped) is generally removed by dialysis.

Aqueous Dispersion

The method essentially based on micro-dispersion of surfactants in aqueous media containing solute(s) for encapsulation or entrapment. Continuous agitation under controlled temperature condition leads to homogenous vesiculation. The dispersion may further be homogenized and ultracentrifuged.

A variation is based on co-dispersion of vesicle forming substance and active drug. The dispersion subsequently homogenized at room temperature followed by continuous bubbling of nitrogen till the vesiculation or hydration is completed. The bubbles possibly provide spherical gas/air at interface for amphiphiles to get organized as per thermo-dynamic stability requirements. Nitrogen is released subsequently and allows the amphiphiles subsequent hydration to form vesicles.

Extrusion

Niosomes were prepared using C16G2 (from L'Oreal) a chemically defined nonionic surfactant by extrusion through a poly-carbonate membrane (0.1 μm nucleopore). The study not only demonstrated the effect of number of extrusion on vesicle size, but also the effect of size on encapsulation of drug. It was found that using extrusion method, vesicles of mean size diameter 136 nm could be prepared. However, on encapsulation of stilbogluconate and calcein in vesicles the resultant mean size of niosomes increased significantly, as it was measured to be 200 nm and 300 nm respectively (Stafford et al., 1988).

Enzymatic Method

Niosomes may also be formed by an enzy-matic process from a mixed micellar solution. In this method, ester links are cleaved by esterases leading to break down products such as cholesterol and polyoxyethylene, which in combination with dicetyl phosphate and other lipids produce multilamellar niosomes. The surfactants used are polyoxyethylene stearyl derivatives and polyoxyethylene cholesteryl sebacetate diacetate.

Single Pass Technique

This is a patented technique involving a continuous process that comprises of the extrusion of a solution or suspension of lipids through a porous device and subsequently through a nozzle. It combines homogenization and high pressure extrusion to produce niosomes with a narrow size distribution in the size range 50–500 nm.

CHARACTERIZATION OF NIOSOMES

Size, Shape and Morphology

Vesicle structure and shape can be characteri-zed by using various microscopic techniques such as optical, freeze fracture electron, surface electron, scanning electron, negative staining transmission electron, cryoelectron, and fluorescence and confocal (Fig. 18.10). The interfacial surface tension of a vesicular system determines the structure of the supramole-cular elements of multilamellar vesicles.

The size and shape of niosomes are depen-dent on drug entrapment, nature of drug and nature of surfactant used. In case of hexadecyldiglyceryl ether-based vesicles, it was observed that percent entrapment of drug tends to increase the size of niosomes. The effect is attributed to the interaction of solute molecules with the polar head group of sur-factants. The net increase in resultant charge and force of repulsion thereby accounted for an increased vesicle size, when complex formation between polar head of surfactant and solute molecule takes place or salting out of surfactant polar heads due to complex formation takes place, hence a local high energy is built. The latter may cause thermo-dynamic instability, which in turn could promote vesicles to aggregate and to form larger vesicles (Yoshioka et al., 1994; Zarif et al., 1993).

Vesicle Charge

Size and charge of vesicles have a significant effect on their stability and drug encapsulation. Size and charge can be assessed using a multifunctional zeta potential analyzer, where size of vesicles is the result of repulsion forces between the bilayers and the entrapped drug. It is found that the size of niosomes loaded with gallidermin was smaller for anionic niosomes than cationic niosomes due to neutralization of their negative charge by the positive charge of entrapped gallidermin. Correspondingly, cationic niosomes were larger due to repulsion of bilayers and also between the positive charges of the niosome and gallidermin.

Bilayer Rigidity and Homogeneity

The biodistribution and biodegradation of niosomes are influenced by rigidity of the bilayer. Inhomogeneity can occur both within niosome structures themselves and between niosomes in dispersion and could be identified using p-NMR, differential scanning calorimetry (DSC) and Fourier transform-infra red spectroscopy (FT-IR) techniques. Recently, fluorescence resonance energy transfer (FRET) was used to obtain deeper insight in the structure, shape and size of the niosomes.

Entrapment Efficiency

This is determined by measuring the difference between the unentrapped and total amounts of drug initially added. Unentrapped drug is separated by various techniques such as exhaustive dialysis, gel filtration and centrifugation. Total amount of drug can be determined by digesting a specific amount of a preparation and analyzing using a suitable analytical method. Percent entrapment can then be calculated in the usual way.

Entrapment efficiency depends mainly upon method of preparation. Nonionic surfactants based vesicles prepared by ether injection method demonstrated higher entrapment efficiency as compared to those prepared by handshaking method. The difference critically related to the vesicles type and size, which in turn were found to be related to the method of preparation. Ether injection method, however produces conventional unilamellar vesicles more uniform in size resulting into higher drug entrapment compared to MLVs. Gradual increase in cholesterol concentration results into relatively low entrapment efficiency.

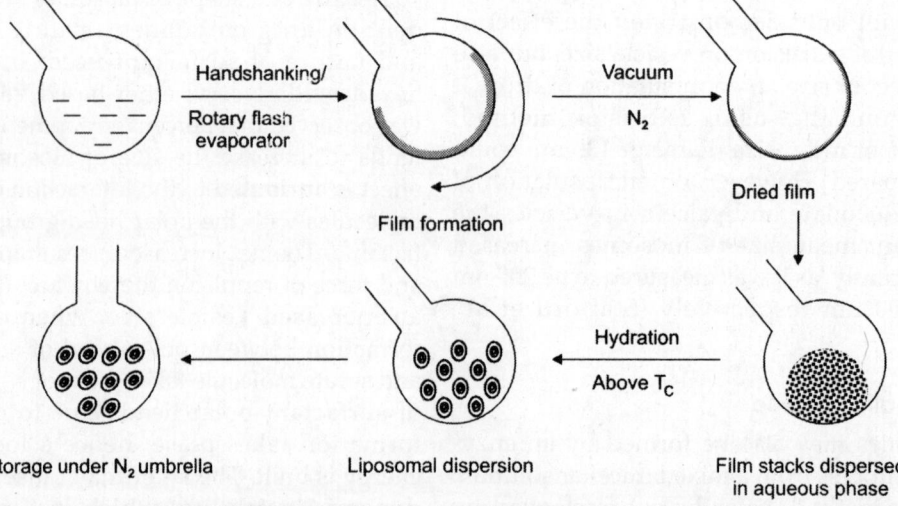

Fig. 18.7: Preparation of dried-reconstituted vesicles (DRVs)

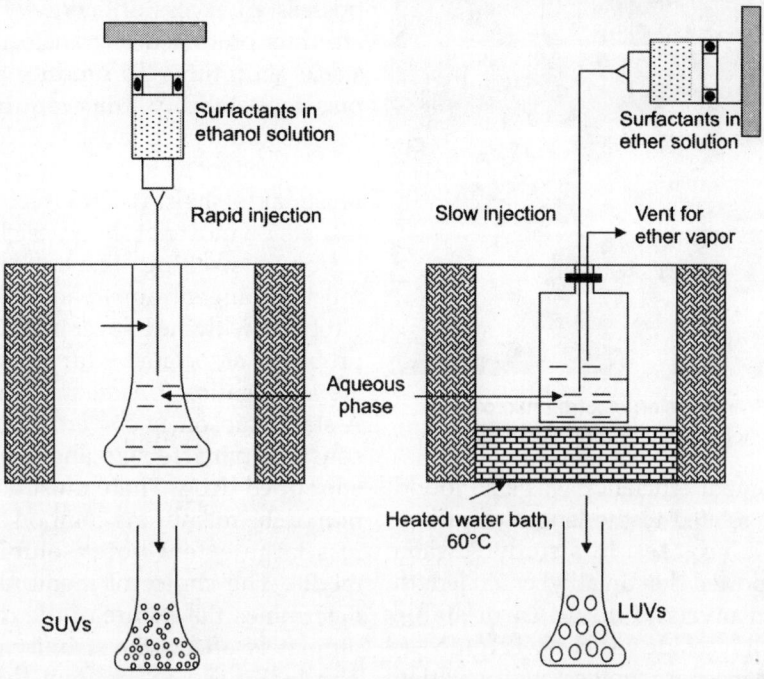

Fig. 18.8: Principle of vesicle formation by solvent dispersion method in which the two phases (aqueous and organic) are miscible with each other and form different types of vesicles

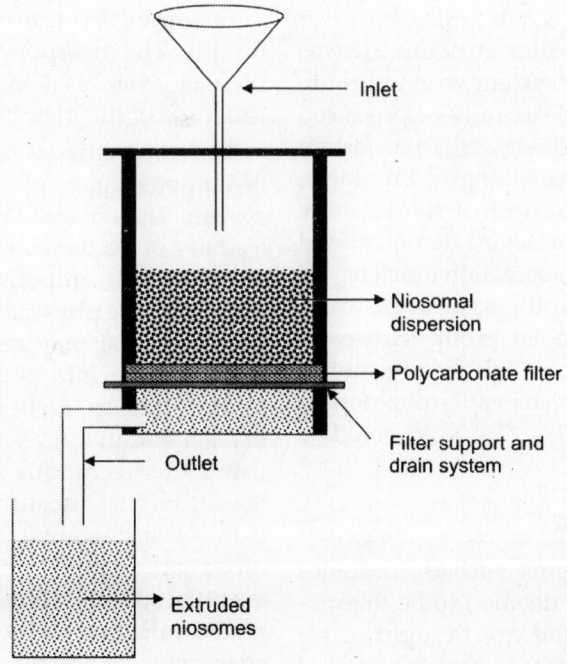

Fig. 18.9: Niosomes preparation using extrusion technique based on polycarbonate filters

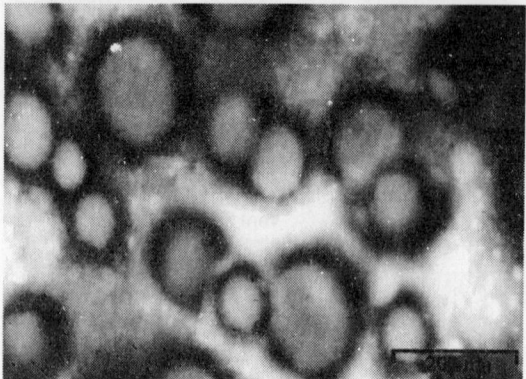

Fig. 18.10: Transmission electron microscope (TEM) photomicrograph of niosomes

The entrapment efficiency was also found to be linearly related to the length of carbon chain in alkylglycosides. In a study Kiwada et al., 1985 reported that an alkyl chain length not less than myristyl could form stable vesicles. Cetylglycoside vesicles with glucose, galactose, and mannose showed encapsulation capacity practically comparable to the phosphatidylcholine liposomes. The shorter length alkyl chain (lauryl, decyl, and octyl) surfactants of alkylglycoside series, however do not form the vesicular structure. It was noted that a vesicular system with optimum encapsulation capacity can only be produced by proper selection of alkylglycosed surfactant of an appropriate chain length. Similarly, modification or alteration of hydrophilic head group of C16 surfactant demonstrated dramatic effect on encapsulation efficiency. It could be attributed to the associated water with sugars used as polar group. However, more detailed studies are required to establish the mechanism via which head group dependent entrapment efficiency by NSVs could be explained.

STABILITY OF NIOSOMES

Hydrated bilayer systems, such as liposomes and niosomes are not deemed to be thermodynamically stable and are thought to represent a metastable state in that the vesicles possess an excess of energy. These particles are thus predicted to transform into bilayer stacks with time. To produce a system with maximal stability, thus requires that these predicted transformations be slowed down to such an extent as to produce a product with a reasonable shelflife. In effect, the colloidal dispersion must not show vesicle aggregation, fusion or swelling. The entrapped material must remain entrapped and show no incompatibility with the bilayer materials. The main problems associated with storage of vesicles are aggregation, fusion and leakage of drug. A stable niosomes dispersion must exhibit a constant particle size and a stable level of entrapped drug. There must be no precipitation of the membrane components, which are to a large extent not insoluble in aqueous media. The choice of membrane surfactant determines the nature of the membrane and ultimately affects the stability of the system. The leakiness of carboxy fluorescin (CF) loaded Span-based niosomes was found to follow the trend Span 80 > Span 20 > Span 40 > Span 60 (Yoshioka et al., 1994) and was determined by the degree of membrane fluidity. The incorporation of cholesterol into these niosomal systems found to decrease the leakiness of the membrane.

The encapsulated drug could also be the major determinant of the fate of any niosomal system. The encapsulation of a polymer will lead to a more stable system as the membrane is sufficiently impermeable to this macromolecule. The physical nature of the encapsulated material may also affect the stability. DOX loading into vesicles using an ammonium sulfate gradient leads to the formation of a gel within the vesicles. Niosomes loaded using this technique was found to be less leaky. High concentrations of detergents (soluble surfactants) are incompatible with niosomal systems and reported to cause eventual solubilisation of the vesicles to form mixed micelles and a host of intermediate aggregates.

Methods to Enhance the Stability

Stability of NSVs is maintained by entropic/entholpic repulsion forces arise as vesicles approach close to each other, thus preventing the flocculation. Dehydration of surface hydrophilic groups generally leads to flocculation. Therefore, salt addition or temperature rise, affect the stability particularly the dispersibility. In a study, the mean hydrodynamic diameter of vesicular aggregates was measured as a function of time and it was observed that niosomes tended to aggregate. However, the nature of aggregation was recorded to be reversible. The vesicles redispersed on shaking. Furthermore, the addition of DCP in a low concentration prevented the aggregation.

In an attempt to improve the stability of NSVs against flocculation, cholesteryl oxyethylene ether was added to NSVs based on surfactant I to increase the hydrophilicity of the exterior surface. One measure of the influence on the surface properties due to incorporation of cholesteryl oxyethylene ether was its effect on electorphoretic mobilities or net surface charge. The effect of 5 mole % addition of solulan C5, C16 and C24 was recorded in terms of electrophoretic mobilities as a function of pH. The increasing length of polyoxyethylene unit adsorbed on the surface pushes the plane of shear farther from the particle and decreases the resutlant charge borne by vesicles, the latter attributes to the selective adsorption of OH ions from the bulk (Uchegbu et al., 1991).

Decreasing the air water interface may prevent the crystallization of these self-assembled surfactant monomers and it may be possible to stabilize niosomes by a variety of methods, such as the addition of polymerised surfactants to the formulation, the use of membrane spanning lipids and the interfacial polymerisation of surfactant monomers in situ. The inclusion of a charged molecule in the bilayer, shifts the electrophoretic mobility making it positive with the inclusion of stearylamine and negative on the inclusion of DCP and also prevents niosome aggregation. In addition, the entrapment of hydrophobic drugs or macromolecular prodrugs also increases the stability of these dispersions.

TYPES OF NIOSOMES

Many types of niosomes are mentioned in the literature including discomes, proniosomes, niosomes reversed vesicles, and surfactant based ethosomes.

Proniosomes

Proniosomes are dry formulations of surfactant-coated carrier, which can be formulated out as needed on rehydrated by brief agitation in hot water. Being dry, they reduce problems associated with the physical stability of niosomes such as aggregation, fusion and leakage, in addition they offer the benefits in terms of transportation, distribution, storage and dosing. Stability of dry proniosomes is expected to be more than a premanufactured niosomal, formulation. In release studies, proniosomes appear to be equivalent to conventional niosomes. Size distributions of proniosome-derived niosomes are somewhat better than those of conventional niosomes, so the release performance in more critical cases turns out to be superior.

Proniosomes are dry powders, which make further processing and packaging possible. Further, the powder form provides optimal flexibility, unit dosing, in which the proniosome powder may be provided in capsule which could be cost effective and beneficial. Proniosomes, hydrated by agitation in an aqueous phase for a short period of time, offer a versatile vesicular delivery system with the potential for drug delivery via the transdermal route. This involves the topical application of proniosomes under occlusive conditions, during which they are converted to niosomes due to hydration by water from the skin itself. Compared to niosomes, a proniosome gel appeared to deliver estradiol efficiently through transdermal route. Similarly, a niosomal gel containing ketoprofen was therapeutically superior to a plain ketoprofen gel. Proniosomes allow the nebulized delivery of cromolyn sodium and provide enhanced controlled drug release and physical stability. A proniosome formulation based on maltodextrin was recently developed that has potential applications in the delivery of hydrophobic or amphiphilic drugs. The better of these formulations used a hollow particle with exceptionally high surface area. The main advantage with this formulation is the amount of carrier required to support the surfactant that could be easily adjusted and proniosomes with very high mass ratios of surfactant to carrier could be prepared.

Discomes

These are the large discoid structures, which exist under certain conditions of the phase diagram of nonionic surfactant vesicles. Ijeoma et al., observed these structures formed during niosomes due to mixed micelles transitions. The structures were noted to exist under certain conditions of phase diagram of niosomes prepared from a hexadecyl diglycerol ether (C16G2), cholesterol, and dicetylphosphate in the molar ratio 69:29:2 by mechanical disruption and sonication method (Uchegbu et al., 1992). Among the other phases, a unique phase termed as 'discome' phase was identified. The vesicles were incubated with polyoxyethylene cholesteryl ether and solulan C24 at 74°C. Turbidity measurements were made at 350 nm. A plot between turbidity and solulan C24 corresponding to change in the phase, was observed specially in regard to lamellar, micellar and discome phase existence. Dispersion in discome phase was noted to be comprised of larger disc like structures (volume distribution diameter 12–60 μm). Discomes were found to entrap water soluble solute effectively. Carboxy fluorescien (CF) aqueous volume entrapment 1.209 ± 0.97 L per mol of surfactant has been reported. From discomes, 50% of the entrapped CF was released in 24 hours when studied for diffusion study.

A C16G2-cholesterol ratio 7:3 favored the formation of discomes. Increasing concentration of cholesterol at and above the stated level, prior to challenge with solulan C24, suppressed the formation of discomes. The low molecular fraction of cholesterol in vesicular system prior to addition of solulan C24 facilitates the formation of discomes by lending bilayer, relatively more permeable to the solulan molecules. Thus, solubilization of niosomes by addition of solulan probably proceeds involving dispersion and surfactant bilayer phases, until a critical level of solulan in bilayer is reached with an eventual formation of discomes. Further, partitioning of solulan C24 beyond its critical phase concentration leads to the breakdown of discomes. Finally, solubilization of vesicles/discomes/aggregates is completed proceeding through mixed micellization.

Discomes differ from the bilayer sheets, which are formed during transition of vesicles to the micelles. The empty discomes incubated with CF for 1 hour, immediately prior to *in vitro* release measurement were noted to have no CF adsorbed on the surfaces. Dialysis of discome system was found not to affect their morphology. Discomes were found to be stable up to 6 months, when stored at 4°C. However, discomes dispersion exhibited a decrease in turbidity, when heated to 37°C indicating their instability. The large volume carrying capacity and minimal opacity of discomes lend them to be novel drug delivery system especially in ophthalmology. However, in order to stabilize discomes at 37°C, further formulation modification studies should be carried out. The nonuniform curvature of nonionic surfactant disc (discomes) could be related to heterogenous dispersion of disc components at molecular level. The same could be a possible explanation for C16G2 vesicles to micelles transition.

Discomes, in addition to their many advantages seem to have a special advantage in ocular administration, where in large size of discomes may prevent their drainage into the systemic pool as well as the 'disc' shape could provide for better fit in the culdesac of the eye. The use of discoidal niosomes for ocular delivery has been studied by Vyas et al. (1998). Timolol maleate, α-blocker used in the treatment of open-angle glaucoma was entrapped in discomes and their use as delivery system in the treatment of open-angle glaucoma was studied. Timolol maleate loaded discomes, were found to release the drug in a controlled fashion over a prolonged period of time. The change in intraocular pressure (IOP) was reported fast in discoidal formulation treated animals as compared to plain drug solution and niosomal timolol maleate treated animals.

Uchegbu and coworkers have reported the solubilization of the lipophilic tubulin inhibitor paclitaxel by using C16G2-cholesterol-solulan C24 in different ratios. This was the first report of its kind, where the solubilization of an extremely hydrophobic compound by C16G2 discomes has been reported. It has been well documented by Uchegbu et al. (1992), that heating of the formulations containing discomes (>35°C) resulted in loss of turbidity due to the transition from a discome phase that also contains spherical and tubular vesicles to a phase containing tubular and spherical vesicles and possibly mixed micelles. It is interesting to note that a change in the structure of the vesicles from discomes to mixed micelles was not accompanied by the precipitation of paclitaxel. This is likely due to the drug in the discome phase is solubilized in the bilayer(s), whereas it becomes solubilized in the hydrophobic core of the mixed micelles at higher temperature.

NSVs Reversed Vesicles

Reverse micelles and reverse emulsion, i.e. o/w and w/o are well known and accepted terms used in the expression of symmetrical pattern. One notable exception is reversed vesicles. Normal vesicles wherein close hydrocarbon compartments separating aqueous interior and exterior, were first described in 1964. These systems, as discussed earlier, also were resulted on the hydration of phospholipids as lamellar liquid crystals dispersed in aqueous phase. The literature on normal vesicular systems, i.e. liposomes and niosomes is abound, whereas reverse vesicle formation is recently reported by Kunieda et al. (1991).

Nonionic surfactant tetraethyleneglycol dodecylether (R12E-04), was dissolved in dodecane to form an isotropic solution. The binary system so constituted was free of any crystal structures. However, addition of small amount of water resulted into split of isotropic structures and as a consequence formation of liquid lamellar crystalline phase. The latter was found to be in equilibrium with an excess of oil phase. The system was noted to resemble a normal vesicular system in which addition of water widens the spacing between hydrocarbon segments. Reversed vesicles are formed spontaneously by hand shaking method on addition of an excess of oil phase. The system exhibited common characteristics of colloidal system, i.e. aggregation on storage or separation of phases. The effective surface of vesicles is with projecting hydrocarbon chain, thus, they are expected to have better barrier penetration efficiency. The potential of such a system in therapeutics is still to be explored and established.

Nonionic Surfactant Vesicle-in-water-in-oil (V/W/O) Systems

Modified versions of vesicular systems have always been the thought of researchers in order to explore their full potential as a drug delivery system. However, there are limitations due to the structural constraints on the formulation constituents of both amphiphile and oil phase.

A newer system employing the use of NSV is the vesicle-in-water-in-oil (V/W/O) system. The system has been patented by Albert and coworkers in the year 1992. The system and its potential as a drug delivery system has been studied exhaustively by Yoskioka et al. (Florence, 1993, Florence et al., 1996). Generally, vesicular systems are used as aqueous suspensions, but there are potential uses for systems in which the external phase is nonaqueous. V/W/O/ systems are those in which the aqueous suspensions of vesicles are dispersed in a continuous oil phase. This type of a system has been studied as a potential immunological adjuvant and as a drug delivery system (Florence et al., 1996). The system has a dual advantage of not only capable of encapsulating water-soluble and insoluble agents, but also the presence of an external nonaqueous barrier through which the encapsulated solute must diffuse.

The system is an emulsion prepared by dispersion of niosomes in water, followed by re-emulsification in oil using a surfactant mixture of low HLB to achieve a stable W/O emulsion. The resulting vesicle-in-water-in-oil system (V/W/O) (Fig. 18.11), is a close analogue of O/W/O emulsions and a concept to microsphers (S)-in-oil-in-water dispersions (S/O/W) (Yoshioko and Florence, 1994) or W/O/W multiple emulsions (Hasida et al., 1980). The major advantage of the system is the use of nonionic surfactant to form the vesicles (NSVs), which is also a component of the stabilizing system used for W/O emulsion. Thus, the migration of the stabilizing surfactant from the o/w interface to the W/O interface and vice versa is arrested thus W/O/W

multiple emulsion (Florence et al., 1989) related stability problem is effectively addressed.

Polymer-coated Nonionic Surfactant Vesicles

Nonionic surfactant vesicles are now being widely studied as an alternative to liposomes, as liposomes pose certain stability-related problems. In order to improve the stability of multilamellar vesicular systems, a novel method has been recently reported by us (Vyas and Venkatesan, 1999). The multilamellar vesicles were coated with poly(phthaloyl-L-lysine) the coating was affected by interfacial condensation polymerization technique using p-phthaloyl dichloride and L-lysine. The polymeric coat was brought about around each bilayer of the multilamellar vesicles. The polymer coated vesicles were found to be stable under various osmotic conditions and released the drug in a controlled fashion. The drug release rate was retarded compared to plain uncoated MLVs.

A similar report for increasing the vesicle stability of unilamellar vesicles was reported by us earlier (Venkatesan and Vyas, 1998). The method involved the use of butylcyanoacrylate to form a polymeric coat on individual discreate ULVs. The polymeric coat was brought about by a pH (5.8–5.5) change induced polymeization. The polymer-coated vesicles were found to be osmotically stable. Polymer-coated vesicles can be used to increase the stability of the vesicles both

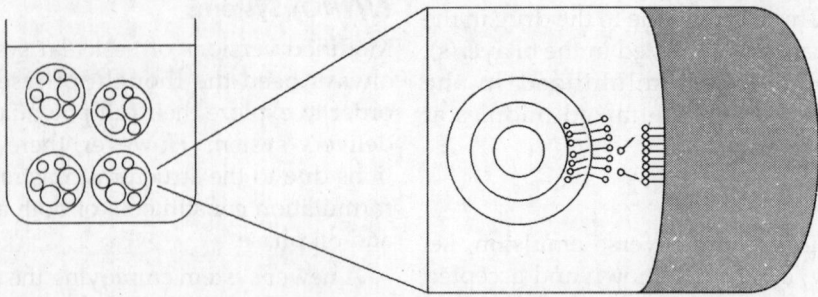

Fig. 18.11: Schematic representation of the V/W/O formulation

in vitro and *in vivo*. The system is further being studied for the triggered delivery of drugs from the vesicles.

Nonionic Surfactant-based Organogels

A novel nonionic organogel has been reported by Murdan and coworkers. A study on V/W/O with Span 60 showed that gelation of hexadecane at surfactant concentrations as low as 1% w/v occurred yielding a smooth white semi-solid gel. *In vitro* drug release studies have shown a controlled release of 5(6)-carboxyfluorescein from the V/W/O based organogel as compared to simple solution, NSVs and anhydrous organogel.

Elastic Niosomes

Elastic niosomes are composed of nonionic surfactants, ethanol, and water. They are superior to conventional niosomes because they enhance penetration of a drug through intact skin by passing through pores in the stratum corneum, which are smaller than the vesicles. In fact, their elasticity allows them to pass through channels that are less than one-tenth of their own diameter. Thus, they can deliver drugs or compounds of both low and high molecular weight. Furthermore, they can provide prolonged action and demonstrate superior biological activity compared to conventional niosomes. The transport of these elastic vesicles is concentration independent and driven by transepidermal hydration.

APPLICATIONS OF NIOSOMES

Niosomes for the Treatment of Leishmaniasis

Niosomes with desirable release profile and stability characteristics can be prepared by tailoring surfactant chemically or via bilayer composition modification. NSVs bearing stilbogluconate an antileishmaniasis agent has been found to be suitable for organ-specific drug delivery. Niosomes were found as effective as liposomes in delivery of loaded drug in experimental leishmaniasis. For drug that has high aqueous solubility, it was assumed that the drug is entrapped in aqueous space of the vesicles. The ability of these aqueous compartments to accommodate and retain the drug, may be a limiting factor of vesicular systems. It was further noticed that chemical characteristics of vesicular components are not of much importance as far as parasite hit or antileishmaniasis activity is concerned. This may be assumed to be attributed to the passive delivery of vesicle and the contents through RES recognition and uptake.

Niosomes in Oncology

Investigations have been carried out with niosomes containing anticancer drugs such as methotrexate, adriamycin, doxorubicin etc. NSVs containing methotrexate exhibited an effect comparable to its liposomal counterpart. Much more consistent plasma levels were obtained, however, methotrexate levels in liver of mice were significantly higher. The study thus suggested that MTX contained in NSVs could be useful in maintaining the blood MTX levels after intravenous administration. Moreover, the administration of MTX in niosomes, minimizes the side effects significantly (Azmin et al., 1985). It was observed that in Span(s) with increased lipophilicity, entrapment efficiency increased. Unilamellar vesicles prepared using Span 80 showed maximum entrapment as well as improved antitumor activity.

The plasma doxorubicin levels were considerably prolonged confirming sustained release characteristics of niosomal preparation. Negligible accumulation of doxorubicin was recorded in liver. Cholesterol free niosomes were generally found to be more effective as the reduced cardiac level or accumulation of drug was noted following their administration.

Treatment of HIV-AIDS

Zidovudine is commonly used to treat patients with AIDS, but is limited by its toxicity and low potency. A noisome formulation may overcome these drawbacks. Zidovudine-loaded niosomes would provide sustained delivery of drug for a more effective AIDS therapy, however it is required that such anticipated potentials, should properly be evaluated.

Pulmonary Delivery

Inhalation therapy is frequently used in asthmatic patients, but is limited by poor permeation of drug through hydrophilic mucus. To overcome this, polysorbate 20 niosomes containing beclomethasone dipropionate, were developed for pulmonary delivery to patients with chronic obstructive pulmonary disease. The niosomes provided sustained and targeted delivery, improved mucus permeation and therapeutic effect as well.

Protein and Peptide Delivery

The delivery of proteins to the systemic circulation after their oral administration is hindered by numerous barriers including proteolytic enzymes, pH gradients and low epithelial permeability. The oral administration of recombinant human insulin in a niosomal formulation was demonstrated in a study involving niosomes based on poly-oxyethylene alkyl ethers. Similarly, vasoactive intestinal peptide (VIP) has been successfully delivered across blood brain barrier through glucose appended niosomes.

Niosomes as Immunological Adjuvant

The ability of niosomes to enhance antibody production in response to bovine serum albumin (BSA) was compared with Freund's complete adjuvant (FCA) in the BALB/c mouse. The adjuvant activity of NSVs was found to be dependent on the BSA entrapped within the preformed vesicles. Analysis of the anti-BSA IgG subclasses induced by NSVs and FCA showed that NSVs are relatively better stimulant of IgG2 than FCA, whereas for IgG1 it was found to be a poorer stimulator. Thus, NSVs were realized as potentially better stimulant for Th1 lymphocyte subset than

FCA and thus by inference, potent stimulator of cellular immunity. The NSVs were believed to be potentially advantageous adjuvant in terms of immunological selectivity, low toxicity and stability (Brawer and Alexender, 1992).

Carrier for Hemoglobin

Hemoglobin carrying niosomes were prepared and studied for functional and physical properties. Hemoglobin niosomes were prepared using Oreal's synthetic lipids by reverse phase evaporation method. The niosomes were unilamellar and were found to be permeable to oxygen, with hemoglobin diffusion/release profile modifiable quite closer to nonencapsulated hemoglobin. Moser et al., (1980) carried out study on niosomal hemoglobin for its compatibility and interaction with blood. It was concluded that agglutination with erythrocytes was dispersible on shaking. Albumin and eventually transferrin were found to adsorb on the surface, however, caused no destabilization of niosomes. With regard to coagulation, insignificant effect of niosomes on prothrombin time and coagulation was recorded. However, extended clotting time was noted, which was considered essentially a consequence of blood dilution. Cellular oxygen consumption, oxygenated metabolite gentration and oxidase activity, were nonresponsive to the contained electric charge on the niosomes.

Niosomes Surfactants and Oral Drug Delivery

Peptidal ergot alkaloids are poorly absorbed on oral administration. The partial intestinal absorption of the alkaloids was increased significantly, when administered in bile duct cannulated rats as micellar solution together with POE-24-cholesteryl ether. *In vitro* diffusion studies suggested that diffusion of ergot alkaloids across the mucous barrier is facilitated by their micellar entrapment.

Yoshida et al., (1992) studied the potential of niosomal carrier system in oral delivery of peptide drugs. The absorption of 9-desglycinamide-8-arginine vasopressin (DGAVP) entrapped in $C_{12}EO_3$, was determined. The absorption studies were conducted *in vitro*. The stability of DGAVP was increased significantly in mucosal fluid on incorporation into the niosomes. No substantial difference between the absorptions of DGAVP was recorded. Thus, the possible penetration enhancing effect of surfactants was excluded. An entirely different in serosal concentration profile of DGAVP was recorded, when niosome encapsulated DGAVP was adminsitered. The increased concentration of DGAVP found in acceptor phase was apparently assumed to be due to the protection of DGAVP against intestinal degradation. Another explanation proposed was the absorption and translocation of the vesicluar system intact into the systemic circulation. The actual mechanism which brings about an enhanced absorption of niosomal DGAVP is still to be explored. Nevertheless, niosomes have great potential as carrier system in safe and successful delivery of peptoidal drugs, however extended studies to define toxicological behavior and *in vivo* performance are desired before they can become clinical reality.

Niosomes for Transdermal Drug Delivery

Niosomes appear to have application in topical and transdermal products both containing hydrophobic and hydrophilic drugs. Besides, niosomes have also been used to encapsulate, lidocaine (Vanhal et al., 1996), estradiol (Vanhal et al., 1996), cyclosporin (Dowton et al., 1993), erythromycin (Jayaraman et al., 1996), alpha-interferon (Niemac et al., 1995), plasmid DNA for the human interleukin-1 receptor (Niemic et al., 1997) for topical and trnasdermal delivery.

Junginger et al., 1991 have observed small (100 nm) vesicular structures between the first and second layer of human corncecytes 48 hours after incubation with niosomes prepared from dodecyl alcohol polyoxyethylene ether and cholesterol. Penetration by niosomes of this upper layer appears plausible as these layers are only loosely packed. However, the same study reports the presence of vesicular structures in the deeper seemingly inaccessible areas of the skin and concluded that there was a recognisation of the niosome membrane into individual monomers which on arriving at these deeper layers reformed into niosomes (Junginger et al., 1991). Vanhal et al., 1996 have performed *in vitro* studies on the transdermal penetration of estradiol using high phase transition sucrose-ester-based niosomes or $C_{18}EO_7$ niosomes and low phase transition $C_{12}EO_7$ niosomes. They found that $C_{12}EO_7$ niosomes are better transdermal carriers. The higher flexibility of these bilayers is said to be responsible for improved transdermal penetration. Reducing the cholesterol content of these niosomes cold increase the transdermal delivery of oestradiol.

The intercellular route is the main route of vesicle penetration across the skin (Schatzlein and Ceve, 1993; Schatzlein and Ceve, 1998, Kuijk-Meuwissen et al., 1998). Ultrafexible vesicles penetrate along irregularties between the intercellular lipid lamellae and adjacent corneocytes envelops (Fig. 18.12). The combination of molecules with suitably differing molecular shapes (Fig. 18.13) can render a membrane flexible. The flexible membrane accommodates stress-induced curvature changes and the vesicle changes the shape easily. Consequently, such vesicles require significantly less (deformation) energy to pass through small pores than rigid membranes. Sufficiently elastic vesicles can penetrate into deeper layers, but the rigid vesicles remain restricted to the loosely packed upper layers.

Niosomes and Diagnostic Imaging

Niosomes can also be used for diagnostic purposes. Korkmaz et al., 2000 formulated DTPA carrying niosomes (hexadecyl triglycerol ether-chol-DTPA 10:1:4) to study the *in vitro* release, radiolabeling act as carrier for radiopharmaceuticals and may be used specifically for spleen and liver imaging.

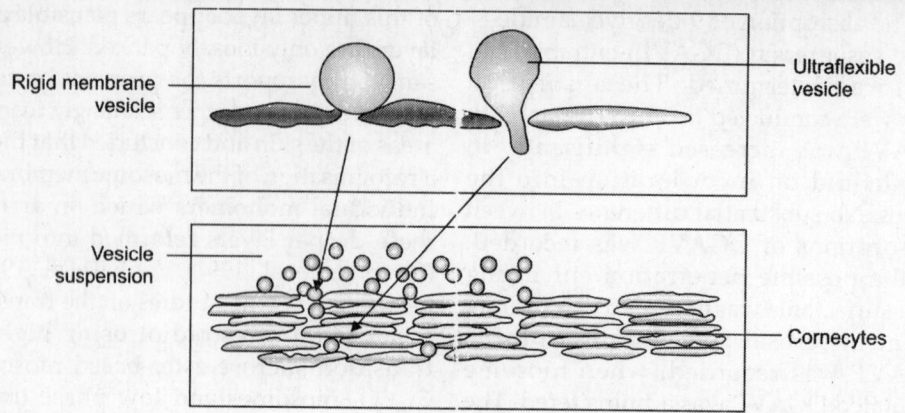

Fig.18.12: Schematic representation of vesicle penetration across the skin via intracellular route

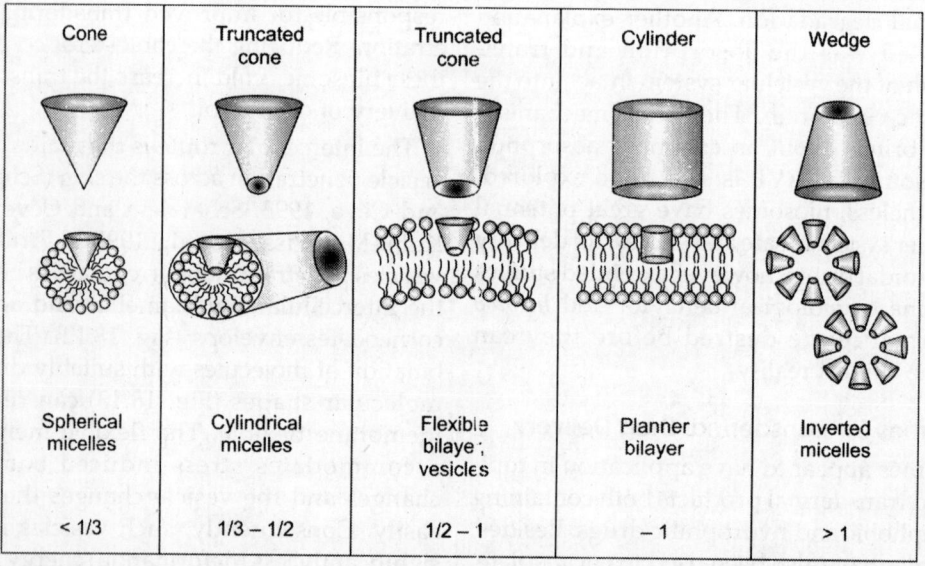

Fig.18.13: Schematic representation of the effective molecular shapes of amphiphiles and the resulting aggregates. The shape of molecule will be determined by the ratio of chain volume to head group

SUGGESTED READINGS

1. Assadullahi TP, Hidler RC and McAuley AJ, *Biochim. Biophys. Acta* 1083, 1991, 271.

2. Azmin MN, Florence AT, Handjani-Vila RM, Stuart JFB, Vanlerberghe G and Whittaker JS, *J. Pharm. Pharmacol.* 37, 1985, 237.

3. Azmin MN, Florence AT, Handjani-Vila RM, Stuart JFB, Vanlerberghe G and Whittaker JS, *J. Pharm. Pharmacol.* 37, 1985, 237–42.

4. Baillie AJ, Coombs GH, Dolan TF and Laurie J, *J. Pharm. Pharmacol.* 38, 1986, 502–505.

5. Baillie AJ, Florence AT, Hume LR, Murihead GT and Rogerson A, *J. Pharm. Pharmacol.* 37, 1985, 863.

6. Bowstra JA, Hofland HEJ, Spies F, Ponec M, Verhoef C and Junginger HE, *Proc. Int. Symp. Control. Rel. Bioact. Mater.* 17, 1990, p 395.

7. Cable C and Florence AT, *J. Pharm. Pharmacol.* 40, 1988, 30P.

8. Cable C Ph.D. Thesis, University of Strathclyde, Glasgow, 1989.

9. Carter KC, Baillie AJ, Alexander J and Dolan TF, *J. Pharm. Pharmacol.* 40, 1987, 370–73.

10. Chabner BA, Allegra CJ, Curt GA and Calabresi, P Antineoplastic agents. In: Goodman and Gilman's The Pharmacological Basis of Therapeutics, ninth edition, 1996, pp. 1265.

11. Chandraprakash KS, Udupa N, Umadevi P and Pillai GK, *Int. J. Pharm.* 61, 1990, R1.

12. Chandraprakash KS, Udupa N, Umadevi P and Pillai GK, *J. Drug. Target.* 1, 1994, 143.

13. Chauhan S and Lawrence MJ, *J. Pharm. Pharmacol.* 41, 1989, pp. 6.

14. Cullis PR, Hope MJ, Bally MB, Madden TM, Mayer LD and Janoff AS In: Ostro MJ (Ed.) Liposomes from Biophysics to Therapeutics, Marcell Dekker, Inc. New York, 1987, pp. 39.

15. Dowton SM, et al., STP Pharma Sciences, 3(5) 1993, 404–407.

16. Duncan R Anti Cancer Drugs 3, 1992, 175–210.

17. Duncan R, Bhakoo M, Riley ML and Tuboku-Metzger A. Soluble polymeric drug carriers: haematocompatibility In: Gomez-Fernandez JC, Chapman D and Packer L (Eds.) Progress in Membrane Biotechnology, Birkhauser Verlag, Basel, 1991, pp. 253–65.

18. Florence AT Non-ionic surfactant vesicles: preparation and characterization. In: Liposome Technology, Vol. II. 2nd ed., Gredoriadis, G. (Ed.), CRC Press, Boca Raton, FL, 1993, 157.

19. Florence AT, Attwood D, Physicochemical Principles of Pharmacy (2nd ed.), Macmillan, London, 1988.

20. Florence AT, Cable C, Cassidy J and Kaye SB In: Gregoriadis G (Ed.), Targeting of Drugs, Plenum Press, New York, 1990, pp. 117.

21. Florence AT, Cable C, Cassidy J and Kaye SB Non-ionic surfactant vesicles as carriers of doxorubicin In: Targeting of Drugs, Fregoriadis, G, Allison AC and Poste G (Eds.), Plenum Pres, New York, 1990, pp. 117–26.

22. Florence AT, Omotosho JA and Whateley TL Multiple w/o/w emulsions as drug vehicles. In: Controlled Release from Drug Polymers and Aggregate Systems, Rosoff, M (Ed.), VCH, New York, 1989.

23. Gebicki JM and Hicks M, *Chem. Phys. Lipids* 16, 1976, 142.

24. Griener J, Reiss JG, Vierlungin P. In: Filler R, Kobayashi Y and Yagopolskii LM (Eds.) *Organofluorine Compounds in Medicinal Chemistry and Biomedical Applications.* Elsevier, Amsterdam, 1993, pp. 339.

25. Guedj G, Pucci B, Zarif L, Coulomb C, Riess JG and Pavia, A. *Chem. Phys. Lip.* 172, 1994, 153.

26. lGuo LSS, Fielding RM, Lasic DD, Hamilton RL and Mufson D, *Int. J. Pharm.* 75, 1991, 45.

27. Handjani-Vila RM, Ribier A and Vanlerberghe, G Liposomes in the cosmetics industry In: Liposome Technology, Gregoriadis, G (Ed.), CRC Press, Boca Raton, 1993, pp. 201–13.

28. Handjani-Vila RM, Ribier A, Rondot B and Vanlerberghe G, *Int. J. Cosmetic Sci.* 1, 1979, 306–314.

29. Haran G, Coben R, Bar LK and Barenholz Y. Biochim. Biophys. Acta 1151, 1993, 201.

30. Haran G, Cohen R, Bar LK, Barenholz Y, Biochim. Biophys. Acta 1151, 1993, 201–215.

31. Harrigan PR, Wong KF, Redelmeier TE, Wheeler JJ and Cullis PR, *Biochim. Biophys. Acta* 1149, 1993, 329.

32. Hashida M, Liao MH, Muranishi S and Sezaki H, *Chem. Pharm. Bull.* 28, 1980, 1659.

33. Hillis LR, Handly JD and Babbitt BP, Utilization of contact sensitive liposome formulations in membrane lytic homogenous immunoassays. In: Liposome Technology. Vol. III, 2nd ed., Gregoriadis, G. (Ed.) CRC Press, Boca Raton, FL, 1993, 301.

34. Hofland HEJ, Bouwstra JA, Verhoef JC, Buckton G, Chowdry, BZ, Ponec M and Junginger HE, *J. Pharm. Pharmacol.* 44, 1992, 287.

35. Israelachvili, J. Intermolecular and Surface Forces. Academic Press, London, 1992.

36. Jayaraman CS et al., *J. Pharm. Sci.,* 85(10) 1996, 1082–4.

37. Kato Y, Hosokawa T, Okubo Y, Hayakawa and Ito K, *Biol. Pharm. Bull.* 16, 1993, 965.

38. Kerr D, Rogerson A, Morrison GJ, Florence AT and Kaye SN, *Br. J. Cancer* 58, 1988, 432–6.

39. Kiwada H, Nakajima I, Matsuura H, Tsuji M and Kato Y, *Chem. Pharm. Bull.* 36, 1988, 1841.

40. Kiwada H, Nimura H and Kato Y, *Chem. Pharm. Bull.* 33, 1985, 2475.

41. Kiwada H, Nimura H, Fujisaki Y, Yamada S and Kato Y, *Chem. Pharm. Bull.* 33, 1985, 753.

42. Koklic T, Trancar J (2012), *BMC Res Notes,* 5(1), 179.

43. Kong F, Zhou F, Ge L, Liu X, Wang Y (2012), *Int. J. Nanomedicine,* 7, 1079–89.

44. Kronberg B, Dahlman A, Carlfors J, Karlsson J and Artusson P, *J. Pharm. Sci.* 79, 1990, 667.

45. Mezei M, Liposomes and the skin. In: Liposomes in Drug Delivery, Gregoriadis G, Florence, AT and Patel HM (Eds.) Harwood, Amsterdam, 1993, 125.

46. Mokhtarieh AA, Cheong S, Kim S, Chung BH, Lee MK (2012), *Biochim Biophys Acta*. [Epub ahead of print]

47. Montero MT, Marti A and Hernandez-Borrel, *J. Int. J. Pharm.* 96, 1993, 157.

48. Mosgoeller W, Prassl R, Zimmer A (2012), *Methods Enzymol*, 508, 325–54.

49. Murtas E, Carafa M, Riccierei E, Santucci E and Alhaique, F. Proc. Int. Symp. Control. Rel. Bioact. Mater. 21, 1994, pp. 857.

50. N Venkatesan and SP Vyas, Polymer coated vesicles: Development and characterization, Drug Delivery 1998: 5(4); 251–5.

51. Neumann R and Ringsdor H, *J. Am. Chem. Soc.* 108, 1986, 487.

52. Niemac S, et al., *Pharmaceutical research* 12(8) 1995, 1184–8.

53. Niemic SM et al., *J. Pharm. Sci.* 86 (60) 1997, 701–707.

54. Niemiec SM, Hu Z, Ramachandran C, Wallach, DFH and Weiner N, *STA Pharm. Sci.* 4, 1994, 145.

55. Okahata Y, Tanamachi S, Nagai M and Kunitake, T, *J. Colloid Interface Sci.* 82, 1981, 401.

56. Omotosho JA, Law TK, Whateley TL and Florence AT Colloids Surf. 20, 1986, 133.

57. Parthasarathi G, Udupa N, Umadevi P and Pillai GK, *J. Drug. Target*. 2, 1994, 173.

58. Pimm MV, Perkins AC, Strohalm J, Ulbrich K and Duncan R, *J. Drug Target*. 3, 1996, 375–83.

59. Pippa N, Pispas S, Demetzos C (2012), *Int. J. Pharm. Apr 1*. [Epub ahead of print]

60. Puglia C, Bonina F (2012), *Expert Opin Drug Deliv,* 9(4); 429–41.

61. Quer CB, Elsharkawy A, Romeijn S, Kros A, Jiskoot W (2012), *Eur J Pharm Biopharm*. [Epub ahead of print]

62. Raja Naresh RA, Singh UV, Udupa N and Pillai GK Indian Drugs 30, 1994, 275.

63. Riber A, Handjani-Vila, RM, Bardez E and Valeur B, *Colloids Surfaces* 10, 1984, 155.

64. Rogerson A, Cummings J, Willmott N and Florence AT, *J. Pharm. Pharmacol*. 40, 1988, 337–42.

65. SP Vyas and N Venkatesan, Poly (phthaloyl-L-lysine)-coated multilamellar vesicles for controlled drug delivery: in vitro and in vivo performance evaluation, Pharm. Acta Helv. 1999: 74; 51–8.

66. SP Vyas, N Mysore, V Jaitely and N Venkatesan, Discoidal niosome based controlled ocular delivery of timolol maleate. Die Pharmazie 1998: 53(7); 466–9.

67. Seymour LW, Ulbrich K, Strohalm J, Kopecek J and Duncan R, *Biochem Pharmacol*. 39, 1990, 1125–31.

68. Stafford S, Baillie AJ and Florence AT, *J. Pharm. Pharmacol* 40, 1988, 26P.

69. Tanaka M, Fukuda H and Horiuchi T, *J. Am. Oil Chem. Soc.* 67, 1990, 55.11.

70. Tohamy AA, Abdel Azeem, AA, Shafaa MW, Mahmoud WS (2012), *Gen Physiol Biophys.,* 31(1), 85–91.

71. Uchegbu IF Ph.D. Thesis, School of Pharmacy, University of London, 1994.

72. Uchegbu IF, Bouwstra JA, Florence AT, *J. Phys. Chem.* 96, 1992, 10548.

73. Uchegbu IF, Double JA, Kelland LR, Turton JA and Florence AT, *J. Drug Target.*

74. Uchegbu IF, Double JA, Kelland LR, Turton JA and Florence AT, *J. Drug Target.* 3, 1996, 399–409.

75. Uchegbu IF, Double JA, Turton JA and Florence AT, *Pharm. Res.* 12 (7), 1995, 1019–1024.

76. Uchegbu IF, Florence, A.T. Adv. Colloid Interface Sci. 58, 1995, 1–55.

77. Uchegbu IF, Gianasi E, Cociancich F, Florence AT and Duncan R, *Proc. Int. Symp. Control. Release Bioact. Mater.* 23, 1996, 182–3.

78. Uchegbu IF, McCarthy D, Schatzlein A and Florence AT, *S.T.P. Pharma Sci.* 6(1), 1996, 33–43.

79. Uchegbu IF, Ringsdorf H and Duncan R, *Proc. Int. Symp. Control. Release Bioact. Mater.* 23, 1996, 791–792.

80. Uchegbu IF, Turton JA, Double JA, Florence AT, *Biopharm. Drug Dispos.* 15, 1994, 691–707.

81. Udupa N, Chandraprakash KS, Umadevi P and Pillai GK, *Drug Develop. Ind. Pharm.* 19, 1993, 1331.

82. Van Hal DA, Ph.D. Thesis, Leiden University, Leiden; 1994.

83. Van Hal, DA, et al., *STP Pharma Sciences*, 6(1) 1996, 72–8.

84. Van Hat, DA et al., *European J. Pharm. Sci.*, 4 (1996), 147–57.

85. Vanlerberghe G, Handjani-Vila RM, Berthelot C, and Sebag, H. In: Chemie Physikalische Chemie and Anwendungstechnik der Grenzflachenaktiven Stoffe. Carl Hanser Verlag, Munchen, 1972, pp. 139.

86. Vemuri S, Yu CD, Wangsatorntanakun V and Roosdorp N, *Drug Devel. Ind. Pharm.* 16, 1990, 2243.

87. Walter A, Vinson PK, Kaplun A and Talmon Y, *Biophys. J.* 60, 1991, 1315.

88. Wang J, Chen J, Ye, N, Luo, Z, Lai, W, Cai, X, Lin, Y. (2012), *Curr Drug Metab.* [Epub ahead of print]

89. Yang FY, Teng MC, Lu M, Liang HF, Lee YR, Yen CC, Liang ML, Wong TT (2012), *Int J Nanomedicine.* 7, 965–74.

90. Yoshika T, Gursel M, Skalko N, Gregoriadis G and Florence AT, *J. Drug. Target.* 2, 1995, 533.

91. Yoshioka T and Florence AT, *Int. J. Pharm.* 108, 1994, 117.

92. Yoshioka T, Sternberg B and Florence AT, *Int. J. Pharm.* 105, 1994, 1.

93. Yoshioko T and Florence AT, *Int. J. Pharm.* 108, 1994, 117–23.

94. Zarif L, Gulik-Krzywicki T, Reiss JG, Pucci B, Guedj C and Pavia A, *Colloids Surfaces* 84, 1993, 107.

19

Solid Lipid Nanoparticles

INTRODUCTION

Solid lipid nanoparticles (SLNs) have attracted increasing scientific and commercial attention as novel colloidal drug carrier for intravenous applications as they have been proposed as an alternative putative particulate carrier system. SLNs were introduced at the beginning of the 1990s; they are basically submicron size colloidal carriers (50–1000 nm) usable for controlled drug delivery. They are composed of physiological lipids (like glycerides of body's fatty acids assure high biocompatibility and biodegradability), dispersed in water or in an aqueous surfactant solution. SLNs as colloidal drug carriers interestingly combine advantages of polymeric nanoparticles, fat emulsions and liposomes simultaneously, address some of their disadvantages. The main features of SLNs include, excellent physical stability, protection of incorporated labile drugs from degradation, controlled drug release (fast or sustained), good tolerability and site-specific targeting. A distinctive advantage of SLNs over polymeric nanoparticles is that the lipid matrix is consisted of physiological lipids, which eliminate the danger of acute and chronic toxicity. In comparison to other particulate carriers, SLNs possess some added benefits as drug delivery system, such as a good biocompatibility and biodegradation. Furthermore, SLNs can be used as a carrier system for both hydrophobic and hydrophilic drugs. Nevertheless, potential disadvantages, such as insufficient loading capacity, drug expulsion after polymorphic transition during storage and relatively high water content of the dispersions (70–99.9%) have been observed. SLNs formulations for various routes of application (parenteral, oral, dermal, ocular, pulmonar, rectal) have been developed and thoroughly characterized *in vitro* and *in vivo* (Fig. 19.1). A product based on SLNs has recently been introduced to the polish market (nanobase, Yamanouchi) as a topical moisturizer.

This chapter highlights the main features of SLNs, including the concept of SLNs, methods of production, and their applications. Furthermore, special emphasis has been paid to the drug incorporation and effect of the heterogeneity of the lipid particle, and the presence of other colloidal species.

ADVANTAGES OF SLNS AS ALTERNATIVE PARTICULATE CARRIER

Some distinctive advantages of SLNs are as below:

- Small size and relatively narrow size distribution provides possibilities for extravasations and hence practical opportunities for site-specific drug delivery.

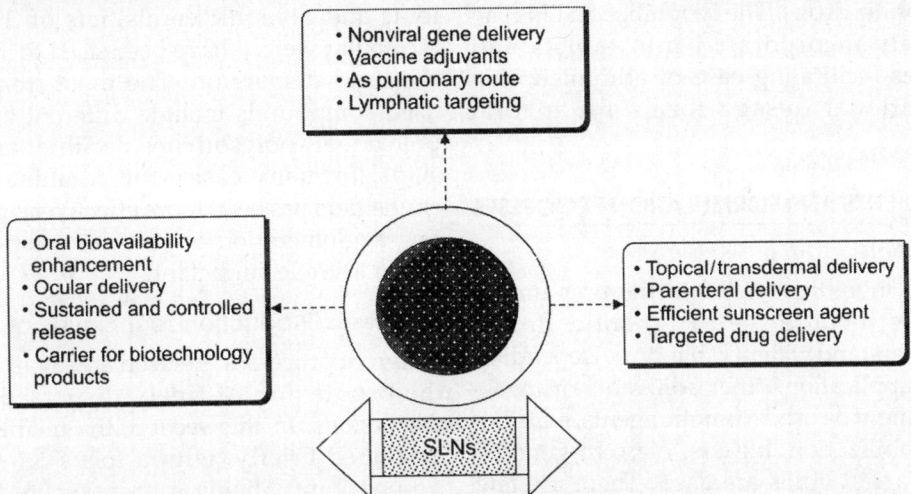

Fig. 19.1: Application of SLNs in various fields of drug/DNA delivery and immunization

- Controlled release of active drug over a long period can be achieved.
- Protection of incorporated drug against bio or biochemical degradation.
- Possible sterilization by conventional methods, i.e. autoclaving or gamma irradiation.
- SLNs can be lyophilized as well as spray dried.
- No toxic metabolites are produced.
- Possible avoidance of use of organic solvents.
- Relatively cheaper and stable.
- Ease of industrial production by hot dispersion technique.
- Incorporation of drug can reduce distinct side effects of drug, e.g. thrombophlebitis that are associated with IV injection of diazepam or etomidate.
- Surface modification can easily be accomplished and hence can be used for site-specific drug delivery.

SLNS VERSUS OTHER COLLOIDAL DRUG CARRIERS

SLNs have been proven to be a better alternative as drug carrier in comparison to conventional O/W emulsion if a prolonged release or protection of drug against chemical degradation is required. Incorporation of the drug into the solid lipid matrix might surely offer a better protection that can be achieved in the oily internal phase of emulsion and liposomes. Prolonged drug release from emulsions does not appear to be feasible, while it can be successfully achieved to an extent using SLNs. Compared to polymeric nanoparticles; the SLNs possess some genuine therapeutic advantages. Apart from the lower cytotoxicity, due to the absence of solvents in the production process, and a relatively low cost for the excipients the major advantage relates to the large-scale production that is possible by using the simple process of high-pressure homogenization. Such equipments are already available for pharmaceutical industry and commonly used for the production of emulsions. Compared to liposomes, the SLNs offer the advantage of offering better protection to drug against chemical degradation, as there is no access of water into the inner core of lipid particles. Depending on the nature of drug, a higher payload could be achieved. SLNs may represent an effective and viable option for resolving these problems owing to their better stability and significant loading capacity for both lipophilic and hydrophilic drugs. The lyophilized SLNs can be easily incorporated into tablets and capsules facilitating ease of administration conventional dosage forms for in oral route.

INGREDIENTS AND FORMULATION PROCESSES

Ingredients

General ingredients used in the preparation of SLNs include the drug, solid lipids, emulsifiers, and water (Table 19.1). Depending on the application, other adjuvants or ingredients might be used (osmotic agents, matrices for lyophilization, buffers, etc.). In general, physiological lipids are used. There are few exceptions, such as amphiphilic calixarenes. The term 'lipid' is generally used in a very broad sense and includes triglycerides (e.g. tristearin), partial glycerides (e.g. monostearate), fatty acids (e.g. stearic acid), steroids (e.g. cholesterol), and waxes (e.g. cetyl palmitate). More attention should be given to the physicochemical properties of the lipid and accordingly, they may be classified on the basis of their interactions with water. The choice of emulsifier depends on the route of administration, especially more limited to parenteral administrations. A large variety of ionic and nonionic emulsifiers of different molecular weight have been used to stabilize the lipid dispersion. The most frequently used compounds include different kinds of poloxamer, polysorbates, lecithin, and bile acids. In many cases, the combination of emulsifiers has been more effective in preventing agglomeration of particles compared to use of a single surfactant.

Processes/Production Techniques of SLNs

Different processes are used and available for the production of finely dispersed SLNs dispersions. In this section, the methods are described briefly, with a focus on scaling up possibility, being a prerequisite for the introduction of a product to the market. To manufacture SLNs, the hot high-pressure homogenization above the melting point of the lipid and subsequent nanomerization is recommended (melt emulsification). However, the cold high-pressure homogenization (high pressure milling of lipid suspensions) for thermolabile drugs is preferred and used. Other production methods for SLNs including the production from microemulsions, the precipitation and dispersion by using ultrasonication yield product with varied particle size distribution.

Table 19.1: List of lipids used for the preparation of SLNs

Triglycerides	Hard fat types	Emulsifiers/coemulsifiers
Trilaurin	Witepsol® (available in different grades	Soybean lecithin
Tristearin	W35, H35, H42 and E85)	Egg lecithin
Trimyristin	Glyceryl monostearate	Phosphatidylcholine
Tripalmitin	Glyceryl palmitostearate	Poloxamer 188
Tribehenin	Cetyl palmitate	Poloxamer 407
Hydrogenated coco-glycerides	Stearic acid	Poloxamer 908
(SoftisanÒ 142)	Palmitic acid	Tyloxapole
	Decanoic acid	Polysorbate 20
	Behenic acid	Polysorbate 60
	Acidan N12	Polysorbate 80
	Sodium cholate	Sodium glycocholate
		Sodium cholate
		Taurocholic acid, taurodeoxycholic acid
		Butanol

High-pressure Homogenization

High pressure homogenization (HPH) has emerged as a reliable and powerful technique for the preparation of SLNs. High-pressure homogenizers push a liquid with high pressure (10 to 200 MPa) through a narrow gap (in the range of few microns). The fluid accelerates on a very short distance to very high velocity (over 1000 km/h). Excessively, high-shear forces disrupt the particles down to the submicron range. Typical lipid contents ranges between 5% to 10% of the fluid and creates no problem in the homogenization. Even lipid concentrations up to 40% can be homogenized to lipid nanodispersions. Two general approaches of the homogenization, viz. the hot and the cold homogenization techniques, can be used for the production of SLNs. In both cases, a preparatory step involves incorporating the drug into the bulk lipid by dissolving or dispersing the drug in the lipid melt solution (Fig 19.2).

Hot Homogenization Technique

The hot homogenization technique schematically shown in Fig. 19.3, can be applied to lipophilic and insoluble drugs. Even many heat sensitive drugs can be processed because the exposure time to high temperatures is relatively short. Hot homogenization is carried out at temperatures above the melting point of the lipid and can therefore be regarded as an equivalent of the homogenization of an emulsion. A pre-emulsion of the drug-loaded lipid melt and the aqueous emulsifier phase (same temperature) is obtained by a high-shear mixing device (Ultra-Turrax). The quality of the pre-emulsion affects the quality of the final product to a large extent, where droplets in the size range of a few micrometers are desirable. The primary product of the hot homogenization is a nanoemulsion resulting from the liquid state of the lipid. Solid particles are expected to be formed on cooling of the dispersion to room temperature or below. Because of the small particle size and the presence of the emulsifiers, lipid crystallization may be effectively retarded, and the sample may remain as a supercooled melt (nanoemulsion) for several months. The technique is found, however unsuitable for loading of hydrophilic drugs into SLNs because of higher partition of drug in water that occurs during homogenization and resulting into low drug(s) entrapment efficiency.

Cold Homogenization Technique

For hydrophilic drug, the cold homogenization technique is the method of choice (Fig. 19.3). The first preparatory step is the same as used in the hot homogenization procedure and includes the solubilization or dispersion of the

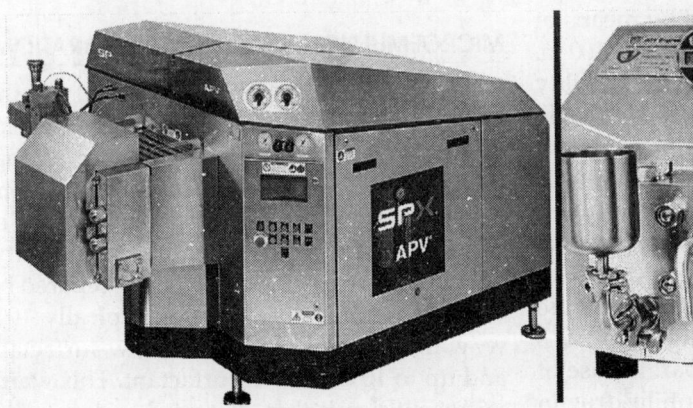
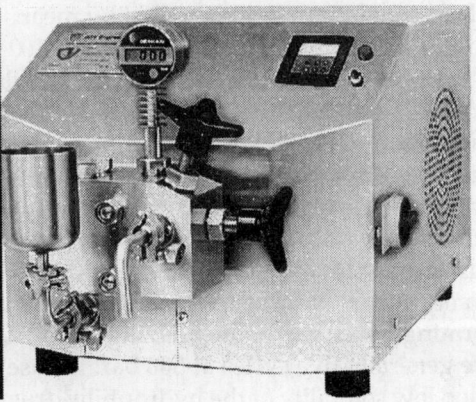

Fig. 19.2: Photographs showing various homogenizers

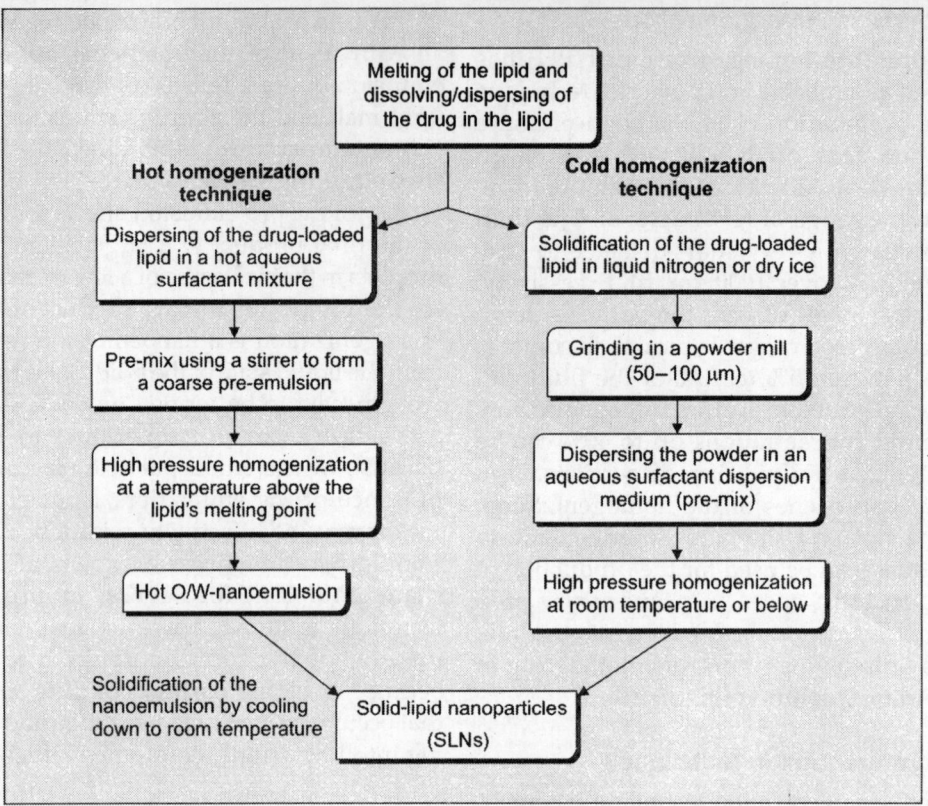

Fig. 19.3: Schematic procedure of hot and cold homogenization techniques for SLNs production

drug in the melt of the bulk lipid. The drug-containing melt is cooled rapidly (e.g. by means of dry ice or liquid nitrogen). The high cooling rate favors a homogenous distribution of the drug within the lipid matrix. The solid (drug-containing) lipid is milled by means of ball or mortar milling in the range of 50–100 m. The lower temperatures increase the fragility of the lipid and, therefore, favor particle disruption. The solid lipid microparticles are dispersed in a chilled emulsifier solution. A presuspension is formed by high speed stirring of the particles in a cold aqueous surfactant solution. This presuspension is then homogenized at or below room temperature forming SLNs; the homogenizing conditions are generally five cycles at 500 bar. In case of a too low solubility of the hydrophilic drug in the melted lipid, surfactants can be used for

solubilization of the drug. This homogenization technique avoids and minimizes melting process of lipid and appears to be a most suitable option for thermosensitive and thermolabile drugs.

MICROEMULSION-BASED SLNS PREPARATIONS

SLNs preparations that are based on the dilution of microemulsions have been developed by Gasco. It should be mentioned that there are different definitions and opinions proposed to the structure and dynamics of microemulsion in the scientific community. Firstly, a warm microemulsion is prepared by stirring, a mixture containing typically 10% w/w molten solid lipid, 15% w/w surfactant and up to 10% w/w cosurfactant. This warm microemulsion is then dispersed under stirring in an excess of cold water (typical ratio 1:50) using an especially developed thermostated syringe. Addition of the microemulsion to the water results into the precipitation of the lipid phase forming fine particles (Fig. 19.4). The excess water is removed either by ultra-filtration or by lyophilization in order to increase the particles population. The effects of experimental factors, such as microemulsion composition, dispersing device, temperature and lyophilization on size and structure of the obtained SLNs have been studied intensively. It is observed critically, that the removal of excess of water from the prepared SLNs dispersion is a difficult step, since it drastically affects the particle size of formed product. Also, high concentrations of surfactants and cosurfactants (e.g. butanol) are required in the process, however their use is less desirable due to regulatory reasons and *in vivo* application (Fig 19.4).

Preparation by W/O/W Double Emulsion Method

Recently, a method based on emulsification and solvent evaporation for the preparation of SLNs loaded with hydrophilic drugs has been introduced to the scientific community. Here, the hydrophilic drug is encapsulated-along with a stabilizer to prevent drug partitioning into the external water phase during solvent evaporation of a W/O/W double emulsion. This technique has been used for the preparation of sodium cromo-glycate-containing SLNs, however, the average size obtained was in the micrometer range (Fig. 19.5).

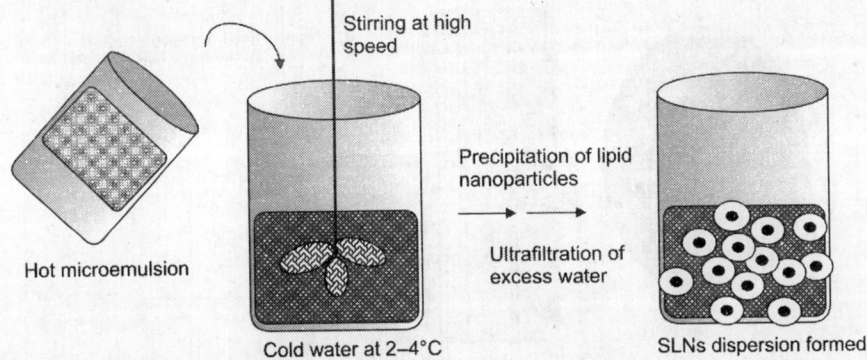

Fig. 19.4: Schematic representation of SLNs dispersion formed via microemulsion method

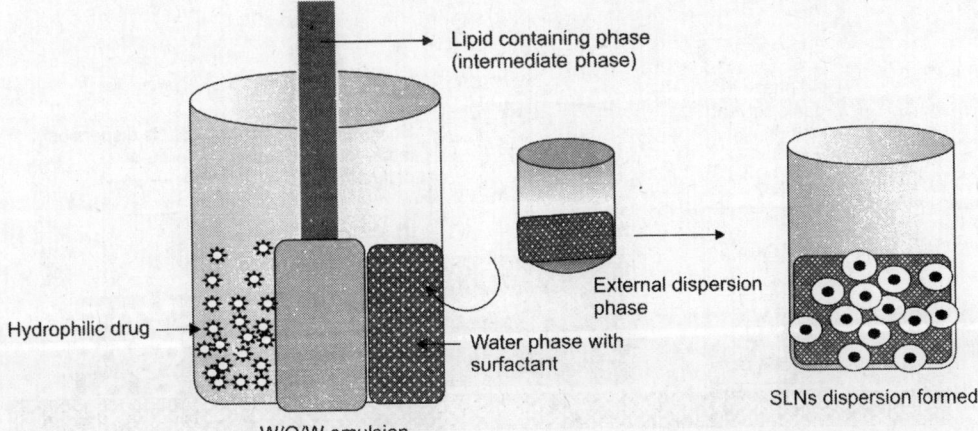

Fig. 19.5: Schematic representation of SLNs dispersion formed via W/O/W double emulsion method

Preparation by Solvent Emulsification Evaporation

In solvent emulsification evaporation method, lipophilic material is dissolved mainly in a water-immiscible organic solvent that is emulsified in an aqueous phase to obtain O/W emulsion. The SLNs dispersion is formed by precipitation of the lipid in the aqueous medium upon evaporation of organic solvent under reduced pressure. Here, particle size of SLNs mainly depends on the type and concentration of lipids, surfactants and co-surfactants in the organic phase. As low lipid content (5% w/w) produces very small particle size 30–100 nm, while as the lipid content increases (more than 5% w/w) particles become larger owing to the higher viscosity of the dispersed phase. The major advantage of this method is the total avoidance of thermal stress and suitability for thermolabile drugs (Fig. 19.6).

Preparation by Solvent Emulsification Diffusion

The SLNs dispersions were prepared from emulsions having partially water-miscible solvents with low toxicity, such as benzyl alcohol or butyl lactate, by a solvent diffusion technique. The process is based on the water miscibility of these solvents. Upon adding O/W emulsion into water, the drug dissolved in the organic solvent solidifies instantly due to diffusion of the organic solvent from the droplets to the continuous phase. Generally, the particle size obtained is below 100 nm with very low polydispersity could be produced (Fig. 19.7).

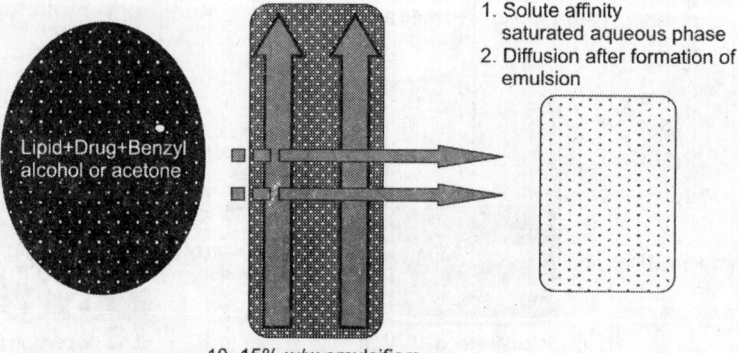

1. Solute affinity saturated aqueous phase
2. Diffusion after formation of emulsion

Lipid+Drug+Benzyl alcohol or acetone

10–15% w/w emulsifiers

Fig. 19.6: Schematic representation of SLNs dispersion formed via solvent emulsification evaporation method

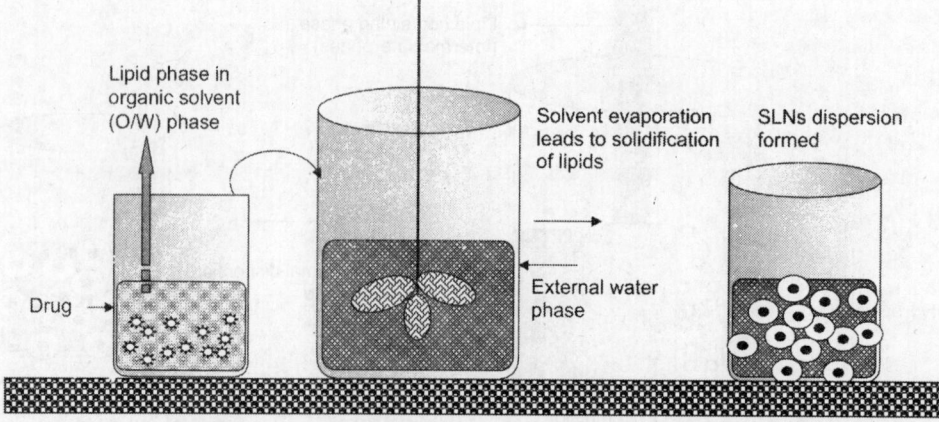

Lipid phase in organic solvent (O/W) phase

Solvent evaporation leads to solidification of lipids

SLNs dispersion formed

Drug

External water phase

Fig. 19.7: Schematic representation of SLNs dispersion formed via solvent emulsification diffusion method

Preparation of SLNs Using a Membrane Contactor

A new process using a membrane contactor is recently introduced for large-scale production of SLNs. Initially, this method was used for the preparation of emulsions and polymeric nanoparticles. In this method, lipid phase is pressed at a temperature above the melting point of the lipid, through the membrane pores allowing the formation of small droplets. The aqueous phase circulates inside the membrane module, and sweeps away the droplets that form at the pore outlets. Cooling of the preparation forms SLNs. Size of SLNs can be influenced by process parameters like aqueous phase and lipid phase temperatures, aqueous phase cross-flow velocity, lipid phase pressure and of course membrane pore size. Large-sized SLNs are obtained with higher lipid phase content. Temperature of aqueous phase below the fusion temperature is preferred for the small size nanoparticles. Lipid phase temperature has profound influence on the SLNs size and lipid flux, as the temperature of lipid phase increases, the particle size decreases. Interestingly, it was found that the size of lipid particles was largely unaffected by membrane pore size. The size of SLNs formed by membrane of pore size 0.1 µm was 175 nm and with 0.45 µm, it was 180 nm, which may be due to influence of interfacial tension. The advantages of this process for the preparation of SLNs are the use of simple apparatus, the control of the SLNs size by an appropriate choice of process parameters and its scaling-up abilities.

Preparation of SLNs by Ultrasonication

Ultrasonication method is very simple and can be easily adapted for the preparation of SLNs of various lipids. In this method, SLNs are obtained by ultrasonication of preformed lipid microparticles. It can be possible to regulate the size of SLNs by altering the frequency and intensity of sonication. Furthermore, this method is modified to improve the stability of the obtained SLNs dispersions by combining high speed stirring and ultrasonication at higher temperature. However, major limitation of this method is the broader particle size distribution ranging into the micrometers and potential metal contamination due to particles from probe materials. The large particle size may lead to physical instabilities such as particle growth upon storage and hence not suited for SLNs intravenous administration.

Preparation of SLNs by Supercritical Technique

Recently, techniques based on supercritical fluid have also been developed for the production of SLNs in which compressed supercritical fluid (SCF) above their critical pressure and temperature are used for the preparation of SLNs. Generally, nontoxic and cheaper SCF like carbon dioxide is used. Organic solvents commonly used have large volumetric expansion coefficients and large diffusion coefficients in SCF, which make the method suitable for the production of nanoparticles. The solute must be soluble in solvent but insoluble in SCF and a growth retardant compound that is at least partially soluble in the SCF with two functional groups in which one is SCF-philic and other SCF-phobic. When solution and SCF come in contact, the solvent diffuses into the SCF causing supersaturation and nucleation of particles comprising the solute material. The rapid expansion of supercritical fluid solution (RESS) and the supercritical fluids anti-solvent (SAS) process are the two most commonly used SCF based preparation techniques. In RESS process, solution of solute in SCF sprayed through a fine nozzle into a low-pressure chamber for supersaturation followed by nucleation and precipitation of the solute due to expansion of solution. This process has limited application due to the low polarizability of SCF like carbon dioxide which make it a poor solvent for most pharmaceuticals and biopolymers with high degree of agglomeration of the precipitated particles. In SAS process, high solubility or miscibility of organic solvents in SCF is utilized for the preparation in which SCF used as an antisolvent. When solute carrying organic solvent is injected into the SCF it extracts organic solvent from the solution causing supersaturation and nucleation of the material, which precipitates in the form of fine particles.

Scale Up Feasibility

For the introduction of a product to the market, scaling up feasibility is of utmost importance. For the two primarily used methods of the preparation of SLNs, HPH and production via microemulsions, scaling up possibilities have been investigated. HPH, a GMP unit for clinical batch production was developed and validated, which can achieve batch sizes between 2 and 10 kg SLNs dispersion. Further, a large scale production line was designed having a capacity of 50–150 kg SLNs dispersion per hour by placing two homogenizers in series. The production of SLNs with these lines can be performed in discontinuous or continuous modes. For the production via microemulsions, a system has been developed allowing the production of 100 ml microemulsion which is then poured into an excess of cold water forming SLNs. The dispersing water ration ranged from 1:1 to 1:10, leading to batch sizes of up to 1.11. Experimental factors, which have been investigated, were the pressure of the pneumatic cylinder, the temperature and the needle gauge of the syringe containing the microemulsion as well as the volume of dispersing water.

INFLUENCE OF INGREDIENT COMPOSITION ON PRODUCT QUALITY

Influence of the Lipid

Using the hot homogenization, it has been found that the average particle size of SLNs dispersions tended to increase with higher temperature melting lipids. These results are in agreement to the general theory of HPH and can be explained by the higher viscosity of the dispersed phase. However, other critical parameters for nanoparticles formation are different for different lipids. Examples include the rate of lipid crystallization, the lipid hydrophilicity (influence on self-emulsifying properties and the shape of the lipid crystals (and therefore the surface area). It is also noteworthy, that most of the lipids used represent a mixture of several chemical compounds. The composition might therefore vary from different suppliers and might even vary for different batches from the same supplier. However, small differences in the lipid composition (e.g. impurities) may even have considerable impact on the quality of SLNs dispersion (e.g. by changing the zeta potential, retarding crystallization processes etc.). For example, lipid nanodispersions made with cetyl palmitate from different suppliers exhibit different particle sizes and storage stabilities despite of the fact, they are prepared using the same preparation conditions (Table 19.2).

The influence of lipid composition on particle size was evaluated on SLNs produced via high-shear homogenization. The average particle size of Witepsol W35 SLNs was significantly smaller (117.0 ± 1.8 nm) than the size of Dynasan118 based SLNs (175.1 ± 3.5 nm). Witepsol W35 contains shorter fatty acid chains and considerable amounts of mono and diglycerides with surface active properties.

Increasing the lipid content over 5–10% in most of the cases produced the particles larger in size (including microparticles) and broader particle size distributions. Both, a decrease in homogenization efficiency and an increase in particles agglomeration may cause this effect which has also been observed for nanoemulsions.

Influence of the Emulsifier

The choice of the emulsifiers and their concentrations are of great impact on the quality of the SLNs dispersion. Investigating the influence of the emulsifier concentration on the particle size of compritol SLNs dispersions, best results were obtained with 5 wt% sodium cholate or poloxamer 188. Batches produced with lower concentrations of the emulsifier contained higher amounts of microparticles. Siekmann et al. reported that 2 wt% tyloxapol was insufficient to stabilize a 10 wt% tripalmitin dispersion. Increasing the tyloxapol concentration to 10 wt% resulted in 85 nm particles with an unimodal size distribution.

High concentrations of the emulsifier reduce the surface tension and thus facilitate the partitioning of drug during homogenization. The decrease in particle increases the surface area. The increase in the surface area during HPH (high pressure homogenization) takes place rapidly. Therefore, kinetic aspects have to be considered. The process of a primary coverage of the new surfaces competes with the agglomeration of uncovered lipid surfaces. The primary dispersion must contain excessive emulsifier molecules, which should rapidly cover the new surfaces. The excessive emulsifier molecules might be present in different forms, e.g. molecular solubilized (emulsifier monomers), in form of micelles (SDS) or liposomes (lecithin). The time scale of the redistribution processes of emulsifier molecules between particle surfaces, water-solubilized monomers and micelles or liposomes is different. In general, SDS and other micelle-forming low molecular weight surfactants will rapidly achieve the new equilibrium. Redistribution processes take relatively a longer time for relatively high molecular weight surfactants (poloxamer) and lecithin.

CHARACTERIZATION OF SLNS

The characterization of the SLNs is a necessity, however it is a difficult requirement due to the submicron size of the particles and the complexity of the system, which also includes dynamic phenomena (Table 19.3). Any particle

Table 19.2: Patents related to SLNs

Patent	Year	Original assignee/inventor	Title
US2004/0081688 A1	2004	Maria Dorly Del Curto, Daniela Chicco, Pierandrea Esposito, Washington DC	Amphiphilic lipid nanoparticles for peptide and/or protein incorporation.
US 2006/008378 A1	2006	V. Prasad Shastri, Eric Sussman, Ashwath Jayagopal. Atlanta, GA.	Functionalized SLNs and methods of making and using same.
US 2006/0222716A1	2006	Joseph Schwarz, Michael Weisspapir, Toronto	Colloidal solid lipid vehicle for pharmaceutical use
US 2007/0053988A1	2007	Audrey Royere, Jerome Bibette, Didier Bazile, Arlington US	Monodisperse solid lipid particle compositions.
US2008/0311214 A1	2008	Kollipara Koteswara Rao, Washington DC	Polymerized solid lipid nano-particles for oral or mucosal delivery of therapeutic proteins and peptides
US 2008/0206341A1	2008	Gasco, Maria Rosa, Roslyn US	Lipid nanoparticles as vehicles for nucleic acids, process for their preparation and use.
Us 2008/0102127 A1	2008	Hai Yan Gao, Joseph Schwarz, Michael Weisspapir, CA	Hybrid lipid-polymer nano-particulate delivery composition
US 2008/0286365A1	2008	Ferro Corporation, Cleveland US	Method for producing solid-lipid composite drug particles
US 2010/0233275A1	2010	Patrick Saulnier, Jean-Pierre Benoit, Nicolas Anton, US	Process for preparing lipid nanoparticles
US 2011/0208161A1	2011	Yehuda Ivri, CA	Intracochlear drug delivery to the central nervous system

Table 19.3: List of SLNs evaluation parameter and their characterization method

Parameter	Characterization method
Particle size and size distribution	Photon correlation spectroscopy (PCS)
	Laser defractometry (LD)
	Transmission electron microscopy (TEM)
	Scanning electron microscopy (SEM)
	Atomic force microscopy (AFM)
Charge determination	Mercury porositometry
	Laser doppler anemometry
	Zeta potential meter
Chemical analysis of surface	Static secondary ion mass spectrometry
	Sorptometer
Carrier-drug interaction	Differential scanning calorimetry (DSC)
SLNs dispersion stability	Critical flocculation temperature (CFT)
Release profile	*In vitro* release characteristics under physiologic and sink conditions
Drug stability	Bioassay of drug extracted from nanoparticles
	Chemical analysis of drug

separating from the aqueous environment or only undergoing dissolution in water could easily lead to misleading results due to particles aggregation and changed samples, especially if stabilizers are removed from the particle surface. Various parameters which are directly related to the stability and release kinetics of SLNs are measurement of physico-chemical properties, particle size and zeta potential, degree of crystallinity and lipid modification as well as analysis of drug release properties of SLNs. Some of the important studies related to characterization of SLNs are summarized in Table 19.4.

Table 19.4: Summary of *in vitro* and/or *in vivo* characterization studies of SLNs carried out by different scientific communities

Nature of SLNs and study	Characterization parameters
Stabilized with poloxamine 908 and poloxamer 407	Phagocytic uptake and cytotoxicity
Formulated with phospholipid and triglyceride	Evidence for phospholipid bilayer formation *in vitro*
To observe function of the lipid matrix and the surfactant	Cytotoxicity study
Effect of autoclaving, storage and lyophilization	Drug retention and stability
Duodenal administration of SLNs	Localization in lymph and plasma
For controlled drug delivery	Drug release and release mechanism
SLNs containing gadolinium(III) complexes	NMR relaxometric investigations
SLNs in aqueous dispersion after addition of electrolyte.	Stability determination
Effect of surfactant and surfactant mixtures	Enzymatic degradation of SLNs
Crystallinity of the lipid phase.	Long-term stability
Based on binary mixtures of liquid and solid lipids	1H-NMR study
Cationic solid-lipid nanoparticles	Transfection plasmid DNA
Effect of surfactants, storage time, and crystallinity	Lipase degradation
Solid lipid nanoparticles derived from amphiphilic cyclodextrins	Scanning electron microscopy and atomic force microscopy imaging
Influence of emulsifiers of SLNs	Crystallization behavior

Contd.

Table 19.4: Summary of *in vitro* and/or *in vivo* characterization studies of SLNs carried out by different scientific communities *(Contd.)*

Nature of SLNs and study	Characterization parameters
Interaction of solid lipid nanoparticles with skin	Skin hydration and viscoelastic study
Tween 80- and poloxamer 188-stabilized solid lipid nanoparticles	Plasma protein adsorption
Investigations on the structure	Photon correlation spectroscopy, field-flow fractionation and transmission electron microscopy
Distribution and modification of sorption sites	Hyperpolarized 129Xe NMR spectroscopy
Surface-modified solid lipid nanoparticles (SLNs)	Influence of lecithin and nonionic emulsifier
Drug-free and drug-loaded solid lipid nanoparticles (SLNs)	DSC and 1H NMR
Surface properties of SLNs	Binding affinity for DNA, streptavidin and biotinylated ligands

Size and Morphology

The particle size is one of the most important parameters of SLNs. Two main techniques are being used to determine the particle size distribution of nanoparticles namely photon correlation PCS and electron microscopy. The electron microscopy includes SEM, TEM and freeze-fracture techniques. It was concluded that results coordinate well with better agreement when freeze-fracturing and PCS are quantitatively compared. The electron microscopy, however could be adopted as an alternative option, which measures individual particle for size and distribution. It is much less time consuming. Additionally, freeze fracturing of particles allows for morphological determination of inner structural details of particles. In combination with freeze fracture procedures, TEM permits differentiation among nanocapsules, nanoparticles and emulsion droplets. Scanning electron microscopy is relatively less time consuming. However, particles being based on organic material are nonconductive, hence require gold coating. The thickness of gold coat may vary from 30–50 nm. Thus, determined size should be denoted as gold-coated particle size rather than as particle size (Fig. 19.8). The most widely used method to characterize the size of SLNs is PCS and LD. PCS (also known as dynamic light scattering) measures the fluctuation of the intensity of the scattered light due to particulate movement and covers a size range from a few nanometers to about

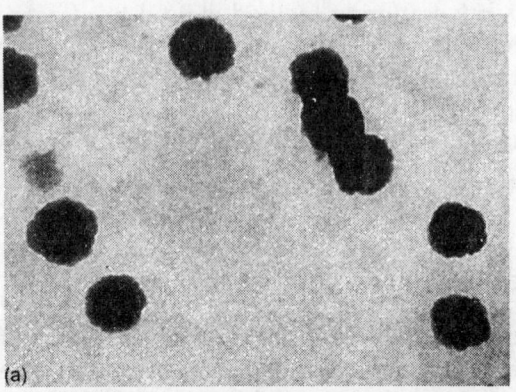 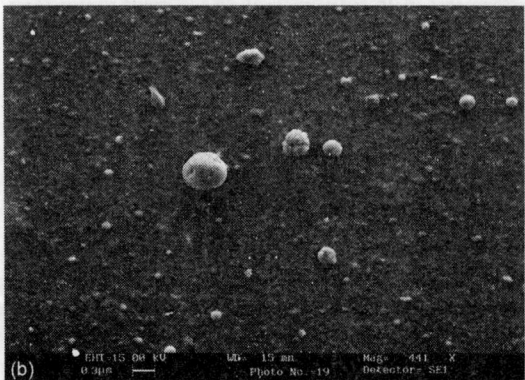

Fig. 19.8: Photomicrographs of SLNs (a) TEM, (b) SEM (adapted from Gupta et al., 2001)

3 m. This method is based on the diffraction angle on the particle radius. Smaller particles create more intense scattering at high angles than do larger ones.

This method requires only very small amounts of sample and is rapid and easy to perform, and also its range of operation falls nominally between a few nanometers to a few micrometers. Thus, it covers the relevant range for lipid nanoparticles based suspensions. PCS analyzes the Brownian motion of the particles in the dispersion medium. Light microscopy is not sensitive to the nanometer size range but gives a fast indication of the presence of microparticles. Electron microscopy provides, in contrast to PCS and LD, a direct information on the particle shape. However, the investigator should pay special attention to possible artifacts, which are co-produced during the sample preparation. Atomic force microscopy (AFM) is an advanced nanoscopic technique that has been applied for the characterization of solid lipid nanoparticles. The AFM images can be obtained in an aqueous medium and for this reason, it is an effective means for the investigation of nanoparticle behavior in biological environment. Mercury porositometry is an equally suitable technique for the sizing of nanoparticulates. The freeze-dried nanoparticles are filled in a dilatometer under vacuum then measured with the help of a mercury pressure porositometer. The method largely measures particulate agglomerates as mercury fails to penetrate to a greater extent within the primary particles.

Zeta Potential

The measurement of the zeta potential allows predictions about the storage stability of colloidal dispersion. In general, particle aggregation is less likely to occur for charged particles (high zeta potential) due to electric repulsion. However, this rule cannot strictly applied for the systems, which contain steric stabilizers, because the adsorption of steric stabilizer decreases the zeta potential due the shift in the shear plane of the particle yet providing physical stability to the system.

Degree of Crystallinity and Lipid Modification

Particle size analysis is a necessary step to characterize SLNs quality. Moreover, the degree of lipid crystallinity and the modification of the lipid parameters are also strongly correlated with drug incorporation and release rate of SLNs. Differential scanning calorimetry (DSC) and X-ray scattering are widely used methods to investigate the properties of the lipid. Lipid modifications possess different melting points, melting enthalpies constitute the basis of use of DSC for the study of lipid modification. Phase transitions are accompanied with free energy changes, and are due to either an alteration in the enthalpy (ΔH) or entropy (ΔS) of the system. Enthalpy changes result in either endothermic or exothermic signals, depending on whether the transition is due to melting of a solid or recrystallization of an isotropic melt. It should be mentioned that the transition from the crystalline to amorphous phase requires a high-energy input. This is in contrast to crystalline to liquid crystalline and liquid crystalline to relatively amorphous transitions as well as changes between different liquid crystalline phases, which all consume low amount of energy. Therefore, care should be taken to ensure that measuring device should be sensitive enough to give a sufficiently low detection limit. X-ray scattering method is used to measure length of the long and short spacing of the lipid lattice in SLNs. Infrared and Raman spectroscopy have also been proposed as useful tools to investigate structural properties of SLNs.

The magnetic resonance techniques, NMR and ESR, are powerful tools used to investigate dynamic phenomena and the characteristics of nanocompartments in colloidal lipid dispersions. Due to the noninvasiveness of both methods, repeated measurements of the same sample are possible.

NMR active nuclei of interest are 1H, 13C, 19F and 35P. Due to the different chemical shifts, it is possible to attribute the NMR signals to particular molecules or their segments. For example, lipid methyl protons give signals at 0.9 ppm while protons of the polyethylene glycol chains give signals at 3.7 ppm. Simple 1H-spectroscopy permits an easy and rapid detection of supercooled melts. It permits also the characterization of liquid nanocompartments in the developed lipid particles, which are made of blends from solid and liquid lipids. This method is based on the different proton relaxation times required in the liquid and semisolid/solid state. Protons in the liquid state give sharp signals with high signal amplitudes, while semisolid/solid protons give weak and broad NMR signals under these circumstances. The great potential of NMR with its variety of different approaches (solid-state-NMR, determination of self-diffusion coefficients etc.) has scarcely been used in the SLNs, although it will provide unique insights into the structure and dynamics of SLNs dispersions.

ESR requires the addition of paramagnetic spin probes to investigate SLNs dispersions. A large variety of spin probes are commercially available. The corresponding ESR spectra give information about the microviscosity and micropolarity. ESR permits the direct, repeatable and noninvasive characterization of the distribution of the spin probe between the aqueous and the lipid phase. Experimental results demonstrate that storage induced crystallization of SLNs leads to an expulsion of the probe out of the lipid into the aqueous phase. Furthermore, using an ascorbic acid reduction assay, it is possible to monitor the time scale of the exchange between the aqueous and the lipid phase. The development of low-frequency ESR permits noninvasive measurements on small mammals. ESR spectroscopy and imaging will give new insights about the fate of SLNs *in vivo*.

Models for Incorporation of Active Compounds

There are basically three different models for the incorporation of active ingredients into SLNs:

   i. Homogeneous matrix model
   ii. Drug-enriched shell model
   iii. Drug-enriched core model

The structure obtained is a function of the formulation composition (lipid, active compound, and surfactant) and of the production conditions (hot *vs.* cold lipid HPH).

A homogeneous matrix with molecularly dispersed drug or drug present in amorphous clusters is thought to be obtained mainly when the cold homogenisation method is applied, however, it also occurs when very lipophilic drugs are incorporated in SLNs using the hot homogenisation method. In the cold homogenisation method, the bulk lipid contains the dissolved drug in molecularly dispersed form, mechanical breaking of lipid phase by high pressure homogenisation produces nanoparticles with homogeneous matrix structure (Fig. 19.9). The same may happen when the oil droplets produced by the hot homogenisation method are cooled and crystallized. The phase separation between lipid and drug does not occur during this cooling process. This model is assumed to be valid and useful for incorporation of the drug such as prednisolone, which can show slow release, i.e. from 1 day up to weeks.

An outer shell enriched with active compound can be obtained, when phase separation

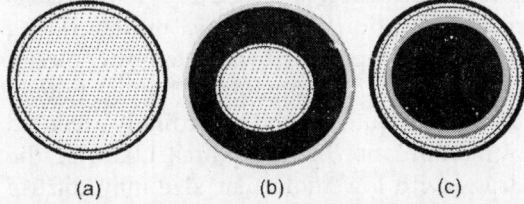

(a)   (b)   (c)

Fig. 19.9: Models of incorporation of active compounds into SLNs—(a) homogeneous matrix, (b) compound-free core with compound enriched outer shell, (c) drug-enriched core with lipid shell

occurs during the cooling process of oil droplets and subsequent formation of SLNs. The lipid can precipitate first forming practically a compound-free lipid core. At the same time, the concentration of active compound in the remaining liquid, lipid increases continuously during the process of lipid core formation. Finally, the compound-enriched shell crystallises. This model assumes, e.g. for coenzyme Q10-where the enrichment leads to a very fast release. A fast release can be highly desired when application of SLNs to the skin is intended to increase the drug penetration, especially when used under occlusive conditions. A core enriched with active compound can be formed when the reverse of the process occurs, which means the active compound starts precipitating first and the shell develop later with distinctly less drug (Fig. 19.9). This leads to a membrane controlled release governed by the Fick's law of diffusion. The three models presented, where each represents for an ideal type. Obviously when, there are mixed types which can be considered as a fourth model. From this, it is inferred that the structure of SLNs, formed clearly depends on the chemical nature of active compound and excipients and also on their interaction thereof.

In addition, the structure can be influenced or determined by the other production conditions.

In Vitro Release

In vitro drug release from SLNs may occur through diffusion of drug through the matrix or degradation of the lipid matrix. Drug diffusion velocity can be affected by choice of manufacturing parameters. The fast release may be attributed to and accordingly executed by manipulation of surface area. Likewise, the drugs with low molecular size may diffuse faster and also the viscosity of the drug solution particularly in the matrix may affect drug diffusion. The shorter distance of diffusion path and lower viscosity of diffusion

may favor the diffusion. This indicates the controlled adjustment of release can be made by chemical modification of the lipid matrix. In addition, surfactant, their concentration, and production temperature also affect the release characterstisc. A study with SLNs prepared with or without surfactant proves that incorporation of a surfactant facilitates drug release. Several factors, which could affect the drug release from the SLNs, using different model drugs were also investigated. The Dynasan 112 SLNs were prepared by hot high-pressure homogenization method bearing either tetracaine or etomidate and stabilized with Lipoid S 75. These SLNs remained in the liquid state for longer time and showed a burst release. The small size of SLNs in combination with surfactant could have contributed to the observed burst release of drug. On the other hand, cholesterol and compritol SLNs containing prednisolone prepared by cold homogenization technique did not show any burst effect, where after 5 weeks, only 83.8% and 37.1% of drug was released respectively. These results can be explained by differences in melting temperature of the lipid and the homogenization temperature, which are important parameters which determine the structure of the SLNs matrix. Prolonged release with lower melting lipids may be due to interactions between drug-lipid molecules, surfactant lipid molecules and solubility of the drug in the molten and solid lipids. Partition coefficient does not affect drug release pattern from SLNs, as drugs with higher partition coefficient sometimes show faster release. These observations suggest that controlled release can be achieved by modification of the chemical nature of the lipid matrix and temperature adjustment.

Storage Stability of SLNs

The SLNs cannot be simply considered as colloidal lipid dispersions with solidified droplets. Basically, the main problems with SLNs dispersions, is the presence of additional colloidal structures (micelles and liposomes) are also present. SLNs have additional features (supercooled particle size should be completely in the submicron melts, different modifications, nonspherical shapes) which are contributing to or determining the stability of the colloidal lipid suspension. But, gelation phenomena, increase in particle sizes and drug expulsion from the SLNs are the major problems encountered on storage. The modification of the lipid, gelation, particle aggregation and drug expulsion are interlinked with each other. A supercooled melt, which is the first product formed after hot homogenization, represent a nanoemulsion. It is characterized by spherical lipid droplets and a high concentration level incorporation of guest molecules. The transformation of the lipid melt to lipid crystals results in an increase of particle surface, decrease of the loading capacity of the lipid and, therefore, it further worsen the stability problems. Stability of the lipid dispersions decreases as stability improvement of the lipid through chemical modification is attempted.

Sterilization of SLNs Formulation

Sterilization of SLNs is a most desirable step needed, especially when they are intended and prepared for parenteral, pulmonary or ocular administration. Researchers investigated the effect of different sterilization techniques like steam sterilization at 121°C for 15 min and at 110°C for 15 min and γ-sterilization on SLNs characteristics. These findings suggested that parameters influencing SLNs characteristics are sterilization temperature and SLNs composition. The choice of the emulsifier is of significant importance as the properties of emulsifier, such as mobility and hydrophobicity are also affected at higher temperatures. It was found that lecithin stabilized SLNs can be sterilized by autoclaving. SLNs can be sterilized by autoclaving, where an almost spherical shape is maintained without any significant increase in size. Steam sterilization of SLNs prepared with poloxamer 188,

induced a significant increase in particle size due to temperature-induced dehydration of the ethylene glycol chains that resulted in a decrease of the thickness of the protecting layer. Literature reported that during autoclaving the high temperatures sterilization presumably forms a hot O/W microemulsion that probably modifies the size of the hot nanodroplets and hence on cooling reformed into SLNs of larger size due to coalescence of nanodroplets. After sterilization, stability of SLNs is also affected and as the concentration of surfactant decreases the zeta potential of SLNs dispersed in water decreases. The temperature can be adjusted with the time in case of different lipids. SLNs dispersions can also be sterilized by filtration like other colloidal carriers as liposome, emulsions etc. but in the liquid state. γ-irradiation could be a better alternative to steam sterilization for temperature sensitive materials. Increase in particle size is not significant in case of γ-sterilization, therefore, SLNs can be preferably produced aseptically without altering their characteristics.

Coating of SLNs with Hydrophilic Substances

In case of systemic use, ideal drug delivery occurs through selective uptake of carrier with the contents by the target organ or accumulation at the site of action with a low systemic level of drug. It is very difficult to obtain this ideal situation in practice, because anatomical barriers limit and govern the distribution of drugs. SLNs which are hydrophobic, are exposed to phagocytic uptake by macrophages. Studies on systemic use of SLNs have focused on improving their circulation time in the blood circulation, since macrophages in RES recognize them as foreign substances and quickly remove them due to their physicochemical properties, mainly particle size, surface charge and surface hydrophobicity. Uptake by phagocytic cells is mediated by blood components, which are called opsonins and specific cell receptors on macrophages that operate independently. The opsonic factors include proteins, such as immunoglobulin G, complement C3b and fibronectin. These factors are adsorbed on nanoparticles, then the particles are immediately cleared by the macrophages of the mononuclear phagocytic system. The surface characteristics of the particles determine whether or not opsonization will take place and which component will be involved. As a consequence, the mechanism of particle-cell interaction will also depend on the nature of the opsonic component and the relevant receptor-mediated process.

To avoid phagocytic uptake and to modulate biodistribution parameters of drugs for their long blood circulation, surface properties of colloidal drug carriers can be modified by using various techniques. Of the many techniques used to enhance the blood circulation time of particles, surface coating with polyethylene glycol (PEG) polymers has been reported to be successful. Previously, it was reported that immunogenicity of bovine serum albumin is decreased by using PEG. This technique is being used to decrease the immunogenicity of proteins including enzymes such as superoxide dismutase and

asparaginase. A decrease was observed in the recognition of PEG-modified proteins by macrophages. The same mechanism was thought to be useful in case of particles to increase their biodistribution. When the particles are coated with PEG, it can favorably modify the surface hydrophobicity of particles and sterically stabilize them, thus suppressing the binding of serum proteins (e.g. apoproteins) and other opsonic factors. Sterically stabilized SLNs have also been referred as stealth SLNs, but conversely nonstealth SLNs by various research groups. PEG derivatives are available of various molecular weights, which are essentially block copolymers; chemically they contain hydrophilic and hydrophobic residues that give them amphiphilic characteristics. In an aqueous PEG-coated SLNs dispersion, soluble hydrophilic residue of PEG turns toward the water phase while insoluble hydrophobic residue is oriented or adsorbed on the lipophilic SLNs forming of a protective shell around it (Fig. 19.10).

Effect of PEG Coating on Physical Properties of SLNs and Bioavailability of Drugs

In general, surface modification of colloidal particles by coating with a hydrophilic

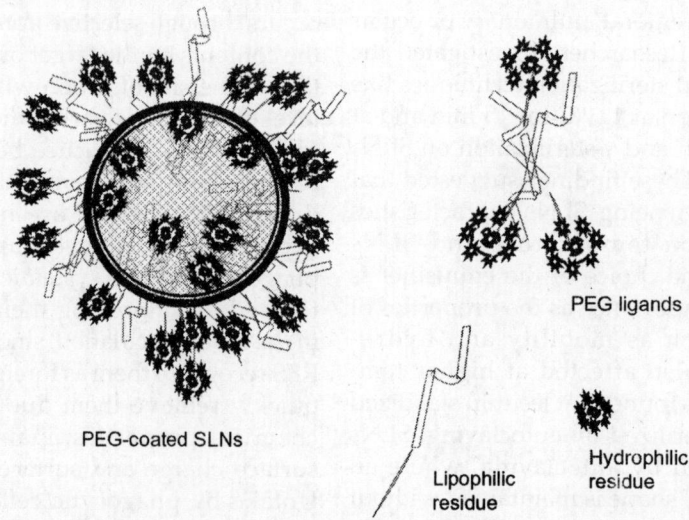

PEG-coated SLNs

PEG ligands

Lipophilic residue

Hydrophilic residue

Fig. 19.10: Schematic representation of SLNs coated with PEG and molecular residue of PEG

substance like PEG has been reported to bring following benefits for:

- Providing good physical stability and dispersability to colloids
- Improving presence of colloids in blood circulation for systemic use
- Increasing stability of colloids in body fluids such as GI fluids
- Acceleration of colloid transport across the epithelium
- Modulation of interaction of colloids with mucosa for specific delivery requirements and drug targeting
- Increasing biocompatibility and decreasing thrombogenicity of drug carriers

Coating materials are mostly adsorbed on the surface of the nanoparticles. Stability of coated particles also depends on the strength of the bond between particle and coating material. In case of PEG, it attaches covalently to the nanoparticle surface and provides a hydrophilic stearic barrier around SLNs. This protective layer prevents agglomeration during the production and/or storage, and subsequently, improves physical stability and dispersability of inner phase. Concentration of stealth agents strongly affects the rate of the phagocytic uptake. There is an inverse relationship between concentration and uptake. Earlier study showed the phagocytic uptake of PEG-coated dipalmitoyl phosphatidylamine and stearic acid based SLNs by murine macrophages.They reported a significant increase in particle size with a linear relation to the PEG concentration used in the formulations and a decrease in murine uptake compared with nonstealth SLNs. Optimum particle size for lymphatic uptake was reported to be between 10 nm and 100 nm. In general, increase in particle size by coating nanoparticles with stabilizing hydrophilic molecules leads to an extended blood circulation of SLNs. Various researchers have also indicated that the colloidal carrier systems are required to possess smaller size, hydrophobicity and strong negative surface charge

for effective penetration into lymphatic interstitium.

Heiati et al. (1998) reported that PEG coating did not change the particle size of azidothymidine-loaded trilaurin SLNs. The hydrophilic character of coating prolonged the release of lipophilic azidothymidine. PEG coating further enhances the blood level of the drug compared to nonstealth SLNs and also decreases the urinary excretion in mice. It was also observed that there was no significant change in the particle size of SLNs. However, the hydrophilic surface characteristic of the particles due to PEG, reduced the phagocytic recognition in rats. Correlation between hydrophobicity and the rate of phagocytosis of colloidal particles was recorded, as reported in various studies. There was a marginal alteration in particle size (from 80 nm to 90 nm), a fivefold enhancement of the doxorubicin peak plasma concentration recorded and a sevenfold enhancement especially in case of stealth SLNs. Maximum drug concentration was observed in the lungs with stealth SLNs. In brain tissues, doxorubicin was determined after administration of stealth SLNs, while no drug was detected in brain in case of plain drug solution and nonstealth SLNs. Surface charge of colloidal particles reportedly influenced and modified biodistribution and clearance rate of drugs. Half-life of negatively charged colloids was generally higher than that of positively charged colloids. However, it should be noted that a strong negative charge or a strong positive charge usually leads to rapid phagocytic uptake compared to particles of weak negative charge. Zeta potential which indicates the surface characteristics, is greatly affected by the nature of coating. A study that investigated the surface modification of PEG-coated SLNs, uncoated tripalmitin SLNs presented a negative charge due to the anionic ingredients in their composition. When they were coated with PEG, the zeta potential showed a less negative value than that of nonstealth SLNs. PEG decreased zeta potential from −50.3 mV to −34.8 mV in the negative range. The presence of PEG on the surface of SLNs partially masked the negative charge of the uncoated particles. This effect is common for PEG-coated nanoparticles due to an extension of the plane of shear of the nanoparticles (Gref et al., 2000). Similar results were found in various studies on drug carriers. Zeta potential of the stealth SLNs (between −38.0 mV and −32.5 mV) was reported to be lower than nonstealth SLNs (−47.5 mV) indicating the presence of PEG chains on the surface.

TOXICITY ASPECTS AND *IN VIVO* FATE OF SLNS

The SLNs are well tolerated in living systems owing to prepared from biodegradable compounds as for them metabolic pathways exist. But, the toxicity of the emulsifiers is considered. Problems are not encountered on peroral or transdermal administration and IM or SC injection, if appropriate surfactants are used. The particle size is not a very significant aspect in case of these routes of administration, because a low content of microparticles might decrease the performance of the SLNs system. Nevertheless, toxic events are minimized. Moreover, the absence of pyrogens must be checked in case of parenteral administration. Problems may arise, because SLNs may interfere with the pyrogen tests (limulus test). Particles size distribution is important for IV injection due to the risk of capillary blockage which could result in death due to fat embolism. The diameter of the fine capillaries is about 9 μm. Hence, considering the safety points, the particle size should be completely in the submicron range. Gelation of the low viscosity SLNs dispersion in the syringe needle might occur that would immediately form a viscous suspension with undesirable particle sizes. Both the solid state of the lipid and the danger of injection-induced gelation are serious hurdles in the development of SLNs dispersions for IV injection in the clinical practice.

The interaction of SLNs with phogocytes has been studied *in vitro* on human granulocytes.

A luminol-based chemoluminescence was used to compare the SLNs with polymeric particles and to assess the relative influence of the SLNs composition on the rate of phagocytosis of poloxamer-stabilized compritol. The rate and extent of phagocytosis in case of cetyl palmitate SLNs was low in comparison to polystyrene nanoparticles. An indirect chemoluminescence assay was developed in order to distinguish the minute differences in phagocytosis of SLNs. The results indicate that poloxamine 908 prevents the uptake of compritol SLNs more efficiently than poloxamer 407. It was previously reported that dipalmitoyl-phosphatidylethanaolamine-PEG and stearic acid-PEG 2000 might successfully be used to produce stealth SLNs. The steric stabilizers reduce the SLNs uptake in murine macrophages to a large extent. The PEG (polyethylene glycol) chains are capable of preventing the interaction of SLNs with human serum albumin. One of the most important aspects to keep drug carriers in the blood circulation for longer is by grafting their surface with certain water soluble polymers with flexible chain, such as PEG. The stealth nature of PEG is mainly depended on the formation of a dense hydrophilic cloud of long flexible chains on the surface of the colloidal particle that reduces their hydrophobic interactions with the RES. The tethered and/or chemically anchored PEG chains can undergo spatial conformations, consequently hinder the interactions of blood components with their surface and reduce the binding of plasma proteins with nanocarriers, thus reduce the opsonization even at a low concentration of the protecting polymer (Fig. 19.11). Therefore, PEGylation apparently improves the blood circulation time of colloidal particles.

APPLICATIONS OF SLNS IN DRUG DELIVERY

SLNs are considered as the next generation of delivery system. Similar to liposomes, they are consisted of biocompatible excipients. The main benefits of SLNs relate to solid state of the particle matrix, their ability to protect

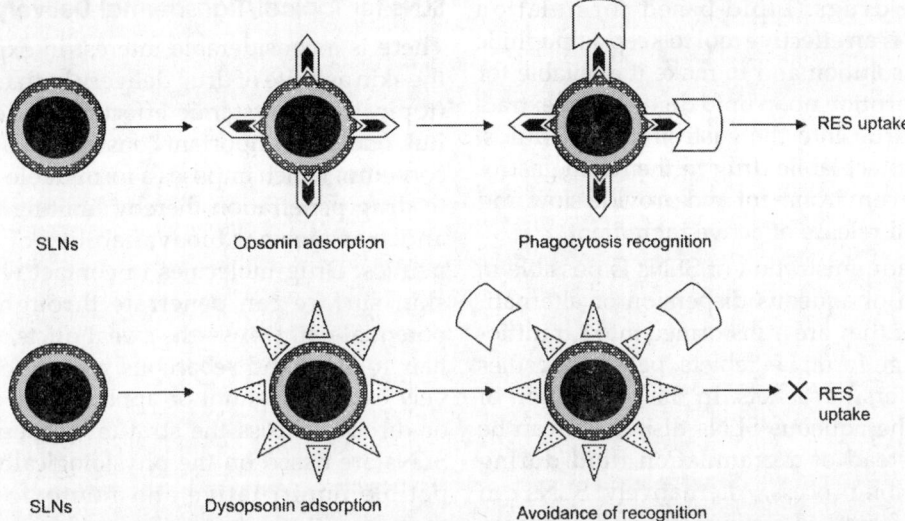

Fig. 19.11: *In vivo* fate of SLNs after adsorption of serum components

chemically labile ingredients against chemical decomposition and the possibility to modulate drug release. SLNs provide platform for development of dosage forms for any predefined routes of delivery like parenteral, oral, topical, rectal, and pulmonary etc.

Parenteral route is widely used for administration of SLNs in clinical practice, as it provides maximum bioavailability of the administered dose. The potential advantages which earn the consideration of SLNs for parenteral route over other drug carriers, especially for lipophilic drugs pertain to the use of natural lipids, which are known to be generally nontoxic. Unlike fat emulsions, which have a fluid core, the solid core of SLNs prolongs the release of the incorporated lipophilic drugs. The intravenously administered SLNs showed higher and prolonged plasma levels of therapeutic moiety. SLNs have successfully been administered intravenously to the animals. Pharmacokinetic studies of doxorubicin-loaded SLNs revealed that higher blood levels were achieved in comparison to a commercial drug solution after IV injection in rats. Concerning the body distribution, SLNs were found to produce higher drug concentrations in lung, spleen and brain, while the drug from solution accumulated more into liver and kidneys. The biodistribution data of camptothecin-loaded SLNs also showed an increased uptake in some organs, especially in the brain. There are many other parenteral applications which appear to be feasible and of therapeutical value; an example is the treatment of arthritis of joints with the lipophilic corticoids incorporated into SLNs.

Oral route has many advantages for drug therapy, as it is relatively safe, convenient for the patient, and allows self-administration. The use of lipid-based systems for oral delivery is seemingly rewarding, as it provides an understanding of the manner in which lipids could enhance oral bioavailability and reduce plasma profile variability and formulation versatility. Moreover, the lipidic excipients are better characterized with scale up possibilities with available technology.

While these systems may provide the maximum flexibility in the modulation of the drug release profile within the GIT, they may also provide protection against chemical degradation for labile drug molecules, e.g.

peptide drugs. Lipid-based formulation strategy is an effective tool to keep a lipophilic drug in solution and to make it available for oral absorption upon lipid digestion or extraction of drug into the gastrointestinal fluids. SLNs protect labile drug in the harsh gastrointestinal environment and provide slow and sustained release of active ingredient.

Oral administration of SLNs is possible in the form of aqueous dispersion or alternatively after they are transformed into a traditional dosage form, i.e. tablets, pellets, capsules or powders in sachets. In the production of tablets the aqueous SLNs dispersion can be used instead of a granulation fluid during granulation process. Alternatively, SLNs can be transferred to a powder (e.g. by spray-drying) and added to the tabletting powder mixture. Similarly in the production of pellets, the SLNs dispersion can be used as wetting agent in the extrusion process. SLNs powders can be used for the filling of hard gelatin capsules; alternatively, the SLNs can be produced directly in liquid PEG 600 and filled into soft gelatin capsules. Sachets are also possible using spray dried or lyophilized powders. In both the cases, it is beneficial to have a higher solid content. For economic reasons spray drying might be a preferred method of drying of SLNs dispersions into powders.

SLNs can be used to improve the bioavailability of drugs, e.g. cyclosporine A. Clozapine, a lipophilic drug, that is rapidly absorbed orally with an improved bioavailability, when administered in SLNs. SLNs have also been found suitable for lymphatic transport and hence for improving oral bioavailability of clozapine. Drug incorporated in SLNs shows enhanced and consistent bioavailability with longer drug retention in plasma. This enhanced bioavailability is due to controlled and optimized release of drug of nanosized particles. Additionally, SLNs are biodegradable and offer cost effective large scale production possibility.

SLNs for Topical/Transdermal Delivery

There is a considerable interest in exploring the skin as a site of drug delivery both for local (topical) and systemic effect (transdermal). But, one most important constraint is stratum corneum, which imposes a formidable barrier to drug penetration thereby limiting topical and transdermal bioavailability of therapeutics. Drug molecules in contact with the skin surface can penetrate through three potential pathways—the sweat ducts, via the hair follicles and sebaceous glands (collectively called the shunt or appendageal route), or directly across the stratum corneum. As SLNs are based on the physiologically compatible nonirritative and nontoxic lipids therefore, they seem to be useful as appropriate topical formulation. Most of the lipids used in SLNs formulation have an FDA approved status or belong to a class of excipients which are conventionally used in commercially available topical cosmetic or pharmaceutical preparations.

With respect to their use as carriers for drugs and cosmetics, favorable properties of SLNs include (i) good local tolerability of many formulation components; (ii) nanometric size of SLNs, which facilitates the contact with stratum corneum, thus enhances drug penetration due to high specific surface area; (iii) sustained drug release properties; (iv) an occlusive effect due to film formation on the skin surface that reduces transepidermal water loss. These factors also favor drug penetration and appear to be desirable in chronic atopic eczema. The solid lipid matrix, of SLNs generally controls the release from these carriers. SLNs as a drug carrier were used for topical delivery of drugs clotrimazole, prednicarbate, betamethasone 17-valerate, glucocorticoids, podophyllotoxin, and isotretinoin. SLNs are introduced as the new generation of carriers for cosmetics, especially for ultraviolet (UV) sunscreening agent (blockers) for use on human skin. SLNs formulation-based safe sunscreen product exhibited showed that SLNs particles have the ability of reflecting and scattering UV radiation on their own, thus leading to photoprotection and further incorporation of a sunscreen agent that may lead to a synergistic effect in photoprotection. The photoprotective effect of sunscreen 2-hydroxy-4-methoxybenzophenone, when incorporated into the SLNs dispersion was found to be threefold better compared to a reference emulsion.

SLNs for Pulmonary Administration

The use of SLNs-based system for pulmonary drug delivery has not yet been fully explored and established, however for pulmonary delivery, aqueous SLNs dispersions may be nebulized, and SLNs powders might be used as dry powder inhalers. SLNs could be spray-dried by using lactose as an excipient in the spray-drying process. Control of the release profile for prolonged release of drug in the lung and a faster degradation of SLNs particles can play a beneficial role in pulmonary delivery of drugs. In addition, SLNs exhibited a high tolerability and may be successfully employed for targeting to lung macrophages. Targeting potential of SLNs is also beneficial with the possiblity for treating infections of the macrophage and RES prominent systems. Macrophages of liver and spleen are relatively more accessible compared to parasites in the lung macrophages.

Cationic SLNs as Novel Transfection Agent

Numerous approaches have been explored for development of carrier systems for gene delivery using both viral and nonviral delivery vehicles. Colloidal carriers, such as SLNs might be an attractive tool for the assembly of multi-component transfection systems, as they can bind DNA, carry targeting residues as well as release additives, such as DNase inhibitors, endosomolytic substances or regulators of transcription. In addition, to already discussed advantages of SLNs as drug carrier one advantage of SLNs pertains to charge of the particles that can be modulated via the composition, thus allowing binding of oppositely charged molecules via electrostatic interactions. Transfection activity seems to be measured by both the cationic lipid and the matrix lipid used. It was previously demonstrated that combination of cetylpalmitate and N-[1-(2,3-dioleoyloxy) propyl]-N,N,N-trimethylammonium chloride have led to the significantly higher transfection efficiencies. For gene transfer, cationic SLNs can be formulated using the same cationic lipids as used in case of liposomal transfection agents. Cationic SLNs form complexes with polyanionic polymers, such as DNA offering excellent stability to the DNA or RNA complexed with SLNs.

SLNs as New Adjuvant for Immunization

Immunization provides protective shield to the body or immunization vaccination, is a prophylactic approach through which the body is protected or made strong enough to fight against any invading pathogenic infection. Several adjuvants, which are frequently used include Freund's complete adjuvant and aluminum hydroxide particles. They however, possess several side effects, therefore new adjuvants have been developed like emulsion system SAF 1 and MF 59. SLNs can also be used as vaccine adjuvant, as they possess long-term physical stability and solid state lipid of SLNs degrade slowly providing longer exposure to the immune system. Further, degradation can also be slowed down by modifying surface properties and additionally, they are sterilizable by autoclaving or sterile filtration. Advantages over the other adjuvants are the biodegradation of SLNs and their good tolerability by the body. Other advantages arising from these systems are their structural variability, low toxicity arising from natural lipids used and possibility of further modification of drug delivery to the specific cells of the organs or tissues.

SUGGESTED READINGS

1. Absolom DR (1986), *Methods Enzymol.*, 132, 281–318.

2. Almeida AJ and Souto E (2007), *Adv Drug Deliv Rev.*, 59, 478–90.

3. Almeida AJ, Runge S, Mu"ller RH (1997), *Int. J. Pharm.*, 149, 255–65.

4. Attama AA (2011), *Recent Pat Drug Deliv Formul.*, 5, 178–87.

5. Bondi ML and Craparo EF (2010), *Drug Deliv.*, 7, 7–18.

6. Bummer PM (2004), *Crit Rev Ther Drug Carr Syst.*, 211–20.

7. Bunjes H, Koch MHJ, Westesen K (2000), *Langmuir*, 16, 5234.

8. Bunjes H (2011), *Current Opinion Coll. Inter Sci.*, 16. 405–411.

9. Bunjes HJ (2010), *Pharm. Pharmacol.*, 62, 1637–45.

10. Bunjes H, Westesen K, Koch MHJ (1996) 129, 159.

11. Cavalli R, Marengo E, Rodriguez L, Gasco MR (1996), *Eur. J. Pharm. Biopharm.*, 43, 110–15.

12. Cevc G (2004), *Adv Drug Deliv Rev.*, 56, 675–11.

13. Das S and Chaudhury A (2010), *AAPS Pharm Sci Tech.*, 12, 62–76.

14. Davis SS (2001), *Adv Drug Deliv Rev.*, 56, 1241–42.

15. Ekambaram P, Sathali AH and Priyanka K (2012), *Sci. Revs. Chem. Commun.*, 2, 80–102.

16. Finsey R (1994), *Adv. Colloid Interface Sci.*, 52, 79.

17. Freitas C, Müller RH Eur. *J. Pharm. Biopharm.*, 47, 125, 1999.

18. Gallarate M, Battaglia L, Peira E and Trotta M. (2011), *Inter J Chem Eng.*, 25, 6.

19. Garti N, Sato K (1988), Crystallization and polymorphism of fats and fatty acids, Marcel Dekker, New York.

20. Gasco MR (1997), *Pharm. Technol.*, 9, 52–8.

21. Harde H, Das M and Jain S (2011), *Expert Opin Drug Deliv.*, 8, 1407–24.

22. Hu FQ, Yuan H, Zhang HH, Fang M (2002), *Int. J. Pharm.*, (2002) 239 121–8.

23. Illum L, Davis SS, Muller RH, Mak E, West P (1987), *Life Sci.*, 40, 367–74.

24. Illum L, Davis SS (1983), *J. Pharm. Sci.*, 72, 1086–1090.

25. Illum L, Davis SS (1984), *FEBS Lett.*, 167, 79–82.

26. Illum L, Davis SS (1986), *Int. J. Pharm.*, 29, 53.

27. Jenning V, Thunemann AF, Gohla SH (2000), *Int. J. Pharm.*, 199, 167–77.

28. Jores K, Mehnert W, Mäder K (2003), *Pharm. Res.*, 20, 1274, 2003.

29. Kaur IP, Bhandari R, Bhandari S, Kakka V (2008), *J. Contr. Rel.*, 127, 97–109.

30. Kreuter J (1983), *Int. J. Pharm.*, 14, 43–58.

31. Kreuter J (1991), *J. Control. Rel.*, 16, 169.

32. Kreuter J (1994), *Eur. J. Drug Metab. Pharmacokinet.* 19, 253–6.

33. Kreuter J, Alyautdin RN, Kharkevich DA, Ivanov AA (1995), *Brain Res.*, 674, 171–4.

34. Kreuter J, Berg U, Liehl E, Soiva M, Speiser PP (1986), *Vaccine*, 4, 125–9.

35. Kreuter J, Haenzel I (1978), *Infect. Immun.*, 19, 667–75.

36. Kreuter J, Liehl E, Berg U, Soiva M, Speiser PP (1988), *Vaccine*, 6, 253–6.

37. Kreuter J, Speiser P (1976), *J. Pharm. Sci.*, 65, 1624–7.

38. Kreuter J, Stieneker F, Lower J (1991), *Proc. Int. Symp. Controlled Release Bioact. Mater.*, 18, 277–8.

39. Lu B, Xiong SB, Yang H, Yin XD, Chao RB (2006), *Eur. J. Pharm. Sci.*, 28, 86–95.

40. Luck M, Schroder W, Paulke BR, Blunk T, Muller, R.H. (1999) *Biomaterials*, 20, 2063–8.

41. Martins S, Sarmento B, Ferreira DC and Souto EB (2007), *Int J Nanomedicine.*, 2, 595–97.

42. Mehnert W and Mader K (2001), *Adv Drug Deliv Rev.*, 47, 165–96.

43. Mei Z, Chen H, Weng T, Yang Y, Yang X (2003), *Eur. J. Pharm. Biopharm.*, 56, 189–196.

44. Meyer O, Kirpotin D, Hong KL, Sternberg B, Park JW, Woodle MC, Papahadjopoulos D (1998), *J. Biol. Chem.*, 273, 15621–7.

45. Middaugh CR, Evans RK, Montgomery DL, Casimiro DR (1998), *J. Pharm. Sci.*, 87, 130–46.

46. Moghimi SM, Muir IS, Illum L, Davis SS, Kolb-Bachofen V (1993), *Biochim. Biophys. Acta*, 1179, 157–165.

47. Moghimi SM, Patel HM (1989), *Biochim. Biophys. Acta*, 984, 379–83.

48. Moghimi SM, Patel HM (1998), *Adv. Drug Deliv. Rev.*, 32, 45–60.

49. Mu"ller RH, Mehnert W, Lucks JS, Schwarz C, zur Mu"hlen A, Weyhers H, Freitas C, Ru"hl D (1995), *Eur. J. Pharm. Biopharm.*, 41, 62–9.

50. Muhlen Zur., Mehnert W (1998), *Pharmazie*, 53 552.

51. Muhlen Zur., Schwarz C, Mehnert W (1998), *Eur. J. Pharm. Biopharm.*, 45, 149–55.

52. Muhlen Zur., Zur Muhlen E, Niehus H, Mehnert W (1996), *Pharm. Res.*, 13, 1411–6.

53. Ogawara K, Yoshida M, Kubo J, Mnishikawa M, Takakura Y, Hashida M, Higaki K, Kimura T (1999), *J. Control. Rel.*, 61, 241–50.

54. Parhi R and Suresh P (2012), *Curr Drug Discov Technol.*, 9, 2–16.

55. Sawant KK and Dodiya SS (2008), *Recent Pat Drug Deliv Formul.*, 2, 120–35.

56. Seyfoddin A, Shaw J, and Al-Kassas R (2010), *Drug Deliv.*, 17, 467–89.

57. Siekmann B, Westesen K (1994), *Pharm. Pharmacol. Lett.*, 3, 225, 1994.

58. Siekmann B, Westesen K (1996), *Eur. J. Pharm. Biopharm.*, 43, 104, 1996.

59. Souto EB and Muller RH (2010), *Handb Exp Pharmacol.*, 197, 115–41.

60. Storhoff JJ, Mirkin CA (1999), *Chem. Rev.*, 99, 1849–62.

61. Trotta M, Debernardi F, Caputo O (2003), *Int. J. Pharm.*, 257, 153–60.

62. Vyas SP, Malaiya A (1989), *J. Microencaps.*, 6, 493–9.

63. Vyas SP, Sihorkar V (2000), *Adv. Drug Deliv. Rev.*, 43, 101–64.

64. Westesen K, Bunjes H, Koch MHJ (1997), *J. Control. Rel.*, 48, 223, 1997.

65. Wissing SA, Kayser O and Muller RH (2004), *Adv Drug Deliv Rev.*, 56, 1257–72.

20

Drug Conjugates

INTRODUCTION

The technology of bioconjugation has attracted interest and attention from nearly every discipline in the life sciences. It includes the chemical-linking of two or more molecules to form a novel complex having the combined properties of its individual components. Natural or synthetic compounds with their individual activities can be chemically combined to create unique substances possessing engineered characteristics. The application of the available cross-linking reactions and reagent systems for creating novel conjugates with peculiar activities, has made possible the assay of minute quantities of substances, the *in vivo* targeting of molecules and the modulation of specific biological processes. Modified or conjugated molecules have been used for purification, detection or localization of specific cellular components, and in the treatment of diseases. Table 20.1 represents the various benefits of bioconjugation in pharmaceutical chemistry.

Cross-linking and modifying agents produced with the help of conjugation techniques, can be applied to alter the native state and function of peptides and proteins, sugars and polysaccharides, nucleic acids and oligonucleotides, lipids and almost any other imaginable molecule that can be chemically derivatized. The structure and function of natural and synthetic molecules can be investigated and mechanism of receptor-ligand interactions can be deduced determined with the help of modification or conjugation strategies.

BIOCONJUGATE TECHNIQUES

Modification and conjugation techniques are based on two interrelated chemical reactions. The reactive functional groups present on the various cross-linking or derivatizing reagents and functional groups present on the target macromolecules to be modified. Reactive functional groups on cross-linking reagents, tag and probe to provide the means to label

Table 20.1: Advantages of bioconjugation in pharmaceutical chemistry		
S. No.	Advantages of bioconjugation in pharmaceutical chemistry	
1.	Stabilization of labile drugs from chemical degradation	
2.	Protection from proteolytic degradation	
3.	Reduction of immunogenicity	
4.	Decreased antibody recognition	
5.	Increased body residence time	
6.	Modification of organ disposition	
7.	Drug penetration by endocytosis	
8.	New possibilities of drug targeting	

specifically certain target groups on ligands, peptides, proteins, carbohydrates, lipids, synthetic polymers, nucleic acids, and oligonucleotides. Knowledge of the basic mechanisms by which the reactive groups couple to target functional groups provides the means to design intelligently a modification or conjugation strategy. By employing the correct reagent systems that can react with the chemical groups available on target molecules, the successful chemical modifications could be imparted. The endogenous or exogenous ligands can be conjugated with either the drug or drug-bearing delivery systems using various noncovalent and covalent techniques.

Covalent Conjugation

Covalent conjugation can be achieved using cross-linking reagents which make the terminal functional groups of one molecule active which can subsequently be conjugated with another target molecule (Table 20.2). Three different cross-linking reagents are used in general:

- Zero-length cross-linkers
- Homobifunctional cross-linkers
- Heterobifunctional (bifunctional and trifunctional) cross-linkers.

Zero-length Cross-linkers

They are smallest available reagent systems for bioconjugation. These compounds mediate the conjugation of two molecules by forming a bond containing no additional atoms. Thus, one atom of a molecule is covalently attached to an atom of a second molecule with no intervening linker or spacer. In many conjugation schemes, the final complex is bound together by using specific chemical components that add foreign structures to the substances being cross-linked, i.e. EDC [1-ethyl-3-(3-dimethylaminopropyl) carbodiimide hydrochloride], NHS (N-hydroxysulphosuccinimide), CMC [1-cyclohexyl-3-(2-morpholinoethyl) carobodiimide], N,N'-carbonyldiimidazole. (Fig. 20.1).

They are used to mediate the formation of amide linkages between a carboxylate and an amine or phosphomidate linkage between a phosphate and an amine. They are the most efficient zero-length cross-linkers in use, being efficient in forming conjugates between two protein molecules, between a protein and a peptide, between oligonucleotides and proteins, between a protein and a delivery system like liposomes and a combination of these with small molecules. A method of NHS

Table 20.2: Various cross-linking reagents used in the bioconjugation of proteins and macromolecules with other target macromolecules or delivery systems

Zero-length cross-linkers	Homobifunctional cross-linkers	Heterobifunctional cross-linkers
Carbodiimide	NHS esters	Bifunctional cross-linkers
EDC	Imidoesterases	Amine reactive and sulfhydryl reactive
EDC and sulfo-NHS	Sulfhydryl reactive cross-linkers	SPDP, LC-SPDP, sulfo-LC-SPDP
DCC	Aldehydes	SMCC and sulfo-SMCC, MBS and sulfo-MBS
Woodward's reagent K	Bis-epoxides hydrazides	Carbonyl reactive and sulfhydryl reactive
N,N'-carbonyldiimidazole	Bis-diazonium derivatives	MPBH, PDPH
Schiff base formation and reductive amination	Bis-alkylhalides	Amine or sulfhydryl or carboxylate or arginate reactive and photoreactive
		NHS-ASA, APDP, ABH, APG
		Trifunctional cross-linkers
		ABNP, sulfo-SBED

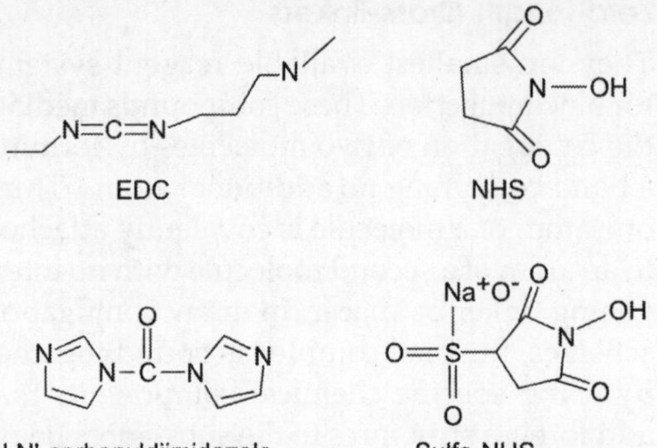

EDC

NHS

N,N'-carbonyldiimidazole

Sulfo-NHS

Fig. 20.1: Structure of some cross-linking agents

ester-mediated protein-carrier conjugation is to create sulfo-NHS esters directly on the carboxylate of the carrier protein using the EDC (Fig. 20.2).

A carbodiimide reaction in the presence of sulfo-NHS activates the carboxylate group on the carrier to form amine reactive sulfo-NHS esters. The activation reaction is conducted at pH 6, since the amines on the protein will be protonated and therefore be less reactive towards sulfo-NHS esters that are formed. In addition, the hydrolysis rate of the esters is dramatically slower at acid pH. Subsequent coupling with an amine-containing carrier creates conjugates through amide bond formation.

Homobifunctional Cross-linkers

They are used for modification and conjugation of macromolecules consisted of bioreactive compounds containing the same functional group at both the ends. Most of these homobifunctional reagents are symmetrical in design with a carbon chain spacer connecting the two identical reactive ends, i.e. formaldehyde, glutaraldehyde, carbohydrazide, DST

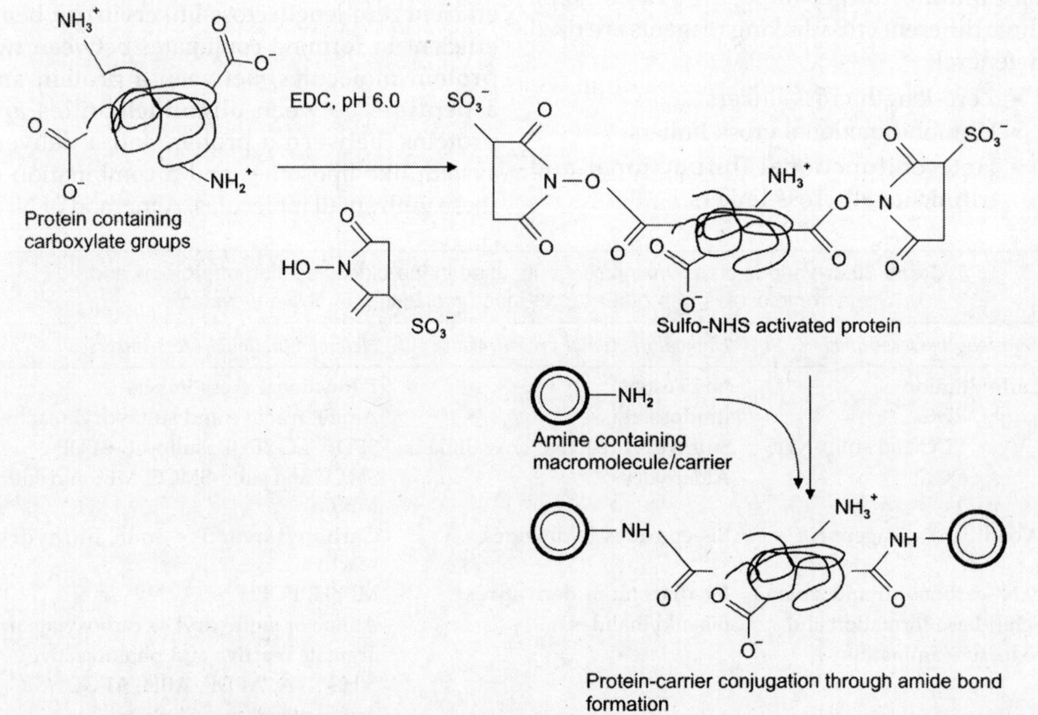

Fig. 20.2: The carbodiimide, EDC, can be used in the presence of sulfo-NHS to create reactive sulfo-NHS ester groups on proteins, which subsequently couple with an amine-containing carrier (or macromolecule) to create conjugates through resultant amide linkage

(disuccinimidyl tartarate) etc. Most of these homobifunctional cross-linkers could tie one protein to another macromolecule or delivery system by covalently reacting with the same common groups on both the molecules (Fig. 20.3).

Two protocols are used for the conjugation using these cross-linkers, i.e. one-step protocol and two-step protocol. Single step protocol involves the addition of all reagents at the same time to the reaction mixtures. This protocol however, provides the least control over the cross-linking process and invariably leads to a multiple of products, only a small percentage of which represents the desired conjugates. In two-step protocols, one of the proteins to be conjugated is reacted with the homobifunctional cross-linker and by products removed. In the second stage, the activated protein is mixed with the other protein or molecule to be conjugated and the final conjugation process occurs. The most commonly employed homobifunctional cross-linkers are NHS esters. They activate

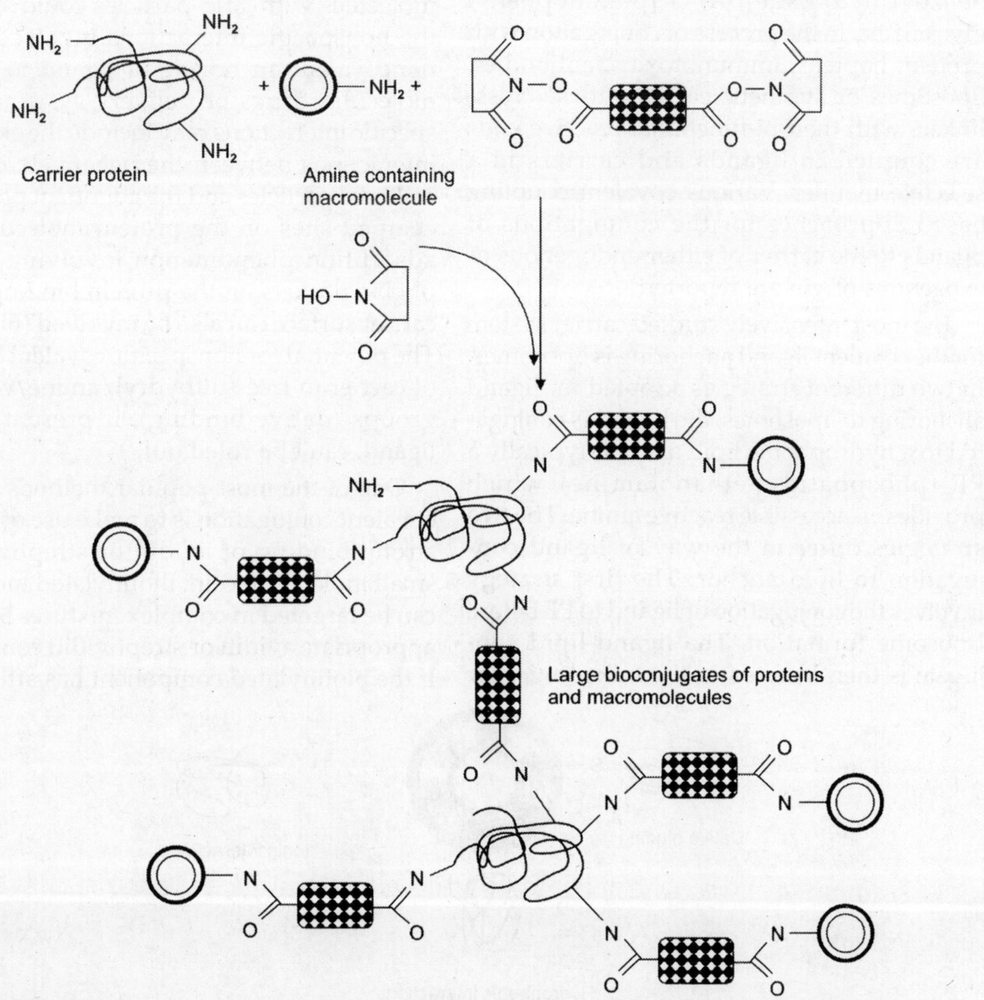

Fig. 20.3: Protein carrier-macromolecule conjugate can be formed using homobifunctional NHS ester cross-linkers

carboxylate groups on the proteins or other moieties to be conjugated with other molecules having amine nucleophiles.

Heterobifunctional Cross-linkers

They contain two different reactive groups that can couple to two different functional targets on macromolecules; the result is the ability to direct the cross-linking reaction to selected parts of target molecules, thus governing better control over the conjugation process, i.e. SPDP [(N-succinimidyl 3-(2-pyridyldithio) propionate], ABH [p-azido-benzoyl hydrazide], APG [p-azidophenyl glyoxal] etc. In the process of conjugation with protein, haptens, immunotoxins, antibodies, liposomes or synthetic carriers, these cross-linkers with their bi-functional reactive ends are coupled to ligands and carriers in a selective manner. Various covalent coupling based approaches for the conjugations of ligands to the carrier of either endogenous or exogenous origin are reported.

The most intensively studied carrier system for the covalent ligand anchoring is liposomes. In two different strategies adopted for ligand anchoring to liposomes, the ligand is conjugated to a hydrophobic lipid anchor, typically a PE (phosphatidyl-ethanolamine) which provides an accessible reactive amine. The two strategies differ in the way of ligand conjugation to lipid anchor. The first strategy involves the conjugation of ligand to PE before liposome formation. The ligand-lipid conjugate is then inserted in the mixed micellar solution of detergent and other lipids by detergent dialysis technique.

Trifunctional cross-linkers are relatively new forms of conjugation reagents, possessing three different reactive or complexing groups per molecule, i.e. 4-azido-2-nitrophenyl-biocytin-4-nitrophenyl ester.

Noncovalent Conjugation

In order to obtain a versatile targeting methodology, noncovalent anchoring of site directing ligands has been appreciated. An interesting observation of labeling of macro-molecules with gold particles could simulate the nonspecific interactions involved in the noncovalent anchoring of ligand to macro-molecular drugs or delivery systems. Non-specific interactions may include the electronic interactions between the negatively charged colloidal particles and the abundant positively charged sites on the protein molecules. An adsorption phenomenon involving hydro-phobic pockets on the protein binding to the carrier surface can also be involved (Fig. 20.4). The potential for nonspecific covalent binding of carrier to free sulfhydryl/amine/carboxyl groups (dative binding), if present on the ligand, can't be ruled out.

One of the most popular methods of non-covalent conjugation is to make use of natural strong binding of avidin or streptavidin to small molecule biotin. Biotinylated molecules can be targeted in complex mixtures by using appropriate avidin or streptavidin conjugates. If the biotinylated component has affinity for

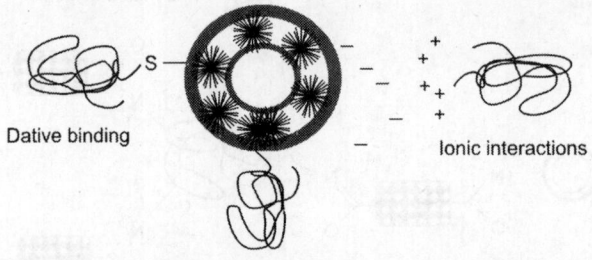

Dative binding

Ionic interactions

Hydrophobic interactions

Fig. 20.4: Hypothetical model to depict nonspecific and noncovalent interactions that could occur between the ligand and the carrier

binding to a particular antigen or receptor then the same can be located by the use of an avidin/streptividin conjugate containing a detecting molecule. A series of avidin or streptividin-biotin interactions can be built upon each other, utilizing the multivalent nature of each tetrameric avidin/streptividin molecule to enhance further the detection capability for the target. The same concept could be exploited with drug carriers as well.

Liposomes with biotin modified lipids can be easily prepared and used to attach a variety of avidin/streptividin linked targeting proteins/ligands. Nonspecific protein based binding ligands (for example, avidin, strep-tividin, protein A or protein G) can be attached to liposomes using covalent conjugation methods. However, the site-directed targeting ligands, more often an antibody or biotinylated antibody, can then be noncovalently conjugated to the liposomes via specific affinity interactions with the nonspecific binding ligands. This however restricts the use of only antitarget immunoglobulin molecules as targeting ligands. Antibodies can be conjugated to liposomes using an indirect approach incorporating an avidinbiotin system. Biotinylated liposomes may be complexed with biotinylated antibodies using avidin as a bridging molecule or may be complexed with an antibody-avidin conjugate (Fig. 20.5).

Bioconjugate Applications

Bioconjugation techniques are used in the preparation of unique conjugates and labeled molecules for use in particular application areas. These include hapten-carrier immunogen conjugates and antibody-enzyme conjugates

Hapten-carrier immunogen conjugates, i.e. carbodiimides-mediated hapten carrier conjugates and glutaraldehyde-mediated hapten carrier conjugates, are used in antibody production, in immune response research and in the production of vaccines.

Antibody-enzyme conjugates, i.e. NHS ester-maleimide-mediated conjugates, glutaral-dehyde-mediated conjugates are used in immunoassays, targeting and detection techniques. Since the development of enzyme-linked immunosorbent assay (ELISA) systems and the ability to make conjugates of specific antibodies with enzymes has provided the means to quantify or detect hundreds of important analytes. The use of enzymes as labels in immunoassay procedures surpassed radioactive tags as the means of detection, primarily due to the long-term stability potential of an enzyme system and the hazards

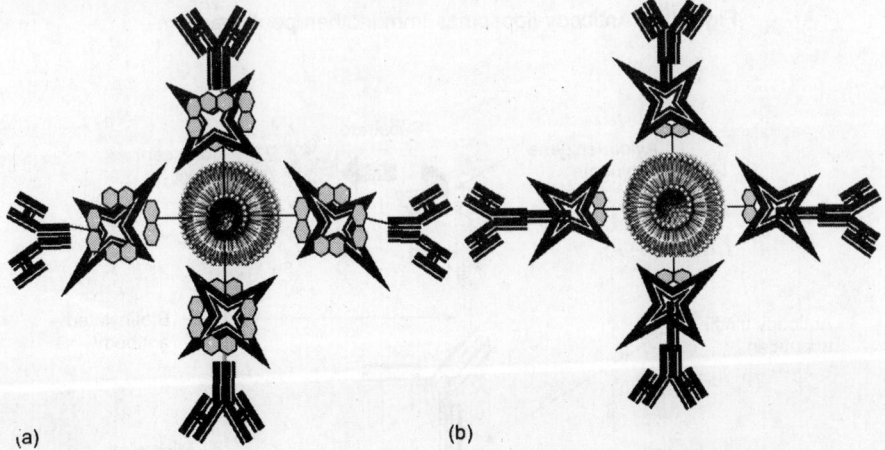

(a)   (b)

Fig. 20.5: Methods of conjugation of proteins/macromolecules/antibodies to liposomal surface. (a) Method depicts the conjugation of biotinylated antibody with biotinylated liposomes using avidin as a bridging molecule. (b) Method depicts conjugation of biotinylated liposomes with an antibody-avidin conjugate

and waste problems associated with radio-isotopes.

In addition to labeling immunoglobulins with enzymes to provide detectability through their catalytic action on a substrate, antibody molecules also can be labeled or tagged with small compounds that can provide indigenous traceable properties. Labeled antibodies, i.e. fluorescently labeled antibodies, radiolabeled antibodies and biotinylated antibodies are also having immense uses in immunoassays, targeting and detection techniques. Antibody-liposomes conjugates may possess encapsulated components that can be used for detection of desired site and targeted therapy. Liposomes conjugating antibodies directed against tumor cell antigens can deliver encapsulated toxins or drugs to the cancer cells, affecting selective toxicity and cell death (Fig. 20.6).

Biotin, avidin, and proteins can also be appended onto the surface of liposomes with the help of various conjugation techniques for various types of therapeutic applications. Avidin or streptavidin conjugates are used in immunoassays. The specificity of antibody molecules provides the targeting ability to recognize and the bind particular antigen molecules. If there are biotin labels on the antibody molecule, it creates multiple sites for binding of avidin and streptavidin. If avidin or streptavidin in turn labeled with an enzyme, fluorophore, etc., then a very sensitive antigen-detection system is created. The potential for more than one labeled avidin to become attached to each antibody through its multiple biotinylation sites is the key to dramatic increase in assay sensitivity over other which use antibodies directly labeled with a detectable tag (Fig. 20.7).

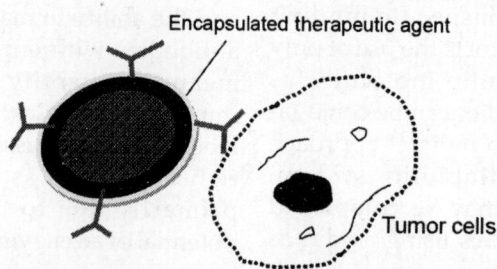

Fig. 20.6: Antibody-liposomes immunotherapeutic system

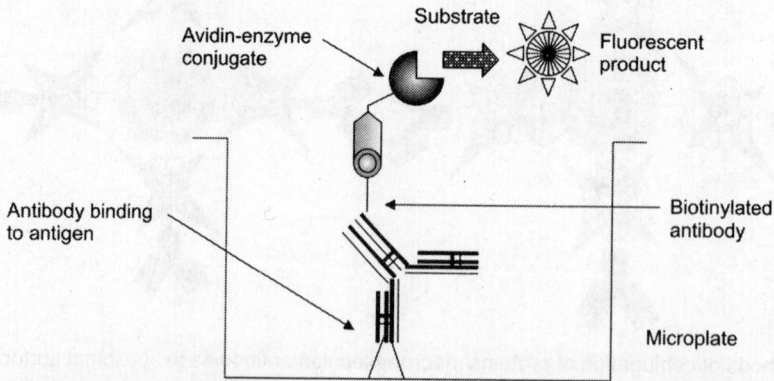

Fig. 20.7: The basic design of the labeled avidin-biotin (LAB) assay system

Enzymatic labeling of DNA and chemical modification of nucleic acids and oligonucleotides can be done effectively using bioconjugation techniques. To modify the unique chemical groups on nucleic acids, the methods have been developed that allow derivatization through discrete sites on the available bases, sugars, or phosphate groups. These conjugation methods can be used to add a functional group or label an individual nucleotide or one or more sites in oligonucleotide probes or full-sized DNA or RNA polymers.

GLUTARALDEHYDE-BASED HAPTEN-CARRIER CONJUGATION

In bioconjugation techniques, glutaraldehyde is used as homobifunctional cross-linking reagent in conjugation procedure to prepare hapten-carrier conjugates. Glutaraldehyde reacts with primary amino groups to create Schiff bases or double-bond addition product. The conjugates formed in the reaction of glutaraldehyde with protein carriers and peptide haptens are usually of high molecular weight and may be precipitated. Various types of procedures are discussed in the literature to form glutaraldehyde conjugates. In some methods, neutral pH environment in phosphate buffer (pH 6.8–7.5) is maintained, while in other procedures alkaline conditions in carbonate buffer (pH 8–9) are maintained and used. In general, the higher pH conditions will be more preferred to form Schiff base intermediates which result in greater

conjugation yields with higher molecular weight cojugates.

CARBODIIMIDE-BASED CONJUGATION TO PHOSPHATIDYLETHANOLAMINE LIPID DERIVATIVES

Liposomal membrane is composed of underivatized phosphatidylethanolamine that contains an amino group that participates in the carbodiimide reaction with carboxylate groups of proteins. Carboxylate groups are activated by water-soluble carbodiimide EDC to form active ester intermediate that can react with phosphatidylethanolamine to form an amide linkage (Fig. 20.8).

Unfortunately, due to abundance of both amide and carboxylates present on proteins, EDC coupling of proteins to the surface of liposomes often results in considerable protein to protein cross-linking. Sometimes, vesicle aggregation also occurs due to protein coupling between liposomes. This polymerization problem can be avoided by first blocking the amino groups of the protein with citraconic acid, which has been used successfully with antibodies.

GLUTARALDEHYDE-BASED CONJUGATION TO PHOSPHATIDYLETHANOLAMINE LIPID DERIVATIVE

Glutaraldehyde, a homobifunctional crosslinker reacts with phosphatidylethanolamine residues present on the liposome surface to form an activated surface reactive aldehyde group. A two-step conjugation reaction using

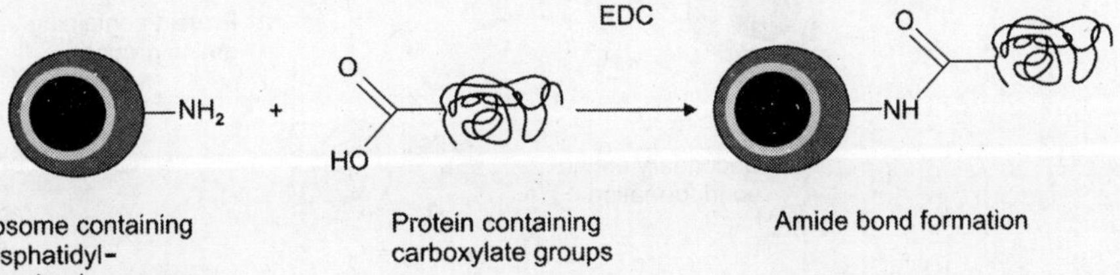

Fig. 20.8: Reaction showing the conjugation of protein with a liposome containing phosphatidylethanolamine groups using a carbodi-imide reaction with EDC

glutaraldehyde is a suitable method when working with liposomes, since precipitated protein would be difficult to remove from suspension of vesicles (Fig. 20.9).

AVIDIN-BIOTIN SYSTEM

Avidin-biotin system is one of the most popular conjugation techniques of non-covalent conjugation, which is used in specific-targeting applications and assay designs. Avidin is a glycoprotein that contains four identical subunits and each subunit contains one binding site for biotin and one for oligosaccharide modification. This interaction may be used to enhance the signal strength of immunoassay systems. The only shortcoming associated is tendency of avidin molecule to bind nonspecifically to components other than biotin due to its high pI (isoelectric point) and carbohydrate content. Streptavidin is another biotin-binding protein isolated from *Streptomyces avidinii* with less or non-specificities for avidin. Streptavidin, similar to avidin contains four subunits, each with a single biotin-binding site. Avidin and streptavidin are used in bioconjugation techniques to conjugate other proteins or label various detection reagents without loss of biotin-binding activity.

There are various basic immunoassays based on avidin-biotin interaction. Biotinylated antibody creates multiple sites for the binding of avidin or streptavidin. If avidin or streptavidin is labeled with enzyme or fluorophore etc. a very sensitive antigen detection system is created. Some of the assay systems are typically labeled avidin-biotin (LAB) assay system, bridged avidin-biotin system (BRAB), and avidin-biotin complex (ABC) system. Similar techniques are used to develop avidin-biotin system for detection of nucleic acid hybridization in which avidin-labeled complexes are used to detect DNA probes labeled with biotin through binding of their complementary DNA target. Avidin-biotin system can also be used in the nonenzyme assay systems in which labeled avidin molecules can be utilized for detection of biotinylated molecule, after it binds to its target. Similarly, in radioimmunoassay designs, radiolabeled avidin can be employed as a universal detection reagent. In the tumor-

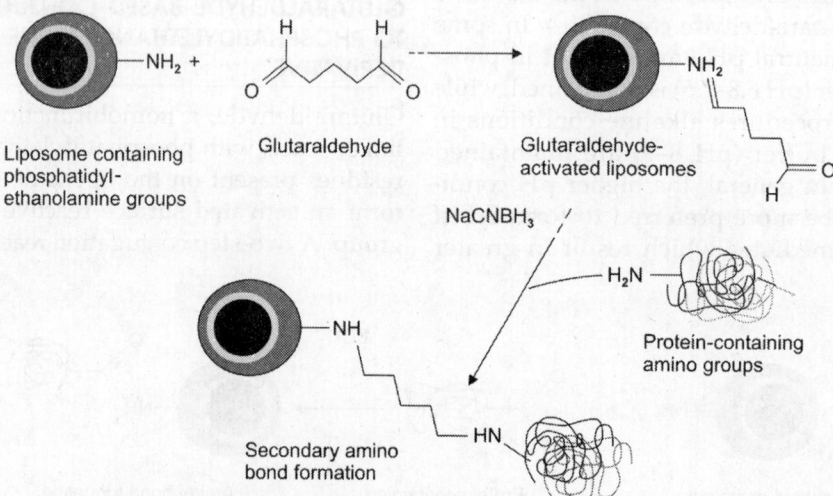

Liposome containing phosphatidyl-ethanolamine groups

Glutaraldehyde

Glutaraldehyde-activated liposomes

NaCNBH₃

Protein-containing amino groups

Secondary amino bond formation

Fig. 20.9: Reaction showing glutaraldehyde activation of phosphatidyl-ethanolamine-containing liposomes used to couple protein molecules

imaging techniques, avidin labeled I_{125} can be used to localize biotinylated monoclonal antibodies directed against tumor cells *in vivo*.

Preparation of Avidin-HRP or Streptavidin-HRP Conjugates

Horseradish peroxidase (HRP) can be conjugated with avidin or streptavidin by periodate oxidation and reductive amination. Periodate oxidation of polysaccharide components of the glycoprotein molecule (HRP and avidin) produces reactive aldehyde groups. Another protein (biotin) can be conjugated with these reactive aldehyde groups by reacting the aldehyde with amines to form Schiff bases with subsequent reduction using sodium cynoborohydride to create stable secondary amino bonds (Fig. 20.10).

PREPARATION OF COLLOIDAL GOLD-LABELED PROTEINS

The labeling of targeting molecules, especially proteins, with gold nanoparticles has been used in the visualization of cellular or tissue components by electron microscopy. Gold labeling of immunoglobulin-binding proteins is used as a universal probe for detection and visualization of any antibody-antigen interaction in tissue sections, cells and blots (Fig. 20.11).

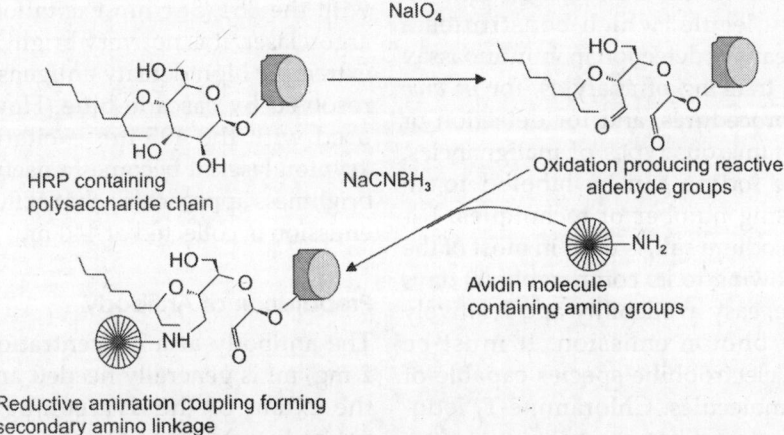

Fig. 20.10: Schematic diagram showing the conjugation of HRP with avidin by the process of reductive amination and periodate oxidation

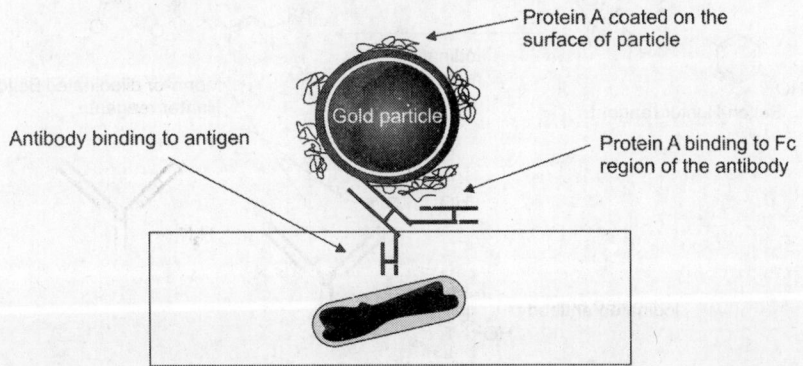

Fig. 20.11: Schematic diagram showing protein A-gold complex for visualization of tissue components in electron microscopy

The labeling of macromolecules with gold particles depends on the several interactions, such as the electrostatic attraction between the positively-charged gold particles and negatively-charged sites on the protein molecule, adsorption phenomenon and covalent binding of gold to free sulfhydryl groups (dative binding). Mono-dispersed colloidal gold suspensions are used for protein labeling, which can be produced by a variety of chemical methods in which reductive processes using chlorouric acid (HauCl$_4$) are used to create the spheroidal gold particles.

RADIOLABELED ANTIBODIES

Radioactive labels can be attached onto an antibody molecule, which constitutes a powerful means of detection in immunoassay procedures, tracking of analytes, for *in vivo* diagnostic procedures, and for detection or therapy of numerous types of malignancies. Radioactive iodine can be labeled to an antibody using number of techniques. I$_{125}$ supplied as sodium salt, is used in most of the procedures owing to its comparably 60 days long half-life, easy availability and relatively low-energy photon emission. It must be oxidized to electrophilic species capable of modifying molecules. Chloramine-T, iodo-beads and iodogen are commonly used as oxidizing agents. It leads to an iodination reaction at available tyrosine residues within the polypeptide chain. Some other cross-linking or modification reagents containing an activated aromatic ring may also be iodinated to label at other conjugation site within protein molecule, if tyrosine can not be labeled. For example, Bolton-Hunter reagent may be used to add radioactive iodine to antibody molecule by modifying the primary amines within the antibody. It can also be used in the absence of tyrosine residue on the molecule (Fig. 20.12).

Cascade Blue Conjugation of Antibodies

Cascade blue, a UV-excitable dye, can be used for immunofluorescence labeling. When used with the 351/361 nm excitation lines of an argon laser, it is not very bright; usually only extremely high density antigens can be well-resolved by cascade blue. However, when used with the 405 nm excitation line of a krypton laser, it becomes a useful dye with a brightness approaching that of fluorescein and emission is collected at 440 nm.

Preparation of Antibody

The antibody at a concentration of at least 2 mg/ml is generally needed and moreover, the extent of the dye conjugation to the antibody may depend on the concentration of

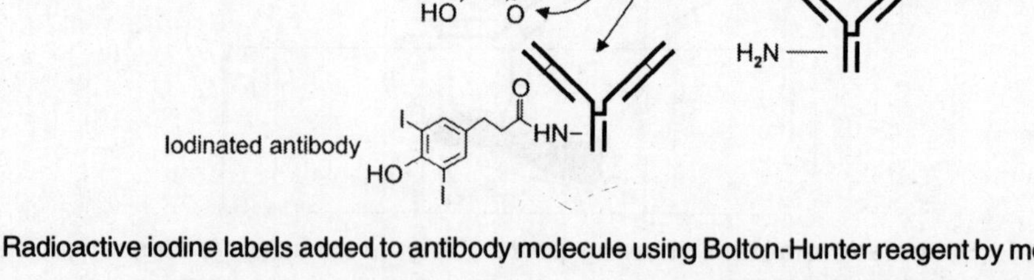

Fig. 20.12: Radioactive iodine labels added to antibody molecule using Bolton-Hunter reagent by modification of amines

antibody in solution. Therefore, a consistent concentration of antibody should be used for stable conjugation.

The reactive cascade blue molecule is unstable. Therefore, the solution of the cascade blue should be used almost immediately. When first conjugating an antibody, a range of cascade blue to antibody concentrations should be compared. The protocol suggests 150 µg per mg of antibody; for a first-time titration of cascade blue, try a range of 40 to 600 µg cascade blue per mg of antibody. Compare each conjugate by staining (a titration of antibody on cells for each reagent to determine the optimal staining concentration should be performed). Then the conjugate is with the brightest 'positive' cells should be chosen.

Phycoerythrin Conjugation of Antibodies

Phycoerythrin (PE) is one of the most commonly used fluorescent dyes for FACS analysis. PE is a large protein (approximate molecular weight 240 kDa) containing 25 fluors. Typically, only one PE molecule is conjugated to an antibody. Nonetheless, by virtue of its huge absorption coefficient and almost perfect quantum efficiency, it is one of the brightest dyes used today. It emits at about 570 nm and can be excited by common argon laser lines. Direct PE conjugates are relatively easy to prepare.

ANTIBODY-TOXIN CONJUGATES

Cell type-specific cytotoxic agents have been constructed in several laboratories by linking highly potent toxins or their subunits to antibody molecules. Most of the toxins (Table 20.3) that have been considered for use in immunoconjugates are composed of two functionally distinct protein moieties, the A chain and the B chain. A chain is a single polypeptide that exhibits enzymatic activity and induces cell killing by shutting down protein synthesis.

The toxins most widely have been used include diptheria toxin (the endotoxin from *Cornebacterium diphtheriae*) and the plant toxins ricin (from *Ricinus communis*) and abrin (from *Abrus precatorius*). Abrin, ricin, and diphtheria toxins are composed of two polypeptide subunits, A and B joined by a disulfide bond. The A chain of the plant toxin ricin, e.g. can inactivate up to 1500 ribosomes per minute by removing a single adenine base from 28S ribosomal RNA. B chains, which may be single polypeptides or several polypeptides held together in loose association, bind to the cell surface and mediate translocation of A chains into the cytosol. Diphtheria toxin, for instance, is endocytosed and when exposed to low pH, hydrophobic domains on the B chain are inserted into the endosomal membrane. This

Table 20.3: Toxins commonly used for construction of immunoconjugates

Toxin	Source	Effect on intact cells	Binding cells	Catalytic effect
Gelonin (monomer)	*Gelonium multiflorum*	Nontoxic	No	Inactivated ribosomes
Pokeweed antiviral protein (monomer)	*Phytolacca americana*	Nontoxic	No	Inactivated ribosomes
Ricin (heterodimer)	*Ricinis communis*	Toxic	Yes	Inactivated ribosomes
Abrin (heterodimer)	*Abrus precatorius*	Toxic	Yes	Inactivated ribosomes
Modeccin (heterodimer)	*Adenia digitata*	Toxic	Yes	Inactivated ribosomes
Diphtheria toxin (heterodimer)	*Corynebacterium diphtheriae*	Toxic	Yes	ADP-ribosylates EF-2
Pseudomonas toxin (single polypeptide)	*Pseudomonas aeruginosa*	Toxic	Yes	ADP-ribosylates EF-2

insertion facilitates the transfer of the A fragment into the cytosol, presumably through pore formation by the B chain. All three toxins have similar mode of cytotoxic action. They bind by means of recognition sites on the B chain to the component of plasma membrane of virtually all cell types in sensitive species of animals; abrin and ricin recognize galactose terminating glycoproteins and glycolipids, whereas the receptor for diphtheria toxins have not yet been identified. The A chain then penetrates (or is transport across) the plasma membrane or the membrane of an endocytotic vesicle and kills the cells by inactivating its machinery for protein synthesis. There are two types of antibody-toxin conjugates with the cell specificity. First is to link the antibody by a disulphide bond to the isolated A chain moiety or alternatively to one of the single chain plant peptides, such as gelonin from glonium multiflorum, whose damaging action on the eukaryotic ribosomes is apperantly identical to that of the A chain of abrin and ricin. The second is to link the intact toxin to the antibody and block the cell recognition site on the B chain to prevent the conjugate from binding to and killing the cells nonspecifically (Fig. 20.13).

PROTEIN CONJUGATES OF FUNGAL TOXINS

Nearly all fetal cases of poisoning by mushrooms in man are due to three Amanita species (*A. phalloides, A. verna,* and *A. virosa*), which contain two families of toxic cyclopeptides, amatoxins and phallotoxins. Conjugation of amatoxins and phallotoxins to protein was performed to obtain a selective killing of cells, which display high uptake of the protein, attached to the toxins.

Phallotoxins Fungal Toxin to Proteins

Using either carbodiimide or mixed anhydrides coupling method, four different phyllotoxins-bovine serum albumin conjugates have been prepared (Table 20.4). Phallacidin (PC) is the most abundant

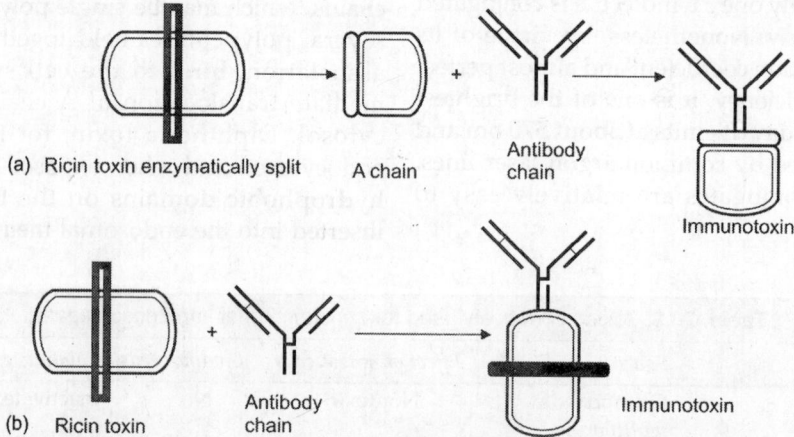

(a) Ricin toxin enzymatically split   A chain   Antibody chain   Immunotoxin

(b) Ricin toxin   Antibody chain   Immunotoxin

Fig. 20.13: Schematic pictures showing the formation of immunotoxin

S.No.	Compounds	Molar ratio	Coupling method	Remarks
	Table 20.4: Phallotoxins coupling to bovine serum albumin by various methods			
1.	Bovine serum albumin-PC	2.7	ECDI	No affinity to actin
2.	Bovine serum albumin-PD-C	9.6	Mixed anhydride (MA)	Affinity to actin 5%
3.	Bovine serum albumin-PD-C	2.4	ECDI, MCDI	Affinity to actin 5%
4.	Bovine serum albumin-PD	2.3	ECDI	–

phallotoxin with a native carboxylic group in side chain, which allows the formation of amide bond with the amine group of the protein, however the carboxylic group, is very close to the peptide backbone, and thus its coupling can affect the biological activity of the toxin. Therefore, a functional group has been introduced into the dihydroxy-L-leucine side chain of phallocidin (PD-C).

POLY-L-LYSINE CONJUGATES

In recent years numerous novel methods have been for reducing the toxic side effects associated with cancer chemotherapeutic agents and other potentially beneficial compounds. Polylysine is used as polymeric carrier and it interacts with many cells in both specific and unusual ways. Earlier studies indicated that polylysine possessed antiviral, antibacterial phage and antibacterial activities (Fig. 20.14). Polylysine also has an affinity for cancerous tissue and is capable of enhancing the uptake of macromolecules into cells, such as albumin and peroxidase. In addition, polylysine shows very specific effects with some types of tumor cells. An additional desirable property of polylysine is its facile degradation by intracellular trypsin. Consequently, polylysine shows many characteristics, which

suggest its use as a drug carrier. It has an affinity for at least some cancer cells, it is readily taken up by endocytosis, and it can be readily cleaved by trypsin, once its conjugates enter cells. The practical use of polylysine as a drug carrier requires additional considerations—(1) toxicity; (2) retention of conjugate integrity until the conjugate reaches the target cell; and (3) the biodegradation of conjugate to an active drug form once the conjugate reaches the target site. The toxicity of polylysine and its neoplastic activity are highly dependent upon molecular weight and concentration. At high molecular weights and high concentrations, polylysine has pronounced effects. At low concentration and low molecular weight, polylysine has minimal or limited effects. Thus, low concentrations of low molecular weight lysine polymers are indicated as drug carriers. Polylysine is an effective drug carrier for various cell types. Several drugs, including methotrexate, daunomycin, and 6-aminonicotinamide, have been attached to polylysine with a retention of drug activity. Methotrexate can be coupled directly to the ε-amino groups of polylysine via its glutamate moiety. Resistance toward methotrexate has been encountered in the treatment of cancer patients. The polylysine conjugates of methotrexate were taken up by cells at a higher rate than free drugs form. This increased uptake can overcome drug resistance. Addition of heparin at a high concentration restores growth inhibitory effect of methotrexate-polylysine (Fig. 20.15).

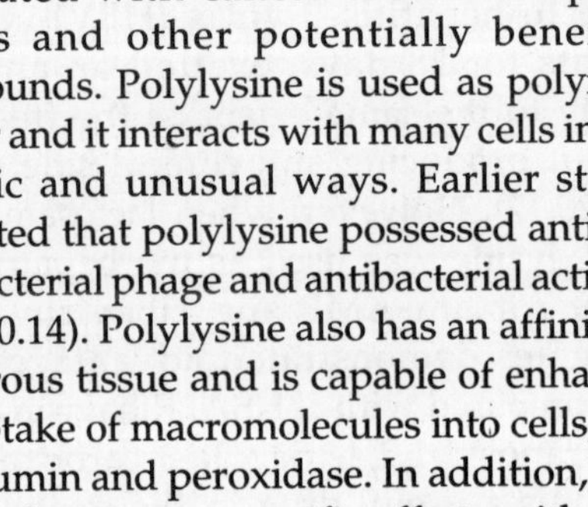

Fig. 20.14: Structure of poly-L-lysine

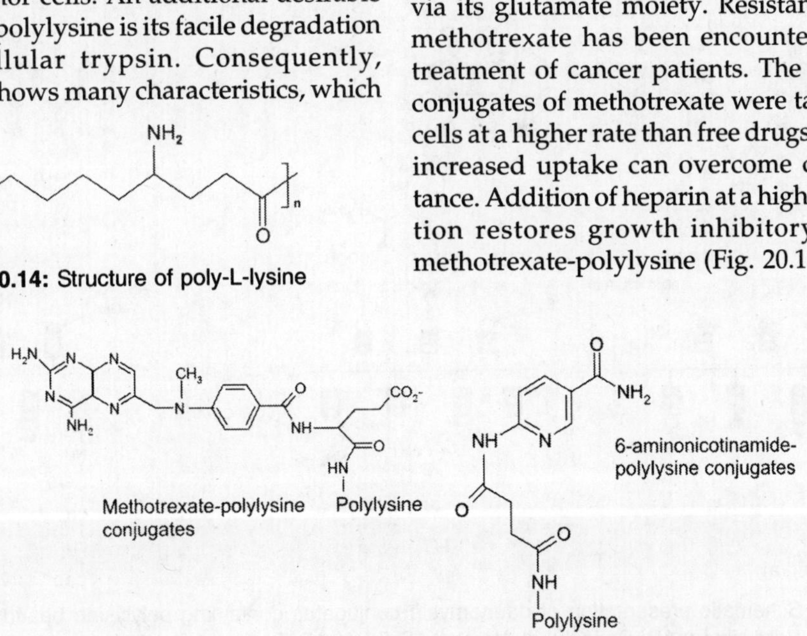

Fig. 20.15: Structure of some polylysine-anticancer drug conjugates

Daunomycin can be coupled to polylysine using a number of spacer groups including succinate and 6-aminonicotinamide can be covalently linked to polylysine via a succinate spacer. Generally, the conjugate possesses only 5–20% of the activity of the free drug. The activity of the conjugate, however, is strikingly different from that of the free drug. The activity of the conjugate is highly dependent upon the target cell type and other constituents present within the target cells. In some cases, the toxicity of the conjugate in animals is decreased relative to the free drug, while beneficial antineoplastic activity is retained. Previous studies indicate that polylysine has potential for 'targeting' drugs to specific cell or tissue sites.

A group of water-soluble drug conjugates in which daunomycin is coupled to cationic, amphoteric or anionic branched polypeptides and a new conjugate containing a cationic polypeptide carrier modified with a cell penetrating octa-arginine are also reported. The results suggested that attachment of polypeptide and cell penetrating peptide to the bioactive agent, depending on the cell line,

could significantly improve the antitumor activity of the drug (Fig. 20.16).

Poly-L-lysine conjugates has been investigated mainly for their role as nonviral gene vector (polycation conjugates) and for antiviral properties of the conjugated nucleoside analogs. In order to reduce the extrahepatic side effects of antiviral nucleoside, analogues in the treatment of chronic viral hepatitis, these drugs are conjugated with galactosyl-terminating macromolecules adenine arabinoside mono-phosphate (ara-AMP), conjugated with lactosaminated human serum albumin (L-HSA, neoglycoconjugate), when administered to hepatitis-B virus (HBV)-infected patients for 28 days, exerted an antiviral activity to the same extent as the free drug without producing any clinical side effects (Fig. 20.17). However, when lactosaminated poly-L-lysine was used as the hepatotropic carrier for ara-AMP and ribavirin, these conjugates demonstrated advantages over those prepared with L-HSA. Ribavirin (l-b-d-ribofuranosyl-1,2,4-triazole-3-carboxamide) (RIBV), is a useful drug in the treatment of chronic type C hepatitis, but displays toxicity

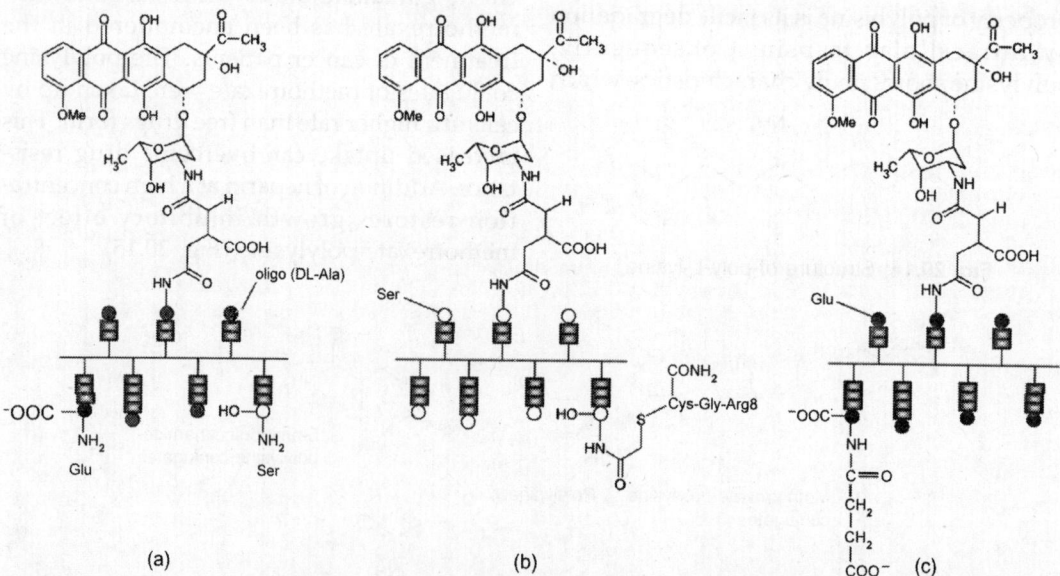

(a) (b) (c)

Fig. 20.16: Schematic presentation of daunomycin conjugates containing polylysine based polypeptide carriers. (a) Polylysine-(cADi-Seri/Glui-dl-Alam) (cAD-SAK/cAD-EAK). (b) Polylysine-(cADj-Glui-dl-Alam)-Cys-Gly-Arg8 (cAD-SAK-Cys-Gly-Arg8). (c) Polylysine-(cADj- SuccGlui-dl-Alam) (cAD-SuccEAK).

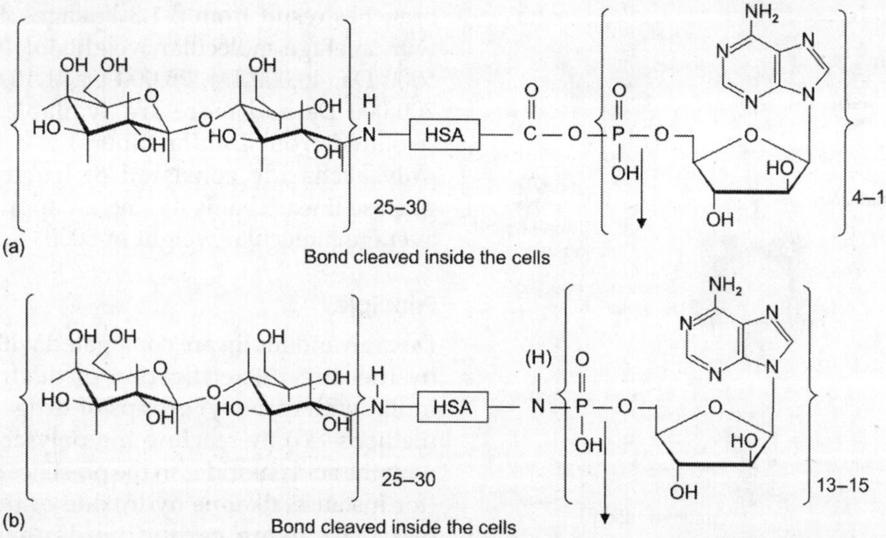

Fig. 20.17: L-HSA conjugates of ara-AMP. (a) The synthesis at pH 5–5.5 produces a phosphoanhydride bond between L-HSA and ara-AMP. (b) The synthesis at pH 7.5 produces phosphoamide bonds between L-HSA and ara-AMP.

for red blood cells, which limits its dosage and necessitates withdrawal in some patients. Studies showed that delivery of RIBV to the liver, reduces the risk of anemia and permits higher hepatocyte drug concentrations with improved therapeutic results. Liver targeting was achieved by coupling the drug to galactosyl-terminating peptides, which specifically enter hepatocytes. The conjugation of RIBV with lactosaminated poly-L-lysine, constitutes a hepatotropic carrier used for intramuscular administration of conjugates. On intramuscular administration to mice, the conjugate was selectively taken up by the liver, where the drug was released in a pharmacologically active form. Poly-L-lysine can also be easily conjugated with biological response modifiers, such as muramyl dipeptide (MDP).

However, the major role of poly-L-lysine conjugates is their ability to act as a nonviral gene vector. Receptor-mediated gene transfer is a promising gene delivery technique. For non-viral gene delivery system a vector should have the ability to make structure compact and mask DNA negative charges. The polylysine could form complex with plasmid DNA and protect DNA from nuclease degradation. It employs a DNA-binding polycation, to compact plasmid DNA to a size that can be taken up by the cells (100–200 nm). To allow internalization by receptor-mediated endocytosis, cell-binding ligands, such as asialoglycoproteins, galactose and transferrin (Fig. 20.18), can be covalently attached to polylysine. Several nonviral gene vectors including fusogenic liposomes, genosomes (DNA-liposomes/lipid complexes) and Lipofection™ (lipid-DNA complex) are investigated as the major gene vectors. Antisense oligonucleotides are a novel class of therapeutic agents known to selectively transform gene expression. High transfection levels can be achieved by using polylysine-based systems *in vitro*. The formation of homogeneous, small, soluble, and stable DNA complexed with poly-L-lysine particles, appears to be an important aspect. The charge ratio of DNA to polylysine, (i.e. the moles of amino groups of polylysine divided by the moles of phosphate groups supplied by DNA), the size of polylysine, the degree of modification of polylysine as well as the conditions used to assemble the complex are some major factors that influence the size and solubility of the resulting DNA complex.

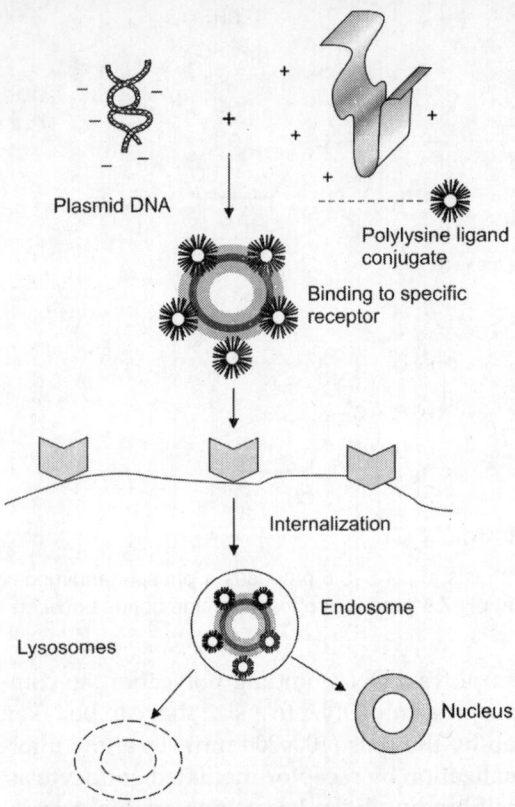

Fig. 20.18: Receptor-mediated endocytosis of DNA-polylysine conjugate

DEXTRAN AND INULIN CONJUGATES AS DRUG CARRIERS

Dextran is a biosynthetic polymer composed of branched glucan (polysaccharide consisting of many glucose molecules) with chains of varying lengths (from 3 to 2000 kilodaltons). The straight chain consists of α-1,6 glycosidic linkages between glucose molecules, while branches result from β-1,3 linkages. Dextran with average molecular weights of 1000 Da, 5000 Da, 40,000 Da, 75,000 Da, 1,10,000 Da, 700,000 Da and more are available. Inulin (isolated from Dahila tubers) is a natural polysaccharide consisted of fructose and glucose linear chains having an approximate average molecular weight of 5000.

Principle

Dextran and inulin are conjugated with drugs by the direct esterification of dextran and inulin with carbonyl groups of drugs by two methods—(i) by reacting the polysaccharide with the acid chlorides in the presence of bases (for instance alkaline hydroxide or pyridine) or (ii) by using carbodiimide, azides or mixed anhydrides, such as chloroacetic or trichloroacetic anhydrides (Fig. 20.19).

LECTIN AS CARRIER

Lectins are a group of proteins with the characteristic ability to bind saccharides moieties at two or more sites on the molecules. This structure endows lectins with the ability to agglutinate red blood cells and cultured cells by agglutinate red blood cells and cultured cells by cross-linking cell surface saccharides structures. The majority of the lectins, which have been characterized, are derived from plant seeds and they have been extensively studies under the name of phytohemagglutinins. Some lectins are used in blood typing a variety of them have been used as experimental tools to investigate biological roles of cell surface glycoproteins.

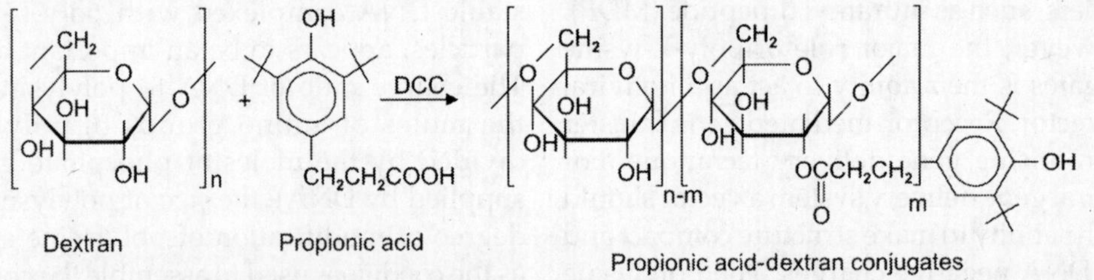

Dextran + Propionic acid $\xrightarrow{\text{DCC}}$ Propionic acid-dextran conjugates

CH_2CH_2COOH

Fig. 20.19: Synthetic scheme for sterically hindered phenol-dextran conjugate

Some lectins (e.g. wheat germ agglutinin, concanavalin A), specifically bind with agglutinate tumor cells but not with normal control cells under defined experimental conditions, thereby providing the valuable tools for investigating biochemical changes associated with oncogenic transformation.

Advantages of Lectins as a Carrier of Drugs and Enzymes

- Lectins are readily purified by simple affinity chromatography techniques that are useful both in the initial isolation of the lectins and in purifying conjugates, which contains lectins.
- Lectins can tolerate higher coupling frequencies without loss of binding activity as compared to antibodies.

Disadvantages of Lectins as a Carrier

- Retention for longer period at the site of injection in a variety of tissues
- Lower specificity
- Many lectins are toxic and potent inducers of inflammation.

GLYCOPROTEINS AS DRUG CARRIERS

Glycoproteins are well-known carrier for drug targeting to specific cell types, by virtue of a range of plasma membrane receptors for glycoprotein. Some of these receptors are listed in the Table 20.5. In general they mediate entry into cells by endocytosis so they are valuable in directing molecules to endosomes, lysosomes, and other structures with which such vesicles fuse. In addition, small permeable molecules may be deposited inside particular cells by such mean and then, after hydrolysis of their carrier, be freed to diffuse throughout the cell, thus reaching cytosolic and other locations nonselectively. Glycoproteins have also found application as spacer molecules, thereby allowing larger amounts of a drug to be linked to antibodies (which are used to target the drugs) than to antibody alone. Glycoproteins may also be used to direct liposomes erythrocyte ghosts or viral envelopes to specific cell types, where they fuse with cell surface, threreby depositing their soluble contents into the interior of the cell.

GALACTOSE TERMINATED FETUIN AS CARRIERS FOR PEPSTATIN

Pepstatin is a group specific inhibitor of aspartic proteinases and has already some well identified clinical applications. Although, directing pepstatin to the liver is not difficult, the first pepstatin glycoprotein carrier, which has been made, asialofetuin (galactose

Table 20.5: Some cellular receptors for glycoproteins and their respective location	
Receptor	*Respective locations*
Serum glycoproteins with carbohydrate termini	Hepatocytes
Galactose terminated glycoproteins	Transferrin
Other serum glycoproteins	Reticulocytes
2-Macroglobulins	Macrophages, fibroblasts
Lysosomal enzymes	
Mannose terminated enzymes	Macrophages
Mannose-6-phosphate terminated enzymes	Fibroblasts
Harmones and growth factors	
TSH	Thyroids
Gonadotropins	Gonadal cells
Cellular growth factors such as epidermal growth factors	Fibroblast
Opsonins	
Complement components	Leukocytes
Antibodies	Leukocytes

terminated)-pepstatin selective towards hepatocytes. The conjugation involves purification of the serum glycoprotein fetuin (from commercial samples) and its enzymatic (or chemical) desialylation to expose terminal galactose residues, for subsequent chemical conjugations.

BIOCONJUGATES WITH PROTEIN DRUGS

The rationale of polymer conjugation to proteins for pharmaceutical applications is widely explored. The attachment of soluble and biocompatible polymers aims at the improvement of protein stability and the modification of their pharmacokinetic profiles. One of the major drawbacks in the use of biologically active proteins in therapy is the common short bioresidence time. They are either rapidly removed by renal ultrafiltration or inactivated by the immunosystem or by plasma enzymes. After polymer conjugation, the stability and the pharmacokinetic profile of a protein is generally improved because, as in the case of low molecular weight drugs, the polymer increases the molecular volume of drug, protects it from enzymatic and hydrolytic degradation and shields its immunological epitopes. Many polymers are being studied for these applications, the most popular are dextran and mPEG, the first is poly-functional, while the second monofunctional. Other mono-functional polymers with properties similar to mPEG are also being studied. Among these, a new form of poly (N-vinyl pyrrolidone) and poly (N-acryloyl morpholine) are also used.

Dextran Protein Conjugates

There are at least 20 polypeptides and proteins conjugated with polysaccharides, mainly dextrans. Streptokinase was the first therapeutic enzyme to be conjugated to a polymer (dextran of 35–50 kDa molecular mass) with significant therapeutic success. Since 1980, after its approval for clinical use in the treat ment of cardiovascular and ophthalmological pathologies caused by thrombosis, it has been produced in Russia, on a large scale, under the trade name of 'Streptodekase®'. This streptokinase conjugate is characterized by long bioresidence time in humans, where it can last for over 3 days. Also the overall toxicity of streptokinase is decreased after dextran conjugation, as demonstrated by reduced hemorrhagic complications, rethromboses and allergic reactions. When the native enzyme is used, these complications are observed in 72%, 16% and 27% of the patients, respectively, while the same problems are reduced to 6%, 5.5% and 2%, respectively, using Streptodekase®. Some other examples related to protein-dextran conjugates, such as plasmin-oxidized dextran, hemoglobin was coupled to a bromo-amino or an aldehyde dextran, aprotinin was coupled to cycloxymethyl dextran.

Poly (Ethylene Glycol) (PEG) Protein Conjugation

The most impressive clinical results with PEG-enzymes were obtained with adenosine deaminase (ADA). The deficiency of this enzyme causes severe immunodeficiency that is inherited as an autosomal recessive trait. It also causes recurrent infections, due to impaired immune function. When ADA was conjugated to PEG of 5 kDa molecular mass, the conjugate was still active and had a longer residence time in the body as compared to the original enzyme. Most importantly, its immunogenicity was dramatically reduced, a property that allows the safe administrations as needed in this life-long disease. PEG-ADA (Adagen®) was approved by the FDA, as was PEG asparaginase (Oncospar®), an antitumor agent, which is specific for the treatment of acute lymphocytic leukemia. Asparaginase is commonly used in free form, but some patients develop an immune based resistance that may be overcome by its PEGylated form. In fact, asparaginase modification with PEG is accompanied by decreased immunogenicity, antigenecity, and proteolytic susceptibility. Figure 20.20 represented that 'Y' shaped

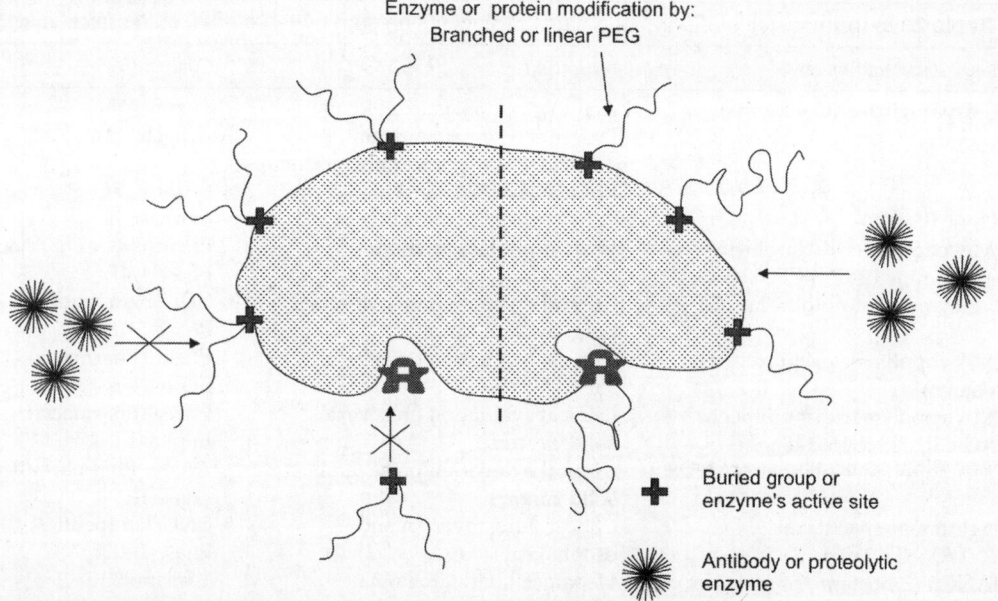

Enzyme or protein modification by:
Branched or linear PEG

Buried group or
enzyme's active site

Antibody or proteolytic
enzyme

Fig. 20.20: Relevance of PEG shape on protein surface coverage or enzyme active site access. The higher steric hindrance of branched PEGs

branched PEG improved the PEG shielding effect on a protein surface, thus being more effective in protecting the conjugated protein from proteolytic enzymes and antibodies.

POLYMER-DRUG CONJUGATES

The field of polymeric drug delivery is fast expanding and rapidly emerging area. It has virtually proved its clinical potential with the launch of many products in the market listed in Table 20.6. Among all approaches, the polymeric drug conjugates have led into a new era of drug delivery systems and widely explored techniques, useful to improve therapeutic properties of peptides, proteins, small molecules or oligonucleotides. Recently, interest in polymer conjugates with biologically active moiety has been demanded remarkably, because such conjugates are preferably accumulated in solid tumors and can reduce systemic toxicity. Along the marketed products already shown in Table 20.6, others are also available for the treatment of different diseases, demonstrating the potentials of the technology.

Helmut Ringsdorf in 1975, proposed a model mainly consists of five components, such as macromolecular polymeric backbone, drug, spacer, targeting moiety and a solubilizing agent (Fig. 20.21).

However, the macromolecular polymers should be ideally water-soluble, nontoxic, and nonimmunogenic, as well as should be degraded and/or eliminated. Finally, the macromolecular carrier should possess suitable functional groups for attaching the respective drug or spacer. The drug can be conjugated directly or via a degradable or nondegradable linker to the polymer backbone to allow a control over the release rate of the active drug from the conjugate at the target site. According to the site and the mode of action, polymer conjugates possess either 'tuned' degradable or nondegradable bonds. In order to obtain such bonds, the strategies generally involve incorporation of amino acids, peptides or small chains as spacer molecules through multiple chemical steps applying protections and deprotections chemistry. A polymeric drug conjugated

Table 20.6: Current status of polymeric drugs conjugates present on the market or in clinical trials

Polymer-drug conjugates	Indication	Company
PEG-asparaginase (Oncaspars)	Acute lymphoblastic leukemia	Enzon
PEG-G-CSF (Pegfilgrastim, neulastas)	Prevention of neutropenia associated with cancer chemotherapy	Amgen
HPMA copolymer-doxorubicin (PK1; FCE28068)	Lung and breast cancers	Pfizer (CRC/Pharmacia) In phase II
HPMA copolymer-doxorubicin-galactosamine (PK2; FCE28069)	Hepatocellular carcinoma	Pfizer(CRC/Pharmacia) Phase I/II
Polyglutamate-camptothecin (CT-2106)	Clinical evaluation on colorectal, lung, ovarian cancer	Cell Therapeutics Phase I/II
HPMA copolymer-paclitaxel (PNU166945)	Clinical evaluation on several solid cancers	Pfizer (Pharmacia) In phase I
HPMA copolymer-camptothecin (MAG-CPT; PNU166148)	Clinical evaluation on several solid cancers	Pfizer (Pharmacia) In phase I
HPMA copolymer-platinate (AP5280)	Clinical evaluation on several solid cancers	Access Pharmaceutical Phase II
Polyglutamate-paclitaxel (XYOTAX; CT-2103)	Cancer, lung, ovarian and esophageal	Cell Therapeutics Phase II/III
SMANCS (Zinostatin, Stimalamer)	Hepatocellular carcinoma	Yamanouchi
PEG-adenosine deaminase (Adagens)	SCID syndrome	Enzon
Linear PEG-interferon α2b (PEG-Introns)	Hepatitis C, clinical evaluation or cancer, multiple sclerosis and HIV/AID	Schering Plough/Enzon
Branched PEG-interferon α2a (Pegasyss)	Hepatitis C	Roche/Nektar
PEG-growth hormone receptor antagonist (Pegvisomant, Somaverts)	Acromegaly	Pfizer (Pharmacia)
PEG-G-CSF (Pegfilgrastim, neulastas) cancer chemotherapy	Prevention of neutropenia associated with	Amgen
Branched PEG-anti-VEGF aptamer (Pegaptanib, MacugenTM)	age-related macular degeneration	Eye Tech Pharmaceuticals
PEG-anti-TNF Fab (CDP870; certolizumab pegol, cimzia)	Rheumatoid arthritis and Crohn's disease	UCB (formerly Celltech)

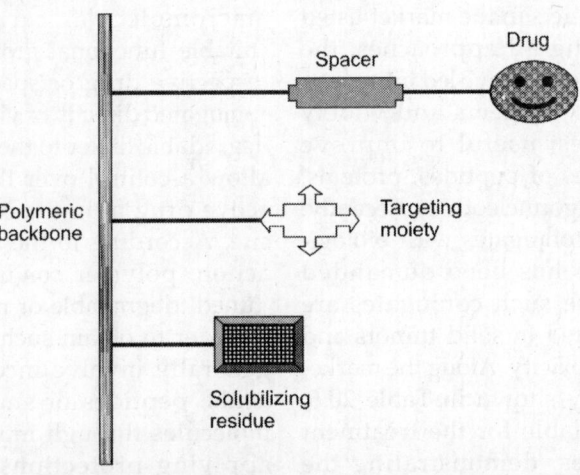

Fig. 20.21: Schematic representation of polymeric drug conjugate model

system exhibited various benefits, such as increased water solubility of poorly soluble bioactive moieties, enhancement of bioavailability, prolonged half-life, higher stability, transport of drug to targeted organ or tissue and intracellular trafficking, favorable pharmacokinetics, reduction in antigenic activity, ability to provide passive or active targeting of the drug specifically to the site of its action. The anticancer polymer-drug conjugates present some advantages as compared to the parent free drug are—(a) passive tumor targeting by the enhanced permeability and retention (EPR) effect; (b) decreased toxicity; (c) increased solubility in biological fluids; (d) ability to overpass some mechanisms that causes drug resistance and (e) ability to elicit immunostimulatory effects.

The designs of polymeric drug conjugates are largely aimed to decrease the steric hindrance exhibited by polymers and the biocomponents. In addition, the reactivity of polymer and drug must be promoted and supported. This is especially true for high molecular weight linear polymers and bulkier unstable drugs, such as steroids and chemotherapeutic agents. Further, it is essential to elucidate the structure activity relationship (SAR) of a drug, when it is conjugated to a polymer using different conjugation sites, as they can affect the efficacy and mechanism of action, when compared with its free form. However, the design and synthesis of new polymeric candidates in view of their biological implications, has just been initiated. Moreover, the various polymers have known as N-(2-hydroxypropyl) methacrylamide copolymer (HPMA), polyglutamic acid (PGA), dextran and poly (ethylene glycol) (PEG) may be employed for designing of polymeric drug conjugates

ADVANTAGES IN THE PREPARATION OF BIOCONJUGATES WITH LOW MOLECULAR WEIGHT DRUGS

One of the main advantages of chemical coupling of low molecular weight drugs to polymers is the modification of pharmacokinetic profile of drugs and, as a consequence, their bioavailability. In fact, in the classic prodrugs approach (as, for example, with acyl moieties) the modification of the drug pharmacokinetic or metabolic profiles is mainly based on a simple slow release of drug in plasma from the low molecular weight carriers by the action of water only or by enzymes, or on biomodification in body disposition. On the other hand, in the bioconjugation technology with high molecular weight polymers, several factors act together to affect the pharmacokinetics and, therefore, the bioavailability of the drug (Table 20.7). Among them, the following points are considered:

1. The shielding effect of the polymer that offers a relevant protection from chemical or enzymatic degradation to the conjugated drug. Similarly, polymers are very effective in masking the antigenic sites of the drugs, as a consequence, their antigenic-immunogenic characteristics that, if present, can be responsible for drug depletion, may be greatly reduced. In the case of PEG, both these phenomena have been correlated to the high mobility, associated with conformational flexibility, and water-binding ability of the polymer chain. These characteristics prevent, the approach of any macromolecule, such as immunoglobulins or degrading enzymes, as well as conjugate adhesion to surfaces.

2. The reduction in renal excretion, due to the large volume of the macromolecular conjugate. This reduction generally occurs when the threshold of serum albumin volume is reached. It is to be noted that, in the case of PEG, the critical point of the albumin hydrodynamic volume is reached at a molecular mass of about one-third of the protein with same mass. This is due to the quasi-random coil conformation of the polymer and its high hydration.

3. In some cases, polymer coupling was demonstrated to promote a targeted deli-

Table 20.7: Patents related to drug conjugates

Patent	Year	Original assignee/inventors	Title
US7374762	2008	Immuno Gen, Inc., Cambridge, US	Drug conjugate composition
US7445764	2008	KTB Tumor Forschungsgesellschaft mbH, Feriburg (DE	Carrier-drug conjugate
US 2005/0276812 A1	2005	Genentech, Inc. US	Antibody-drug conjugates and methods
US7282590	2007	The Research Foundation of State University of New York	Drug conjugates
US 5514794	1996	Eli Lilly and Company, Ind.	Antibody-drug conjugates
US 2011/0064752 A1	2010	Centrose, LLC, US	Extracellular targeted drug conjugates
US 2010/0240883 A1	2010	Nian Wu, Brian Charles Keller, CA (US)	Lipid-drug conjugates for drug delivery
US 2010/0298495 A1	2010	Iulian Bobe, Naoya Shibata, Hiroyuki Saito, Mitsunori Harada, Japan	Block copolymer for drug Conjugates and pharmaceutical composition
US 5502037	1996	Neuromed Technologies, Inc., Silver Spring, MD	Procytotoxic drug conjugates for anticancer therapy
US 2011/0117009 A1	2011	Felix Kratz, Rainer Haag, Marcelo Calderon, Berlin	Drug conjugates with polyglycerols

very of drugs to body sites characterized by an increased capillary permeability as, for example, inflamed tissues. This phenomenon is referred as enhanced permeability and retention (EPR) effect. EPR allows the specific localization of a drug at the level of cancer tissue due to the higher permeability of blood capillaries in that area, accompanied by a reduced lymphatic drainage. Both these phenomena permit the accumulation of the drug-polymer at the level of the tumor tissue through an ultrafiltration process.

4. The macromolecular characteristic of the bioconjugates is responsible for the exploitation of a totally new pathway for the entrance of drug into the cell that can only be based on adsorption or receptor-mediated endocytosis. This new pathway has been exploited even more thoroughly by the design of specific linkages arms between polymer and drug. This linkage has to be stable in blood while cleavable only intracellularly, because of the acidic environ-ment of endosomes or by means of the rich enzymatic machinery of the lysosomes. The esters or amide conjugates with a double bond carrying bicarboxylic acids, labile at low pH, while stable at physiological conditions, were found to be a useful approach for targeted-drug delivery.

LIMITATIONS IN THE CONJUGATION OF POLYMERS TO LOW MOLECULAR WEIGHT DRUGS

Despite the advantages of bioconjugation, many problems still have to be overcome before an ideal polymeric construct can be realized. Most of the problems are technical that still need to be optimized. Among the goals to be achieved, we ought to remember:

1. To improve the chemistry of binding in order to find out conditions of activation and conjugation that are mild enough not to affect the stability of the polymer, since chain cleavage with reduction of molecular mass does sometimes occur, and this reaction is not easy to detect.

2. To develop suitable chemical approaches that allows those sites in the drug molecule, which are involved in its receptor binding to remain accessible or unmasked. This task, even if not trivial, is more easily achieved through modification of poly-peptides and proteins that carry several different sites, which are potentially suitable for polymer anchoring.

3. To develop analytical methods for the characterization of the constructs as a whole and of their individual components, after proper degradation and separation.

4. To obtain well-characterized polymers, possibly with low polydispersivity.

5. To choose the polymers, which have already been approved by the FDA, or alternatively, which are highly likely to be so.

POLYGLUTAMIC ACID (PGA)-E-(C(RGDFK)2)-PACLITAXEL CONJUGATE

Recently, the PGA-PTX-E-[c(RGDfk)2] desi-gned with the hope that a combination of a PGA conjugate containing RGD peptidomi-metic motifs with an anti-angiogenic agent might enhance the effects as seen for PGA-paclitaxel (PGA-PTX) alone. In situations, where tumor is well vascularized, but vasculature permeability is poor, this strategy might be essential since the tumor endothelial cells are directly exposed to the conjugate in the blood circulation. Paclitaxel (PTX) is a potent cytotoxic insoluble drug; however, it is hydrophobic and causes side effects such as neutropenia, neuropathies, and when solubilized in cremophor EL causes hyper-sensitivity reactions. PGA-PTX conjugate is currently undergoing phase, three clinical trials showing promising results. PGA is a water-soluble, biocompatible nontoxic and biodegradable polymer that accumulates in the tumor bed by an enhanced permeability and retention (EPR) effect, when it is used at a nano-scaled size of 10–150 nm. It was seen that conjugated PGA with PTX and a targeting moiety, the cyclic RGD peptidomimetic, E-[c(RGDfk)2], could actively target the con-jugate to the proliferating tumor endothelial cells overexpressing AVB3 integrin. The resulting PGA-[c(RGDfk)2]-PTX nanocon-jugate was measured of a diameter size of ~30 nm. The ester linker between the polymer and the drug is hydrolytically labile and PTX release occurs under lysosomal acidic pH while the PGA itself is degradable by lyso-somal enzymes, such as cysteine proteases, particularly cathepsin B. PGA-E-[c(RGDfk)2]-PTX nanoconjugate inhibited the proliferation of endothelial cells, their migration towards vascular endothelial growth factor (VEGF) and their formation as capillary-like tubular structures. The adhesion of endothelial cells to fibrinogen-coated wells was inhibited by PGA-E-[c(RGDfk)2]-PTX, but not affected by PGA-[c(RADfk)]-PTX control conjugate (Fig. 20.22). These results advocate for this conjugate as a novel targeted anti-angiogenic anticancer therapy.

PGA-drug conjugates derived from mono-disperse PGA are expected to be more reproducible and predictable in regard to their in vivo pharmacological behavior. However, in case of solid tumor therapy, it was more appreciable to use the polydispersed PGA-drug conjugates to maximize the EPR effect. Recombinant DNA technology may be more suitable for producing fusion protein products linking PGA of a defined size to therapeutic proteins, such as interferon-α^2 and granulocyte colony stimulating factor. Conjugation of drug molecules to PGA can affect the overall biodegradation of the PGA polymer, i.e. introducing p-nitroanilide through tripeptide spacers to the side-chains of PGA decreased the degradability of the polymer conjugates. Depending on the nature of the bonds used to link drug molecules to PGA, the degrada-tion of the polymer backbone may not necessa-rily always lead to the release of free drug.

The carboxyl groups on the side-chains of PGA offer attachment points for the conjuga-tion of chemotherapeutic agents to the polymeric carrier. Several drug conjugates have also been described using derivatives of

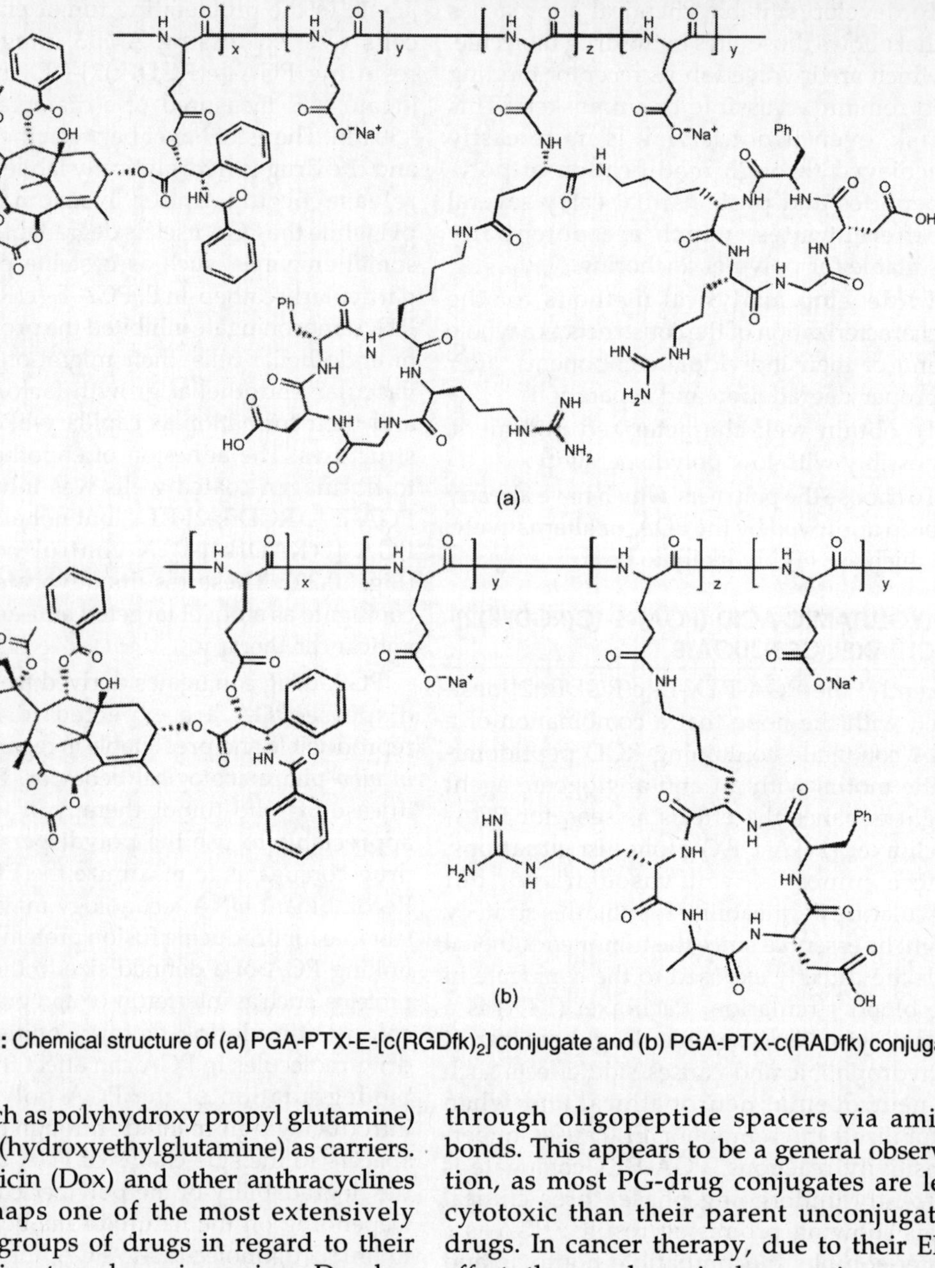

(a)

(b)

Fig. 20.22: Chemical structure of (a) PGA-PTX-E-[c(RGDfk)₂] conjugate and (b) PGA-PTX-c(RADfk) conjugate

PGA, such as polyhydroxy propyl glutamine) and poly(hydroxyethylglutamine) as carriers. Doxorubicin (Dox) and other anthracyclines are perhaps one of the most extensively studied groups of drugs in regard to their conjugation to polymeric carriers. Dox has been conjugated to PGA under the assumption that greater selectivity may be achieved if the conjugates only degrade and release Dox after they are endocytosed by tumor cells. Thus, Dox was conjugated to PGA either directly or through oligopeptide spacers via amide bonds. This appears to be a general observation, as most PG-drug conjugates are less cytotoxic than their parent unconjugated drugs. In cancer therapy, due to their EPR effect, these polymeric drug conjugates are retained at tumor site and then release the drug molecules over a prolonged period of time at the tumor site and ultimately presented better therapeutic efficacy as compared with conventional therapy.

N-(2-HYDROXYPROPYL) METHACRYLAMIDE (HPMA)-BASED POLYMERIC DRUG CONJUGATES

Polymer drug conjugates based on N-(2-hydroxypropyl) methacrylamide (HPMA) copolymers have been widely studied over the last 30 years. Most of these drug conjugates were developed for the treatment of tumors, with a special focus on the site-specific delivery of anticancer and anti-inflammatory agents into tumor tissues or cells. Proper selection of the molecular weight and the spacer between the drug and carrier is essential for achieving an effective tumor or tumor cell-specific drug targeting followed by controlled drug release, which is important for the subsequent anti-tumor activity of the drug. The most frequently studied HPMA-based conjugates contain oligopeptide spacers (e.g.

GFLG sequences) between the drug and carrier designed for enzymatic drug release by lysosomal enzymes. In the last decade, the synthesis and properties of HPMA-based conjugates (Fig. 20.23), in which the drug is bound to a carrier by pH-sensitive hydrazone bonds, have been intensively studied.

While the hydrazone bond is relatively stable at neutral pH, which corresponds to the blood environment, the drug is released under mildly acid conditions, such as in endosomes or lysosomes of tumor cells, with half-lives in hours. These conjugates are highly cytotoxic for cancer cells *in vitro* and exhibit an enhanced accumulation in solid tumor tissue and expressed superior antitumor activity. Furthermore, macromolecules are more selectively accumulated in solid tumors due to the EPR effect. The extent of passive

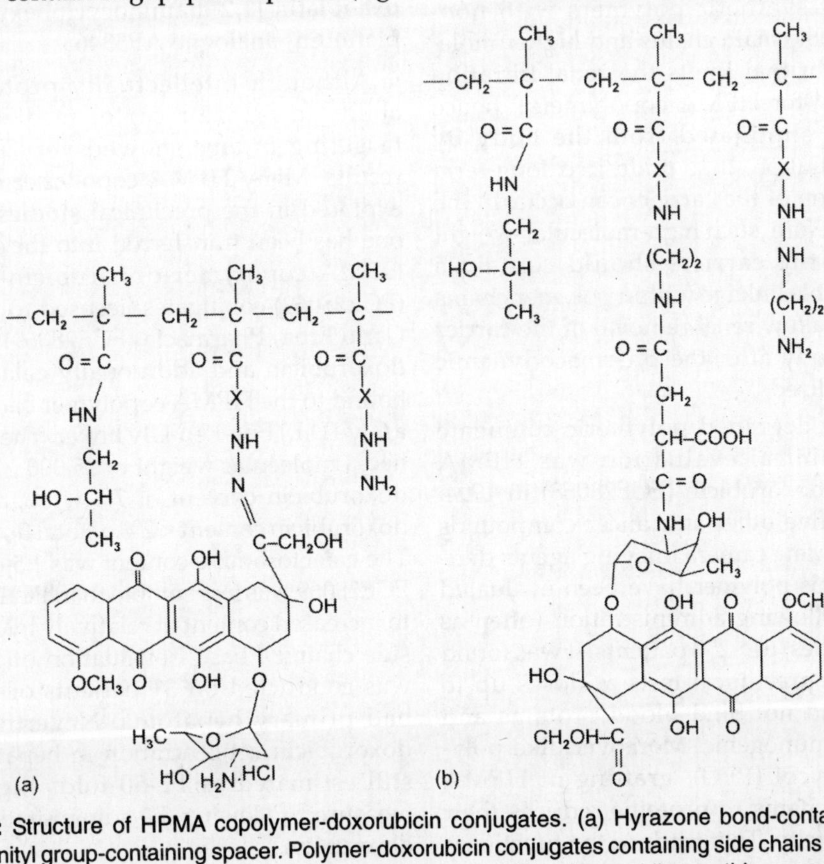

Fig. 20.23: Structure of HPMA copolymer-doxorubicin conjugates. (a) Hyrazone bond-containing spacer. (b) Cis-aconityl group-containing spacer. Polymer-doxorubicin conjugates containing side chains of hydrazone-bound doxorubicin moieties were attached via single-amino-acid or longer oligopeptide spacers

accumulation of macromolecules in solid tumors strongly depends on their size and molecular weight. The EPR effect was observed for HPMA-based copolymers with molecular weights higher than 2×10^4. The EPR effect was recorded to be predominant with increasing molecular weight of polymers. The antitumor activity of HPMA-based conjugates can be improved by either introducing targeting moieties, e.g. monoclonal antibody or oligopeptides, or by enhancing their passive targeting due to the EPR (enhanced permeability and retention) effect.

The high-molecular-weight of polymer conjugates prevents fast clearance of the drug from the organism by renal filtration and in this way, ensures prolonged blood circulation and retention of the drug in the body. Probably most polymeric conjugates are essentially synthetic polymers with non-biodegradable main chains and higher molecular weight that limits the renal filtration (ca. 5×10^4 for HPMA copolymers); hence cannot be eliminated from the body by kidneys filtration, thus undesired long-term accumulation of the carriers can occur in the body. Therefore, such high-molecular-weight polymer drug carriers should contain a biodegradable linkage within polymer chains in order to allow renal removal of the carrier from the body after the pharmacodynamic effect is realized.

The first degraded polymeric conjugate to enter clinical evaluation was HPMA copolymer-doxorubicin (FCE28068) in 1994. Since then five other anticancer compounds and two gamma camera imaging agents derived from this polymer have been evaluated clinically following administration (often as multiple cycles) to > 250 patients. It was found nontoxic in preclinical tests at doses up to 30 g/kg, did not bind blood proteins and was nonimmunogenic. Moreover, like polyethylene glycol (PEG), grafting of HPMA copolymer chains to proteins reduces their immunogenicity. To introduce the functiona-

lity needed for drug conjugation, and also to insert biodegradable linkers for drug release, HPMA copolymers were prepared. There are several polymeric conjugates used for solid tumor therapy via passive targeting, already entered in clinical phases. For example, HPMA copolymer-doxorubicin (FCE28068, licensed to Farmitalia Carlo Erba/Pharmacia), HPMA copolymer-paclitaxel (PNU 166945, developed by Pharmacia) with the specific aim of improving drug solubility to enable more convenient administration with subsequent controlled release of paclitaxel. Other polymeric conjugates include HPMA copolymer-camptothecin (PNU 166148, developed by Pharmacia) and HPMA copolymer-platinates (AP5280, AP5346, licensed to Access Pharmaceuticals Inc.). These compounds are typically carboplatinum analogue AP5280 and an oxaliplatin [1,2-diaminocyclohexyl (DACH) platinum] analogue AP5346.

Although intellectually protected, the ability to realize receptor mediated tumor targeting *in vivo* showed very promising results. Many HPMA copolymer conjugates explored in the preclinical studies, but only one has been transferred into the clinic. The HPMA copolymer-doxorubicin-galactose (FCE28069) conjugates licensed to Farmitalia Carlo Erba/Pharmacia (FCE28069) contained doxorubicin and additionally galactosamine bound to the HPMA copolymer backbone via a Gly-(D,L) Phe-Leu-Gly linker. The conjugate had a molecular weight of 25,000 g/mol with doxorubicin content of 7.5 wt.%, and a free doxorubicin content < 2% of total doxorubicin. The galactosamine content was 1.5–2.5 mol%. FCE28069 was less soluble than FCE28068 due to increased content of relatively hydrophobic side chains. Phase I evaluation of FCE28069 was conducted on 31 patients of which 23 had primary hepatoma. Nevertheless the doxorubicin concentration in hepatoma was still estimated as 12–50 folds higher than measured following the administration of free doxorubicin.

POLYETHYLENE GLYCOL (PEG)-BASED POLYMERIC DRUG CONJUGATES

Through the pioneering research in 1970s, Davis, Abuchowski and colleagues developed the concept of polyethylene glycol (PEG)-protein conjugation (PEGylation), and since then the continuing entry of PEGylated proteins into routine clinical use has been a paradigm shift in the acceptance of polymerbased macromolecular medicines. This technique is used to increase protein solubility and stability, and reduce protein immunogenicity; moreover, polymer conjugation prolongs plasma half-life through prevention of renal elimination and avoidance of receptor-mediated protein uptake by cells of the reticuloendothelial system (RES). Consequently, polymer-conjugated therapeutics requires less frequent dosing, which is a great benefit to the patient. For optimized synthesis of a polymer-protein conjugate, a semi-telechelic polymer (one with a single reactive group at one terminal end) is required to avoid protein crosslinking during conjugation; furthermore, the linker used must be chosen carefully to ensure that the linking chemistry will not generate toxicity or immunogenicity. The synthetic approach requires reproducible, site-specific protein modification. Linear and branched PEGs with molecular masses of 5000–40000 g/mol have been used to create protein conjugates, and the chosen PEG molecular mass shown a great impact on their pharmacokinetics. In some cases, multiple PEGs have been attached per protein molecule.

There are several examples for PEG-protein conjugation as the PEG-L-asparaginase (Oncaspar) was the first antitumor PEGylated protein approved for clinical use in 1994. This conjugate contains multiple PEG chains (molecular mass 5000 g/mol) linked to the enzyme, and it is used in the treatment for acute lymphoblastic leukemia (ALL), a disease that has an essential requirement for the amino acid L-asparagine. The native enzyme induces hypersensitivity reactions and has a relatively short plasma half-life (8–30 hrs), which necessitates daily administration for 4 weeks, whereas the PEG-L-asparaginase conjugate has a plasma half-life of 14 days and can, therefore, be administered as 1 hour infusion every 2 weeks. Currently, other PEGylated enzymes are undergoing clinical development such as PEG-recombinant arginine deaminase (rhArg) is being developed as a treatment for hepatocellular carcinoma as a single agent, which depletes arginine, and also in combination with 5-fluorouracil (5-FU). Another PEG-granulocyte colony stimulating factor (PEG-GCSF) (Neulasta/PEG-filgrastim), is currently used to prevent severe cancer chemotherapy induced neutropenia. It was reported that administration of one dose of PEG-GCSF (100 μg/kg), by subcutaneous injection on day 2 of each chemotherapy cycle, gives the equivalent neutrophil support when compared with GCSF (5 μg/kg/day) given by daily injection throughout the chemotherapy cycle. The half-life of PEG-GCSF is longer (15–80 hr) compared with that of the native protein (1.3–7.2 hrs). Although, some allergic reactions have been seen following administration of GCSF, whilst none was observed in clinical trials in case of PEG conjugate.

PEG has been successfully used for protein modification and currently also employed in case of low molecular weight of anticancer drugs. Basically, to circumvent the concerns of the nonspecificity and high systemic toxicity associated with chemotherapy, many researchers have proposed anticancer drug PEG conjugation. PEG-drug conjugates are attracting increasing interest as novel anticancer agents providing unique disposition characteristics in the body, such as an extended half-life in blood, specific organ targeting, and sustained release at the injection site. However, the low molecular weight drugs present a crucial limit, the low drug payload accompanying the available methoxy or diol forms of this polymer. In the case of PEG, the use of larger polymer does not correlate well with an increase in the amount of drug selectively delivered into the tumor, because large PEGs are disadvantageous polymer in regard to drug ratios particularly in case of low molecular weight drugs. In the case of PEG, the number of available groups for drug coupling does not change with the length of polymeric chain.

Recently, PEG conjugates containing anticancer drugs, such as doxorubicin, paclitaxel, and camptothecin have been described. Most of the PEG low molecular weight drug conjugates that entered the clinical trials are from the camptothecin family, namely camptothecin itself, SN38 and irinotecan. The PEG-camptothecin (PROTHECAN or Pegamotecan) Pegamotecan (Enzon Pharmaceuticals, Inc.) is a prodrug obtained by coupling two molecules of camptothecin to a diol PEG of 40 kDa. In phase I trial, the maximum tolerated dose of the conjugate, administered for 1 hour IV every 3 weeks, was determined to be 7000 mg·m^{-2}, both for heavily and minimally pretreated patients. This amount and administration schedule was also the recommended dose for phase II studies. Furthermore, the conjugate appeared better tolerated, with a low incidence of toxicities with respect to irinotecan. Nonetheless, the toxicological profile of the conjugate is similar to that of the native drug and this is probably due to quick *in vivo* hydrolysis of the ester linkage between camptothecin and PEG with the release of the free drug. A new PEG-SN38 (EZN-2208) product is designed by the use of multi-arm PEG. The most advanced conjugate, conjugated with one of these PEGs entered recently phase I clinical trials. This compound was obtained by coupling a 4arm-PEG of 40 kDa with the camptothecin derivative SN38, through a glycine spacer. It was established that, EZN-2208 showed a 207-fold higher exposure to SN38 compared to irinotecan in treated mice, with a tumor to plasma drug concentration ratio increased over the time during a four day long pharmacokinetic and biodistribution studies. The conjugates demonstrated promising antitumor activity *in vitro* and *in vivo*. In mouse xenograft models of MX-1 breast, MiaPaCa-2 pancreatic or HT-29 colon carcinoma, treatment with the conjugate, administered either as a single dose or multiple injections, showed better results than plain irinotecan.

PEG-irinotecan (NKTR-102) is another multi-arm PEG that was also exploited for the preparation of PEG-irinotecan (NKTR-102) by Nektar therapeutics. The drug has been covalently bound to a 4arm-PEG. The conjugate showed prolonged pharmacokinetic profiles with a half-life of 15 days as compared to 4 hours as obtained with free irinotecan.

SUGGESTED READINGS

1. Annemiek JML, van Rensen, Wauben MHM, Stulemeyer MCG, van Eden W, Cromelin DJA (1999), *Pharm. Res.*, 16, 198.
2. Avrilionis K, Boggs JM (1996), *Cell. Immunol.*, 168, 13.
3. Bartling GJ, Brown HD, Chattopadhyoy SK (1973), *Nature*, 243, 432–344.
4. Casi G and Neri Dario (2012), *J. Contr. Rel.*, In press.
5. Chu BCF, Kramer FR, Orgel LE (1986), *Nucleic Acid Res.*, 14, 5591.
6. Ducry L, and Stump B (2010), *Biocon Chem.*, 21, 5–13.
7. Duncan R (2006), *Nat Rev Cancer.*, 6, 688–01.
8. Gao X, Huang L (1996), *Biochem.*, 35, 1027.
9. Garagiola DM, Huard TK, Lo Buglio AF (1979), *Blood*, 54, 84.
10. Ghose SS, Kao PM, Kwoh DY (1989), *Anal. Biochem.*, 178, 43–51.
11. Ghose SS, Kao PM, Mecue AW, Chappelle HL (1990), *Bioconjugate Chem.*, 1, 71–6.
12. Haag R and Kratz F (Int. Ed. 2006). *Angew Chem.*, 45, 1198.
13. Haag R, Kratz F, Angew (2006), *Chem Int Ed Engl.*, 45, 1198–215.
14. Haisma HJ, Boven M, Vanmuijen M, Dejong J, Vander Vijgh WJF, Pinedo HM (1992), *Br. J. Cancer*, 66, 474.
15. Hartman FC, Wold F (1966), *J. Am. Chem. Soc.*, 88, 3890.
16. Hearn MJW, Bethell GS, Ayers JS and Hancock WS (1979), *J. Chromatogr.* 185, 463–70.
17. Hege KM, Daleke DL, Waldmann TA, Matthay KK (1989), *Blood*, 74, 2043.

18. Hermanson GT (1996), *Bioconjugate Techniques,* New York, Academic Press, 10.
19. Hoare DG, Ksohland DE (1966), *J. Am. Chem. Soc.,* 88, 2057.
20. Iyer U and Kadambi VJ (2011), *J Pharmacol Toxicol Methods.,* 64, 207–12.
21. Kedar E, Rutkowski Y, Braun E, Emanuel N, Barenholz Y (1994), *J. Immunother. Emphasis Tumor Immunol.,* 16, 47.
22. Kejik ZK et al., (2011), *Bioorg Med Chem Letters.,* 21, 5514–20.
23. Khaw BA, Torchilin VP, Vural I, Narula J (1995), *Nature Med.,* 1, 1195.
24. Kim YW, Fung MSC, Sun NC, Sun CRY, Chang NT, Chang TW (1990), *J. Immunol.,* 144, 1257.
25. Kinsky SC (1972), *Biochim. Biophys. Acta.,* 265, 1.
26. Kitagawa T, Aikawa T (1976), *J. Biochem.,* 79, 233.
27. Komath SS, Bhanu K, Maiya BG, Swamy MJ (2008), *Biosci Rep.,* 20, 265.
28. Kotite NI, Staros JV, Cunningham LW (1984), *Biochem.,* 23, 3099–104.
29. Kraehenbuhl JP, Galardy RE, Jamieson JD (1979), *J. Exp. Med.,* 139, 208.
30. Králova J, Kejík Z, Pouc kova P, Kral A, Martásek P, Kral VJ (2010), *Med Chem.,* 53, 128.
31. Ludwig FR, Jay FA (1985), *Eur. J. Biochem.,* 151, 83–7.
32. Oda Y, Yanagisawa M, Maruyama M, Hattori K, Yamanoi T (2008), *Bioorg Med Chem* 16, 8830.
33. Peng L, Calton GJ, Burnett JW (1987), *Appl. Biochem. Biotechnol.,* 14, 91–9.
34. Polson AG, Williams M, Gray AM, Fuji RN, Poon KA, and McBride J (2010), *Leukemia,* 24, 1566–73.
35. Senter PD (2009), *Chem Bio,* 13, 235–44.
36. Senter PD (2009), *Curr. Opin. Chem. Biol.,* 13, 235–44.
37. Sheehan JC, Preston J, Cruickshank PA (1965), *J. Am. Chem. Soc.,* 87, 2492–3.
38. Sheehan JC, Cruickshank PA, Boshart GC (1961), *J. Org. Chem.,* 26, 2525–8.
39. Tan Y, Sun X, Xu, M, An, Z., Tan, X., Han, Q., Miljkovic DA, Yang M, Hoffman RM (1998), *Protein Extra. Puruf.,* 12, 45.
40. Tanaka T, Kaneo Y, Miyashita M (1996), *Biol. Pharm. Bull.,* 19, 774.
41. Till MA, Ghetie V, Gregori T, Patzer EJ, Porter JP, Uhr JW, Capon DJ, Vitetta ES (1988) *Science,* 242, 1166.
42. Tokihiro K, Irie T, Uekama K (1997), *Chem. Pharm. Bull.,* 45, 525.
43. Vicent MJ (2007), AAPS J, 9(2): E200–E207.
44. Vitetta ES (1990), *J. Clin. Immunol.,* 10, 515.
45. Wagner E, Curiel D, Cotton M (1994), *Adv. Drug Deliv. Rev.,* 14, 113.
46. Wagner E, Zatloukal K, Cotton M, Kirlappos H, Mechtler K, Curiel DT (1992), *Proc. Natl. Acad. Sci.,* 89, 6099.
47. Webb S (2011), *Nat Biotechnol.,* 29, 297–298.
48. Weissner JH, Hwang KJ (1982), *Biochim. Biophys. Acta.,* 689, 490.
49. Wright S, Huang L (1989), *Adv. Drug Deliv. Rev.,* 3, 343.
50. Wu D, Yang J, Pardridge WM (1997), *J. Clin. Invest.,* 100, 1804.
51. Wu M, Fan J, Gunning W, Ratnam M (1997), *J. Membr. Biol.,* 159, 137.

21

Cyclodextrin Complexes

INTRODUCTION

Cyclodextrins (CD) are natural cyclic oligo-saccharides. They typically contain 6(α-CD), 7(β-CD), or 8(γ-CD) glucopyranose units. This cyclic orientation provides a truncated cone structure, that is hydrophilic on the exterior and lipophilic on the interior. CD complexes are formed, when a guest molecule is partially or fully contained in the interior of the cavity. The parent CD structure has been chemically modified to generate a parenterally safe CD-derivative. The modifications are typically made at one or more of the 2, 3, or 6 position hydroxyls (Fig. 21.1). Amphiphilic CDs are obtained by the chemical per-modification of natural CD (β-CD or γ-CD) by the selective substitution of aliphatic chains of varying length (2C to 18C), structure (linear or branched) linked with different bonds (ester, ether, amide, thio, fluoro) of high purity.

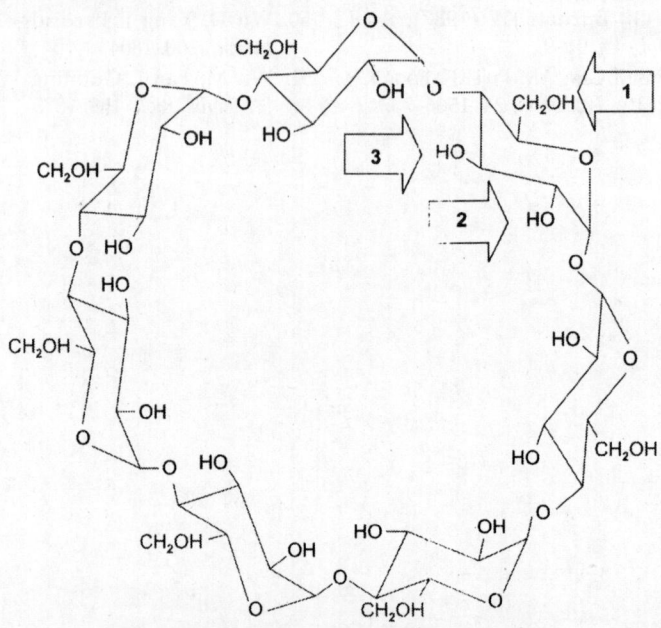

Fig. 21.1: Structure of cyclodextrin complex

The most important attribute of CD is the ability to create inclusion complexes with a large number of molecules or their portions; however, not all molecules (drugs) can form stable complexes. There are some limitations, like very high aqueous-soluble substances, generally cannot be included. Recently, it has been reported that high aqueous soluble drug substances could be resulted with CD rather an association compound in which drug interacts with the hydrophilic outer surface of CD (hydroxyls at position 3).

CYCLODEXTRIN-BASED PRODUCTS

It was very first time discovered and presented by Cramer and coworkers, that the CD possesses ability to form inclusion complexes. By the early 1950s, the basic physicochemical characteristics of CD had been discovered, including their ability to solubilize and stabilize drugs. The first CD-related patent was issued in 1953 to Freudenberg, Cramer and Plieninger. The first CD-containing pharmaceutical product was marketed in Japan. Later CD-containing products appeared on the European market in 1997 and also in the US. More than 30 different pharmaceutical products containing CD are now available in the market worldwide (shown in Table 21.1).

Dissociation of the inclusion complex is a relatively rapid process usually driven by a large increase in the number of water mole-

Table 21.1: CD-containing marketed pharmaceutical products (adapted from Loftsson and Duchene, 2007)

Drug/cyclodextrin	Trade name	Formulation	Country
α-Cyclodextrin			
Alprostadil (PGE1)	Prostavastin, Rigidur	IV solution	Japan, Europe, USA
OP-1206	Opalmon	Tablet	Japan
Cefotiam hexetil HCl	Pansporin T	Tablet	Japan
β-Cyclodextrin			
Benexate HCl	Ulgut, Lonmiel	Capsule	Japan
Cephalosporin (ME 1207)	Meiact	Tablet	Japan
Chlordiazepoxide	Transillium	Tablet	Argentina
Dexamethasone	Glymesason	Ointment	Japan
Diphenhydramin HCl, Chlortheophyllin	Stada-Travel	Chewing tablet	Europe
Iodine	Mena-Gargle	Solution	Japan
Nicotine	Nicorette, Nicogum chewing gum	Sublingual tablet	Europe
Nimesulide	Nimedex	Tablet	Europe
Nitroglycerin	Nitropen	Sublingual tablet	Japan
Omeprazol	Omebeta	Tablet	Europe
PGE2	Prostarmon E	Sublingual tablet	Japan
Piroxicam Brexin,	Flogene, Cicladon	Tablet, suppository	Liquid Europe, Brazil
Tiaprofenic acid	Surgamyl	Tablet	Europe
2-Hydroxypropyl-β-cyclodextrin			
Cisapride	Propulsid	Suppository	Europe
Itraconazole	Sporanox	Oral and IV solutions	Europe, USA
Mitomycin	Mitozytrex	IV infusion	Europe, USA
Methylated-β-cyclodextrin			
Chloramphenicol	Clorocil	Eyedrop solution	Europe
17 β-Estradiol	Aerodiol	Nasal spray	Europe
Sulfobutylether-β-cyclodextrin			
Voriconazole	Vfend	IV solution	Europe, USA
Ziprasidone mesylate	Geodon, Zeldox	IM solution	Europe, USA

cules in the surrounding environment. The resulting concentration gradient shifts the equilibrium. In highly dilute and dynamic systems like the body, the guest has difficulty in finding another cyclodextrin to reform the complex and is released in solution.

ADVANTAGES

There are several benefits of drug-CD complexation in drug delivery systems. They are as follows:

- The rate of dissolution and the solubility may be enhanced by using the CD-drug complexes, resulting in high and significantly improved bioavailability. As, due to poor or limited solubility of drug, the bioavailability of drug is also poor, the CD complexes, however improve the bioavailability. The bioavailability is typically expressed as a change in an area under the plasma concentration *vs.* time curve (AUC) value, a change in the time to

reach maximum plasma levels of the given compound (T_{max}), and/or the maximum plasma level achieved (C_{max}). Earlier study stated that albendazole on complexation with HP-β-CD resulted in an increase in AUC 1.4 times and C_{max} 1.2–2.8 mg/ml in comparison to pure drug (Fig. 21.2).

- Drugs such as voriconazole (antifungal) and ziprasidone (anti-schizophrenia agent) possess poor water solubility, a major obstacle in development of parenteral formulation. But sulfobutylether-β-cyclodextrin (captisol) is nowadays being used to obtain their parenteral formulations.
- The CD-based inclusion complexes may be successfully utilized for development of sublingual tablet or a chewing gum to mask or abate astringent, irritating and bitter taste of many therapeutically active compounds. CD entraps such compounds molecularly and thus complexed molecules cannot

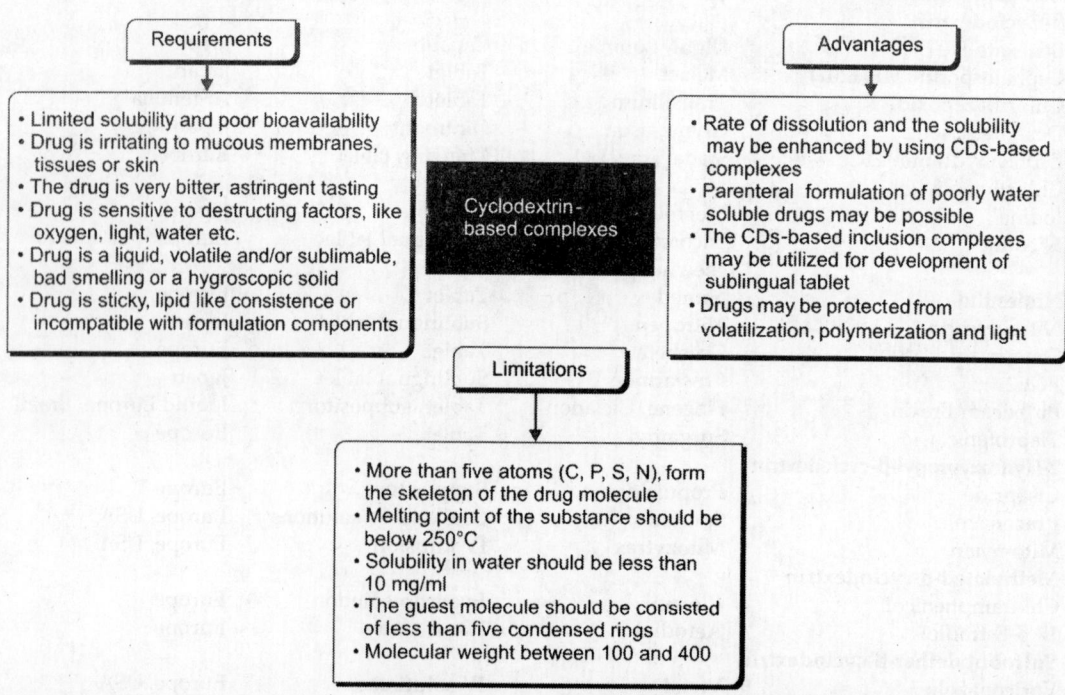

Requirements

- Limited solubility and poor bioavailability
- Drug is irritating to mucous membranes, tissues or skin
- The drug is very bitter, astringent tasting
- Drug is sensitive to destructing factors, like oxygen, light, water etc.
- Drug is a liquid, volatile and/or sublimable, bad smelling or a hygroscopic solid
- Drug is sticky, lipid like consistence or incompatible with formulation components

Cyclodextrin-based complexes

Advantages

- Rate of dissolution and the solubility may be enhanced by using CDs-based complexes
- Parenteral formulation of poorly water soluble drugs may be possible
- The CDs-based inclusion complexes may be utilized for development of sublingual tablet
- Drugs may be protected from volatilization, polymerization and light

Limitations

- More than five atoms (C, P, S, N), form the skeleton of the drug molecule
- Melting point of the substance should be below 250°C
- Solubility in water should be less than 10 mg/ml
- The guest molecule should be consisted of less than five condensed rings
- Molecular weight between 100 and 400

Fig. 21.2: Schematic illustration showing the requirements, benefits and limitations associated with CDs

access taste buds in the buccal cavity, therefore bitter taste is not perceived, i.e. if cetirizine is administered in saturated-CD solution it possesses no bitter taste.

- Drugs (amlodipine), phytoconstituent (astaxanthin) and compounds like vanillin, bisphenol, cinnamaldehyde, volatile oils (clove oil), flavoring agents (lemon and orange peel oil) are rapidly lost due to volatilization, oxidation, polymerization, photo reactions (photo degradation). But, it was investigated that their complexation with different CD derivatives could overcome the problems to the satisfactory level.

- For many potent therapeutically active entities, preparation of suitable dosage form is a challenge because of their sticky, lipid like consistency, incompatibility with formulation components etc. CD complexation is one of the most promising solutions to such problems.

LIMITATIONS

All the categories of drugs are not suitable options for CD-based complexation. Drug molecule to be complexed with CD, should have certain characteristics. These characteristics are generally favored for pharmaceutical and medicinal benefits, however exceptions cannot be neglected.

- More than five atoms (C, P, S, N) form the skeleton of the drug molecule.
- Melting point of the substance should be below 250°C.
- Solubility in water should be less than 10 mg/ml.
- The guest molecule should consists of less than five condensed rings.
- Molecular weight between 100 and 400.

Basically, inorganic compounds are not appropriate for complexation. However, halogens, non-dissociated acids (H_3PO_4, HI, etc.), gases (Xe, CO_2 etc.) are exceptions. Too large molecules (protein, peptides, enzymes, etc.) and strongly hydrophilic compounds generally cannot be complexed.

The large water soluble molecules with side chains capable of forming complex react with CD in aqueous solutions, resulting in improved solubility and stability (e.g. the stability of an aqueous solution of insulin, or many other peptides, proteins, hormones, enzymes, is significantly improved in presence of an appropriate CD). Usually, mass of tablets and capsules lies in the range of 500–800 mg and CDs have high molecular weight. So, drugs having molecular weight 100–400 Da are more suitable options for complexation, so that they can be easily molded into most favored oral dosages.

MECHANISM OF DRUG CYCLODEXTRIN COMPLEXATION

Various molecules can be fitted into the cavities of CD to form supramolecular inclusion complexes, which have been extensively studied as models for understanding the mechanism of molecular recognition. The unique capability of forming inclusion complexes in the inner cavities of CD and many other favorable physicochemical and biological properties, natural CD and their derivatives have been applied in drug delivery systems to enhance the solubilization, stabilization, and absorption. The kinetics of drug-CD interaction and subsequent complexation could be explained on the basis of hydrophilic and hydrophobic interaction, possibilities of CD interaction with water and drug molecules respectively.

- The displacement of polar water molecules from the apolar CD cavity.
- The increased number of hydrogen bonds formed as the displaced water returns to the larger pool.
- A reduction of the repulsive interactions between the hydrophobic guest and the aqueous environment.

The ability of a CD to form an inclusion complex with a guest molecule depends on two key factors. The first is steric and depends on the relative size of the CD of the guest molecule or certain key functional groups within the guest. The size-geometric factor of the molecule is most important because it decides whether the molecule is able to form stable inclusion with α, β and γ-CD (Table 21.2).

If a molecule has adequate properties, it interacts with CD inside cavity without forming covalent bonds; this interaction is guest/host type. CD inclusion complex is mainly formed via the substitution of included water by the appropriate guest molecule. Release of the enthalpy-rich water molecules from the cavity decreases the energy of the system. A decrease in the energy of the system is due to reduced contact surface area between the solvent and solute as well as solvent (highly polar water) and imperfectly solvated (hydrophobic) CD cavity. Some other factors, such as hydrogen bonding, changes in surface tension, van der Waals' interactions, and ring strain release, also can have some influence on the complex formation. The complexation is usually a concentration-dependent process and the molar ratio (1:1, 1:2, 2:1, 2:2) can depend on the guest/host proportion. It is possible that in solution the molecule interacts with the outer surface of CD and CD complexes may agglomerate (self-association). The second critical factor is the thermodynamic interactions between the different components of the system (CD, guest, solvent), where a favorable net energetic driving force is essential to pull the guest into the CD. While this initial equilibrium to form the complex is very rapid (often within minutes), the final equilibrium can take much longer to reach. Once inside the CD cavity, the guest molecule makes conformational adjustments to take maximum advantage of the weak van der Waals' forces that exist.

The association/dissociation equilibrium in aqueous solution is one of the most characteristic features of inclusion. Drug release from the CD complex is mainly caused by dissociation due to dilution in fluids. However, in topical applications, such as ocular, nasal, rectal, or dermal, with minimal or no dilution mechanism, the potential mechanism of drug release from CD complex is preferential drug uptake by tissue. The drug substances possess physicochemical properties that allow it to penetrate into or through biological membranes (skin, mucosa,

Table 21.2: Cyclodextrin characteristics

Cyclodextrin type	Alfa	Beta	Gamma
Number of glucose units	6	7	8
Cavity diameter (Å)	4.7–5.3	6.0–6.5	7.5–8.3
Cavity height (Å)	7.9	7.9	7.9
Cavity volume (Å3)	174	262	427
Appearance	Crystalline White Powder	Crystalline White powder	Crystalline White powder
Molecular weight	973	1135	1297
Bulk density, g/cm^3	0.4–0.7	0.4–0.7	0.4–0.7
Water solubility (25°C), g/100 mL	14.5	1.8	23.2
Content (dry basis)	>98%	>98%	>98%
Specific rotation in aqueous solution	+147° to +152°	+160° to +164°	+174° to +180°
Water	<10%	<14%	<11%
Heavy metals	<5 ppm	<5 ppm	<5 ppm
Residue on ignition	<0.1%	<0.1%	<0.1%
Volatile organics	<20 ppm	<5 ppm	<50 ppm

or cornea), then the tissue acts as a sink causing dissociation of the complex. Only a free fraction of drug that is in equilibrium with the complexed fraction may be available for absorption, thus CDs are able to increase bioavailability rather by delivering the drug substance to absorption site and by minimization of drug hydrophobicity than permeation by itself. The penetration into or permeation through the biological membranes of inclusion complex and CDs are questionable because of their large mass (>1000 Da) and hydrophilicity.

Recently, CD-based polyrotaxanes and polypseudoro taxanes, the inclusion complexes composed of multiple CD rings threaded on a polymer chain with or without bulky end-caps, have led to interesting developments of supramolecular biomaterials such as hydrogels and biodegradable polyrotaxanes (Fig 21.3). These biomaterials could be used for controlled drug delivery based on mechanisms, which are different from the conventional systems. Over the last decade, cationic polymers have been receiving growing attention as gene delivery carriers. CD was used to modify and functionalize cationic polymers, or serve as a core or template for synthesis of new cationic polymers with star architectures. Cationic polyrotaxanes, supramolecules with multiple cationic CD threaded and end-capped on a polymer chain were also developed as a new class of gene delivery vectors

INCLUSION AND NONINCLUSION COMPLEXES

It is generally accepted that in aqueous solutions, CDs form 'inclusion complexes', where water molecules located within the lipophilic central cavity, are replaced by a lipophilic guest molecule or a lipophilic moiety on, e.g. a drug molecule. However, the hydroxy groups on the outer surface of the CD molecule, are able to form hydrogen bonds with other molecules and CD can, like noncyclic oligosaccharides and polysaccharides, form water soluble complexes with lipophilic water-insoluble compounds. It has been shown that α-CD forms both inclusion and noninclusion complexes with dicarboxylic acids and that the two types of complexes

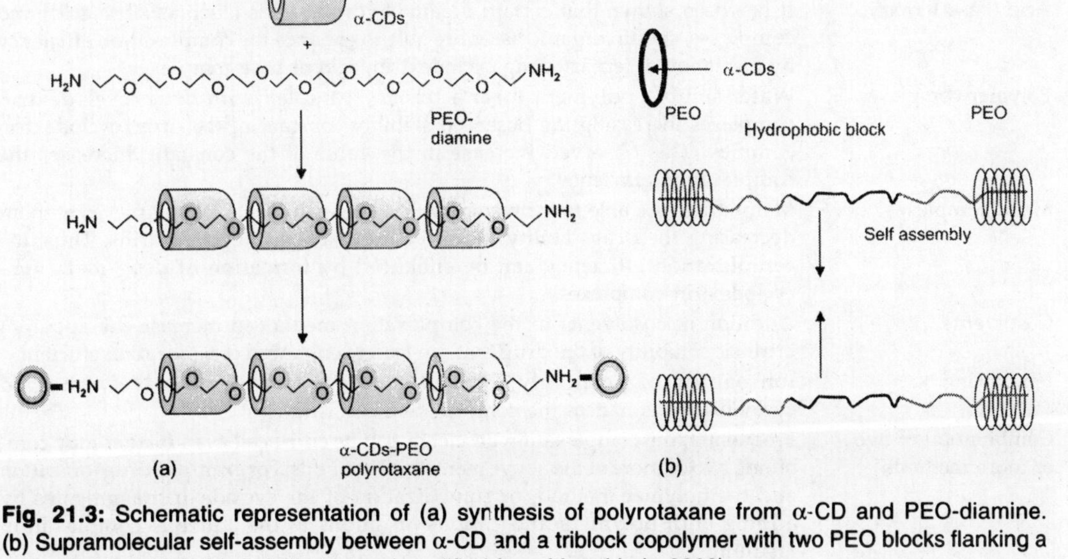

Fig. 21.3: Schematic representation of (a) synthesis of polyrotaxane from α-CD and PEO-diamine. (b) Supramolecular self-assembly between α-CD and a triblock copolymer with two PEO blocks flanking a hydrophobic middle block (adapted and modified from Li and Loh, 2008)

coexist in aqueous solutions. In saturated aqueous solutions guest/cyclodextrin complexes frequently consist of a mixture of inclusion and noninclusion complexes.

METHODS TO ENHANCE THE COMPLEXATION EFFICIENCY

There are number of methods available to be used to enhance the complexation efficiency (or rather the solubilization efficiency) of CD. Formation of CD complexes is an equilibrium process, where free guest molecules are in equilibrium with molecules in the complex. Increasing the solubility of the guest through ionization, salt formation, formation of metal complexes and addition of organic cosolvents to the aqueous complexation media would lead to enhance the complexation efficiency (e.g. enhanced solubilization) in aqueous CD

solutions saturated with the guest. The application of supercritical fluids to prepare complexes is also partly based on enhancement of the intrinsic solubility (Table 21.3).

TOXICOLOGICAL ASPECTS

CD Aggregates

CD and CD-based complexes self-associate to form nanoscale aggregates that interact with water soluble polymer or organic acids and bases. The formed structures can be made visible by Cryo-TEM micrographs. The size and shape of β-CD aggregates in water have been shown to depend on the CD concentration and other external factors. Other investigations have indicated that the aggregate diameter is much smaller, ranges from 3 to 5 nm.

Table 21.3: Various methods that have been applied to enhance the complexation efficiency (or rather the solubilization efficiency) of CDs in pharmaceutical formulations

Effect	Consequences
Drug ionization	Unionized drugs do usually form more stable complexes than their ionic counterparts. However, ionization of a drug increases its apparent intrinsic solubility resulting in enhanced complexation.
Salt formation	It is sometimes possible to enhance the apparent intrinsic solubility of a drug through salt formation, i.e. forming a more water-soluble salt of the drug without significantly reducing its ability to form CDs complexes.
Acid/base ternary complexes,	It has been shown that certain organic hydroxy acids (such as citric acid) and certain organic bases are able to enhance the complexation efficiency by formation of ternary drug cyclodextrin/acid or base complexes.
Polymer complexes	Water-soluble polymers form a ternary complex with drug/cyclodextrin complexes increasing the observed stability constant of the drug/cyclodextrin complex. This observed increase in the value of the constant, increases the complexation efficiency.
Metal complexes	Many drugs are able to form somewhat water-soluble metal complexes without decreasing the drugs ability to form complexes with cyclodextrins. Thus, the complexation efficiency can be enhanced by formation of drug metal ion-cyclodextrin complexes.
Cosolvents	Addition of cosolvents to the complexation media can increase the apparent intrinsic solubility of the drug that can lead to enhanced complexation efficiency.
Ion pairing	Ion pairing of positively charged compounds with negatively charged cyclodextrins enhances the complexation efficiency.
Combination of two or more methods	Frequently, the complexation efficiency can be enhanced even further may combining two or more of the above mentioned methods. For example, drug ionization and the polymer method, or solubilization of the cyclodextrin aggregates by adding both polymers and cations or anions to the aqueous complexation medium.

DRUG AVAILABILITY FROM CD-CONTAINING PRODUCTS

Natural CDs are regarded as a nonirritant to skin, eyes, and mucosa upon inhalation. However, α-CD may cause some noncorrosive eye irritation. Among CD derivatives, HP-β-CD (HP-hydroxypropylated) is regarded as safe and nonirritating, while methylated CD can cause serious irritations and even corrosion to the eye. Cytotoxicity of CD on corneal membranes may be due to its inter-action with membranes components, such as cholesterol, phospholipids, and proteins. For evaluation of the influence of CD on membrane irritation, damage or induced cytotoxicity, hemolysis data are useful. The hemolytic effect depends on the type (for parent CD, it is in following order—β-CD > α-CD > γ-CD) and concentration (strongly) of CD, and that of methylated CD is much higher than other CD. Previously, it was reported that CD extracts the lipids from membrane without entering into the membrane. The CD forms a new lipid containing compartment in the aqueous phase that equilibrates freely with the cell surface. α-CD is able to solubilize phospholipids rather than sterols, while β-CD interacts mainly solubilizing cholesterol and proteins. It was stated that derivatisation has a significant influence on CD ability to solubilise membrane ingredients.

Application of CD solution directly onto the mucosa (nasal, buccal or vaginal) is regarded as safe for hydrophilic and natural CD in a wide range of concentrations, while for methylated CD derivatives, the concentration and the application time should be controlled. Methylated β-CD can be regarded as safe below concentrations of 5%, furthermore, *in vivo* conditions-dilution and mucociliary clearance will decrease of CD concentration and irritation on application site. Calidiol, a nasal spray contains estradiol and RM-β-CD and is applied in the treatment of osteoporosis in postmenopausal women. It provides very fast drug diffusion into the tissue cells

resulting in a pulsative therapy. Also HP-β-CD as hydrophilic natural CD is regarded as nonirritant to the mucosa and has no direct influence on mucosa integrity, however it can increase the activity of a lipophilic absorption enhancer. β-CD, applied under occlusion condition onto the skin surface in humans, does not induce irritation or allergenic reaction. All tested CDs were well tolerated by the stratum corneum, with the exception of dimethylated derivatives, where changes in corneoxenometry were observed, which indicate disruption in the lipid bilayers. Overall, natural CDs and their hydrophilic derivatives are not able to permeate skin barrier in significant amounts; thus they are safe for localized topical applications.

Generally, all types of above-discussed CD can be safely used in skin and mucosal formulations without risk of irritation; even methylated CD in low concentrations can be safely applied. Only for aqueous solution/suspension containing high concentration of CDs, there is some probability that methylated CD will interact with the stratum corneum lipids (cholesterol, triglycerides) and tem-porarily may affect the membrane integrity. As a consequence of low β-CD aqueous solubility (1.85% at room temperature), they cannot affect membrane structure when administrated as solution. For eye preparation γ-CD, HP-β-CD and SBE-β-CD are recom-mended.

REGULATORY STATUS

The regulatory status of CD is continuously evolving. The natural β-CD can be found in a number of pharmaceutical formulations in numerous countries throughout the world. Under certain conditions it is generally recognized as safe (GRAS) by the FDA and is listed in both the European Pharmacopoeia and US Pharmacopoeia as well as in the Japanese Pharmaceutical Codex. In fact, all three natural cyclodextrins are listed and all three have been approved as food additives. α-CD is listed in European Pharmacopoeia and 2-hydroxypropyl-β-cyclodextrin is listed in both European Pharmacopoeia and US Pharmacopoeia. 2-hydroxypropyl-β-cyclodextrin is cited in the FDA's list of inactive pharmaceutical ingredients. Consensus appears to be building among regulators that cyclodextrins are excipients and not part of the drug substance, which is logical based on their physicochemical properties as drug solubilizers and stabilizers.

PATENTS

The first cyclodextrin-related patent entitled 'Verfahren zur Herstellung von Einschlu β verbindungen physiologisch wirksamer organischer Verbindungen' was issued in Germany in 1953. This patent describes the basic properties of α-, β- and γ-CD complexes, their precipitation in aqueous solutions and how the complexation enhances the chemical stability of biologically active compounds, increases their duration of activity and improves their taste. It contains four claims on preparation of cyclodextrin complexes. However, this patent never found any industrial application.

Current cyclodextrin patents fall into four categories. First, certain methods for production of cyclodextrins are patent protected. For example, the cyclodextrin producing companies have patents on certain production techniques for producing α-, β- and γ-CD and some of their derivatives. Second, there are patents on pharmaceutical applications of certain CD derivatives. For example, Johnson and Johnson has patent on pharmaceutical applications of 2-hydroxypropyl-β-CD in the US and CyDex has a patent on sulfobutylether β-CD. Third, there are patents on methods to improve the performance of CD. For example, certain formulation techniques for improving the solubilizing effects of cyclodextrins through addition of hydroxyacids or water-soluble polymers. Finally, there are patents on specific drug-CD combinations. More than one-third of all CD-related patents fall into this last category. Table 21.4 shows the list of various patents.

Table 21.4: Patents related to β-CD complex

Patent	Year	Original assignee/inventor	Title
4352794	1982	Jurgen Koch, Germany	β-CD as antiacne agent
4555504	1986	Burroughs Wellcome Co., NC	Inclusion complex of β-CD and digoxin
US 2002/0010106A1	2002	Uchiyama Hirotaka, et al., US	Compositions comprising CD
US 2006/0199785A1	2006	Pinnacle Pharmaceuticals, US	β-CD derivatives as antibacterial agents
7202231	2007	The Johns Hopkins University School of Medicine, Baltimore, MD	β-CD compositions, and use to prevent transmission of sexually transmitted diseases
US20090005343	2008	Innovative Biologics, Inc., Los Angeles	β-CD derivatives and their use against anthrax lethal toxin
7851457	2010	Innovative Biologics, Inc., Los Angeles	β-CD derivatives
7700579	2010	Chiesi Farmaceutici S.P.A., Italy	Process for the preparation of piroxicam: β-CD inclusion compounds
US 2011/0237540 A1	2011	Thomas C. Crawford et al., US	CD-based polymers for therapeutic delivery
US 2011/0218247 A1	2011	Curtis Wright, Daniel B. Carr, Fred H. Mermelstein, US	Formulations of low dose diclofenac and β-CD

PHARMACEUTICAL APPLICATIONS OF DRUG-CD COMPLEXES

CDs increase the water solubility of poorly soluble drugs and improve their bioavailability. Light, thermal and oxidative stability of actives can be improved through the formation of CD complexes. CDs have also been used to reduce dermal, gastrointestinal or ocular irritation, mask unpleasant tastes or odors, prevent adverse drug-ingredient interactions and convert oils/liquids into powders to improve handling. There have been a lot of developments of drug delivery systems based on CD, which were used in nasal drug delivery, in peptide and protein delivery, in ophthalmic drug delivery, and in many other areas. The most stable three-dimensional structure of CD is a toroid with the larger and smaller openings presenting hydroxyl groups to the external environment and mostly hydrophobic functionality lining the interior of the cavity (Fig. 21.4). It is this unique configuration that gives CDs their interesting properties and creates the thermodynamic driving force needed to form host-guest complexes with apolar molecules and functional groups.

Drug Solubility and Dissolution

The CD-based inclusion complexation or solid dispersion can significantly improve drug solubility or dissolution of poorly water-soluble drugs. The drugs with inadequate molecular characteristics for complexation, CDs act as hydrophilic carriers, or as tablet dissolution enhancers for drugs with high dose, e.g. paracetamol. Commercially available CDs, such as methylated CDs with a relatively low molar substitution appear to be the most powerful solubilizers. Reduction of drug crystallinity on complexation or solid dispersion with CDs also contributes to the increased apparent drug solubility and dissolution rate. CDs may be able to enhance drug dissolution even when there is no complexation. CDs can also act as release enhancers, e.g. β-CDs enhanced the release rate of poorly soluble naproxen and ketoprofen from inert acrylic resins and hydrophilic swellable [high-viscosity hydroxypropyl methyl cellulose (HPMC)] tableted matrices.

Bioavailability Enhancement

Drugs with poor bioavailability typically have low water solubility and/or tend to be highly crystalline. As shown, cyclodextrins are water-soluble and form inclusion complexes with apolar molecules or functional groups in water insoluble compounds. The resulting complex hides most of the hydrophobic functionality in the interior cavity of the cyclodextrin, while the hydrophilic hydroxyl groups on its

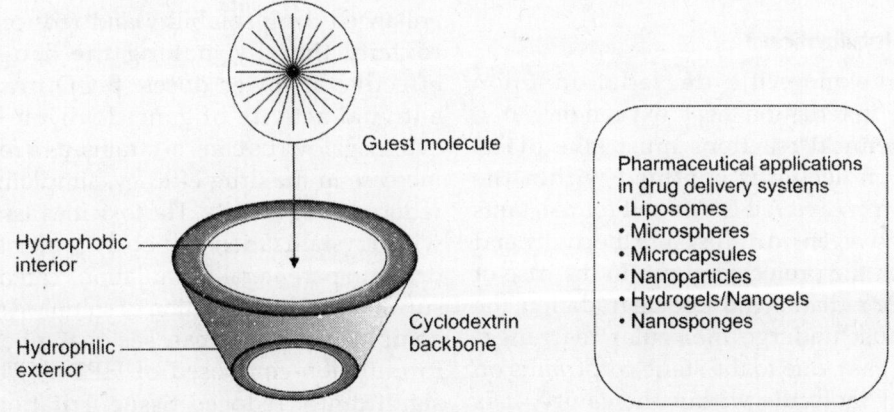

Guest molecule

Hydrophobic interior

Hydrophilic exterior

Cyclodextrin backbone

Pharmaceutical applications in drug delivery systems
• Liposomes
• Microspheres
• Microcapsules
• Nanoparticles
• Hydrogels/Nanogels
• Nanosponges

Fig. 21.4: Multiple benefits exist for CD complexes in pharmaceutical formulations

external surface remain exposed to the environment. The net effect is being a water-soluble cyclodextrin-drug complex. In addition to solubility improvement of drugs, CDs also prevent crystallization of active ingredients by complexing individual drug molecules, so that they can no longer self-assemble into a crystal lattice.

In case of hydrophobic drugs, CDs also enhance the permeability by increasing drug solubility, dissolution and thus making the drug more accessible at the surface of the biological barrier, from where it partitions into the membrane without disrupting the lipid layers of the barrier. There are four possible mechanisms affecting the absorption and thus enhancing bioavailability of CD-complexed drugs by various routes of administration which have been extensively studied and are summarized as follows: (a) CDs increase the solubility, dissolution rate, and wettability of poorly water-soluble drugs; (b) CD prevents the degradation or disposition of chemically unstable drugs in gastrointestinal tracts as well as during storage; (c) CD perturbs the membrane fluidity to lower the barrier function, which consequently enhances the absorption of drugs including peptide and protein drugs through the nasal and rectal mucosa; and (d) competitive inclusion complexation with third components (bile acid, cholesterol, lipids, etc.) to release the included drug.

Active Stabilization

For active molecule degradation upon exposure to radiation, heat, oxygen or water, some chemical reactions must take place. When a molecule is confined within the cyclodextrin cavity, it is difficult for reactants (water or oxygen) to diffuse into the cavity and react with the protected guest. In the case of thermal or radiation induced degradation, the active must undergo molecular rearrangements. Again, due to the steric constraints on the guest molecule within the cavity, it is difficult for the active to fragment upon exposure to heat or light or if it does fragment, the fragments do not have the mobility needed to separate and react before a simple recombination takes place.

Odor or Taste Masking

Through encapsulation within the cyclodextrin cavity, molecules or specific functional groups that cause unpleasant tastes or odors, are isolated from the sensory receptors. The resulting formulations have no or little taste or odor and are much more agreeable to the patient.

Compatibility Improvement

Often one would like to combine multiple ingredients or drug actives within a single formulation due to the potential for synergistic benefits. However, different drugs are often incompatible with each other or another inactive ingredient within a formulation. Encapsulating one of the incompatible ingredients within a cyclodextrin molecule stabilizes the formulation by physically separating the components and prevents chemical interaction.

Drug Safety

CDs have been used to improve the irritation caused by drugs. The CD-based complexes might improve the drug efficacy and potency (i.e. reduction of the dose required for optimum therapeutic activity) due to enhanced drug solubility and reduced drug toxicity thereby making the drug more effective at lower doses. β-CD raised the antiviral activity of ganciclovir on human cytomegalovirus clinical strains, as a resultant increase in the drug efficacy, simulatneously reduced drug toxicity. The toxicities associated with crystallization of poorly water soluble drugs in parenteral formulations can often be surmounted by formation of soluble drug-CD complexes. As we can see that phenytoin formulation composed of HP2-β-CD offers significantly reduced tissue irritation compared to a commercial injection of the drug in a BALB/c mouse model. Further, CD entrapment of drugs at the molecular level prevents their direct contact with biological membranes and thus reduces the side effects and local irritation with no drastic loss of therapeutic benefits.

Controlled Drug Release

In oral delivery, two types of control on drug release may be possible, such as rate-controlled release and the time-controlled release. Basically, the hydrophobic CDs, such as ethylated and acylated CDs with low aqueous solubility may be frequently employed as prolonged-release carriers for water-soluble drugs. Among the various acylated CDs, perobutanoyl-β-CD (TB-β-CD), has the prominent release retarding effect on water soluble drugs, owing to the mucoadhesive property and appropriate hydrophobicity that differ from those of other derivatives having shorter or longer chains. The combined use of CD complex and CD conjugate will be useful for designing various kinds of time-controlled type oral drug delivery preparations (Fig. 21.5).

The drug release from the drug/CD complex after oral administration presented a typical delayed-release behavior. Obviously, a repeated-release preparation may be designed by combining the CD complex as a fast releasing fraction, while a combined preparation of the complex with a slow-releasing fraction may offer the prolonged release preparation. These modified-releases by means of the combination were demonstrated for the ketoprofen/β-CD complex. The coadministration of the CD conjugate and the fast-dissolving ketoprofen/HP-β-CD complex

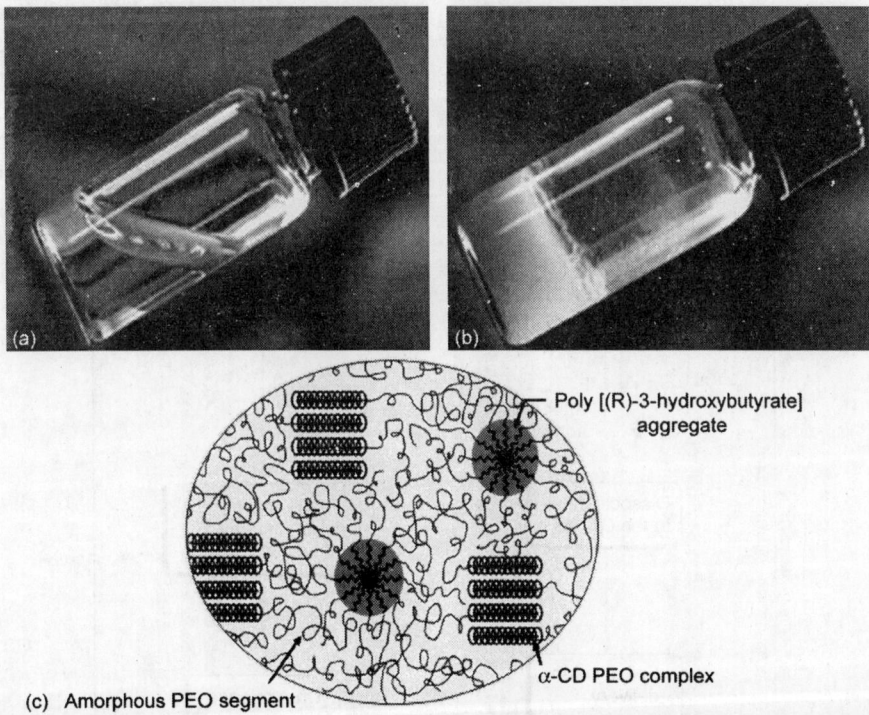

Fig. 21.5: (a) and (b) Optical images of PEO–PHB–PEO (5000–1750–5000) triblock copolymer aqueous solution (c) α-CD–PEO–PHB–PEO (5000–1750–5000) supramolecular hydrogel, the schematic illustration of the structure of α-CD–PEO–PHB–PEO supramolecular hydrogel that provides controlled release (adapted from Li and Loh, 2008)

showed a typical repeated release profile after oral administration. Since pharmaceutical preparations are usually composed of considerable amounts of pharmaceutical excipients and additives to maintain the efficacy and safety of the drug molecules, suitable combination of the CD complex and the third component adjuvant can markedly extend the actions of CD for the design of advanced drug release formulations.

Site-specific Drug Delivery

Drug targeting to specific organ or tissues by drug/CD complex sometimes creates a problem relating to the complex dissociation before it reaches targeting site. Such problem can be overcome by binding of drug covalently to CD. CDs are known to be scarcely capable of being hydrolyzed and only slightly absorbed in passage through the stomach and small intestine; however, they are fermented to small saccharides by colonic microflora and get absorbed as maltose or glucose in the large intestine. Hence, this biological property of CD can be well exploited for site-specific delivery of drugs to colon. The CD conjugates

of biphenylylacetic acid and ketoprofen, n-butylic acid, prednisolone, and 5-fluorouracil, as new candidates have emerged as options for colon-specific delivery among them prednisolone/CD conjugate is particularly employed for colon-specific delivery owing to the alleviation of systemic side effects of prednisolone, while maintaining the anti-inflammatory effect. Colon targeting is essentially classified as a delayed release with fairly long lag time, because the time required for reaching the colon after oral administration is expected to be about 8 hours. When a CD based complex is orally administered, it readily dissociates in the gastrointestinal fluid, depending on the magnitude of the stability constant. This indicates that CD complex is not suitable for colon-specific delivery as the drug is released, because of the dilution and competitive inclusion effects, before it reaches the colon. One of the advantages of the CD-drug conjugate is that it can survive passage through stomach and small intestine, while the drug release is specifically triggered by enzymatic degradation of cyclodextrins in the colon (Fig. 21.6). CD-based colon-targeting

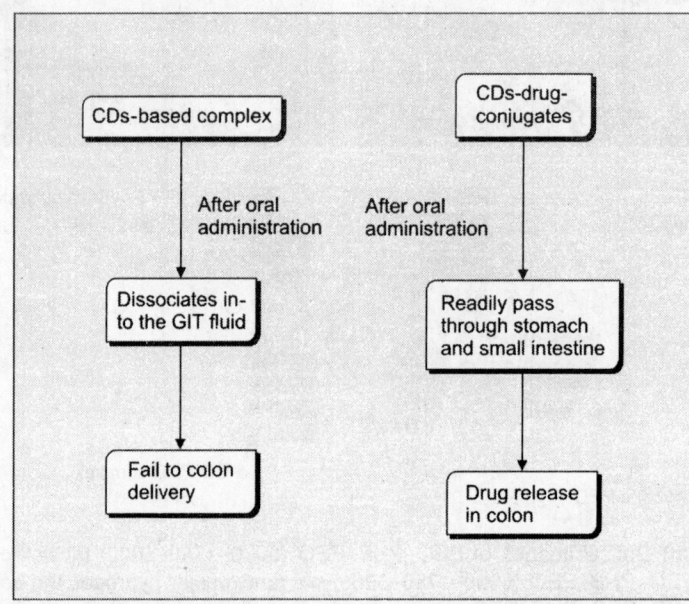

Fig. 21.6: Schematic representation is showing the colon-specific drug delivery

prodrugs can be characterized as follows: In the case of ester type conjugates, drug release is triggered by the ring-opening of cyclodextrins, which consequently provides the site-specific drug delivery in the colon. On the other hand, the amide conjugates do not release the drug even in the cecum and colon, despite of the ring opening of cyclodextrins. The amide linkage of the small saccharide-biphenyl acetic acid conjugates may be resistant to the bacterial enzymes and poorly absorbable from the intestinal tracts due to high hydrophilicity. Therefore, the ester type conjugates are preferable as a delayed release prodrug, which can release a parent drug selectively in cecum and colon.

CD USED IN THE DESIGN OF DELIVERY SYSTEMS

Liposome

CD can be used to improve lipophilic drug entrapment in the aqueous liposomal phase and thus results in a new double-carrier system of drugs-in-CD-in-liposome formulations. For example, such system was investigated for the transdermal delivery of ketoprofen. It was observed that improvement in drug entrapment for ketoprofen/HP-β-CD complex resulted on equimolar ratio. Encapsulation efficiency increased with CD concentration; however, high concentration destabilised liposomal membrane. Liposomal formulations resulted in slower and prolonged drug permeation through membrane (about 40% drug permeated after 24 hours), in comparison to drug solution (60% after 4 hours). The CD interaction with liposomes, lipid membrane depends on the type of CD, complexed drug substance and lipids (Table 21.5).

Microspheres

The role of cyclodextrins in microparticles preparation was firstly studied out by Loftsson and their coworkers. Complexation may not

Table 21.5: Novel drug delivery systems incorporating CD-drug complex

CD type	Drugs	Delivery system	Purpose
β-CD, HP-β-CD	Ketoprofen	Liposomes	Transdermal drug delivery
β-CD, HP-β-CD	Niclosamide	Dendrimers	Solubility enhancement and controlled release
β-CD	Poly (propylene glycol) bisamine	Hydrogel	Biomedical materials for tissue engineering and drug carriers with controlled release
β-CD	Dexamethasone, Flurbiprofen, Doxorubicin hydrochloride	Nanosponges	Nanoparticulate system as drug carriers
2-HP-β-CD	Glutathione	Microparticles	Oral sustained-release delivery systems for tripeptide with reduced peptide degradation
HP-β-CD, HP-β-CD	Triclosan, Furosemide	Nanoparticles	Transmucosal delivery of hydrophobic compounds
β-CD,-β-CD,β-CD	Insulin insulin/CD	Pegylated Polypseudoro taxanes	Polypseudorotaxanes as sustained release system
2-HP-β-CD	Insulin	Nanoparticles	Oral insulin delivery
HP-β-CD	Insulin	Large porous particles	Dry powders for the sustained release used for pulmonary delivery
β-CD hydrate	Amlodipine	Liposomes	Stability against photodegradation
HP-β-CD	Saquinavir	Nanoparticles	Improve oral delivery
HP-β-CD	Itraconazole	Vaginal cream	Developed mucoadhesive vaginal cream

improve the drug dissolution rate from microspheres even in the presence of a high percentage of highly soluble hydrophilic excipients. Nifedipine release from chitosan microspheres was slowed down on complexation with HP-β-CD in spite of the improved drug-loading efficiency; this can be attributed to lesser drug availability from the complex and also due to formation of hydrophilic chitosan/CD matrix layer around the lipophilic drug that further decreases the drug matrix permeability.

Nanoparticles

The safety and efficacy of nanoparticles are limited by their very low drug loading and limited entrapment efficiency that may lead to excessive administration of polymeric material. The applications of CD have been found promising in the design of nanoparticles: one is increasing the loading capacity of nanoparticles and the other is spontaneous formation of either nanocapsules or nanospheres by nanoprecipitation of amphiphilic CDs diesters. Both the techniques were reported to be useful due to great interest of nanoparticles in oral and parenteral drug administration. For example, HP-β-CD increased saquinavir loading into poly (alkyl cyanoacrylate) nanoparticles by providing a soluble drug reservoir in polymeric medium.

Hydrogels

Polymeric hydrogels have attracted interest in biomedical applications because of their favorable biocompatibility in general, high in immense water content; they are attractive for delivery of delicate bioactive agents, such as proteins. For example, chemically cross-linked poly (ethylene oxide) (PEO) polymers were extensively studied for this purpose. Linear water-soluble polymers, such as PEO can penetrate the inner cavity of α-CD to form inclusion complexes with supramolecular structure. The precipitation of the inclusion complexes of α-CD and PEO from aqueous solutions indicates that the resulting complexes are self-assembled into larger supramolecular structures with altered hydrophilicity. As the first example of the hydrogel formation between CDs and polymers the supramolecular self-assembly was initiated and affected through a part of the chain of high molecular weight PEO, which resulted in a sol-gel transition of the α-CD-PEO aqueous solutions. Since both CDs and PEO are known to be biocompatible and bioabsorbable, a new class of injectable drug delivery systems based on the supramolecular hydrogels was emerged. The supramolecular hydrogels were found to be thixotropic and reversible. The viscosity of the hydrogel greatly decreased on agitation. This property renders the hydrogel formulations to be injectable even through a fine needle. The diminished viscosity of the hydrogels eventually restored towards its original value, in most cases within hours, on withdrawal of agitation. These thixotropic and reversible properties of the gel offered us with a unique injectable hydrogel drug delivery system. The various bioactive agents, such as drugs, proteins, vaccines, or plasmid DNAs are incorporated into the gel in a syringe at room temperature without any contact with organic solvents. The drug-loaded hydrogel formulation can then be injected into the tissue under pressure; because of the thixotropic property, and they form a depot for controlled release (Fig. 21.7).

Sunscreen Creams

CDs are helpful in controlling skin penetration of topically applied sunscreen agents and other chemicals. Sunscreens and some topically applied substances should stay onto skin surface without further cutaneous penetration; thus, lowering their release from the carrier is a beneficial feature. Additionally, sunscreen agents under solar radiation generate a variety of decomposition products that can be harmful to DNA, such as free radicals and active oxygen species, and thus decrease its UV-protection. As an example, HP-β-CD significantly reduced the release and

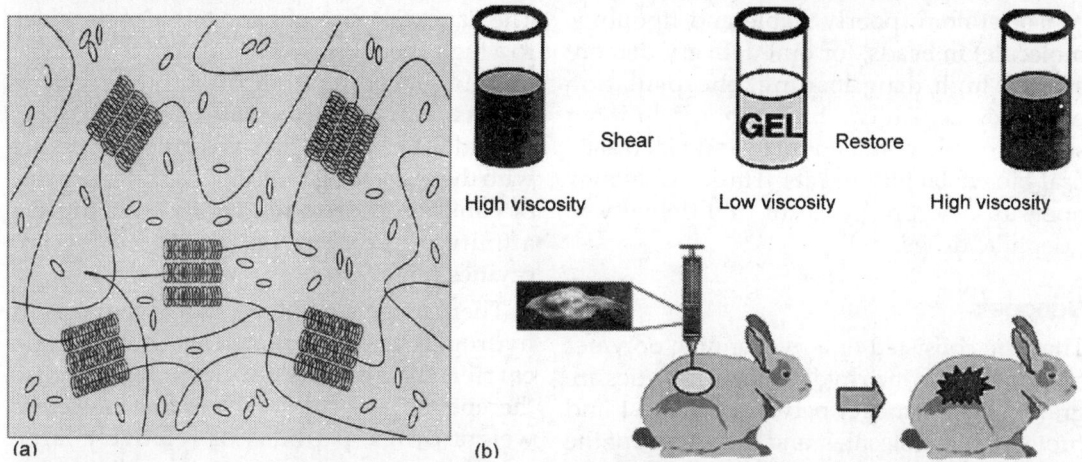

(a)   (b)

Fig. 21.7: Schematic representation (a) Partial inclusion complexation of high molecular weight PEO with α-CD leading to formation of a supramolecular hydrogel. (b) Injectable drug delivery system based on supramolecular hydrogels formed between α-CD and PEO (adapted and modified from Li and Loh, 2008)

membrane permeation of oxybenzone without suppressing the UV-absorbing properties of this chemical. It was demonstrated that skin flux of oxybenzone is related to the CD concentration. The maximum flux occurred at 10% HP-β-CD, while 20% CD excess decreased both skin absorption and permeation. By adding excess of CDs, it is possible to form a drug reservoir on the skin surface.

CD as Skin Penetration Co-enhancers

As skin penetration enhancement is difficult by using only CD and as the influence on drug flux depends not only on CD and drug substance properties, but also on other formulation components. Recently, CDs have been applied with good efficacy as co-enhancers or in combination with other methods viz.; supersaturation, electroporation, or iontophoresis.

Beads

The particulate 'beads' are made of safe and well-known materials: α-CD and soybean oil demonstrated potential to surmount the problems such as poor stability of liposomes in the gastrointestinal tract, use of organic solvents in manufacture of micro/nanocapsules. Beads can be prepared by using soft conditions

(no organic solvent, no cross-linking or surface-active agents, moderate heating). Morphologically, these beads appear as minispheres consisting of a partial crystalline matrix of CD surrounding microdomains of oil (Fig. 21.8).

Beads can be prepared by continuous external orbital shaking of a mixture of an α-CD aqueous solution and soybean oil at room temperature. α-CD is employed for its ability to interact with components of vegetable oil and more especially with triglycerides, whereas the high oil content offers interesting prospects for the microencapsulation of lipophilic drugs. For example, encapsulation

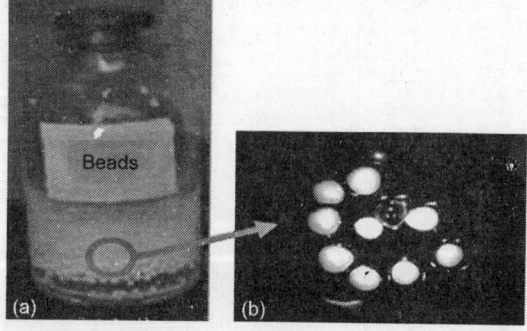

(a)   (b)

Fig. 21.8: Photograph of beads: (a) at the end of the fabrication process. (b) Zoom of beads after washing (adapted from Bocho et al., 2007)

of isotretinoin (poorly stable and lipophilic molecule) in beads, for oral delivery demonstrated high drug loading/encapsulation efficiency, which can be attributed to inner structure (microdomains of oil) and increased oral bioavailability in rats. Thus, beads may open up new prospects for oral delivery of lipophilic drugs.

Nanogels

They are consisted of a hydrophilic polymer backbone, on which hydrophobic moieties are grafted. The nanogel network can host and protect drug molecules, and the release of the drug molecules from the nanogels can be regulated by the incorporation of high-affinity functional groups, stimuli-responsive conformations or biodegradable bonds into the polymer network. The hydrophilicity of the nanogels enables them to be easily disperseable in aqueous media forming free flowing opalescent solutions. Thus, nanogels can be easily administered in liquid dosage form, e.g. parenteral or mucosal administration.

The nanoscale size of nanogels also provides to a high specific surface area that is available for the bioconjugation of active targeting agents. Nanogels in water form CD-rich colloidal networks that are able to interact with the guest drug molecules and are capable of controlling drug release by utilizing the affinity of the drug molecules for the CD cavities (Fig. 21.9).

The nanogels combine the advantages of hydrogels and nanoparticles into a single carrier that can be tailored for specific therapeutic molecules, such as low molecular weight drugs, peptides or relatively large proteins, and target them to specific tissues or cells. Alternatively, CDs can be grafted onto free polymeric chains to play a dual role: as a cross-linking agent and as a host for the guest drug. To perform both the functions, certain CD cavities can be involved in forming complexes with the hydrophobic groups of adjacent polymeric chains, acting as tie up junctions or cross-linking points, while the other CDs interact with the drug molecules.

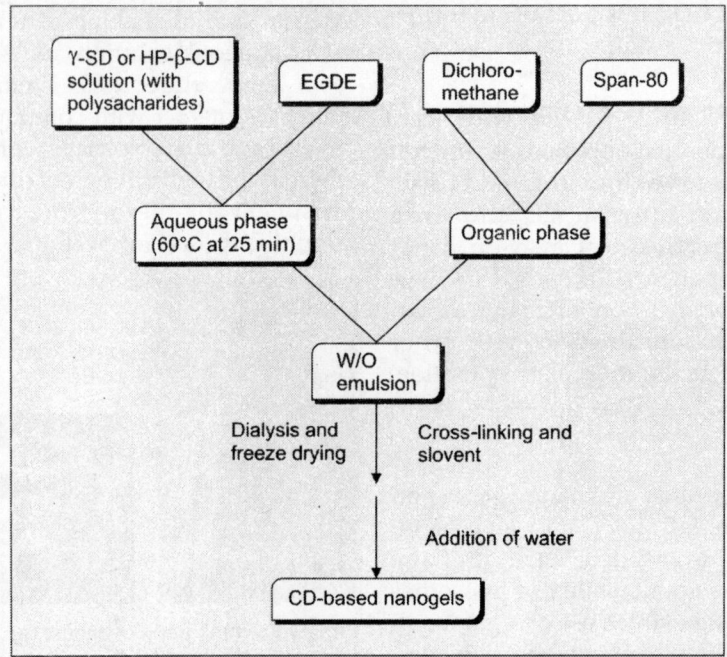

Fig. 21.9: Schematic presentation for the preparation of CD-based nanogels

The nanogels preparation method can be classified as (i) key-lock interactions among preformed chains, with some bearing CDs and others possessing groups that fit into the CDs, (ii) direct covalent cross-linking of CD units by condensation with suitable bi/multifunctional agents, (iii) polymerization of CD monomers bearing acrylic or vinyl moieties (Fig. 21.10). Moreover, CD-based nanogels provide useful functionalities, such as effective bioconjugation, good adhesion to surfaces, controlled complexation and the relatively rapid release of drugs, in addition to their utility as cosmetic ingredients, dyes or antimicrobial agents.

CD-containing Polymers

CD-containing polymers are now being explored as vehicles for delivering nucleic acids into cells. The structures of the CD-containing polycations affect the nucleic acid transfection efficiencies and their toxicities. The CD-containing polymers reveal lower toxicities than polymers that lack the CD. The CD-containing, cationic polymers were able to provide effective DNA delivery to cultured cells with low toxicity. Numerous CD-containing cationic polymers are currently available. Recently, developed methodologies showed that the polyplex (CD-containing polymers and DNA) surface was modified to provide modified polyplexes appropriate for systemic application as gene delivery vehicles. As an example of this methodology, adamantane was conjugated to PEG (polyethylene glycol) and the resulting compound was exposed to CD-containing cationic polymers-based polyplexes for self-assembly between the adamantane and the CD. This methodology can provide particles that are appropriate for systemic gene delivery.

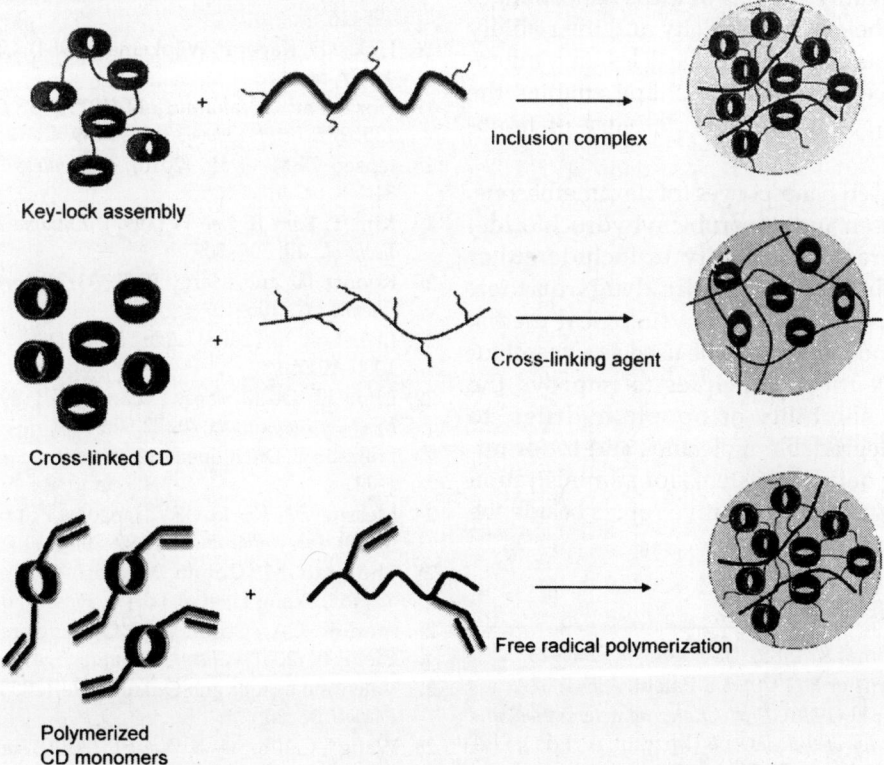

Fig. 21.10: Schematic methods for the preparation of CD-based nanogels

Nanosponges

Nanosponges belong to a new class of materials represented by microscopic particles with cavities a few nanometers wide, characterized by the capacity to encapsulate a large variety of substances that can be transported through aqueous media. In the recent years, β-CD based nanosponges have been synthesized for their potential application in drug delivery, water purification, cosmetics, agriculture etc. In the pharmaceutical field, they could be employed as solubilizing agents or nanocarriers. The nanosponges contain β-CD as building blocks, linked with carbonate groups to form a high cross-linked network. The final nanosponge structure contains both CD lyphophilic cavities and carbonate bridges, leading to a network of more hydrophilic channels. Nanosponges are solid, insoluble in water, and rather crystalline. The important and innovative aspects of these nanosponges include their lack of toxicity and their ability to combine in spherical particles on a micrometric scale. Their tiny shape enables the pulmonary and venous delivery of nanosponges.

CD-based nanosponges (of dexamethasone, flurbiprofen and doxorubicin hydrochloride) demonstrated the ability to include either lipophilic or hydrophilic drugs or their subsequent slow into physiological media. Thus, nanosponges can be used as a vessel for pharmaceutical principles to improve the aqueous solubility of lipophilic drugs, to protect degradable molecules and to formulate drug delivery systems for administration through various alternative routes beside the oral one.

SUGGESTED READINGS

1. Ammeraal R (1988), US Patent, 4, 738, 923.
2. Armbruster F (1970), US Patent, 3, 541, 077.
3. Bender H (1986), *Production, characterization, and application of cyclodextrins* (Mizrahi, A., Eds.), Liss, New York, pp. 31–71.
4. Biwer A, Antranikian G, Heinzle E (2002), *Enzymatic production of cyclodextrins. Appl Microbiol Biotechnol.*, 59, 609–17.
5. Blackwood A, Bucke C (2000), *Enzyme Microb Technol.*, 27, 704–8.
6. Bochot A, Trichard L, Le Bas G, Alphandary H, Grossiord JL, Ducheˆne D, Fattal E (2007).
7. Brunet C, Lamare S, Legoy M (1998), *Biocatal Biotransfor.*, 16, 317–27.
8. Buschmann H, Knittel D, Jonas C et al. (2001), *Lebensmittelchemie.*, 55, 54–6.
9. Cal K, Centkowska K (2008), *Eur. J. Pharm. Biopharm.* 68, 467–78.
10. Chen M, Diao G and Zhang E (2006) , *Chemosphere*, 63, 522–9.
11. Choi J, Lee J, Choi K (1996), US Patent, 5, 492, 829.
12. Figueiras A, Ribeiro L, Teresa M, Veiga VF (2007), *J. Incl Phenom Macrocycl Chem.*, 57, 173–7.
13. Gornas P, Neunert G, Baczynski K and Polewski K (2009), *Food Chem.*, 114, 190–96.
14. Grull, D., Stifter, U. (2001) US Patent, 6, 235, 505.
15. He Y, Fu P, Shen Z, Gao H (2008), *Micron.*, 39, 495416.
16. Hokse H, Kaper F, Wijpkema J (1984), US Patent, 4, 477, 568.
17. Horikoshi K, Nakamura N (1979), US Patent, 4, 135, 977. *Int. J. Pharm.* 339, 121–9.
18. Jensen CEM. et al., (2010), *Molecules*, 15, 4067–84.
19. Kim T, Kim B, Lee H (1997), *Enzyme Microbial Technol.*, 20, 506–509.
20. Koontz JL, and Marcy JE (2003), *J Agricul Food Chem.*, 51, 7106–10.
21. Li J, Loh XJ (2008), *Adv. Drug Deliv. Rev.* 60, 1000–1017.
22. Lima H, De Moraes, F Zanin, G (1998), *Appl Biochem Biotechnol.*, 70/72, 789–804.
23. Loftsson T, Duchˆene D (2007), *Int. J. Pharm.* 329, 1–11.
24. Messner M, Kurkov SV, Jansook P, Loftsson T (2010), *Int. J. Pharm.* 387, 199–208.
25. Shulman M, Cohen M, Soto-Gutierrez A, Yagi H, Wang H, et al. (2011), *Plosone*, 6, e18033.
26. Stanier CA, Connell MJO, Anderson HL, Clegg W (2001), *Chem. Commun.*, 5, 493–4.
27. Valentino J, Stella and Quanren He. (2008), *Toxicol Pathol.*, 36, 30.
28. Wang J, Cao Y, Sun B, Wang C (2011), *Food Chem.*, 124, 1069–75.

22

Multifunctional Nanomedicines

INTRODUCTION

Nanomedicines hold the promise of greater localization of therapies to the diseased tissue or organ, while introducing perhaps thousands times fewer drugs into the body which greatly reduces the possibility of side effects. Every biological level of organization presents various barriers which include target specific localization, enhanced clearance, selectivity and permeability of biological membranes, metabolizing enzymes and endosomal or lysosomal degradation. As drug delivery research has progressed, nanotechnology has brought a variety of new possibilities into biological discovery and clinical practice. Currently, comprehensive strategies, such as the use of multifunctional delivery systems have emerged. Through a synergistic effect, multifunctional nanomedicines are capable of overcoming distinct physiological barriers and delivering therapeutic moiety and/or image contrast enhancement agents to target sites in the body. Due to the unique properties of nanoscale matter, the diversity of available materials, and infinite design schemes, nanocarriers have emerged as ideal platforms for achieving multi-functionalization. In this context, the design of multifunctional nano-particles could significantly improve the characteristics of already existing nanoparticles and these nanocarriers might be able to combine different functionalities in a single stable construct. For example, a core particle could be linked to a specific targeting function that recognises the unique surface signatures of their target cells. Simultaneously, the same particle can be modified with an imaging agent to monitor the drug transport process, a function to evaluate the therapeutic efficacy of a drug, a specific cellular penetration moiety and a therapeutic agent.

The potential 'theranostics' possess a high surface area-to-volume ratio, which provides for a high loading capacity of active cargoes that can include drugs, molecular targeting ligands (e.g. tumor-specific antibodies, peptides, small molecules, etc.), cell internalization agents, and/or pharmacokinetic stabilizers (Fig. 22.1).

During the past decades, the multifunctional nanocarriers have been explored for the delivery of genes, drugs, and imaging modalities showing the promising results for therapy in areas, such as cancer and neuropathologies. These flexible platforms consist of polymeric and lipid systems that combine different modalities and stimuli-responsive release properties. Surface modification of pharmaceutical nanocarriers is normally used to control their biological properties in a desirable fashion and simultaneously perform various therapeutically or diagnostically

489

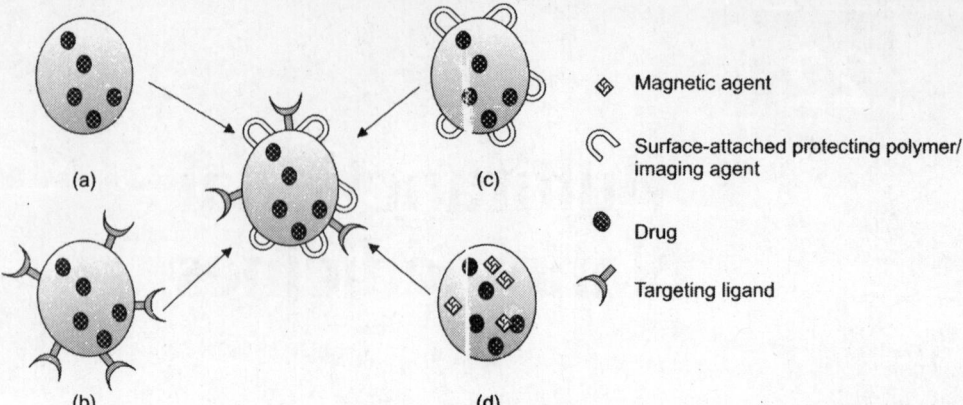

Fig. 22.1: The schematic of assembly of the multifunctional pharmaceutical nanocarrier. Traditional 'plain' nanocarrier (a) drug loaded into the carrier; (b) specific targeting ligand, usually a monoclonal antibody, attached to the carrier surface; (c) surface-attached protecting polymer (usually PEG) allowing for prolonged circulation of the nanocarrier in the blood or contrast nanocarrier for imaging purposes; (d) magnetic particles loaded into the carrier together with the drug and allowing for the carrier sensitivity towards the external magnetic field and its use as a contrast agent for magnetic resonance imaging

important functions. The most important results of such modification include an increased stability and half-life of nanocarriers in the circulation, required biodistribution, passive or active targeting into the required pathological zone, responsiveness to local physiological stimuli, such as pathology-associated changes in local pH and/or temperature, and ability to serve as imaging/contrast agents for various imaging modalities (gamma-scintigraphy, magnetic resonance imaging, computed tomography, ultra-sonography). The multifunctional nanomedicines can indeed be functionalized with drugs as well as fluorescent substances therefore their diagnostics and therapeutic potentials are enormous. However, from a broader perspective, the nanocarriers incorporated with multiple diagnostic, therapeutic or targeting molecules can pave the way to successful treatment and management of a large range of other diseases. Multifunctional nanomedicine integrates target labeling, drug delivery and reporting abilities, allowing diseases to be monitored and treated simultaneously. It holds considerable promise as

next generation of medicine, and attained much attention of researchers in recent years. Certain inorganic nanoparticles with unique optical properties such as colloidal gold, iron oxide nanocrystals, especially quantum dots, can greatly improve the ability to detect diseases at much earlier stages, and offer a new opportunity for development of novel multifunctional drug formulations.

DESIGNING OF MULTIFUNCTIONAL NANOMEDICINES

The diagnostic and/or therapeutic aims of a multifunctional nanocarrier system direct and demand the design of a formulation. The literature is available abound wherein; an algorithm of different types of nanocarrier formulations for the diagnosis, imaging, and treatment of a wide spectrum of diseases has been discussed. These multifunctional nanocarriers basically consist of three main design components.

  a. A platform (core) material

  b Encapsulated payload/biologically active agents

  c. The targeting/surface properties

Figure 22.2 schematically presents the composition of multifunctional nanocarriers. Nanocarrier platforms can be categorized as organic-based, inorganic-based or a hybrid combination of the organic and inorganic. Organic nanoplatforms include polymeric nanocarriers, lipid-based nanocarriers (e.g. liposomes and nanoemulsions), dendrimers, and carbon-based nanocarriers (e.g. fullerenes and carbon nanotubes). Inorganic nano-platforms include metallic nanostructures, silica nanoparticles, and quantum dots. An example of a hybrid platform is colloidal gold encapsulated in liposomes or superpara-magnetic iron oxide particles encapsulated in polymeric nanoparticles. Selection of the core material is highly dependent on the properties of the biologically active agents. Inherent and dynamic properties of the biological agents, such as therapeutic index, lipophilicity, charge, and size should be considered.

As the availability of biologically active agents continues to expand, there can be innumerable therapeutic combinations. When combining therapeutic agents with each other, with an imaging/diagnostic modality, or with delivery of energy, the interaction of system components, (i.e. synergy, quenching, enhanced toxicity) and release kinetics should also be considered. Surface properties represent third design component of multifunctional nanocarriers. A common surface modification technique that decreases reticuloendothelial system (RES) clearance and imparts *in vivo* longevity is the physical or covalent attachment of poly (ethylene glycol) (PEG) chains to the nanocarrier platform. For example, in case of tumor microvasculature, which is known to be highly fenestrated, colloidal particles can accumulate through enhanced permeability and retention (EPR) effect.

PEG surface modification increases circulatory residence time, which increases the probability of their accumulation at the target. Block copolymers of poly (ethylene oxide) (PEO) and poly (propylene oxide) (PPO) (e.g. Pluronics®) have also been used as surface conjugates to enhance circulation and achieve passive targeted delivery.

Further more, the developments of the concept of pharmaceutical nanocarriers involves the attempt to add the property of the specific target recognition ability to the carriers vis-a-vis long circulation. Simultaneously, both the

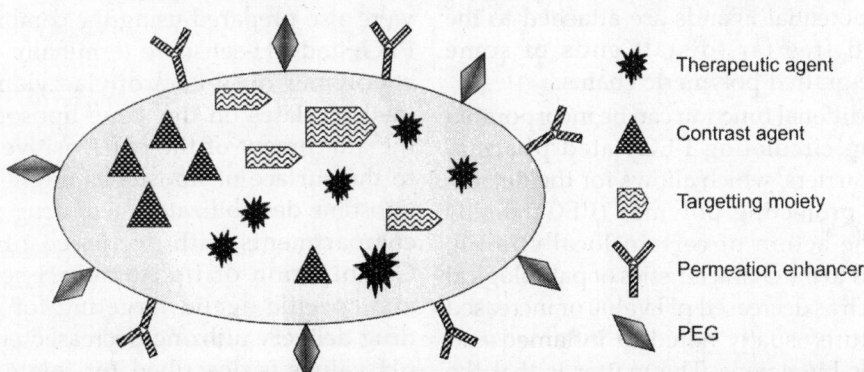

Fig. 22.2: Schematic illustration of multifunctional nanocarrier system. The core material of the nanocarrier can be organic (e.g. liposomes and polymeric nanoparticles), inorganic (e.g. quantum dots) or a fusion combination of organic and inorganic materials. Therapeutic drugs or DNA, imaging agents (such as contrast enhancers), and therapeutic adjuvants can be incorporated. Surface modification can consist of poly (ethylene glycol) (PEG) residues with targeting ligands

protecting polymer and the targeting moiety can be attached on the surface of the nanocarrier. Targeting of drug carriers with an aid of ligands specific to cell surface-receptors allows for the selective drug delivery to those cells. To obtain 'simple' targeted nanocarriers, a variety of methods have been developed to chemically attach corresponding vectors (antibodies, peptides sugar moieties, folate, and other ligands) to the carrier surface. There are evident reasons for the design of ligand-coated long-circulating drug carriers: (a) ligand (an antibody, another protein, peptide or carbohydrate) attached to the carrier surface may enhance the rate of its elimination from the blood and uptake in the liver and spleen, and the presence of the sterically-protecting polymer may block RES uptake. (b) longevity of the specific ligand-bearing nanocarrier may allow for its successful accumulation even in the targets which receive limited and low blood supply or with low density of the surface receptors. For example, to achieve better selective targeting by PEG-coated liposomes or other particulates, targeting ligands could be attached to nano-carriers via the PEG spacer arm, so that the ligand is extended outside of the dense PEG brush excluding steric hindrances for its binding to the target receptors. With this as an aim, potential ligands are attached to the activated free far (distal) ends of some liposome-grafted polymeric chains.

An additional function can be incorporated onto long circulating PEGylated pharmaceutical carriers, which allows for the detachment of protecting polymer (PEG) chains under the action of certain local stimuli, attributed to the characteristics of pathological areas, such as decreased pH value or increased temperature usually noted in inflamed and neoplastic bioregions. The matter is that the stability of PEGylated nanocarriers may not always be favorable for drug delivery. In particular, if drug containing nanocarriers accumulate within the tumor, where they should easily release the drug to kill the tumor cells. Likewise, if the carrier has to be taken up by cell via an endocytic pathway, the presence of the PEG coat on its surface may preclude the contents from escaping the endosome and being delivered in the cytoplasm. In order to solve these problems, e.g. in the case of long-circulating liposomes, the chemistry was developed to detach PEG from the lipid anchor in the therapeutically desired conditions. Labile linkage that would degrade only in the acidic conditions characteristic of the endocytic vacuole or the acidotic tumor mass can be based on the diortho esters, vinyl esters, cysteine-cleavable lipopolymers, double esters and hydrazones that are quite stable at pH around 7.5, but hydrolyzed relatively fast at pH values of 6 and below. Polymeric components with pH sensitive (pH-cleavable) bonds are used to produce stimuli-responsive drug delivery systems that are stable in the circulation or in normal tissues, however, acquire the ability to degrade and release the entrapped drugs in low areas or cell compartments with lowered pH, such as tumors, infarcts, inflammation zones or cell cytoplasm or endosomes. A variety of liposomes and polymeric micelles have been described that include the components with acid-labile bonds. Serum-stable, long-circulating PEGylated pH sensitive liposomes were also prepared using the combination of PEG- and pH-sensitive terminally alkylated copolymer of N-isopropylacrylamide and methacrylates on the same liposome, since the attachment of the pH-sensitive polymer to the surface of liposomes might facilitate liposome destabilization and drug release in compartments with decreased pH values. Combination of liposome pH-sensitivity and specific ligand targeting for cytosolic drug delivery utilizing decreased endosomal pH values is described for folate targeted liposomes.

Surface modifications of superparamagnetic nanoparticles (Fig. 22.3), are considered as promising strategy for drug delivery into regional lymph nodes and for diagnostic

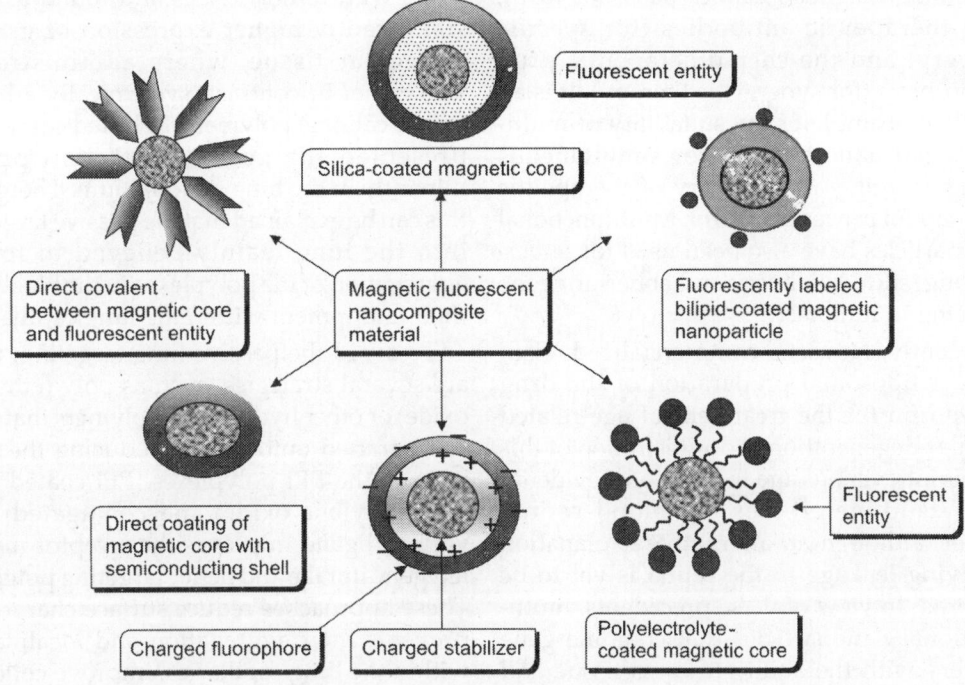

Fig. 22.3: Some magnetic fluorescent nanocomposites

imaging purposes. Similarly, other nano-carriers, PEG-modified magnetite nano-spheres demonstrated an increased colloidal stability and improved localization of drug/marker probe in lymph nodes.

Design of Intelligent Multifunctional Nanocarriers

The design of functional nanocarriers that combine several properties is an elaborate process that requires different steps, such as the depositing of metal layers onto a supporting nanoparticle core, modifying the biocompatible polymer used to stabilize the nanoparticle and the use of different linkers. Furthermore, these different properties of multifunctional nanoparticles have to be integrated, so that they operate in an orchestrated way and indeed provide the desired functionalities. An elegant example is of nanoparticles which had specific targeting and cell-internalisation functions, under normal conditions (i.e. when not bound specifically to the target), the specific target function is exposed, providing a long circulation life and specific delivery, whereas the cell-internalisation function remains hidden. In this manner, the cell-internalisation function does not interfere with the nanoparticle circulation. When specific binding occurs, subsequent to the binding at the low pH of the pathological environment, the penetration function becomes activated, facilitating penetration of nanoparticle within the cell.

APPLICATIONS

Multifunctional Nanocarriers for Drug and Gene Delivery

Multifunctional delivery nanosystems are just emerging, but earlier research performed on *in vivo* studies with multifunctional nanoparticles, serves to emphasize the promising future of these novel nanomaterials. Researchers have developed a multifunctional nanosystem combining magnetic nanocrystals (for MRI), with therapeutic antibodies (for specific delivery) and the chemotherapeutic drug doxorubicin (for synergistic therapy). It is an excellent example of the suitability of multifunctional nanoparticles for simultaneous *in vivo* imaging and delivery of therapeutic products for cancer treatment. Multifunctional nanoparticles have also been used for *in vivo* imaging, siRNA delivery and abberrant gene silencing in tumors.

Recently, Novartis commercialized Visudyne, a liposomal preparation of the drug verteporfin for the treatment of age-related macular degeneration. Administration of this drug is intravenous and there is some evidence that Visudyne crosses the blood-retinal barrier, although an alternative explanation involving leakage to the retina is yet to be explored. In view of these precedents, multifunctional nanoparticles that combine gene delivery with the ability to cross tissue and membrane barriers could constitute ideal non-viral vectors for gene therapy. One of the first indications of the potential of multifunctional platforms for gene delivery, has been transferring genes to the retina. Intravenously administered liposomes could effectively cross the blood-retinal barrier mediated through anti-insulin antibody and could carry along the rDNA construct for expression of target gene in the eye for retinal delivery. Multifunctional vehicles based on nanorods, dendritic polymers and quantum dots constitute other examples of nanosystems designed for gene delivery.

Polyethyleneimine (PEI) has been popularly employed as a most efficient cationic polymer-based gene transfer system for pDNA and siRNA delivery. Various PEI based formulations studied as PEI anticancer gene formulations are competent to achieve tumor regression through a combination of gene transfer and an intrinsic antiproliferative activity. To bypass the systemic barriers, PEI-based gene delivery complexes have been administered locally for lung, liver and brain along with tumor tissues and found to elicit significantly higher expression of gene in particular tissue, where administration was done. In contrast, systemically administered cationic polymer PEI based complexes presented the gene transfection predominantly in the lung endothelium. Therefore, this can be explained that the passive targeting into the lung mainly believed to follow aggregation of the polyplexes in the blood and their entrapment within the lung capillaries.

To avoid the passive lung targeting, there are several strategies, such as poly (ethylene oxide) or other hydrophilic polymers that have been grafted onto PEI, or reducing the N/P ratio of the PEI polyplexes. PEI coated with poly(ethylene oxide) and conjugated with various ligand improves the receptor mediated gene uptake and better targeting potential. These approaches reduce surface charge and prevents their aggregation and localization within the lung capillaries, improve colloidal stability, while the transfection efficiency was still comparable to that of PEI. This occurs largely due to poor cellular uptake of the poly (ethylene oxide) covered polyplex by cells. Hence, it is thus obligatory that along with poly (ethylene oxide) coating, the ligand conjugation on the carriers surface, promotes receptor-mediated uptake if overcome the problem relating to poor cellular uptake (Fig. 22.4).

Medical Diagnostics

In Vitro Diagnostic

In vitro diagnosis for medical applications, has traditionally been a laborious task; blood and other body fluids or tissue samples are sent to a laboratory for an analysis, which could take hours, days or even weeks, depending on the technique used, and is highly labor intensive. Several disadvantages include sample deterioration, cost, lengthy waiting times (even for urgent cases), inaccurate results for small sample quantities, difficulties in integrating parameters obtained by a wide variety of methods and poor standardisation of sample collection.

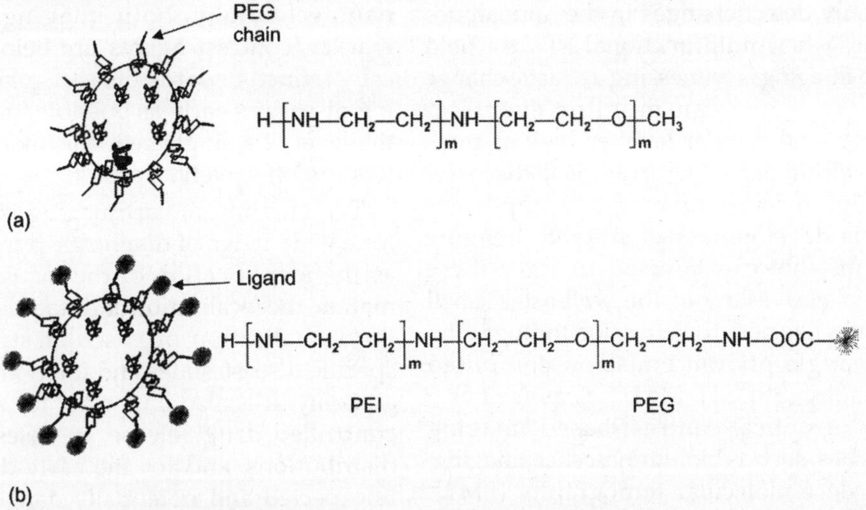

Fig. 22.4: Schematic representation of (a) PEG grafted and (b) Ligand conjugated PEI polymeric nonviral nanocarriers for DNA or RNA delivery

Steadily, miniaturisation, parallelisation and integration of different functions on a single device, based on techniques derived from the electronics industry, have led to the development of a new generation of devices that are smaller, faster and cheaper, do not require special skills, and provide accurate readings. These analytical devices require much smaller samples and will deliver more complete (and more accurate) biological data from a single measurement. The requirement for smaller samples also means less invasive and less traumatic methods of extraction. Nanotechnology enables further refinement of diagnostic techniques, enabling to high throughput screening (to test one sample for numerous diseases, or screen large numbers of samples for one disease) and ultimately point-of-care (POC) diagnostics.

In Vivo Diagnostics

In vivo diagnostics refer not only in general to imaging techniques, but also cover implantable devices. Nanoimaging includes several approaches using techniques for the study of *in vivo* molecular events and molecules manipulation. Imaging techniques cover advanced optical imaging and spectroscopy, nuclear imaging with radioactive tracers, magnetic resonance imaging, ultrasound, optical and X-ray imaging, all of which depend on identifying tracers or contrast agents that have been introduced into the body to mark the diseased site. The goal of *in vivo* diagnostics research is to create highly sensitive, highly reliable detection agents that can also deliver and monitor therapy. This is the 'find, fight and follow' concept of early diagnosis and therapy control that is encompassed in the concept of theranostics. With this strategy, the tissue of interest can firstly be imaged, using target specific contrast nanostructures. Then, combined with a pharmacologically active agent, the same targeting strategy can be used for applying therapy. Finally, monitoring of treatment effects is possible by sequential subsequent imaging.

Imaging

Molecular imaging and image guided therapy is now a basic tool for monitoring of a disease and in developing almost all the clinicodiagnostic applications of *in vivo* nanomedicine. Originally, imaging techniques could only detect changes in the appearance of tissues when multifunctional NPs, the field of brain imaging is witnessing a drastic change in the ways one can monitor events at molecular and cellular level as well as track the development of neurological diseases, cancerous formations etc. One important aspect is development of suitable imaging platforms that can be used to trace these agents *in vivo*. Many of the well-established modalities like positron emission tomography (PET), single photon emission computed tomography (SPECT), MRI, CT, as well as a variety of optical-contrast-based imaging approaches, such as bioluminescence imaging, fluorescence molecular tomography (FMT), and optoacoustic tomography, have gained considerable interest and applicability in neurological research (Fig. 22.5).

Later, contrast agents were introduced to more easily identify and map the locus of a disease. Today, through the application of nanotechnology, both imaging tools and marker/contrast agents are being dramatically refined towards the end goals of detecting disease as early as possible, eventually at the level of a single cell, and monitoring the therapy effectively.

Targeted molecular imaging is important for a wide range of diagnostic purposes, such as the identification of the locus of inflammation, the localisation and staging of tumors, the visualisation of vascular structures or specific disease states and the examination of anatomy. It is also important for research on controlled drug release, in assessing drug distributions, and for the early detection of unexpected and potentially dangerous drug accumulations. The convergence of nanotechnology and medical imaging opens the doors to a revolution in molecular imaging (also called nanoimaging) in the foreseable future, leading to the detection of a single molecule or a single cell in a complex biologi-

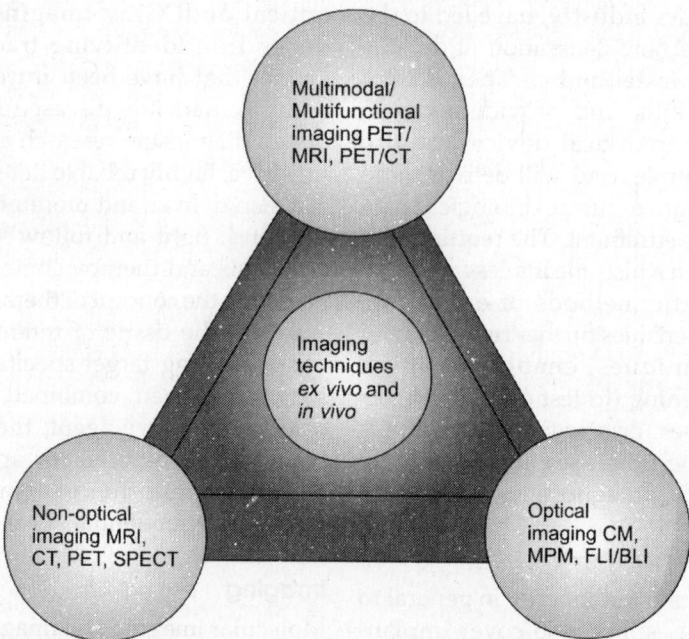

Fig. 22.5: Various applications of imaging technique; confocal microscopy (CM), multiphoton microscopy (MPM), fluorescence imaging and bioluminescence imaging (FLI/BLI), magnetic resonance imaging (MRI), computing tomography (CT), positron-emission tomography and single-photon-emission computed tomography (PET/SPECT), and confocal Raman microscopy (CRM)

cal environment. Nanotechnology can successfully be explored for specific identification of diseased cells in the body and enables its visibility. For example, antibodies that identify specific receptors over-expressed in cancerous cells can be coated with nanoparticles such as metal oxides which produce a high contrast signal on magnetic resonance images (MRI) or computed tomography (CT) scans. Once inside the body, the antibodies on these nanoparticles will bind selectively to cancerous cells, effectively lighting them up for the scanner. Similarly, gold particles could be used to enhance light scattering for endoscopy techniques like colonoscopies. Nanotechnology will enable the visualisation of molecular markers that identify specific stages and types of cancers, allowing physicians to see cells and molecules undetectable through conventional imaging.

Implants and Sensors

Implantable devices are mainly used for *in vivo* diagnostics (Fig. 22.6). Nanotechnology also has many implications for *in vivo* diagnostic devices, such as the swallowable imaging pill and new endoscopic instruments. Monitoring of circulating molecules is of great interest in case of some chronic diseases, such as diabetes or AIDS.

Continuous, measurement of glucose or blood markers of infection constitutes a real value for implantable devices. Miniaturisation for mild invasiveness, combined with surface functionalization and 'biologicalisation' of instruments with autonomous power, self-diagnosis, remote control and external transmission of data are other considerations in the development of these devices. Nanosensors, for example used in catheters, will also provide data to the surgeons. Nanoscale entities could identify pathology/defects; and the subsequent removal or correction of lesions by nano-manipulation could also set a future vision.

The surface/volume ratio of particles becomes very large, when size decreases, so that nanocarriers have a huge surface suitable for chemical interactions with biomolecules, for instance. Moreover, (bio) chemical reaction time is much shorter (it decreases sharply with sample size) and accordingly analytical devices are faster and more sensitive. The ultra small size of the sensing part of a (macro- or micro-) analytical device, with nanopillars, nanobeads, can be possibly exploited for device miniaturisation. Smaller devices offer a lower degree of invasiveness and can even be implanted within the body. Another advantage of the ultraminiaturisation of the sensing part lies in the ultra small size of the biological sample required for measurement. This becomes a key feature for analysing rare samples like some biopsies.

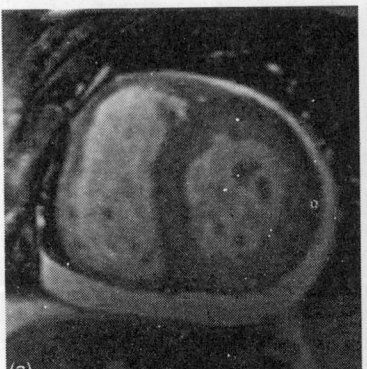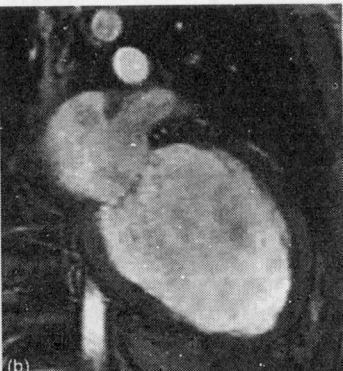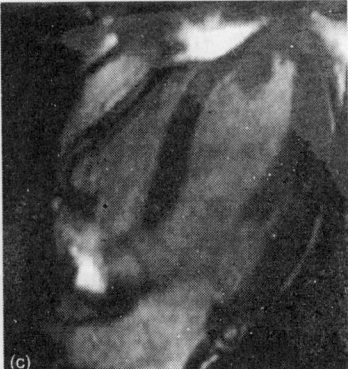

Fig. 22.6: Magnetic resonance image of (a) pericarditis, (b) akinesis (c) intracardiac thrombi (cardiac diseases)

Theranostics, Combined Techniques

Nanobiotechnology offers significant inputs to the improvement of detection devices and for tagging of disease indicators administered *in vivo*, leading to advancement in imaging. Potent driving forces include synergies, such as those between *in vitro* diagnostics (probes and markers) and *in vivo* imaging techniques and those between contrast agents/probe development (in drug delivery and/or toxicology studies) and imaging technology (medical instrumentation).

The combination of *in vitro* diagnostics techniques and *in vivo* nanoimaging could lead to targeted tumor disruption or removal. Tagging tumor cells with functionalised nanoparticles, which react to external stimuli, allows for in situ, localised 'surgery' (breaking up or heating of particles by laser, magnetic fields, microwaves, etc.) without invasiveness within the human body (Fig. 22.7). The capacity of some nanoparticles to carry contrast agents and drugs opens new ways for therapy. Theranostic, used as a combination of therapy and diagnostics, can be looked at differently. Imaging can be used to trace the delivery of drug within the body. But imaging can also be used to activate the drug release from outside, by an external stimulus. Such external stimuli can be laser light, temperature or ultrasounds. All in all, the smart probes represent new concepts for clinical practice.

Novel Carriers as Multifunctional Agents

Microspheres

Magnetic microspheres are supramolecular particles, which are small enough to circulate through capillaries without producing embolic occlusion (<4 µm), but are sufficiently susceptible (ferromagnetic) to be captured in microvessels and dragged into the adjacent tissues by magnetic fields of 0.5–0.8 tesla (T). Magnetic microspheres are prepared by mainly two methods namely phase separation emulsion polymerization (PSEP) and continuous solvent evaporation (CSE). The amount and rate of drug delivery via magnetic responsive microspheres can be regulated by varying size of microspheres, drug content, magnetite content, hydration state and drug release characteristic of carrier. The amount of drug and magnetite content of microspheres needs to be delicately balanced in order to design an efficient therapeutic system. Magnetic microsphere are characterized for different parameters, such as particle size analysis including size distribution, surface topography, and texture etc. using scanning

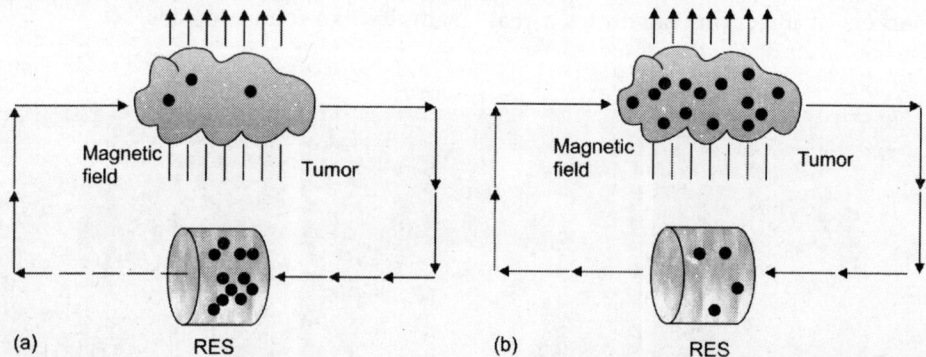

Fig. 22.7: Schematic showing enhanced magnetic tumor targeting hypothesis. (a) For a typical MNP, administered nanoparticles are quickly removed from the circulation by the RES, as indicated by the dashed line (–). Such a phenomenon results in limited tumor exposure of the administered dose and, thus, limited targeting success, (b) Conversely, long circulating MNPs, that avoid RES sequestration, would pass through tumor vasculature many times over, improving MNP exposure to the magnetic field and bettering the probability for enhanced tumor delivery of nanoparticle

electron microscopy (SEM), drug entrapment efficiency, percent magnetite content, and *in vitro* magnetic responsiveness and drug release. Targeting by magnetic microspheres, i.e. incorporation of magnetic particles into drug carriers (polymers) and using an externally applied magnetic field is one way to physically guided/direct this magnetic drug carriers to a desired site. The TiO_2 nanoparticles are consisted of core-shell microsphere, the outermost can act as photocatalyst to decompose organic dyes in wastewater (Fig. 22.8).

Polymeric Micelles

Polymeric micelles are emerging as a powerful, multifunctional nanotherapeutic platform for imaging and therapeutic applications (Fig. 22.9). The unique architecture of polymeric micelles allows for the incorporation of multiple functional components within a single micelle. By combining tumor targeting, stimulated release of therapeutics, and the delivery of imaging agents, multiple interventions against a tumor can be integrated into one platform. Such a 'theranostic' entity has been defined as a nanomedicine platform that can diagnose, deliver targeted treatment in a controlled manner, as well as monitor response to the cancer therapy.

Functionalization of polymeric micelles enables ligand-targeted systems to be developed for cell- specific targeting. A prerequisite for the development of such actively targeted micelles is an effective synthetic method for end-functionalization of the amphiphilic polymers and conjugation of ligands to the ends of the hydrophilic segments. A variety of PEG-PLA block copolymers having amino/saccharide end functional groups have been prepared. Such micelles with peptide/sugar receptors on cell surface for cell specific targeting of drugs. Stability of micelles is a critical factor for effective drug delivery *in vivo*. The micelles target the cells must dissociate to release the entrapped drug at the target site.

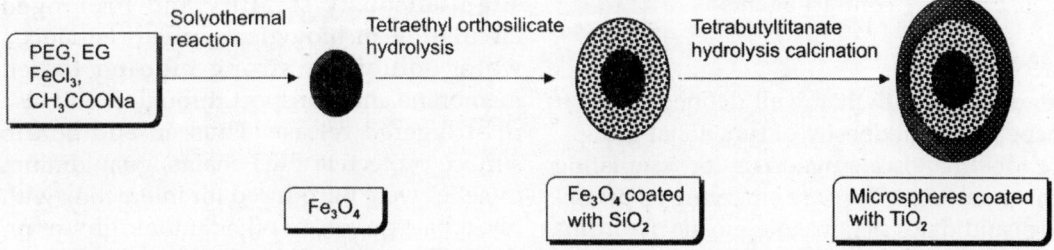

Fig. 22.8: Schematic representation of synthesis of Fe_3O_4 containing TiO_2 core-shell microspheres

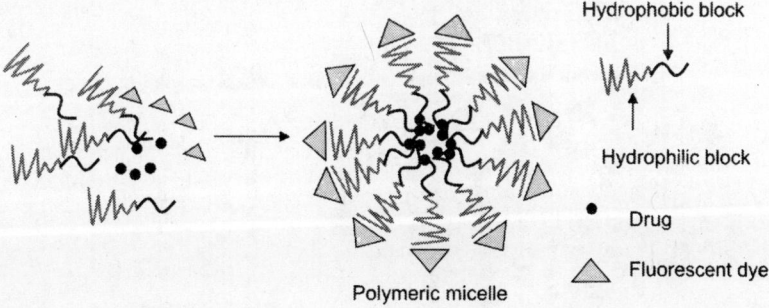

Fig. 22.9: Polymeric micelle with hydrophobic drug encapsulated in the core and fluorescent dye on the surface

Medical imaging modalities, such as magnetic resonance imaging (MRI), computed tomography (CT), single photon emission computed tomography (SPECT), positron emission tomography (PET), and ultrasonography play vital roles in diagnosis and monitoring of therapy. Currently, the field of nanomedicine is converging with medical imaging to further increase contrast specificity between healthy and tumor tissues.

Several micellar platforms have been established for use in MR imaging. Presently, gadoliniums (Gd)-based contrast agents (e.g. Magnevistt) are clinically used, where image contrast is increased by shortening the T_1 relaxation time of water protons. Incorporation of Gd complex on the surface of polymeric micelles can effectively increase the T_1 relaxivity and sensitivity of detection. Polymeric micelles have also been explored for cancer imaging using CT and SPECT. Iodine containing PLL-PEG polymer micelles have been developed having an average diameter of 100 nm and iodine content of 45% (w/w) for use as a CT contrast agents.

Dendrimers

Dendrimers, with their well-defined globular shape and high density of functional groups, are ideal nanoscale materials for templating sensor surfaces. They are emerging as promising candidates as novel diagnostic platforms with stable, dense, well organized, and close-packed arrays on substrate surfaces, and they are able to incorporate multiple branch ends, which can be available for consecutive conjugation reactions. Dendrimers have a larger capture area than linear analogues with consequently high capture probability. They can act as a versatile platform for capturing biomarkers with improved sensitivity and specificity. Dendrimers have been utilized in dip-pen nanolithography, DNA and protein arrays, nanocatalyst-base electrochemical immunosensors, biosensors based on dendrimer-encapsulated Pt nanoparticles and renewable affinity biosensing surfaces. Multifunctional dendrimers and hyperbranched polymers have been designed and synthesized to afford drug delivery systems that can be loaded with bioactive compounds either covalently or noncovalently (Fig. 22.10).

A model system of multifunctional dendrimeric nanocarrier was prepared using diaminobutane poly (propylene imine) with 64 amino endgroups. The designed and prepared carrier was intended to address simultaneously stability and prolonged circulation in biological milieu, enhanced water solubility, strong binding to cell membrane and transport through it and also pH-triggered release. Thus, in addition to surface protective PEG chains, guanidinium moieties were introduced for interacting with phosphate groups or other anionic groups on the cell surface, the binding of which is

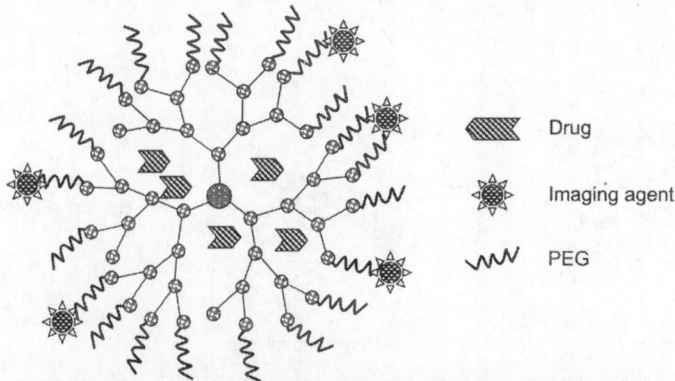

Drug

Imaging agent

PEG

Fig. 22.10: Multifunctional dendrimers designed for DDS loaded with bioactive compounds

amplified owing to multivalency effects. Simultaneously, the accumulation of guanidinium groups on the surface of the dendrimer can also facilitate its transport through cell membrane in a manner analogous to oligoarginine peptides. In addition, owing to the polyamine character of the nanocavities, it is possible to tune the release of the encapsulated ingredient by pH changes. Finally, toxicity decrease is anticipated due to reduction in the number of toxic amino groups.

Following initial studies, where simple functionalization was performed, investigations were undertaken, which, under proper selection of basic dendritic scaffolds and application of multifunctionalization strategy, led to drug delivery systems that are simultaneously biodegradable and nontoxic, show relative stability in the biological environment, show specificity to certain cells and, in certain cases, can penetrate cell membrane. In addition, owing to the molecular features of the interior of dendritic polymers, it is possible to encapsulate a diversity of compounds, the release of which can be controlled and/or tuned in the biological environment, for example by pH or ionic strength. Analyzing these properties further, it was possible through partial functionalization of the surface groups with PEG chains to enhance water solubility, decrease toxicity and increase stability of dendritic nanocarriers in the biological milieu. On the other hand, targeting ligands attached to the dendritic scaffold, for example folate moiety, or RGD peptides, and enhance carriers specificity. Furthermore, their binding to cell receptors is amplified by taking advantage of the multivalent effect, which enhances the effectiveness of binding of nanocarriers to the cells, as more than one of the cell receptors can bind to multiple complementary groups on the surface of a dendritic polymer. Transport through cell membranes has also been facilitated by attaching molecular transporting moieties on nanocarriers. Introduction of cell-penetrating peptides, such as arginine-rich derivatives enhances translocation ability of dendritic nanoparticles. In addition, other structural features fine-tune the transport of dendritic carriers and even determine their subcellular destination. A drug delivery system should have appropriate size and degree of functionalization, flexibility of the functional moiety and an appropriate balance between hydrophilic and hydrophobic moieties on the dendritic surface. These parameters should be taken into consideration in designing multifunctional dendritic systems in order to be internalized, together with their drug load, to specific subcellular sites. Multifunctional dendrimeric nanocarrier can facilitate its transport through cell membrane. In addition, owing to the polyamine character of the nanocavities, it is possible to design and programme the release of the encapsulated ingredient by pH changes. High density surface groups of dendrimers make this system ideally suited for a multitude of uses. The primary amino groups on the surface of the fifth generation dendrimer can be neutralized through partial acetylation, providing enhanced solubility to the dendrimer and preventing nonspecific interactions during targeted delivery. An imaging agent (like fluorescein isothiocyanate), targeting ligand (like folic acid) and drugs (like chemotherapeutic agents) can be conjugated to the remaining nonacetylated primary amino groups of a fifth generation dendrimer for targeted delivery to the cells.

Multifunctional Nanoparticles

The design of nanoparticles that combine several properties requires different steps, such as the depositing of metal layers onto a supporting nanoparticle core, modifying the biocompatible polymer used to stabilise the nanoparticle and the use of different linkers. Furthermore, these different properties have to be coordinated indeed to provide the desired functionalities. For example, the nanoparticles had specific targeting and cell-internalisation functions. Under normal conditions (i.e. when not bound specifically to the target), the specific target function is exposed, providing a long circulation life and specific delivery, whereas the cell-internalisation function remains hidden. In this manner, the cell-internalisation function does not interfere with the nanoparticle circulation. When specific binding is achieved by the nanoparticle to the target cell, the penetration function is exposed and activated, facilitating penetration of nanoparticles within the cell (Fig. 22.11).

Gold nanoparticles provide useful optical signals for specific molecular information. They can be used as optical probes for early detection of oral cancer and can be conjugated to antibodies or peptides through electrostatic interaction or coordinate bonding to probe for specific cellular biomarkers (EGFR) with high specificity and affinity. Nanoparticles with contrast agents are being developed for tumor detection purposes. Labeled and nonlabeled nanoparticles are already being tested as imaging agents in diagnostic procedures, such as nuclear magnetic resonance imaging. Such nanoparticles are paramagnetic, consisting of an inorganic core of iron oxide may be coated with polymers like dextran. There are two main groups of nanoparticles:

1. Superparamagnetic iron oxides with diameter size is greater than 50 nm
2. Ultra small supermagnetic iron oxides nanoparticles smaller than 50 nm

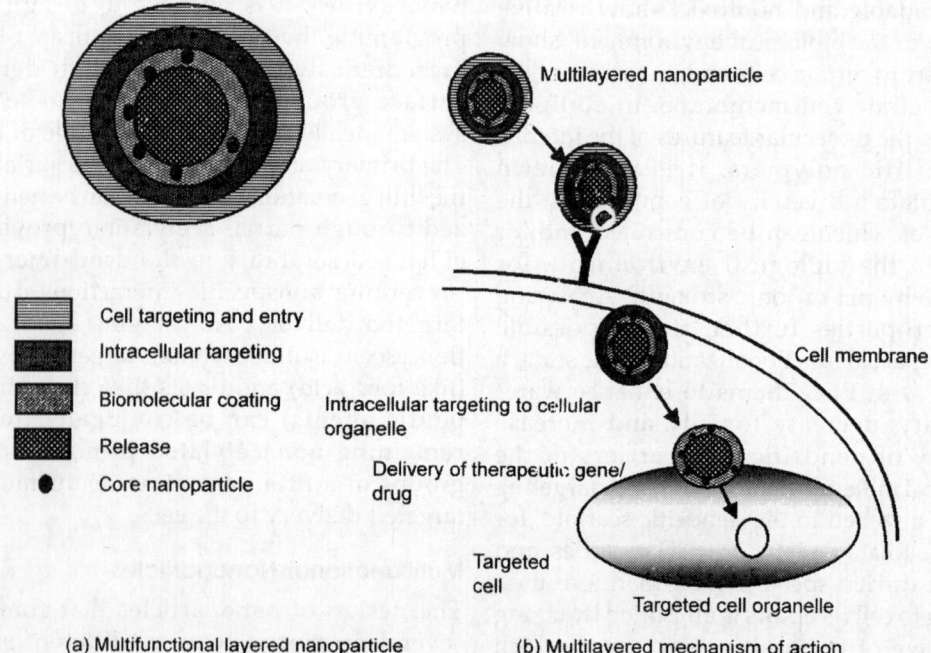

(a) Multifunctional layered nanoparticle

(b) Multilayered mechanism of action

Fig. 22.11: (a) Multilayered nanoparticle system containing targeting, biosensing and drug delivery molecules that release a layer at a time. This produces a nanoparticle system that results in molecular programming, an ordered series of events, for drug/gene delivery. Biosensing molecules allow the feedback-controlled release of drugs, or expression of therapeutic gene sequences, at the individual cell level, (b) general sequence of at least four steps for nanomedical systems (NMS) viz.; interacting with the targeted cell of interest: nanoparticles in the extracellular environment, attachment to the cell membrane and its proper entry, intracellular targeting to desired site of action, and delivery of drugs or production of therapeutic genes at the desired site

Nanocomposite is composed of a dielectric silica core and a thin Au shell. By varying the relative core and shell thickness of the Au nanoshells, their surface plasmon resonance (SPR) effect can be varied across a broad wavelength range that extends from the visible to the NIR region. Silica NPs can be grown in a range of sizes by the Stober method. Au has attracted extensive attention due to the low reactivity, high chemical stability, biocompatibility, and good affinity for binding to amine ($-NH_2$) or thiol ($-SH$) terminal groups of the outer Au layer. The therapeutic procedures use NPs, wherein a hyperthermia is applied to raise the temperature of a region of the body affected by malignancy or other growths, with the advantage that it allows heating to be restricted to the tumor area. Thermal therapeutics are relatively simple to perform and have the potential of treating tumors embedded in vital regions where surgical resection is not feasible. Furthermore, it has been demonstrated that macromolecules and small particles (size range up to 400 nm) could penetrate through blood vessels into tumor due to enhanced permeability and could remain in the tumor for an extended period of time due to poor lymphatic drainage (enhanced permeability, retention effect, and EPR effect).

Magnetic iron oxide nanoparticles (MNPs) have been investigated in both brain tumor diagnostics (primarily in magnetic resonance imaging or MRI) and drug delivery. These potential 'theranostics' possess a high surface area-to-volume ratio, which provides for a high loading capacity of functional cargoes that can include drugs, molecular targeting ligands (e.g. tumor-specific antibodies, peptides, small molecules, etc.), cell internalization agents, and/or pharmacokinetic stabilizers.

Indeed, the combination of antitumor drug(s) and functionalities that enhance drug delivery onto a single platform could substantially improve therapeutic indices, even for macromolecular agents. In addition to targeting relying on the enhanced permeability and retention (EPR) effect and with tumor specific molecular ligands, the magnetic responsiveness of MNPs to an external magnetic field can be used for 'magnetic targeting' of nanoparticles to tumors (Fig. 22.12). Magnetic targeting is especially attractive and affective for brain tumors, as it is noninvasive and does not interfere with normal brain functions.

Hyperthermia

Hyperthermia based cancer therapy relies on the localized heating of tumors above 43°C for about 30 min. MNPs can generate heat under alternating magnetic fields due to energy losses in traversing through magnetic

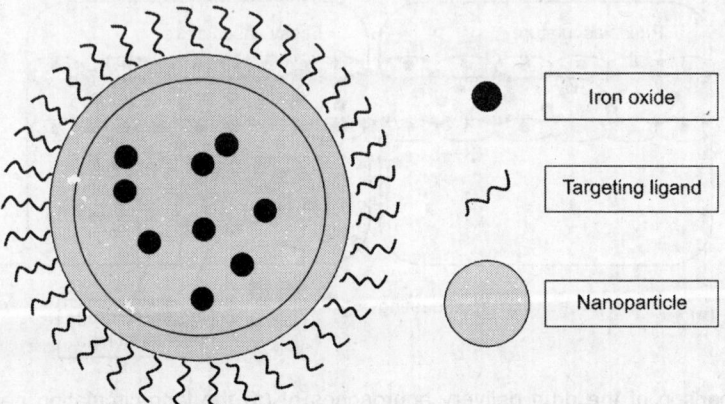

Fig. 22.12: Targeting ligand coated magnetic nanoparticle

hysteresis loop. Generation of different degrees of heat depends on the magnetization properties of specific MNP formulations and magnetic field parameters. Selectivity to tumors was considerably improved through the use of silane coatings and through functionalization approaches. For example, MNPs conjugated with antibodies to cancer-specific antigens/receptors could improve selectivity of MNP uptake by tumors during hyperthermia therapy. Magnetic hyperthermia using magnetic cationic liposomes has been used in a combination approach with TNF-α gene therapy and stress-inducible Gadd 153 promoter, resulting in a dramatic arrest in tumor growth (Fig. 22.13).

Temperature Responsive Synthetic Vectors for Gene Delivery

The gene delivery system should possess a balance between complex formation capa-bilities with gene, its stabilization before the uptake by the cells, however it should disso-ciate following entry inside the cell. The continuous efforts of scientists proposed an intelligent carrier system to control complex formation-dissociation by various stimuli. The stimuli may be light, temperature, magnetic field and pH. These stimuli control the complex formation-dissociation and optimize the complex status for each intracellular process.

The benefits for using these intelligent polymeric gene delivery systems, such as higher transfection efficiency and selective gene expression (by utilizing site, timing and duration period) that might be achieved at a very successful rate. In this context, the thermoresponsive cationic polymeric gene carriers were prepared (e.g. copolymerization of DMAEMA and N-isopropylacrylamide) and evaluated for transfection efficiency in ovarian cancer cells. The finding revealed that

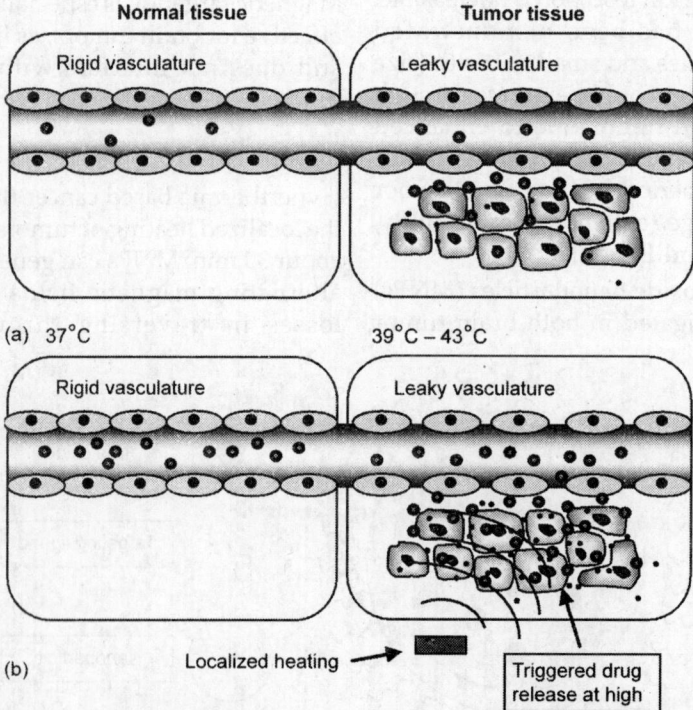

Fig. 22.13: Comparison of the drug delivery approaches of (a) the long-circulating nanoparticles, and (b) the thermosensitive nanoparticles

high molecular weight copolymers were efficient at compacting DNA into particles and transfected ovarian cancer cells efficiently. Further, a variety of temperature-responsive polymeric vector system were developed and evaluated which showed lower critical solution temperature (LCST) at 32°C, such as hydrogels and polymeric micelles as drug carriers (Fig. 22.14).

Magnetic Resonance Imaging (MRI)

MNP-enhanced MRI is based on the superior superparamagnetic qualities of iron oxide MNPs. Several dextran-coated MNP formulations have been approved for clinical use as MRI contrast agents, including ferumoxides, ferumoxtran and ferucarbotran. Experimental studies show that MNP-enhanced MRI is distinctly superior to other noninvasive methods of identifying lymph node metastases from solid tumors and histologically

positive lymph nodes outside of the usual scope of resection. MNP application in delineating primary tumors and detecting metastases, in imaging angiogenesis and mapping vascular supply to primary tumors has a realistic translational potential. Macrophage-specific MNP labeling protocols are used to image inflammatory pathologies, including atherosclerosis, multiple sclerosis and rheumatoid arthritis. Long-term MRI-guided *in vivo* cell tracking of CNS regeneration became possible with the use of grafted MNP-labeled stem cells and neuroprotective glia (Schwann cells and olfactory ensheathing cells). FITC-conjugated MNPs have been used by surgeons to delineate gliomas both pre-operatively, based on their MRI modality, and intraoperatively, based on fluorescent tag. This is particularly valuable since certain tumors, such as gliomas, can shift the position during surgery.

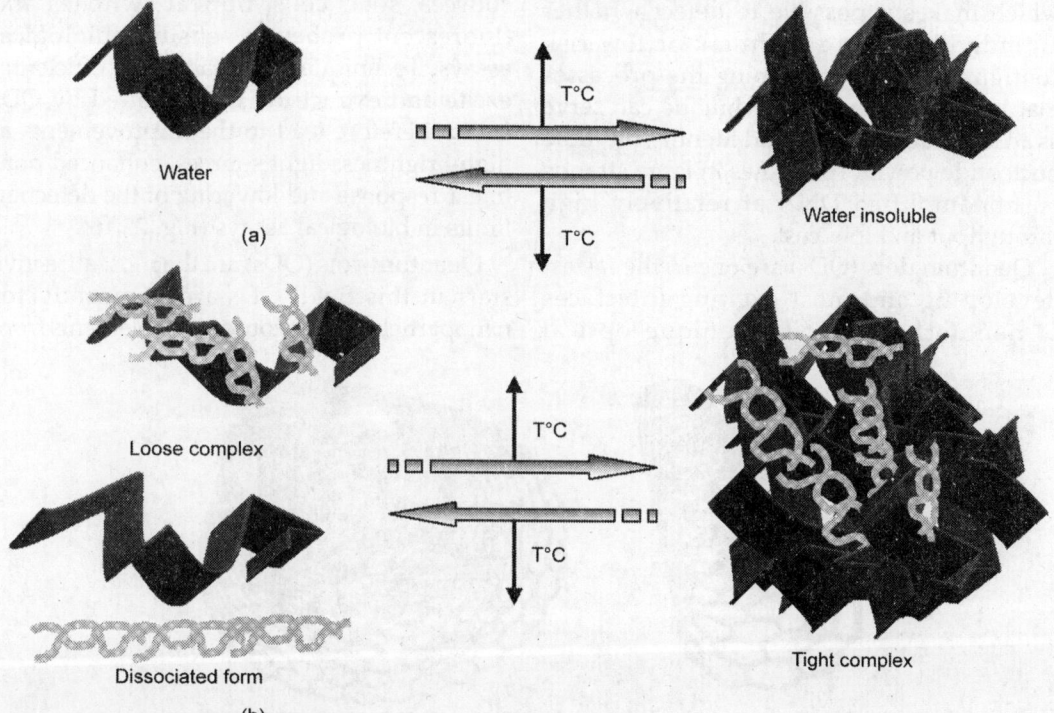

Fig. 22.14: Schematic illustration is showing the concept of temperature-responsive DNA or RNA carriers. (a) temperature-responsive polymer (b) tightly complex formed between the carrier polymer and the DNA is above the transition temperature (T°C)

Other Nanocarriers

Carbon nanocomposites have attracted great attention due to their intrinsic electronic and magnetic properties, allowing their use for improved magnetic tapes, sensors, nanoprobes and electromagnetic shielding coatings. Carbon nanotubes occur in two general forms: SWCNTs and multiwalled carbon nanotubes MWCNTs (Fig. 22.15). SWCNTs can generally be visualized as a single sheet of graphene that has been rolled into a hollow tubular shape. The orientation of the graphene sheet on rolling will dictate the resulting structure of the CNT. SWCNTs can have diameters as small as 0.4 nm and normally no larger than 2 nm. MWCNTs can be viewed as several concentric SWCNTs with outside diameters that range between 5 nm and 100 nm. The interlayer spacing of MWCNTs is approximately 0.34 nm. Carbon nanotubes scan down DNA and look for single nucleotide polymorphism, which makes it possible to detect whether an individual has a high-risk or low-risk configuration for developing the processes that lead to cancer. This technique can serve as an alternative to PCR and identify multiple nucleotide polymorphic sites in large strands on nonamplified DNA at relatively high throughput and low cost.

Quantum dots (QDs) are one of the fastest developing and most exciting interfaces of nanotechnology. The unique optical properties of QDs make them appealing as *in vivo* and *in vitro* fluorophores in a variety of biological investigations, in which traditional fluorescent labels based on organic molecules fall short of providing long-term stability and simultaneous detection of multiple signals. The ability to make QDs water soluble and target them to specific biomolecules has led to promising applications in cellular labeling, deep-tissue imaging, assay labeling and as efficient fluorescence resonance energy transfer donors. QDs derive their unique optical properties, such as a broad absorption spectrum, narrow, size-tunable emission spectrum, high photostability, quantum efficiency and strong nonlinear response from quantum confinement effects. These attributes, coupled with the ability to functionalize QDs with organic molecules and render them compatible with other material systems, has made them important candidates for light sources, solar cells, optical switches and fluorescent probes in sensitive biological assays. Techniques that can more efficiently excite and extract the light emitted by QDs could therefore lead to the improvements in high-brightness light sources, enhanced nonlinear response and lowering of the detection limits in biological assays (Fig. 22.16).

Quantum dots (QDs) are the most attractive stars in this field. QDs are semiconductor nanoparticles (NPs) comprising elements from

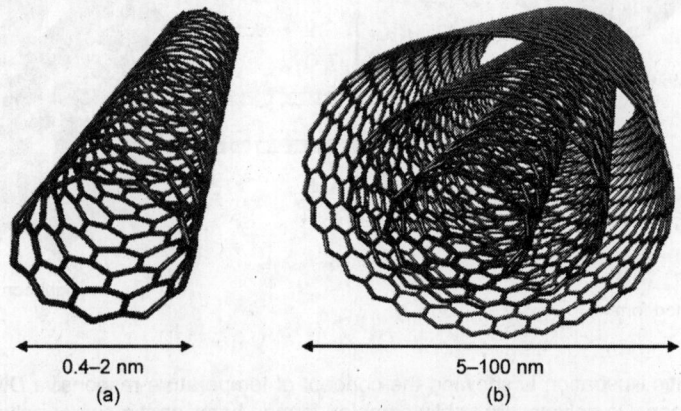

| 0.4–2 nm | 5–100 nm |
| (a) | (b) |

Fig. 22.15: Two CN variants—(a) SWCNT and (b) MWCNT

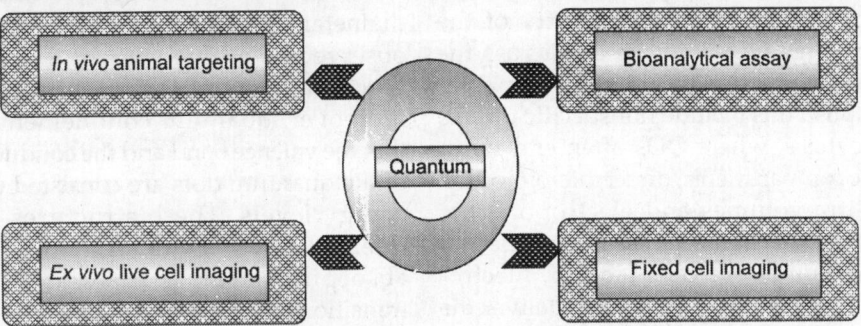

Fig. 22.16: Application of quantum dots

the periodic groups II–VI or III–V. They being the nanoscale crystals of a semiconductor material, such as cadmium selenide, can be used to measure levels of cancer markers, such as breast cancer marker Her-2, actin, micro fibril proteins and nuclear antigens. Up to now, lot of researchers have developed florescent nanoprobes and evaluated them on animal model.

QD assay labeling uses QDs for *in vitro* assay detection of DNA, proteins and other biomolecules. DNA-coated QDs have been shown as sensitive and specific DNA labels as probes for human metaphase chromosomes, and in single-nucleotide polymorphism and multi-allele DNA detection. Conversely, DNA linked to QD surfaces has been used to code and sort the nanocrystals. These results demonstrate that DNA-con-

jugated QDs specifically bind their complements both in fixed cells and *in vitro*. QDs may also be useful for tracking cancer cells *in vivo* during metastasis. A multifunctional QD probe has been developed linked with tumor-targeting antibodies. *In vivo* studies in mice expressing human cancer showed that these QD probes accumulated at the tumor sites (Fig. 22.17). Cellular labeling is the field, where use of QD has made the remarkable progress and attracted the greatest interest. A clear differentiation can be made between labeling of live or 'fixed' cells (dead, with chemically cross-linked components to maintain cellular architecture). Fixed cells can be treated 'harshly' to facilitate entry of the QD reagent by chemically creating pores. For labeling live cells, the process has to be handled judiciously to maintain cellular

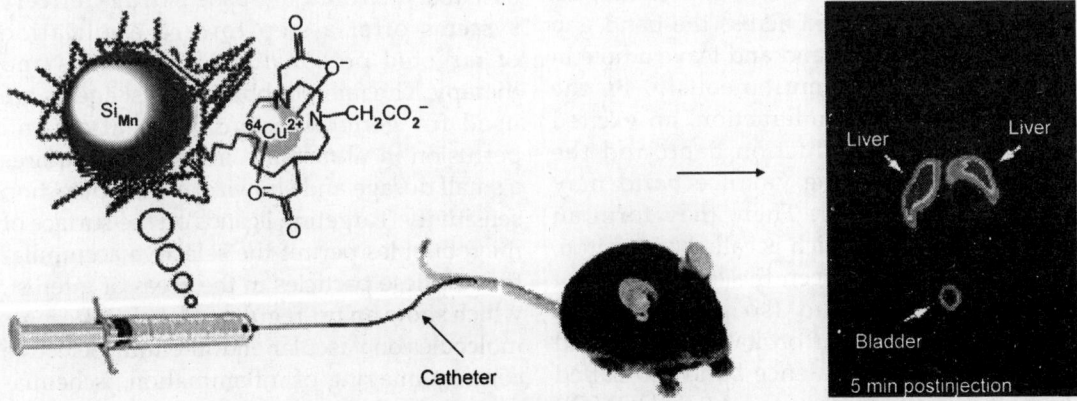

Fig. 22.17: Imaging and biodistribution of silicon quantum dots in mice

viability. The major hurdle is entry of the relatively large QDs into the cell across the cellular membranes' lipid bilayer. Strategies to accomplish this include nonspecific uptake by endocytosis, where QDs often end up in endocytic compartments, direct microinjection of nanolitre volumes and electroporation. Direct microinjection is a tedious work and limits the number of cells labeled. Electroporation uses charge to physically deliver the QDs through the membrane and mediated/targeted uptake. Mediated uptake uses reagents such as lipofectamine 2000, with encapsulated QDs within lipid vesicles to facilitate entry into the cell. Targeted uptake exploits the cells' propensity to recognize and internalize QDs labeled with specific peptides (for example, HIV-derived TAT peptide) and even deliver them to specific cellular compartments, such as the nucleus. Nano-Bio-Chip sensor technique is a promising new diagnostic tool for early detection of oral cancer.

Quantum mechanics can be understood using the emission spectrum of QDs and very tiny clusters of atoms of a semiconductor (ours are indium phosphide) only nanometers in radius. Because of their tiny sizes and simple structures, these systems have been compared to artificial atoms. QDs absorb and emit light at wavelengths determined by their radius, allowing them to be manufactured to have interesting optical and electronic properties. In semiconductor materials, an electron can be excited across the band gap into the conduction band and leave a hole in the valence band simultaneously. By the attractive Coulomb interaction, an excited electron in the conduction band and the resulting hole in the valance band may approach each other. Then, they form an electron-hole pair which is called an exciton. The energy gap between the lowest level of the conduction band (so called lowest unoccupied molecular orbital (LUMO)) and the highest of the valence band (so called highest occupied molecular orbital (HOMO)) increases with a decrease in the quantum dot

diameter. Experimentally, this effect can be observed as a blue shift in the absorption spectrum with decreasing quantum dot size. Moreover, quantum confinement suggests that the valence band and the conduction band of the quantum dots are consisted of discrete energy levels. These structures are often referred to as 'artificial atoms'. The first absorption peak is associated with the transition energy between the LUMO and the HOMO band of quantum dots. A broadening of the absorption spectrum at the blue side as well as at the red side of the first absorption peak is due to size dispersion of quantum dots. Based on these absorption spectra, it is clear that the absorption spectrum shifts to shorter wavelengths as the mean size of the quantum dots decreases. The blue shift proves that the LUMO-HOMO energy gap for small quantum dots is wider than large quantum dots. The absorption spectrum gives information about the required efficient wavelengths to excite the quantum dots. Moreover, the absorption spectrum can also be used to determine the quantum efficiency of quantum dots. To quantify the absorption and emission behavior spectrometers are used, that measure the amount of light absorbed by the sample. The fraction of light absorbed or emitted is plotted against wavelength to give absorption/emission spectrum.

Microbubble targeting and ultrasound-assisted microbubble-based drug-delivery systems offer a step toward application of targeted personalized diagnostics and therapy. The microbubble contrast agents are used for general tissue delineation and perfusion in ultrasound imaging. It requires a small dosage and shows excellent detection sensitivity. Targeting ligands on the surface of microbubbles permit the selective accumulation of these particles in the areas of interest, which show an up-regulated level of receptor molecules on vascular endothelium. Selective contrast imaging of inflammation, ischemia-reperfusion injury, angiogenesis, and thrombosis has been achieved in animal models.

Table 22.1: List of various nanocarriers used as multifunctional ligand

	Size	Structural characteristic	Composition	Drug entrapment
	2–10 nm	Macromolecular tree-like structure	Hyperbranched polymer chain	Covalent conjugation requiring functional group
	100–200 nm	Spherical bilayer structure	Phospholipid cholesterol membrane lipids	Covalent conjugation requiring functional group
	<10 nm	Macromolecular structure	Water soluble	Noncovalent encapsulation/hydrophobic interaction
	10–100 nm	Spherical supramolecular core shell structure	Amphiphilic diblock and triblock copolymers	Noncovalent encapsulation/hydrophobic interaction

Ultrasound-assisted drug delivery and activation, performed by combining microbubble agent containing drug substances or coadministered pharmaceutical agents (including plasmid DNA for transfection), has been implicated in multiple model systems *in vitro* and *in vivo*. Ultrasound and microbubbles-based targeted acceleration of the thrombolytic enzyme action already have reached clinical trials.

List of various nanocarriers used as multifunctional legands is shown in Table 22.1.

SUGGESTED READINGS

1. Bertorelle F (2006), *Langmuir.*, 22, 5385–91.
2. Chertok B, Moffat BA, David AE, Yu F, Bergemann C, Ross BD, Yanga VC (2008), *Biomater.*, 29, 487–96.
3. Chomoucka J, Drbohlavova J, Huska D, Adam V, Kizek R, Hubalek J (2010), *Pharmacol Res.*, 62, 144–9.
4. Chou SW, Shau YH, Wu PC, Yang YS, Shieh DB, Chen CC (2010), *J. Am. Chem. Soc.*, 132, 13270–8.
5. Corchero JL, Villaverde A (2009), *Trends Biotechnol.*, 27, 468–76.
6. Eustis S and el-Sayed MA (2006), *Chem. Soc. Rev.*, 35, 209–17.
7. Gao J, Liang G, Cheung JS, Pan Y, Kuang Y, Zhao F, Zhang B, Zhang X, Wu EX, Xu B (2008), *J Am Chem Soc.*, 130, 11828–33.
8. Gazeau F, Le´vy M, Wilhelm C (2008), *Nanomed.*, 3, 831–44.
9. HG Suh, JS Huh, YM Haam S (2008), *Adv Funct Mater.*, 18, 258–64.
10. Hao R, Xing RJ Xu ZC, Hou Y, Gao S, Sun SH (2010), *Adv Mater.*, 22, 2729–42.
11. Koppolu B, Rahimi M, Nattama S, Wadajkar A, Nguyen KT (2010), *Nanomed NBM.*, 6, 355–61.
12. Liu R, Fraylich M, Saunders BR (2009), *Colloid Polym Sci.*, 287, 627–43.
13. McCarthy JR (2007), *Nanomed.*, 2, 153–67.
14. Medeiros SF, Santos AM, Fessi H, Elaissari A, (2011), *Int J Pharm.*, 403, 139–61.
15. Montet X (2006), *Neoplasia.*, 8, 3214–22.
16. Pisanic TR (2007), *Biomater.*, 28, 2572–81.
17. Purushotham S, Ramanujan RV (2010), *Acta Biomater.*, 6, 502–10.
18. Sosnovik DE and Weissleder R (2007), *Curr. Opin. Biotechnol.*, 18, 4–10.
19. Wilhelm C and Gazeau F (2008), *Biomater.*, 29, 3161–74.

23

■ Floating Drug Delivery System(s)

INTRODUCTION

Floating systems can float on the gastric contents owing to their low bulk density. Usually, floating formulations are prepared from hydrophilic matrices that either have a density lower than one or their density drops below one after immersion in the gastric fluids owing to swelling. Cellulose ether polymers are often used as the floating matrices, and low-density fatty acids can be incorporated as well to decrease hydrating rate and increase buoyancy. The use of various film-coating techniques and incorporation of a floating chamber that is filled with harmless gas or a liquid that gasifies at body temperature are some sophisticated techniques used to develop floating drug delivery system (FDDS). These forms are often called 'hydrodynamically balanced systems' (HBS), as they can maintain low density and keep floating even after hydration. When a floating dosage form is administered with food, the device remains buoyant on the surface of the gastric contents in the upper part of the stomach and moves down toward the pyloric sphincter when the meal empties. The reported gastric retention time (GRT) of such floating devices varies from 4 to 10 hours. The active drug is progressively released from the formulation matrix and gets introduced into the proximal intestine, where it can be absorbed. Various

techniques have been proposed as floating devices, and their performances have been mostly assessed by *in vitro* methods to evaluate their floating and drug release properties. Several approaches are currently utilized in the prolongation of the GRT, including FDDS, swelling and expanding systems, polymeric bioadhesive systems, modified-shape systems, high-density systems, and other delayed gastric emptying devices. The problem arises when the stomach is completely emptied of gastric fluid. In such situation, there is nothing to float on. Floating systems can be based on the following:

1. *Effervescent systems:* Gas-generating materials, such as sodium bicarbonates or other carbonate salts are incorporated. These materials react with gastric acid and produce carbon dioxide, which gets entrapped in the colloidal matrix and causing it to float.

2. *Low-density systems:* Systems having density lower than that of the gastric fluid, so they are buoyant.

3. *Bioadhesive or mucoadhesive systems:* These systems permit a given drug delivery system (DDS) to be incorporated with bio/mucoadhesive agents, enabling the device to adhere to the stomach (or other GI) walls, thus resisting gastric emptying. However, the mucus on the walls of the

stomach is in a state of constant renewal, resulting in unpredictable adherence.

4. *High-density systems:* Sedimentation has been employed as a retention mechanism for pellets that are small enough to be retained in the rugae or folds of the stomach near the pyloric region, which constitutes the part of the organ with the lowest position in an upright posture. Dense pellets (approximately 3 g/cm³) trapped in rugae also tend to withstand the peristaltic movements of the stomach wall. With pellets, the GI transit time can be extended from an average of 5.8–25 hours, depending more on density than on diameter of the pellets, although many conflicting reports stating otherwise also abound in literature.

LOW DENSITY SYSTEM OR FLOATING DRUG DELIVERY SYSTEM (FDDS)

This approach exploits the floating property of substances with density lower than the fluid medium. Floating drug delivery systems either float due to their low density than stomach contents or due to the gaseous phase formed inside the system after they come in contact with the gastric environment. Various floating dosage forms are reported in the literature (Fig. 23.1).

Floating Tablets

A floating dosage unit is useful for drugs acting locally in the proximal gastrointestinal tract (GIT). The systems are also useful for drugs that are poorly soluble or unstable in

intestinal fluids. The floating properties of these systems help to retain them in the stomach for a long time. Various attempts have been made to develop floating systems. After the release of a drug, the remnants of the system are emptied from the stomach. A floating tablet can be said to keep its hydro-dynamically balanced system (HBS). This system is based on the principle that an object of less specific gravity than the gastric fluid will float on the gastric fluid in the stomach and thus it is kept in the stomach for a long period. Consequently, gastrointestinal resi-dence time increases. This system is applicable to drugs that suffer degradation in the intestine, have a higher pH than the stomach, and are poorly absorbed from the lower part of the small intestine. Diazepam, captopril, and morphine are candidate drugs for this type of system. These drugs are mixed with gel-forming hydrocolloids, such as HPMC and fillers of low density to form a tablet. Therefore, the hydrocolloids also retain drug molecules with the tablet matrix by decreasing the diffusion rate of drug molecules from the gel matrix resulting into slow release profile.

Floating Capsules

A billeted floating capsule is consisted of two layers in a capsule—a release layer and a floating layer. The floating layer may be consis-ted of Methocel K4M, lactose, Aerosil 200, magnesium stearate, etc. The release layer may be consisted of various combinations of Methocel K4M, K100, drug, HPMC, and Pharmacoat 606 and 603. A large quantity of high-viscosity polymer is also incorporated to form a strong viscous layer. This helps in maintaining the integrity of the floating layer for a longer time. The drug-release layer consisted of a gelling agent. This avoids disintegration and prevents delivery of large particles containing drug into the intestine, thus reducing side effects. The drug release from capsules consists of a biphasic rapid- and sustained-release formulation. A lipophilic

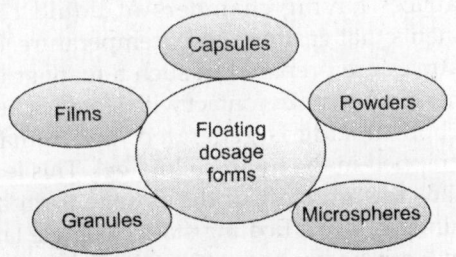

Fig. 23.1: Various floating dosage forms

drug, such as propranolol may be dissolved in oleic acid. Initial rapid release of the drug-oleic acid solution is followed by subsequent sustained release of drug components from a solid erodible matrix based on a Gelucire of low hydrophilic lipophilic balance (HLB) with melting point above 37°C.

CLASSIFICATION OF FDDS: CLASSIFICATION OF SINGLE UNIT FDDS

Depending upon the working principle of single unit FDDS, they are classified into two main categories—noneffervescent and effervescent FDDS.

Noneffervescent FDDS

The FDDS belonging to this class are usually prepared using gel-forming or highly swellable cellulose type hydrocolloids, polysaccharides or matrix forming polymers like polyacrylate, polycarbonate, polystyrene and polymetha-crylate. In one approach, gel-forming hydro-colloid swells, when it comes in contact with gastric fluid after oral administration and maintains a relative integrity of shape and bulk density less than unity within gastric environment. The air thus trapped by the swollen polymer imparts buoyancy to the dosage form. Nevertheless, the gel structure acts as a reservoir for sustained drug release. When these dosage forms come in contact with an aqueous medium, the hydrocolloids imbibe water and hydrate thereby forming a gel at the surface. The resultant gel layer subse-quently controls the diffusion of drug out and passage of solvent into the dosage form. With the passage of time, the exterior surface of the dosage form goes into solution and immediate adjacent hydrocolloid layer becomes hydrated and maintains the gel structure. The drug in dosage form dissolves in and diffuses out with the diffusing solvent forming a 'receding boundary' within the gel structure. Figure 23.2 illustrates the working principle of a hydro-dynamically balanced system (HBS).

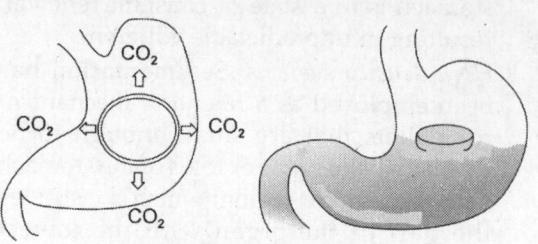

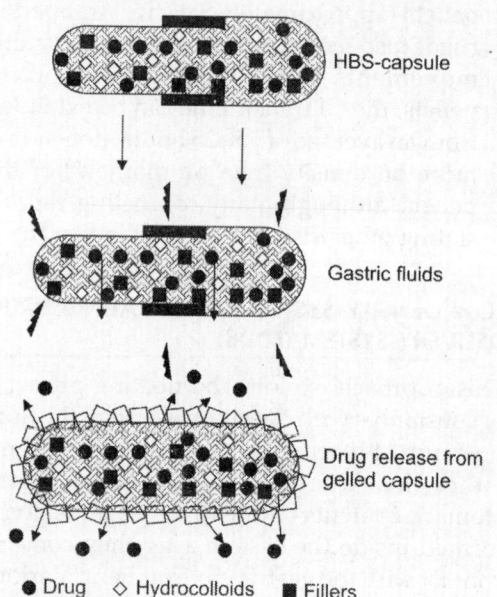

Fig. 23.2: Functioning of hydrodynamically balanced system (HBS)

Effervescent FDDS (Gas Generating Systems)

These FDDS employ matrices from swelling polymers like Methocel® or chitosan and effervescent components, such as sodium bicarbonate and tartaric or citric acid or matrices having chambers of liquid com-ponents that gasify at body temperature. The matrices are prepared in such a manner that when they come in contact with stomach fluid, carbon dioxide is generated, and remains entrapped in the hydrocolloid gel. This leads to an upward drift of the dosage form and maintains it in a floating state. A single layer tablet can be produced by intimately mixing the carbon dioxide generating component in tablet matrix. A bilayer tablet may be compressed in which gas liberating component is present in hydrocolloid layer whilst the drug is compressed in other layer for sustained release. The concept has been judiciously utilized to develop floating capsule consisting of a mixture of sodium alginate and sodium bicarbonate. Recently, a multiple unit-floating pill has been developed based on the concept of effervescence. In this system carbon dioxide gas is generated from reaction of sodium bicarbonate and tartaric acid. The system consisted of sustained release pill surrounded by an effervescent layer. This system is further coated with swellable polymers like polyvinyl acetate and purified shellac. Moreover, the effervescent layer is divided into two sublayers, which prevent direct contact between tartaric acid and sodium bicarbonate.

CLASSIFICATION OF MULTIPLE UNIT FDDS

In spite of extensive research and development in the area of HBS and other floating dosage forms, these systems suffer from an important drawback of high variability of gastrointestinal transit time, when orally administered, because of their all-or-no gastric emptying nature. In order to overcome the above problem, multiple unit floating systems have been developed, which reduce the inter-subject variability in absorption and also reduce the probability of dose-dumping. Reports are abound on the development of both noneffervescent and effervescent multiple unit systems. Much research has been focused and the scientists are still exploring the field of hollow microspheres, capable of floating on the gastric fluid with improved gastric retention properties.

Multiple unit FDDS can be classified as

1. Noneffervescent systems
2. Effervescent systems (gas-generating systems)
3. Hollow microspheres (microballoon)

1. *Noneffervescent systems:* Very few reports are available in the literature on non-effervescent multiple unit systems, as compared to the effervescent systems. However, few attempts have been made exploring the possibility of developing system containing indomethacin, using chitosan as the polymeric excipient. A multiple unit HBS containing indomethacin as a model drug prepared by extrusion process is reported. A mixture of drug, chitosan and acetic acid is extruded through a needle, and the extrudate is cut and dried.

Chitosan hydrates and floats in the acidic media. Furthermore, the required drug release could be obtained by modifying the drug-polymer ratio.

2. *Effervescent systems (gas-generating systems):* There are reports on sustained release floating granules containing tetracycline hydrochloride. The granules are a mixture of drug granulates of two stages A and B, of which A contains 60 parts of HPMC and 40 parts of polyacrylic acid and B contains 70 parts of sodium bicarbonate and 30 parts of tartaric acid. 60 parts by weight of granules of stage A and 30 parts by weight of granules of stage B are mixed along with a lubricant and filled into a capsule. In dissolution media, the capsule shell dissolves and liberates the granules, which showed a floating time of more than 8 hours and sustained drug release characteristics of 80% of incorporated drug released in about 6.5 hours. Floating minicapsules of pepstatin having a diameter of 0.1–0.2 mm have been reported. These minicapsules contain a central core and a coating. The central core consists of a granule composed of sodium bicarbonate, lactose and a binder, which is coated with HPMC. Pepstatin is coated on the top of the HPMC layer. The system floats because of the CO_2 release in gastric fluid and the pepstatin resides in the stomach for prolonged period. Alginates have received

intense attention in the development of multiple unit systems. Alginates are non-toxic, biodegradable linear copolymers composed of L-glucuronic and L-mannuronic acid residues. A multiple unit system was prepared comprised of calcium alginate core and calcium alginate/PVA membrane, both separated by an air compartment. In the presence of water, the PVA leaches out and increases the membrane permeability, maintaining the integrity of the air compartment. Increase in molecular weight and concentration of PVA, resulted in improved floating properties of the system.

Freeze-drying technique is also reported for the preparation of floating calcium alginate beads. Sodium alginate solution is added dropwise into the aqueous solution of calcium chloride, causing the instant gelation of the droplet surface, due to the formation of calcium alginate. The obtained beads are freeze-dried resulting in a porous structure, which aid in floating. The authors studied the behavior of radio-labeled floating beads and compared with non-floating beads in human volunteers using gamma scintigraphy. Prolonged gastric residence time of more than 5.5 hours was recorded for capsule with a floating bead. The nonfloating beads had a shorter residence time with a mean onset emptying time of 1 hour.

A new multiple unit of floating dosage system has been developed having a pill in the core, composed of effervescent layers and coated with swellable membrane layers. The inner layer of effervescent agents based on sodium bicarbonate and tartaric acid was divided into two sublayers to avoid direct contact between these two agents. These sublayers were coated using swellable polymer membrane polyvinyl acetate and purified shellac. When it is immersed in the buffer at 37°C, it settled down and the solution permeated into the effervescent layer through the outer swellable membrane. The CO_2 gas was generated due to neutralization reaction between the sodium bicarbonate and tartaric acid (effervescent agents), producing swollen pills (like balloons) with a density less than 1.0 g/ml.

3. *Hollow microspheres (microballoon):* Hollow microspheres are considered as one of the most promising multiple unit buoyant systems, as they possess the unique advantages of multiple unit systems as well as better floating properties, because of central hollow space in the microsphere (Fig. 23.3). The general techniques involved in their preparation include simple solvent evaporation and solvent diffusion and evaporation. The drug release and better floating properties mainly depend on the type of polymer, plasticizer and the solvents employed for the preparation. Polymers such as polycarbonate, Eudragit® S and cellulose acetate were used in the preparation of hollow microspheres, and the drug release can be modulated by optimizing the polymer quantity and the polymer-plasticizer ratio. Sustained release floating microspheres using polycarbonate have been prepared, employing solvent evaporation technique. Aspirin, griseofulvin and p-nitroaniline were used as model drugs. A dispersed phase containing polycarbo-

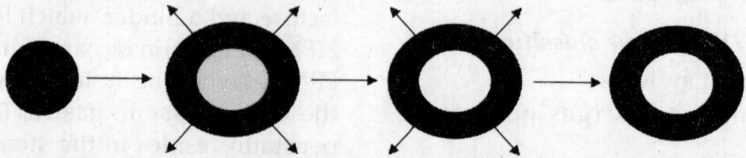

Fig. 23.3: Formulation of floating hollow microsphere or microballoon

nate solution in dichloromethane, and micronized drug, was added to the dispersion medium containing sodium chloride, polyvinyl alcohol and methanol. The dispersion was stirred for 3–4 hours to assure the complete solvent evaporation, and the microspheres obtained were filtered, washed with cold water and dried. The spherical and hollow nature of the microspheres was confirmed by scanning electron microscopic studies. The microspheres showed a drug payload of more than 50%, and the amount of drug incorporated is found to influence the particle size distribution and drug release. The larger proportion of bigger particles was seen at high drug loading, which can be attributed to the increased viscosity of the dispersed phase.

RAFT FORMING SYSTEMS

Raft forming systems have received much attention for the delivery of antacids and drug delivery for gastrointestinal infections and disorders. The basic mechanism involved in the raft formation includes the formation of viscous cohesive gel upon contact with gastric fluids, wherein each portion of the liquid swells forming a continuous layer called a raft. The raft floats because of the buoyancy created due to the formation of CO_2 and acts as a barrier to prevent the reflux of gastric contents like HCl and enzymes into the oesophagus. Usually, the system contains a gel forming agent and alkaline bicarbonates or carbonates responsible for the formation of carbon dioxide to make the system less dense and float on the gastric fluids.

INGREDIENTS USED IN PREPARATION OF FDDS

1. *Polymers:* The following polymers are used in the preparation of FDDS drugs:
   HPMC K4 M, calcium alginate, Eudragit S100, Eudragit RL, propylene foam, Eudragit RS, ethyl cellulose, polymethyl methacrylate, methocel K4M, polyethylene oxide, β cyclodextrin, HPMC 4000, HPMC 100, CMC, polyethylene glycol, polycarbonate, PVA, polycarbonate, sodium alginate, HPC-L, CP 934P, HPC, Eudragit S, HPMC, Metolose SM 100, PVP, HPC-H, HPC-M, HPMC K15, Polyox, HPMC K4, acrylic polymer, E4 M and carbopol.

2. *Inert fatty materials (5–75%):* Edible, inert fatty material of specific gravity less than one can be used to decrease the hydrophilic property of formulation and hence increase buoyancy, e.g. beeswax, fatty acids, long chain fatty alcohols, Gelucires 39/01 and 43/01.

3. *Effervescent agents:* Sodium bicarbonate, citric acid, tartaric acid, Di-sodium glycine carbonate (Di-SGC), citroglycine (CG).

4. *Release rate accelerants (5–60%):* For example, lactose, mannitol.

5. *Release rate retardants (5–60%):* For example, dicalcium phosphate, talc, magnesium stearate.

6. *Buoyancy increasing agents (up to 80%):* For example, ethyl cellulose.

7. *Low-density material:* Polypropylene foam powder (Accurel MP 1000).

LIST OF DRUGS EXPLORED FOR VARIOUS FLOATING DOSAGE FORMS

Table 23.1 shows various drugs used in floating dosage forms.

Microspheres tablets/pills: Chlorpheniramine maleate, aspirin, griseofulvin, acetaminophen, p-nitroaniline, acetylsalicylic acid, ibuprofen, amoxycillin trihydrate, terfenadine, ampicillin, tranilast, atenolol, theophylline, captopril, isosorbide di-nitrate, sotalol, isosorbide mononitrate.

Films: P-aminobenzoic acid, cinnarizine, piretanide, prednisolone, quinidine gluconate.

Granules: Cinnarizine, diclofenac sodium, diltiazem, indomethacin, fluorouracil, prednisolone, isosorbide mononitrate, isosorbide dinitrate.

Table 23.1: List of the drugs used in the formulation of FDDS

Dosage form	Drugs
Floating tablets	Acetaminophem, acetylsalicyclic acid, ampicillin, amoxycillin, atenolol, captopril, cinnerazine, chlorpheniramine, ciprofloxacin, diltiazem, fluorouracil, isosorbide dinitrate, p-aminobenzoic acid, prednisolone, nimodipine, sotalol, theophylline, verapamil.
Floating capsules	Chlordiazepoxide, diazepam, furosemide, L-dopa, benserazide, nicardipine, misoprostol, propranolol, pepstatin.
Floating microspheres	Aspirin, griseofulvin p-nitroaniline, ibuprofen, terfenadine, tranislast
Floating granules	Diclofenac sodium, indomethacin, prednisolone.

Powders: Riboflavin, phosphate, sotalol, theophylline.

Capsules: Verapamil HCl, chlordiazepoxide HCl, diazepam, furosemide and benserazide misoprostol, propranolol HCl, ursodeoxycholic acid, nicardipine.

APPROACHES TO DESIGN FDDS

The following approaches have been used for designing floating dosage forms of single and multiple unit systems.

Single-unit Dosage Forms

In low-density approach, the globular shells possess relatively low density compared to gastric fluid; hence they are used as drug carriers for controlled release. A buoyant dosage form can also be obtained by using a fluid-filled system that floats in the stomach. In coated shells; popcorn, poprice, and polysterols have been exploited as drug carriers. Sugar polymeric materials, such as methacrylic polymer and cellulose acetate phthalate have been used to undercoat these shells. These are further coated with a drug-polymer mixture. The polymer of choice can be either ethyl cellulose or hydroxypropyl cellulose depending on the desired drug release desired. Finally, the product floats on the gastric fluid while releasing the drug gradually over a prolonged duration.

Fluid-filled floating chamber type dosage forms include incorporation of a gas-filled floatation chamber into a microporous component that houses a drug reservoir. Apertures or openings are made in the top and bottom walls through which the gastrointestinal tract fluid enters into and dissolves the drug. The other two walls in contact with the fluid are sealed, so that the undissolved drug remains therein. The fluid present could be air (under partial vacuum) or any other suitable gas, liquid, or solid having an appropriate specific gravity and an inert character. The device is swallowable in size, remains afloat within the stomach for a prolonged time, and after the complete release of drug the shell disintegrates, passes into the intestine, and finally eliminated. Hydrodynamically balanced systems (HBS) are designed to prolong the stay of the dosage form in the GIT and aid in enhancing the absorption. Such systems are best suited for drugs having better solubility in acidic environment and also for the drugs having specific site of absorption in the upper part of the small intestine. To remain in the stomach for an extended period of time, the dosage form must have a bulk density less than 1. It should stay in the stomach, maintain its structural integrity, and release drug constantly. The success of HBS capsule as a better system is best exemplified with chlordiazeopoxide hydrochloride. The drug classically suffers solubility problem wherein it exhibits a 4000-fold difference in solubility while travelling down from pH 3 to 6 (the solubility of chlordiazepoxide hydrochloride is 150 mg/ml and is ~0.1 mg/ml at neutral pH).

HBS of chlordiazeopoxide hydrochloride had comparable blood level time profile as of three 10 mg commercial doses of capsules. HBS can either be formulated as a floating tablet or capsule. Many polymers and polymer combinations with wet granulation as a manufacturing technique have been explored to yield floatable tablets.

Various types of tablets (bilayered and matrix) are reported to have floatable characteristics. Some of the polymers used are hydroxypropyl cellulose, hydroxypropyl methylcellulose, crosspovidone, sodium carboxymethyl cellulose and ethyl cellulose. Self-correcting floatable asymmetric configuration drug delivery system employs a disproportionate 3-layer matrix technology that essentially controls drug release. The 3-layer principle has been further improved by development of an asymmetric configuration drug delivery system in order to modulate the release extent and achieve zero-order release kinetics by initially maintaining a constant area at the diffusing front with subsequent dissolution/erosion toward the completion of the release process. The system was designed in such a manner that it floated over extended period with gastric residence time *in vivo*, resulting in longer total transit time within the GI environment with maximum absorptive ability and consequently greater bioavailability. This particular characteristic would be applicable to drugs that have pH-dependent solubility, a narrow window of absorption and are absorbed by active transport from either the proximal or distal portion of the small intestine. Single-unit formulations are associated with problems such as sticking together or being obstructed in the GIT, which may have a potential danger of producing irritation and gastrointestinal obstruction.

Multiple-unit Dosage Forms

The purpose of designing multiple-unit dosage form is to develop a reliable formulation that has all the advantages of a single unit form and also is devoid of any of the above mentioned disadvantages of single-unit formulations. In pursuit of this endeavor many multiple-unit floatable dosage forms have been designed. Microspheres have high loading capacity, wherein many polymers have been used such as albumin, gelatin, starch, polymethacrylate, polyacrylamine, and polyalkyl cyanoacrylate. Spherical polymeric microsponges, which are commonly referred to as 'microballoons', are prepared. Microspheres have a characteristic internal hollow structure and show an excellent *in vitro* floatability. In carbon dioxide-generating multiple-unit oral formulations several devices with features that extend, unfold, or are inflated by carbon dioxide generated in the devices after administration have been described in the recent patent literature. These dosage forms are excluded from the passage of the pyloric sphincter, if a diameter of ~12 to 18 mm in their expanded state is exceeded (Fig. 23.4).

Practical Approaches in Designing FDDS

The concept of FDDS was first described in the literature as early as 1968, when Davis

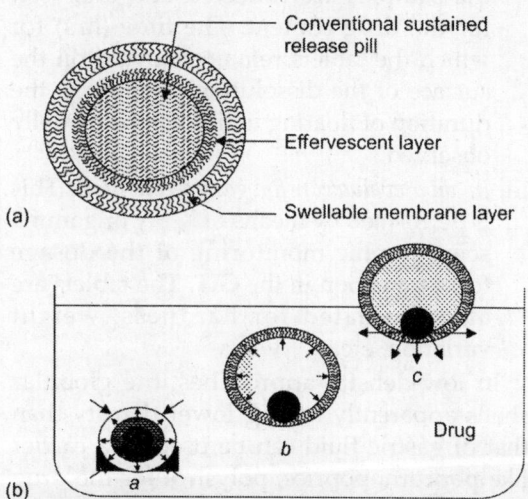

Fig. 23.4: (a) Multiple-unit oral FDDS. (b) Working principle of effervescent floating delivery system— (*a*) penetration of water, (*b*) generation of carbon dioxide and buoyancy (*c*) swellable layer

(1968) disclosed a method to overcome the difficulty experienced by some persons of gagging or choking after swallowing medicinal pills. The author suggested that such difficulty may possibly be overcome by providing pills having a density less than 1.0 g/cm³, so that pills tend to float on water surface. Since then several approaches have been used to develop an ideal FDDS.

Approaches to Design Single- and Multiple-unit Dosage Form

The following approaches have been used for the design of floating dosage forms of single and multiple unit systems.

For Single-unit Dosage Forms (Tablets)

i. *Floating lag time:* It is the time taken by the tablet to emerge onto the surface of dissolution medium and is expressed in seconds or minutes.

ii. *In vitro drug release and duration of floating:* This is determined by using USP II apparatus (paddle) stirring at a speed of 50 or 100 rpm at $37 \pm 0.2°C$ in simulated gastric fluid (pH 1.2 without pepsin). Aliquots of the samples are collected and analysed for the drug content. The time (hrs) for which the tablets remain buoyant on the surface of the dissolution medium is the duration of floating which can be visually observed.

iii. *In vivo evaluation for gastro-retention:* This is performed by means of X-ray or gamma scintigraphic monitoring of the dosage form transition in the GIT. The tablets are also evaluated for hardness, weight variation, etc.

In low-density approaches, the globular shells apparently having lower density than that of gastric fluid can be used as a carrier like popcorn, poprice, polystrol for the drug for its controlled release. The polymer of choice can be either ethyl cellulose or HPMC, depending on type of release desired. Finally, the product floats on the gastric fluid while releasing the drug gradually over a prolonged duration. Fluid filled floating chambers as dosage forms include incorporation of a gas filled floatation chamber into a microporous component that houses as a reservoir with an aperture present at top and bottom walls through which the GI fluid enters to dissolve the drug.

For Multiple-unit Dosage Forms Microspheres)

Apart from the *in vitro* release, duration of floating and *in vivo* gastro-retention tests, the multiple-unit dosage forms are also evaluated for:

i. Morphological and dimensional characters with the help of scanning electron microscopy (SEM). The size can also be measured using an optical microscope.

ii. *In vitro floating ability (Buoyancy %):* A known quantity of microspheres is spread over the surface of a USP (type II) dissolution apparatus filled with 900 ml of 0.1 N HCl containing 0.002% v/v Tween 80 and agitated at 100 rpm for 12 hours. After 12 hours, the floating and settled layers are separated, dried in a dessicator and weighed. The buoyancy is calculated from the following formula:

Buoyancy (%) = $W_f/(W_f + W_s) \times 100$

where W_f and W_s are the weights of floating and settled microspheres respectively.

iii. *Drug-excipient (DE) interactions:* This is done using FTIR. Appearance of a new peak, and/or disappearance of original drug or excipient peak indicates the DE interaction. Apart from the above mentioned evaluation parameters, granules are also evaluated for the effect of aging with the help of differential scanning calorimeter (DSC) or hot stage polarizing microscopy.

Multiparticulate dosage forms are gaining much favor over single-unit dosage forms. The potential benefits include increased bioavailability; predictable, reproducible and generally short gastric residence time, no risk of dose dumping; reduced risk of local irritation and the flexibility to blend pellets with different compositions or release patterns. Because of their smaller particle size, these systems are capable of passing through the GI tract easily, leading to less inter- and intra-subject variability. However, potential drug loading of a multiparticulate system is low because of the proportionally higher need for excipients (e.g. sugar cores). Most multiparticulate pulsatile delivery systems are coated with a polymeric layer that acts as reservoir device. Upon water ingress, drug is released from the core after rupturing of the surrounding polymer layer, due to pressure build-up within the system. The pressure necessary to rupture the coating is achieved with swelling agents, gas producing effervescent excipients or increased osmotic pressure. Water permeation and mechanical resistance of the outer membrane are major factors affecting the lag time. Water soluble drugs are mainly released by diffusion; while in case of water insoluble drug, the release is dependent on dissolution of drug.

FORMULATION DEVELOPMENT AND MECHANISM OF FDDS

Comprehensive knowledge about GI dynamics, such as gastric emptying, small intestinal transit, colonic transit, etc., is key for the optimum design of an oral controlled release dosage form. Knowledge about the rate and extent of drug absorption from different sites of GI tract and factors, which govern the absorption may further assist the design of dosage form. For instance, drugs, which are predominantly absorbed from the upper part of GI tract, such as furosemide, alberterol and theophylline, are worth considering candidates for improving and prolonging their limited oral bioavailabilities. The advent of scintigraphy revolutionized the development process of oral controlled release dosage forms by making it possible to understand various physiological and pharmacological factors involved in oral drug delivery.

Selection of excipients is an important strategic decision in designing of a dosage form with consistence and controlled residence in the stomach. Water soluble cellulose derivatives represent a typical class of polymers best suited for such purposes. It has been suggested that higher molecular weight polymers and slower rates of polymer hydration are usually associated with better floating behavior. Therefore, high molecular weight and less hydrophilic polymers are expected to improve floating properties of delivery systems.

Three major requirements for FDDS formulations are:

i. It must form a cohesive gel barrier
ii. It must maintain specific gravity lower than gastric contents (1.004–1.01 g/cc)
iii. It should release contents slowiy to serve as a reservoir

FDDS have a bulk density less than gastric fluids and hence remain buoyant in the stomach without affecting the gastric emptying rate for a prolonged period of time. While the system is floating on the gastric contents, the drug is released slowly at the desired rate from the system. After release of drug, the residual system is emptied from the stomach. This results in an increased GRT and a better control of the fluctuations in plasma drug concentration. However, besides a minimal gastric content is needed to allow the proper achievement of the buoyancy, a minimal level of floating force (F) is also required to keep the dosage form reliably buoyant on the surface of the meal. To measure the floating force kinetics, a novel apparatus based weight float has been reported in the literature. The apparatus operates by measuring continuously the force equivalent to F (as a function of time) that is required to maintain in the submerged state. The object floats better if F is on the higher positive side. This apparatus helps in optimizing FDDS with respect to stability and durability of floating forces produced in order to prevent the drawbacks of unforeseeable intragastric buoyancy related variations.

$$F = F_{buoyancy} - F_{gravity} = (D_f - D_s)\, gv$$

where, F = total vertical force

D_f = fluid density

D_s = object density

v = volume

g = acceleration due to gravity

IN VITRO AND IN VIVO EVALUATION

There are different studies reported in the literature, which indicate that pharmaceutical dosage forms exhibiting gastric retention *in vitro* floating behavior show prolonged gastric residence *in vivo* as well. However, it has to be pointed out that good *in vitro* floating behavior alone is not sufficient proof for efficient gastric retention *in vivo*. The effects of the simultaneous presence of food and of the complex motility of the stomach are difficult to estimate. Obviously, only *in vivo* studies can provide definite proof that prolonged gastric residence is obtained.

1. *Measurement of buoyancy capabilities of the FDDS:* The floating behavior is evaluated with resultant weight measurements. The experiment may be carried out in two different media, deionised water in order to monitor possible difference. The apparatus and its mechanism are explained earlier. The results showed that polymers of higher molecular weight have slower rate of hydration and better floating behavior. It is also observed that buoyancy in fact is in simulated meal medium rather than deionized water.

2. *Floating time and dissolution:* It is determined by using USP dissolution apparatus containing 900 ml of 0.1 mol/lit HCl as the dissolution medium at 37°C. The time taken by the dosage form to float is termed as floating lag time and the time for which the

dosage form floats is termed as the floating or flotation time. A more relevant *in vitro* dissolution method was proposed to evaluate a floating drug delivery system (for tablet dosage form). A 100 ml glass beaker is modified by adding a side arm at the bottom of the beaker, so that the beaker can hold 70 ml of 0.1 mol/lit HCl dissolution medium and allow collection of samples. A burette is mounted above the beaker to deliver the dissolution medium at a flow rate of 2 ml/min to mimic gastric acid secretion rate. The performance of the modified dissolution apparatus has been compared with USP dissolution apparatus 2 (paddle): The problem of adherence of the tablet to the shaft of the paddle was observed with the USP dissolution apparatus. The tablets however, do not stick to the agitating device in the proposed dissolution method. Similarity of dissolution curves was observed between the USP method and the proposed method at 10% difference level (f2=57) an incorporate. The proposed test may show good *in vitro–in vivo* correlation, since an attempt was made to mimic the *in vivo* conditions such as gastric volume, gastric emptying, and gastric acid secretion rate.

3. *Drug release:* Dissolution tests are performed using a dissolution apparatus. Samples are withdrawn periodically from the dissolution medium with replacement and then analysed for their drug content after an appropriate dilution.

4. *Content uniformity, hardness, friability:* For tablets only.

5. *Drug loading, drug entrapment efficiency, particle size analysis, surface characterization:* (for floating microspheres and beads) Drug loading is assessed by crushing accurately weighed sample of beads or microspheres in a mortar and added to the appropriate dissolution medium which is then centrifuged, filtered and analysed by

various analytical methods like spectrophotometry. The percentage drug content is calculated by dividing the amount of drug in the sample by the weight and simulated meal, total beads, or microspheres. The particle size and the size distribution of beads or microspheres are determined in the dry state using optical microscopy method. The external and cross-sectional morphology (surface characterization) is studied by scanning electron microscope (SEM).

6. *X-ray/gamma scintigraphy:* X-ray/gamma scintigraphy is a very popular evaluation parameter for floating dosage form. It helps to locate dosage form in the GIT, which helps in predicting and correlating the gastric emptying time and the passage of dosage form in the GIT. Here the inclusion of a radio-opaque material into a solid dosage form enables it to be visualized by X-rays. Similarly, the inclusion of a γ-emitting radionuclide in a formulation allows indirect external observation using a γ-camera or scinti-scanner. In case of γ-scintigraphy, the γ-rays emitted by the radionuclide are focused on a camera, which helps to monitor the location of the dosage form in the GI tract.

7. *Pharmacokinetic studies:* Pharmacokinetic studies constitute the *in vivo* studies and several works have been reported. The pharmacokinetics studies of verapamil, from the floating pellets containing drug, filled into a capsule, was compared with the conventional verapamil tablets of similar dose (40 mg). The t_{max} and AUC 0-infinity) values (3.75 hours and 364.65 ng/ml h, respectively) for floating pellets were comparatively higher than those obtained for the conventional verapamil tablets (t_{max} value 1.21 hour, and AUC value 224.22 ng/ml h). The difference was recorded was insignificant between the C_{max} values of both the formulations, suggesting the improved bioavailability of the floating pellets compared to the conventional tablets. An improvement in bioavailability has also been observed in case of piroxicam hollow polycarbonate microspheres administered in rabbits. The microspheres showed about 1.4 times more bioavailability, and the elimination half-life was increased approximately 3 times compared to the free drug.

ADVANTAGES OF FDDS

1. The principle of HBS can be used for any particular medicament or a class of medicament.

2. The HBS formulations are not restricted to medicaments, which are principally absorbed from the stomach. These are equally efficacious for medicaments, which are absorbed from the intestine, e.g. chlorpheniramine maleate.

3. The HBS are advantageous for drugs absorbed through the stomach, e.g. ferrous salts and for drugs meant for local action in the stomach and treatment of peptic ulcer, e.g. antacids.

4. The efficacy of the medicaments administered utilizing the sustained release principle of HBS has been found to be independent of the site of absorption of the particular medicaments.

5. Administration of a prolonged release floating dosage form in the form of tablet or capsule will result in dissolution of the drug in gastric fluid. After emptying of the stomach contents, the dissolved drug is available for absorption in the small intestine. It is therefore, expected that a drug will be fully absorbed from the floating dosage form if it remains in solution form even at alkaline pH of the intestine.

6. When there is vigorous intestinal movement and a short transit time as might be noticed in certain type of diarrhea, poor absorption is expected under such circumstances and it may be advantageous to keep the drug in floating condition in stomach to get a relatively better response.

7. Gastric retention will provide advantages in case of drugs with narrow absorption windows in a small region of intestine.

8. Many drugs prescribed as once-a-day delivery have demonstrated to have suboptimal absorption due to dependence on the transit time of the dosage form, thus render traditional extended release development challenging. Therefore, a system designed for longer gastric retention will extend the time within which drug absorption occurs is in the small intestine.

9. Certain types of drugs can be benefitted by formulating them with gastro-retentive character. These include:

   a. Drugs acting locally in the stomach
   b. Drugs that are primarily absorbed in the stomach
   c. Drugs that are poorly soluble at an alkaline pH
   d. Drugs with a narrow window of absorption
   e. Drugs absorbed rapidly from the GI tract
   f. Drugs that degrade in the colon.

DISADVANTAGES OF FDDS

1. There are certain situations, where gastric retention is not desirable. Aspirin and non-steroidal anti-inflammatory drugs are known to cause gastric lesions, and slow release of such drugs in the stomach is unwanted.

2. Drugs that may irritate the stomach mucosa or are unstable in its acidic environment should not be formulated in gastro-retentive systems.

3. Furthermore, other drugs, such as isosorbide dinitrate, that are absorbed equally well throughout the GI tract have no additional benefit from their incorporation into formulation for a gastric retention system.

MARKETED PRODUCTS OF FDDS

The last three decades of intensive research work resulted in the development of five commercial FDDS. Madopar® HBS (Prolopa® HBS) is a commercially available product used in Europe and other countries, but not available in the US. It contains 100 mg levodopa and 25 mg benserazide, a peripheral dopa decarboxylase inhibitor. This CR formulation consists of a gelatin capsule that is designed to float on the surface of the gastric fluid. After the gelatin shell dissolves, a mucus body is formed that consists of the active drugs and other substances. The drug diffuses successively as hydrated boundary layers of the matrix dissipate. Some of the marketed floating drug delivery formulations are enlisted in Table 23.2.

Table 23.2: List of the marketed FDDS based formulations

Brand name	Delivery system	Drug (dose)
Valrelease	Floating capsule	Diazepam (15 mg)
Madopar HBS (Prolopa HBS)	Floating CR capsule	Benserazide (25 mg) and L-Dopa (100 mg)
Liquid Gaviscon	Effervescent floating liquid alginate preparations	Al hydroxide (95 mg), Mg carbonate (358 mg)
Topalkan	Floating liquid alginate preparation	Al-Mg antacid
Almagate flot coat	Floating dosage form	Al-Mg antacid
Conviron	Colloidal gel forming FDDS	Ferrous sulfate
Cytotech	Bilayer floating capsule	Misoprostol (100 µg/200 µg)
Cifran OD	Gas-generating floating form	Ciprofloxacin (1 gm)

Valrelease® is another example of a capsule, marketed by Hoffmann-LaRoche, which contains 15 mg diazepam; the latter is more soluble at low pH. Diazepam (pK = 3.4) absorption is more desirable in the stomach, not in the intestine, where it is practically insoluble and is poorly absorbed. The HBS system maximizes the dissolution of the drug by prolonging the GRT. Moreover, pharmacokinetic data has demonstrated the blood level equivalence of once per day dosing with the HBS capsule to 3 times daily dosing of conventional, 5 mg Valium® tablets.

Floating liquid alginate preparations, e.g. Liquid Gaviscon, are used to suppress gastroesophageal reflux and alleviate the symptoms of heart burn. The formulation consists of a mixture of alginate, which forms a gel of alginic acid, and a carbonate or that drug releases via diffusion mechanism. Bicarbonate component (e.g. sodium bicarbonate), reacts with gastric acid and evolves CO_2 bubbles. The gel becomes buoyant by entrapping the gas bubbles, and floats on the gastric contents as a viscous layer, which has a higher pH than the gastric contents.

Topalkan® is aluminum-magnesium antacid that involves antacid properties and also an even greater degree the availability of alginic acid in its formula. It has antipeptic and protective effects with respect to the mucous membrane of the stomach and esophagus, and provides, together with the magnesium salts, a floating layer of the preparation in the stomach. Almagate FlotCoat® is another novel antacid formulation that confers a higher antacid potency together with a prolonged GRT and a safe as well as extended delivery of antacid drug.

APPLICATIONS OF FDDS

Floating drug delivery offers several applications for drugs having poor bioavailability because of the narrow absorption window in the upper part of the gastrointestinal tract. It retains the dosage form at the site of absorption and thus enhances the bioavailability. These are summarized as follows.

Sustained Drug Delivery

HBS systems can remain in the stomach for long period and hence can release the drug over a prolonged period of time. The problem of short gastric residence time encountered with an oral controlled release formulation can be overcome with these systems. These systems have a bulk density of <1, as a result of which they can float on the gastric contents. These systems are relatively large in size and thus their passage through the pyloric opening is restricted.

Recently, sustained release floating capsules of nicardipine hydrochloride were developed and were evaluated *in vivo*. The formulation was compared with commercially available MICARD capsules in rabbits. Plasma concentration time curves showed a longer duration of administration (16 hours) in the case of sustained release floating capsules as compared with conventional MICARD capsules (8 hours).

Absorption Site-specific Drug Delivery

These systems are particularly advantageous for drugs that are specifically absorbed from stomach or the proximal part of the small intestine, e.g. riboflavin and furosemide. Furosemide is primarily absorbed from the stomach followed by the duodenum. It has been reported that a monolithic floating dosage form with prolonged gastric residence time was developed with enhanced bioavailability. AUC obtained with the floating tablets was approximately 1.8 times compared to those of conventional furosemide tablets.

A bilayer-floating capsule was developed for local delivery of misoprostol, which is a synthetic analogue of prostaglandin E1 used as a protectant of gastric ulcers caused due to frequent administration of NSAIDs. By targeting slow delivery of misoprostol to the stomach, desired therapeutic levels could be achieved and drug dosage could be reduced.

Absorption Enhancement

Drugs that have poor bioavailability because of site specific absorption from the upper part of the GIT are potential candidates to be formulated as floating drug delivery systems, thereby maximizing their absorption.

A significant increase in the bioavailability of floating dosage forms (42.9%) could be achieved as compared with commercially available LASIX tablets (33.4%) and enteric coated LASIX-long product (29.5%).

Miyazaki et al. conducted pharmacokinetic studies on floating granules of indomethacin prepared with chitosan and compared the peak plasma concentration and AUC with the conventional commercially available capsules. It was concluded that the floating granules prepared with chitosan were superior in terms of peak plasma concentration and maintenance of drug in plasma.

FDDS also serves as an excellent drug delivery system for the eradication of *Helicobacter pylori,* which causes chronic gastritis and peptic ulcers. The treatment requires high drug concentrations to be maintained at the site of infection that is within the gastric mucosa. By virtue of floating ability, these dosage forms can be retained in the gastric region for a prolonged period, so that the drug can be targeted.

Yang et al. developed a swellable asymmetric triple-layer tablet with floating ability to prolong the gastric residence time of triple drug regimen (tetracycline, metronidazole, clarithromycin) of *Helicobacter pylori*-associated peptic ulcers using HPMC and PEO as the rate-controlling polymeric membrane excipients. Results demonstrated that sustained delivery of tetracycline and metronidazole over 6 to 8 hours could be achieved while the tablets remained floating. It was concluded that the developed delivery system had the potential to increase the efficacy of the therapy with improved patient compliance.

Floating drug delivery is associated with certain limitations. Drugs that irritate the mucosa, those that have multiple absorption sites in the gastrointestinal tract, and those that are not stable at gastric, pH are not suitable candidates to be formulated as floating dosage forms.

Floatation as a retention mechanism requires the presence of liquid on which the dosage form can float on the gastric contents. To overcome this limitation, a bioadhesive polymer can be used to coat the dosage form, so that it adheres to gastric mucosa, or the dosage form can be administered with a full glass of water to provide the initial fluid for buoyancy. Also single unit floating capsules or tablets are associated with an 'all or none concept', but this can be overcome by formulating multiple unit systems like floating microspheres or microballoons.

The use of large single-unit dosage forms sometimes poses a problem of permanent retention of rigid large-sized single unit especially in patients with bowel obstruction, intestinal adhesion, gastropathy, or a narrow pyloric opening (mean resting pyloric diameter 12.8 ± 7.0 mm). Floating dosage form should not be given to a patient just before going to bed as the gastric emptying of such a dosage form occurs randomly, when the subject is in supine posture. One drawback of HBS is that this system, being a matrix formulation, consists of a blend of drug and low-density polymers. The release kinetics of drug cannot be changed without changing the floating properties of the dosage form and vice versa.

Enhanced Bioavailability

The bioavailability of riboflavin CR-GRDF is significantly enhanced in comparison to the administration of non-GRDF CR polymeric formulations. There are several different processes, related to absorption and transit of the drug in the gastrointestinal tract, that act concomitantly to influence the magnitude of drug absorption.

Minimized Adverse Activity at the Colon

Retention of the drug in the HBS systems in the stomach minimizes the amount of drug that reaches the colon. Thus, undesirable activities of the drug in colon may be prevented. This pharmacodynamic aspect provides the rationale for GRDF formulation for betalactam antibiotics that are absorbed only from the small intestine, and whose presence in the colon leads to the development of microorganism's resistance.

Reduced Fluctuations of Drug Concentration

Continuous input of the drug following CRGRDF administration produces blood drug concentrations within a narrow range compared to the immediate release dosage forms. Thus, fluctuations in drug effects are minimized and concentration dependent adverse effects that are associated with peak concentrations can be prevented. This feature is of special importance for drugs with a narrow therapeutic index.

Miscellaneous

1. Recent study indicated that the administration of diltiazem floating tablet twice a day might be more effective compared to normal tablets in controlling the blood pressure of hypertensive patient.
2. Madopar® HBS-contains L-dopa and benserazide-the drug is released and absorbed over a period of 6–8 hours and maintains substantial plasma concentration for Parkinson's patients.
3. Cytotech®-containing misoprostol is a synthetic prostaglandin-E1 analog and is used for prevention of gastric ulcers caused by nonsteroidal anti-inflammatory drugs (NSAIDS). As it provides high concentration of drug within gastric mucosa, it is used to eradicate pylori (a causative organism for chronic gastritis and peptic ulcers).
4. 5-Fluorouracil has been successfully evaluated in patients with stomach neoplasm.
5. Developing HBS dosage form for tacrine provides better delivery system and reduces its GI associated side effects in Alzheimer's patients.

6. Alza Corporation has developed a gastro-retentive platform for the OROS® system, which showed prolong residence time in dog model as the product remained in the canine stomach at 12 hours post dose and was frequently remained up to 24 hours.

PHARMACEUTICAL ASPECTS

In designing of FDDS, following characteristics should be sought: (i) retention in the stomach according to the clinical demand; (ii) convenient intake; (iii) ability to load substantial amount of drug with different physicochemical properties and release them in a controlled manner; and (iv) complete matrix integrity of the SR formulation in the stomach, inexpensive industrial manufacturing, optimization between the buoyancy time and release rate (buoyancy time increases by increasing drugpolymer ratio, but release retards by increasing polymer level), lag time, i.e. the time taken by the dosage form to float should be low (Wong P S L et al., 2000).

Most of the floating systems reported in literature are single-unit systems; these systems are unreliable and irreproducible in prolonging residence time in the stomach when orally administered, owing to their unpredictable emptying process. On the other hand, multiple-unit dosage forms appear to be better option, since they reduce the inter-subject variability in absorption and lower the probability of dose dumping. Table 23.3 enlisted some of the patents related to FDDS.

FUTURE PERSPECTIVES IN FDDS

Among the drugs currently in clinical use are several narrow absorption window drugs that may be benefited when compounded and formulated into a FDDS. Replacing parenteral administration of drugs to oral pharmaco-therapy would substantially improve the treatment. It is anticipated that FDDS may enhance this possibility. Moreover, it is expected that the FDDS approach may be used

Table 23.3: List of patents related to FDDS

S.No.	Cited patent	Issue date	Original assignee	Title
1.	US4101650	1978	Zaidan Hojin Biseibutsu Kagaku Kenkyu Kai	Pepstatin floating minicapsules
2.	US4772473	1988	Norwich Eaton Pharmaceuticals, Inc.	Nitrofurantoin dosage form
3.	US4777033	1988	Teijin Limited	Oral sustained release pharmaceutical preparation
4.	US4844905	1989	Eisai Co., Ltd.	Granule remaining in stomach
5.	US5091184	1992	Ciba-Geigy Corporation	Coated adhesive tablets
6.	US7776345	2010	Sun Pharma Advanced Research Company Ltd	Gastric retention controlled drug delivery system
7.	US6340475	2002	DepoMed, Inc	Extending the duration of drug release within the stomach during the fed mode
8.	US5651985	1997	Bayer Aktiengesellschaft	Expandable pharmaceutical forms

for many potentially active agents with narrow absorption window, whose development has been halted due to lack of appropriate pharmaceutical FDDS technologies. Combination therapy to treat *H. Pylori* infection in a single FDDS needs to be developed. Further investigation may concentrate on the following concepts:

- Identification of a minimal cut-off size above which dosage forms to be retained in the human stomach for prolonged period of time. This would permit a more specific control over desired in gestroretentivity.
- Design of an array of FDDS, each having a narrow GRT for use according to the clinical need, e.g. dosage and state of disease. This may be achieved by co-compounding polymeric matrices with various biodegradation properties.
- Study of the effect of various geometric shapes, in a more extended manner than previous studies, extended dimensions with high rigidity on gestroretentivity.
- Design of novel polymers in accordance to clinical and pharmaceutical need.

SUGGESTED READINGS

1. Amrutkar PP, Chaudhari PD and Patil SB (2012), *Colloids and Surfaces B: Biointerfaces.* 89, 182–7.
2. Badve SS, Sher P, Korde A and Pawar AP (2007), *Eur. J. Pharm. Biopharm.,* 65, 85–93.
3. Goole J, Deleuze F, Vanderbist K Amighi A (2008), *Eur. J. Pharm. Biopharm.,* 68, 310–18.
4. Hashim H, Lee Wan Po A (1987), *Int J. Pharm.* 35, 201.
5. Hilton AK, Deasy PB (1992), *Int. J. Pharm.* 86.
6. Ichikawa M, Watanave S, Miyake Y (1991), *J. Pharm. Sci.* 80, 1062.
7. Ingani HM, Timmermans J, Moes AJ (1987), *Int. J. Pharm.* 35, 157.
8. Ritschel WA, Menon A, Saki A (1991), *Exp. Clin. Pharmacol.* 13, 629.
9. Rouge N, Allemann E, Gex-Fabry M, Balant L, Cole ET, Buri P, Doelker E (1998), *Pharm. Acta Helv.* 73, 1998, 81.
10. Sheth PR Tossounian JL (1984), *Drug Dev. Ind. Pharm.* 10, 313.
11. Streubel A, Siepmann J, Bodmeier R (2003), *Eur. J. Pharm. Sci.* 18, 37.
12. Rajinikanth PS, Balasubramaniam J and Mishra B (2007), *Int. J. Pharm.,* 335, 114–22.
13. Tadros MI, (2010), *Eur. J. Pharm. Biopharm.,* 74, 332–39.
14. Sungthongjeen S, Paeratakul O, Limmatvapirat S and Puttipipatkhachorn S (2006), *Int. J. Pharm.,* 324, 136–43.
15. Pornsak S, Srisagul S and Satit P (2006), *Carbohydrate Poly.,* 67, 436–45.
16. Hascicek C, Rossi A, Colombo P, Massimo G, Strusi OL and Colombo G (2011), *Eur. J. Pharm. Biopharm.,* 77, 116–121.
17. Sandra S, Tâmara A, Renata VC, Hendrik M and Karsten M (2008), *Eur. J. Pharm. Biopharm.,* 69, 708–17.

18. Tang Y, Venkatraman SS, Boey YC and Wang L (2007), *Int. J. Pharm.*, 336, 159–65.

19. Srisagul S, Pornsak S and Satit P (2008), *Eur. J. Pharm. Biopharm.*, 69, 255–63.

20. Ninan M, Lu X, Qifang W, Xiangrong Z, Wenji Z, Yang L, Lingyu J and Sanming L (2008), *Int. J. Pharm.*, 358, 82–90.

21. Rajinikanth PS, Balasubramaniam J and Mishra B (2007), *Int. J. Pharm.*, 335, 114–22.

22. Liandong H, Wei L, Jianxue Y, Yanhong J, Chuang S and Hongxin X (2011), *Eur. J. Pharm. Biopharm.*, 42, 99–105.

23. Tadros MI (2010), *Eur. J. Pharm. Biopharm.*, 74, 332–39.

24. Hamdani J, Moës AJ and Karim A (2006), *Int. J. Pharm.*, 322, 96–103.

25. Srikanth MV, Rao NS, Sunil SA, Ram BJ and Murthy Kolapalli (2012), *Acta Pharmaceutica Sinica B.*, 2, 60–69.

26. Muniyandy S and Boddapati A (2011), *Carbohydrate Poly.*, 85, 592–8.

27. Ninan M, Lu X, Qifang W, Xiangrong Z, Wenji Z, Yang L, Lingyu J and Sanming L (2008), *Int. J. Pharm.*, 358, 82–90.

28. Panagiotis B, Kyriakos K and Emanouil G (2011), *Eur. J. Pharm. Biopharm.*, 77, 122–31.

29. Yao H, Yao H, Zhu J, Yu J and Zhang L (2012), *Int. J. Pharm.* 422, 211–19.

30. Amrutkar PP, Chaudhari PD and Patil SB (2012), *Colloids and Surfaces B: Biointerfaces.* 89, 182–7.

31. Sungthongjeen S, Paeratakul O, Limmatvapirat, S and Puttipipatkhachorn S (2006), *Int. J. Pharm.*, 324, 136–43.

32. Pornsak S, Srisagul S and Satit P (2006), *Carbohydrate Poly.*, 67, 436–45.

33. Badve SS, Sher P, Korde A and Pawar AP (2007), *Eur. J. Pharm. Biopharm.*, 65, 85–93.

34. Hascicek C, Rossi A, Colombo P, Massimo G, Strusi OL and Colombo G (2011), *Eur. J. Pharm. Biopharm.*, 77, 116–121.

35. Sandra S, Tâmara A, Renata VC, Hendrik M and Karsten M (2008), *Eur. J. Pharm. Biopharm.*, 69, 708–17.

36. Tang Y, Venkatraman SS, Boey YC and Wang L (2007), *Int. J. Pharm.*, 336, 159–65.

37. Srisagul S, Pornsak S and Satit P (2008), *Eur. J. Pharm. Biopharm.*, 69, 255–63.

38. Vyas SP and Khar RK (2000), In: Controlled Drug Delivery, Concept and Advances, 1st Ediion, Vallabh Prakashan, New Delhi. 322, 96–103.

39. Goole J, Deleuze F, Vanderbist K Amighi A (2008), *Eur. J. Pharm. Biopharm.*, 68, 310–18.

Index

A

Achievement of the buoyancy 519
Acrolein 261, 278
Adsorption theory of mechanism of bioadhesion 57
Agglomerates 157
Aggregation of amphiphile(s) 290
Albumins 261
Alkyl amides 397
Alkyl esters 396
Alkyl ethers 395
Alzet® 209
Amphiphilic dendrimers 382
Angle of contact of microparticles 271
Aqueous dispersion method 401
Atomic force microscopy (AFM) 219
AUC 472
Avidin-biotin system 448
Azobond prodrugs 109

B

Bacterial adhesion 66
Balloon catheters 212
Bilayer rigidity and homogeneity 402
Bioactives 289
Bioadhesion 17
Bioadhesive 16
Bioadhesive polymers 54
Bioconjugation 440
Biofate 289
Buffers 418

C

Capsule-based osmotic pumps 35
Carbohydrate 59
Carrageenan 262
Chemoembolization 284
Chiral dendrimers 382
Chitosan microspheres 276
Collagen 261
Colon-specific drug delivery system 17
Column chromatography 248
CT imaging of liposomes 259
Confocal laser scanning microscopy (CLSM) 270
Contraceptive implants 210

Controlled release of drug 3
Convergent dendrimer growth 382
Cosurfactant 420
cRGD 226
Critical micellization concentration (CMC) 18
Critical packing parameter (CPP) 238
Cross-linkers 441, 442
Crystallization 157
Cubosomes 235
Cyclodextrins 470

D

DEAE cellulose 262
Dehydration-rehydration vesicles 239
Dendrimer drug conjugate 387
Dendrimer toxicity 385
Dendritic boxes 390
Dendron 379
Desferroxamine 285
Desolvation 291, 292
Diffusion controlled release 5
Diffusion theory 56
Discomes 406
Divergent dendrimer growth 382
Double emulsification 83
Drug targeting 2

E

Eagle's medium 206
Effervescent systems 510
Efflux 332
Elastic niosomes 409
Electron spectroscopy for chemical analysis (ESCA) 270
Electronic theory 57
Elementary osmotic pump 37
Emulsion 262
Endotoxin 451
Enhanced permeability and retention effects 24
Entrapment efficiency 348
Enzymatic degradation 17
Enzyme immobilization 90
Everted sac technique 71
Extrusion 401
Extrusion techniques 241

Fluorescein isothiocyanate (FITC) 230
5-fluorouracil (5-FU) 467
Flux regulators 43
Forster resonance energy transfer (FRET) 224
Fracture theory 57

G

Gelatin 261, 272, 273
Gene library 89
Glass transition temperature (T_g) 139

H

HeLa cells 230
HEPES buffer 277
Hexasomes 235
High-pressure homogenization 290
Higuchi–Leeper osmotic pump 36
Higuchi–Thweeues osmotic pump 37
Homogenization 300
Horseradish peroxidase 98, 99
Hybrid dendrimers 382
Hydrodynamically balanced system 16
Hydrogel 45
Hydrophilic-lipophilic balance (HLB) 222
Hyperthermia 312

I

Immunoliposomes 239
Implantable devices 196
Implantable infusion pump 199
Inclusion complexes 471
Intrauterine devices (IUDs) 209
Isoelectric point 270

L

Lacrisert 205
Large unilamellar vesicles (LUVs) 235
Leachable substances 206
Lectins 60
Lipid 418, 419, 420, 422
Liquid crystalline dendrimers 382
L-lysine-based dendrimers 381
Luciferase 216
Luteinizing-hormone-releasing hormone
 (LH-RH) 264
Lyophilization 280

M

Matrix 7
Membrane emulsification technique 85

Metallo dendrimer 382
Micellar dendrimers 382
Microcapsule 90
Microchannel emulsification 85
Microflora 96
Microneedles 150
Minimum effective concentration (MEC) 1
Mitochondrial targeting 27
Monoclonal antibodies (MABS) 283
Mucoadhesion 63
Multidrug resistant (MDR) 227
Multilamellar vesicles (MLVs) 235, 239
Multilayer-core osmotic systems 34
Multiple emulsions 17

N

Nanoprecipitation 290, 301
Nanosponges 488
Nonbirefringence 365
NSVs reversed vesicles 407

O

Ocufit 205
Ocusert® 199, 204, 207
Optical clarity 365
Organogels 359
Organogelators 360
Osmogens 43
Osmosis 31
Osmotic pumps 31
Oxygen substitute 89

P

PAMAM dendrimers 381
Peripheral drug targeting 350
Peristaltic pumps 196
P-glycoprotein (Pgp) 227
pH-responsive nanoparticles 20
pH sensitive liposomes 239
Phallotoxins 452
Phase inversion method 173
Phase separation coacervation technique 266
Pilosebaceous targeting 356
Pluronic F127® 189
Poloxamer 418
Poly-(lactide-co-glycolide) (PLGA) 222
Polymethylmethacrylate (PMMA) 296
Polyvinyl alcohol (PVA) 264
Poly-(glycolic acid) (PGA) 274
Poly-(ε-caprolactone) (PCL) 222
Polyethyleneglycol (PEG) 216

Polymer-coated nonionic surfactant vesicles 408
Polysorbate 418
PPI dendrimers 381
Prodrug-based approaches 108
Proniosomes 405

Q

Quantum dots 506

R

Receptor-specific legands 124
Resealed erythrocytes 18
Reservoir type diffusion sustained system 7
Resistance 15
Reticuloendothelial system (RES) 318

S

Solvation 291
Scanning electron microscopy (SEM) 219
Single pass technique 401
Small unilamellar vesicles, SUVs 235
Solenoid pump 200
Solubility of drug 10
Solubilizing agents 42
Solvent emulsification evaporation 422
Spray drying and spray congealing 267
Starch 261
Stealth liposomes 239
Supercritical fluid (SCF) 423
Supergelators 367
Surface engineered dendrimers 387
Surfactants 43
Sustained released action 82
Systemic lupus erythematosus (SLE) 221

T

Temperature-responsive nanocarriers 20
Transcellular delivery 356
Transdermal delivery 145, 343
Transdermal drug delivery systems 17
Transfersomes 344
Transmission electron microscopy (TEM) 219
Trilaurin 418
Tumor targeted drug delivery 23

U

Ultrasonication method 423
Unilamellar vesicles (ULVs) 239
Unique flow chamber technique 70

V

Vaccine adjuvant 91
Vaccine delivery 29
Vapor pressure powered devices 196, 199
Viscoelasticity 365

W

Wetting theory 56
Wicking agents 42
Wilhelm plate technique 67
Witepsol® 418

Z

Zero-length cross linkers 441
Zero-order release kinetics 326
Zeta potential 86

Introduction to Novel Drug Delivery Systems